Orthopaedic Study Guide Series

Series editors

Nikolaos K. Paschos
Department of Orthopedic Surgery
Division of Sports Medicine
Boston Children's Hospital
Harvard Medical School
Boston, MA, USA

George Bentley
Royal National Orthopaedic Hospital
Stanmore, United Kingdom

Orthopaedics has many different specialisations such as trauma, spine, sports medicine, arthroplasty, oncology, paediatric orthopaedics, hand surgery and microsurgery to name just a few. This means that residents preparing for their exams have a broad field to study and to remember. In addition, orthopaedics is a surgical specialty, thus knowledge of orthopaedic techniques is necessary and is tested during these exams. To cover all these fields and aspects of orthopaedics, this book series has volumes dedicated to each study area and provides a guide for all orthopaedic residents in preparation for residency and fellowship exams.

More information about this series at http://www.springer.com/series/13489

Gazi Huri • Nikolaos K. Paschos
Editors

The Shoulder

Springer

Editors
Gazi Huri
Orthopaedics and Traumatology Department
Hacettepe University
Ankara
Turkey

Nikolaos K. Paschos
Department of Orthopedic Surgery
Division of Sports Medicine
Boston Children's Hospital
Harvard Medical School
Boston, MA
USA

ISSN 2520-1115 ISSN 2520-1123 (electronic)
Orthopaedic Study Guide Series
ISBN 978-3-319-51977-7 ISBN 978-3-319-51979-1 (eBook)
DOI 10.1007/978-3-319-51979-1

Library of Congress Control Number: 2017946755

Printed on acid-free paper

This Springer imprint is published by Springer Nature
The registered company is Springer International Publishing AG
The registered company address is: Gewerbestrasse 11, 6330 Cham, Switzerland

To my daughter Alin Defne, my wife Pınar, and to the peace of the world

Gazi Huri, M.D.

To my teachers that dedicated their life to medical education
To my orthopedic residents that are always an inspiration to strive for excellence
To my family for their endless support all these years

Nikolaos K. Paschos

Series Preface

The vision behind the conception of "Orthopaedic Study Guide Series" was to create a book series that will cover the need of effective and focused revision study for all young orthopedic surgeons. This is a study guide that is the spiritual child of FORTE, the Federation of Orthopedic Trainees in Europe.

The main goal is to highlight some key issues for exam and stimulate young colleagues for additional study. Following these principles, this study guide was built with a unique format incorporating text with concise information, review questions, key points, description of case studies, mnemonic tricks, and references/suggestions for additional study.

The editors would like to thank FORTE for their continuous support in this project, and Springer for their commitment towards the study guide series.

More importantly, we would like to thank the authors and editors for their substantial contribution to this series and their dedication towards orthopedic education and training.

Contributor Preface I

It is an honor and a pleasure for me to write the introduction to the inaugural edition of FORTE (Federation of Orthopaedics Trainees in Europe) Book series. Dr. Huri was a research fellow at our institution in the Division of Shoulder and Elbow Surgery, and despite being a brilliant person, a hard worker, and a good friend, he always seemed to understand and empathize with all of the trainees at our institution. He was a master at teaching and helping the students, residents, and clinical fellows conceptualize and understand the shoulder from the basic anatomy, to the biomechanics, to the examination, the interpretation of radiographs, the treatment options, and how to weigh what was best for the patient. He was always thinking of ways to make knowledge of shoulder conditions and treatments easier to understand to be applied in a practical way to shoulder practice. The result of that interest and awareness was the creation of the International Shoulder Club, which was designed to make it easier for those interested in shoulders to have an organization which would appeal to them. This organization was aimed at the trainee but also the younger generation of providers with an interest in shoulders.

The second product of his interest in shoulders and in helping educate other health care providers was this book. Dr. Huri has recruited an amazing group of contributors who not only have experience in shoulders but are close enough to their training to understand what is important to know at every level. The result is a book of value not only to people new to the shoulder challenges but also to the seasoned veteran who wishes to have a quick and handy guide to the up-to-date concepts and knowledge of shoulder conditions and treatment.

The book is very concise and well organized by topic. Unlike many shoulder books this book gives solid advice and guidance about the nonoperative treatment of most shoulder conditions. There is enough information here for the novice and the expert in a concise and easy-to-understand format. In the theme mentioned above of thoughtfulness about those training in shoulder surgery or in orthopedics in general, each chapter is followed by multiple choice type questions to assist in preparing for boards or for the gruffy attending at your throat.

I can recommend this book without any reservation and it should become a best seller for those within orthopedics and in shoulders particularly.

Baltimore, MD, USA — Edward G. McFarland

Contributor Preface II

Over the past decade, the field of orthopedic surgery has become significantly competitive from the perspective of orthopedics residents. Most residents are interested in pursuing a career in orthopedic surgery and become a good surgeon. The FORTE book series is designed to provide orthopedics residents and trainees a resource to enable them to be more proactive about their intra-operative learning. This book offers a roadmap for the most common orthopedic operative procedures in shoulder surgery. Each chapter presents the basic science, anatomy, biomechanical features of shoulder, principles of physical examination, and an algorithmic approach to shoulder disorders.

This book covers the contents of what an orthopedics and traumatology resident need to know about current trends and concepts about the shoulder.

I hope that this book assists all the trainees in optimally improving their shoulder knowledge and increase the success in board exams.

Thank you very much indeed to Dr. Gazi Huri for his outstanding effort in editing this book and inviting me to participate in this nice work.

Ankara, Turkey — Mahmut Nedim Doral

Editor's Preface

The medical field is continuously changing and growing—aiming to perfect treatments and create better experiences for patients. Today, there are simple procedures for conditions which were very challenging to treat years before. Like other focuses of medicine, orthopedics has also changed for a great deal over the years and has become an area which treats an endless array of conditions. A hundred years ago, orthopedic surgery was in its infancy and orthopedic residency did not even exist. Orthopedics practice was learned in a traditional master and journeyman relationship, or most of the time, just by trial and error. But today, we have several modern and rapid ways of learning and practice. In addition to several educational materials in orthopedics, I believe that this book will be a good reference source that would provide the knowledge base needed for competent orthopedics practice. This book covers the contents of what an orthopedics and traumatology resident need to know with a primary focus on shoulder.

This book is one of the educational projects of Federation of Orthopaedics Trainees in Europe (FORTE) with outstanding international efforts underneath. In this book, we aimed to create a reference which is based on European Education Platform (EEP) core curriculum for preparing for European Board of Orthopaedics and Traumatology (EBOT) Exam. Based on that, this book contains 30 chapters discussed by outstanding experts in the shoulder field. Among these experts, I would like to express my deepest appreciation to Prof. Mahmut N. Doral, Prof. Edward G. McFarland, Prof. Ofer Levy, Prof. Young L. Moon, Prof. Uma Srikumaran, Dr. Ehud Rath, Dr. Filippo Familiari, and all other valuable contributors from all over the world such as the USA, Turkey, the United Kingdom, Israel, Italy, Greece, France, and Korea.

Furthermore I would like to thank my friends Dr. Enis Guryel, Dr. Bram Hentenaar, Dr. Nikolaos Paschos, and Dr. Joao Vide as the FORTE presidents for their great motivation and support. Also I would like to convey my sincere thanks to Ms. Liz Pope for her great patience and encouragement during the project. It was a great pleasure for me to collaborate with her in that long trip.

Finally, I would like to thank my biggest supporters, my daughter Alin Defne and my wife Pınar. Thank you for understanding me even when I worked till mornings and unable to spend time with you. Thank you for loving me. Thank you for being in my life.

Enjoy the book!

Yours sincerely

Gazi Huri

Contents

Editors' Biographies

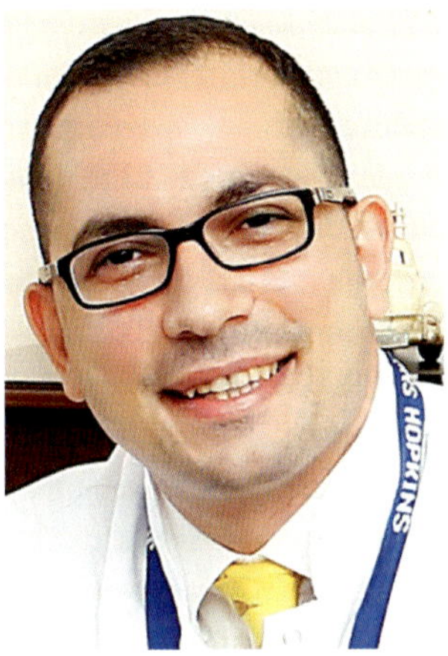

Gazi Huri, M.D. is an Associate Professor at Hacettepe University School of Medicine Department of Orthopaedics and Traumatology, Ankara, Turkey.

He did his residency at Hacettepe University Orthopaedics and Traumatology Department between 2003 and 2008. Consequently he has worked at Johns Hopkins University School of Medicine, Department of Orthopaedics and Traumatology, Division of Sport Medicine, Baltimore, MD, USA, as a fellow "Shoulder Surgeon" between 2012 and 2014.

He has taken several positions in international professional associations and organizations. He is the Turkey representative of the European Board of Orthopaedics and Traumatology (EBOT), which is the most qualified organization on Orthopaedics Education in Europe. In addition he was the former president (2014–2015) of Federation of Orthopaedics Trainees in Europe (FORTE) which represents the young orthopaedics surgeon in Europe and currently he is still keeping the educational committee "President" position in the same organization.

He has an international patent (USA, European PO, Japan, and Turkey) about orthopedics and traumatology which is awarded "the Best Patent Award" and "Best Academic Invention" by the International Federation of Inventors' Associations (IFIA) during the International Inventions Fair 2016. He has more than ten awards for his academic researches and more than 50 papers in international books and journals as well. He is one of the coordinators of the European Union ERASMUS Plus project titled as ESTRO/ European School for Training in Orthopaedics.

He is married and has a child.

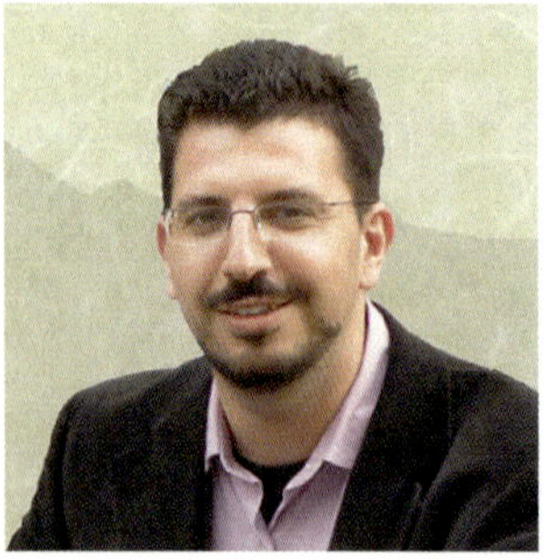

Nikolaos K. Paschos

Dr. Paschos's interdisciplinary background spans the fields of orthopedics, sports medicine, emergency medicine, biomechanics, and regenerative medicine. He is committed for continuous education and training towards improving quality of life of patients. Originally from Greece, Dr. Paschos completed his medical education and residency training at the University of Ioannina, and after spending some time in the UK and Ireland he moved to the USA. He holds a Ph.D. in biomechanics and tissue engineering, and he has worked at the University of California Davis. He is currently working in the Department of Orthopedic Surgery, Division of Sports Medicine at the Boston Children's Hospital, Harvard Medical School. Since 2010, he serves in the Executive Board of Directors of FORTE (Federation of Orthopaedic Trainees in Europe) where he served as the President of FORTE from 2013 to 2014. During that time he initiated the process that led to the birth of the Orthopaedic Study Guide Series.

Contributors

Antoine Adam, M.D. Orthopedic, Traumatology, and Hand Surgery Unit, Nano medicine Research, CHRU Besancon, University of Bourgogne—Franche Comte, Besancon, France

Sercan Akpinar, M.D. Department of Orthopaedics and Traumatology, Medline Hospital, Adana, Turkey

Grassi Alberto, M.D. Istituto Ortopedico Rizzoli, University of Bologna, Bologna, Italy

Mesut Atabek, M.D. Orthopaedics and Traumatology Division, Liv Hospital, Ankara, Turkey

M. Baybars Ataoğlu, M.D. Faculty of Medicine, Department of Orthopaedics and Traumatology, Gazi University, Ankara, Turkey

Ran Atzmon, M.D. Department of Orthopaedic Surgery, Assaf Harofe Medical Center and the Sackler Faculty of Medicine, Tzrifin, Israel

Matthew Baker, M.D. Department of Orthopaedic Surgery, The Johns Hopkins University, Lutherville, MD, USA

Emmanuel Baudouin, M.D. Centre Hospitalier de Chambéry, Place Lucien Biset, Chambéry, France

Nilgün Bek, P.T., Ph.D. Department of Physiotherapy and Rehabilitation, Faculty of Health Sciences, Hacettepe University, Ankara, Turkey

Alex Bitzer, M.D. Division of Shoulder Surgery, Department of Orthopaedic Surgery, The Johns Hopkins University, Baltimore, MD, USA

Etienne Boyer Orthopedic, Traumatology, and Hand Surgery Unit, Nano medicine Research, CHRU Besancon, University of Bourgogne – Franche Comte, Besancon, France

Yusuf Bora Bozduman, M.D. Orthopaedics and Traumatology Department, Hacettepe University School of Medicine, Ankara, Turkey

Aydin Budeyri, M.D. Department of Orthopaedics and Traumatology, SANKO University, Faculty of Medicine, Gaziantep, Turkey

Kadir Büyükdoğan, M.D. Steadman Philippon Research Institute, Vail, Colorado, USA

Kyubo Choi, M.D. Division of Shoulder Surgery, Department of Orthopaedic Surgery, The Johns Hopkins University, Lutherville, MD, USA

Pascal Clappaz, M.D. Clinique Convert, Bourg-en-Bresse, France

Serdar Demirci, P.T., M.Sc. Department of Physiotherapy and Rehabilitation, Hacettepe University, Ankara, Turkey

Mahmut Nedim Doral, M.D. Department of Orthopaedics and Traumatology, Hacettepe University, Ankara, Turkey

Irem Duzgun, P.T., Ph.D. Department of Physiotherapy and Rehabilitation, Hacettepe University, Ankara, Turkey

Atoun Ehud, M.D. Faculty of Health Science, Ben Gurion University, Barzilai Medical Center Campus, Ashkelon, Israel

Leyla Sumeyye Eraslan, P.T., M.Sc. Department of Physiotherapy and Rehabilitation, Hacettepe University, Ankara, Turkey

Cem Zeki Esenyel, M.D. Department of Orthopaedic Surgery, Giresun University Medical Faculty, Giresun, Turkey

Filippo Familiari, M.D. Department of Orthopaedic and Trauma Surgery, Magna Græcia University, Catanzaro, Italy

Raggi Federico, M.D. Istituto Ortopedico Rizzoli, University of Bologna, Bologna, Italy

Olimpio Galasso, M.D. Department of Orthopaedic and Trauma Surgery, Magna Græcia University, Catanzaro, Italy

Nickolas G. Garbis, M.D. Loyola University Medical, Maywood, IL, USA

Giorgio Gasparini, M.D. Department of Orthopaedic and Trauma Surgery, Magna Græcia University, Catanzaro, Italy

Seyedali R. Ghasemi, M.D. Division of Shoulder Surgery, Department of Orthopaedic Surgery, The Johns Hopkins University, Lutherville, MD, USA

Lullini Giada, M.D. Istituto Ortopedico Rizzoli, University of Bologna, Bologna, Italy

Marcheggiani Muccioli Giulio Maria, M.D., Ph.D. Istituto Ortopedico Rizzoli, University of Bologna, Bologna, Italy

Carbone Giuseppe, M.D. Istituto Ortopedico Rizzoli, University of Bologna, Bologna, Italy

Ugur Gonc, M.D. Orthopaedics and Traumatology Division, Liv Hospital, Ankara, Turkey

Gazi Huri, M.D. Department of Orthopaedics and Traumatology, School of Medicine, Hacettepe University, Ankara, Turkey

Jacob Joseph, B.A. Division of Shoulder Surgery, Department of Orthopaedic Surgery, The Johns Hopkins University, Lutherville, MD, USA

Saygin Kamaci, M.D. Department of Orthopaedic Surgery, University of Louisville Hospital, Kentucky, USA

Ulunay Kanatlı, M.D. Faculty of Medicine, Department of Orthopaedics and Traumatology, Gazi University, Ankara, Turkey

Dogac Karaguven, M.D. Department of Orthopaedics and Traumatology, Ufuk University, Ankara, Turkey

Mehmet Kaymakoğlu, M.D. Department of Orthopaedics and Traumatology, School of Medicine, Hacettepe University, Ankara, Turkey

Kelly G. Kilcoyne, M.D. Johns Hopkins Orthopaedic Surgery, Johns Hopkins University School of Medicine, Baltimore, MD, USA

T. Lascar, M.D. Centre Hospitalier Princesse-Grace, Monaco, France

Ofer Levy, M.D., M.Ch.(Orth.), F.R.C.S. Shoulder and Elbow Centre Reading Shoulder Unit, Berkshire Independent Hospital, Reading, UK

François Loisel, M.D. Orthopedic, Traumatology, and Hand Surgery Unit, Nano medicine Research, CHRU Besancon, University of Bourgogne – Franche Comte, Besancon, France

Edward G. McFarland, M.D. Division of Shoulder Surgery, Department of Orthopaedic Surgery, The Johns Hopkins University, Lutherville, MD, USA

Gauthier Menu Orthopedic, Traumatology, and Hand Surgery Unit, Nano medicine Research, CHRU Besancon, University of Bourgogne – Franche Comte, Besancon, France

Young Lee Moon, M.D. 3D Medical Application Work Group, IEEE-SA, Milano, Italy

3D Printing Work Group, ISO-TC 261, Berlin, Germany

American Shoulder and Elbow Surgeons, San Diego, CA, USA

Orthopaedic Department, Chosun University Medical Research Center, Chosun University Hospital, Gwangju, South Korea

Ersin Mutlu, M.D. Orthopaedics and Traumatology Department, Hacettepe University School of Medicine, Ankara, Turkey

Laurent Obert, M.D. Orthopedic, Traumatology, and Hand Surgery Unit, Nano medicine Research, CHRU Besancon, University of Bourgogne – Franche Comte, Besancon, France

Tsvieli Oren, M.D. Ma'ayanei Hayeshua Medical Center, Bnei-Brak, Israel

Osman Orman, M.D. Orthopaedic and Traumatology/Hand Surgery, Baltalimani Metin Sabancı Bone and Joint Diseases Education and Research Hospital, Istanbul, Turkey

Mustafa Özer, M.D. Meram Medical Faculty, Department of Orthopaedics and Traumatology, Necmettin Erbakan University Medical School, Konya, Turkey

Ashnaa Rao, M.D. Johns Hopkins School of Medicine, Baltimore, Maryland, USA

Mustafa Rashid, MB, ChB, MRCS, M.Sc. Nuffield Department of Orthopaedics, Rheumatology, and Musculoskeletal Sciences (NDORMS), Oxford, UK

Ehud Rath, M.D. Department of Orthopaedic Surgery, Tel Aviv Soursky Medical Center and the Sackler Faculty of Medicine at Tel Aviv University, Tel Aviv, Israel

Severin Rochet, M.D. Orthopedic, Traumatology, and Hand Surgery Unit, Nano medicine Research, CHRU Besancon, University of Bourgogne – Franche Comte, Besancon, France

Danny Ryan, MA, MB, BChir (Cantab), PGCME, FRSA, MRCSEng Trauma and Orthopaedic Surgery, Gloucestershire Royal Hospital, Gloucester, UK

Rachid Saadnia, M.D. Orthopedic, Traumatology, and Hand Surgery Unit, Nano medicine Research, CHRU Besancon, University of Bourgogne – Franche Comte, Besancon, France

Roberti di Sarsina Tommaso, M.D. Istituto Ortopedico Rizzoli, University of Bologna, Bologna, Italy

Zachary T. Sharfman, M.D. Department of Orthopaedic Surgery, Tel Aviv Soursky Medical Center and the Sackler Faculty of Medicine at Tel Aviv University, Tel Aviv, Israel

Uma Srikumaran, M.D., M.B.A. Johns Hopkins Orthopaedic Surgery, Johns Hopkins University School of Medicine, Baltimore, MD, USA

Zaffagnini Stefano, M.D. Istituto Ortopedico Rizzoli, University of Bologna, Bologna, Italy

Julien Uhring, M.D. Orthopedic, Traumatology, and Hand Surgery Unit, Nano medicine Research, CHRU Besancon, University of Bourgogne – Franche Comte, Besancon, France

Ahmet Yildirim, M.D. Department of Orthopaedics and Traumatology, Selcuk University Medical School, Konya, Turkey

Taha Ibrahim Yildiz, P.T., M.Sc. Department of Physiotherapy and Rehabilitation, Hacettepe University, Ankara, Turkey

Part I

Basic Science

Shoulder Anatomy

1

Nickolas G. Garbis

The shoulder is a complex joint that is essential to daily function. It serves as the connection of the axial skeleton to the upper extremity. It has an essential function in positioning the upper extremity in space, to allow us to interact with the environment, and to manipulate our surroundings. In this chapter, we will present an overview of the basic anatomy of the shoulder

Bones and Joints

There are four bones which comprise the shoulder girdle. The sternum, the clavicle, the scapula, and the humerus. Going over the specifics of these individual bones will assist in understanding the relationships between them and the rest of the body. In addition, there are several articulations considered when evaluating the shoulder girdle. These are the sternoclavicular (SC) joint, acromioclavicular (AC) joint, and the glenohumeral joint. Although not technically "joints," we also take into consideration certain articulations or potential spaces, namely the subacromial space and the scapulothoracic bursa.

N.G. Garbis, M.D.
Loyola University Medical Center,
Maywood, IL, USA
e-mail: ngarbis@lumc.edu

Sternum

The sternum is derived from the Greek word στέρνον which means chest. It serves as the connection point of the appendicular skeleton to the axial skeleton [1]. The sternum is composed of three parts: the manubrium (Latin: handle), the body, and the xiphoid process. The sternum at its most cephalad portion has a notch which is a depression between the two sternoclavicular joints [2]. The sternoclavicular articulation consists of shallow notches at the superolateral corners of the manubrium that articulate with the medial ends of the clavicles (Fig. 1.1). The manubrium and body also serve as the insertion point of the costal cartilages for ribs 1–7. While the majority of orthopedic surgeons will not perform any surgical procedures on the sternoclavicular joint, it is important to understand it's role in the biomechanics of shoulder motion.

Clavicle

The clavicle is a curved bone that spans from the sternum medially to the acromion laterally. It has a flattened shape near the lateral third but a convex shape medially [2]. It is the first bone in the body which begins to ossifymm in utero at 5 weeks of life. The medial epiphysis is also the last bone to fuse at age 23–25 [3]. At the sternal end, the clavicle is approximately 23 mm × 22 mm in cross section, 12 mm × 12 mm in the diaphy-

G. Huri, N.K. Paschos (eds.), *The Shoulder*, Orthopaedic Study Guide Series,
DOI 10.1007/978-3-319-51979-1_1

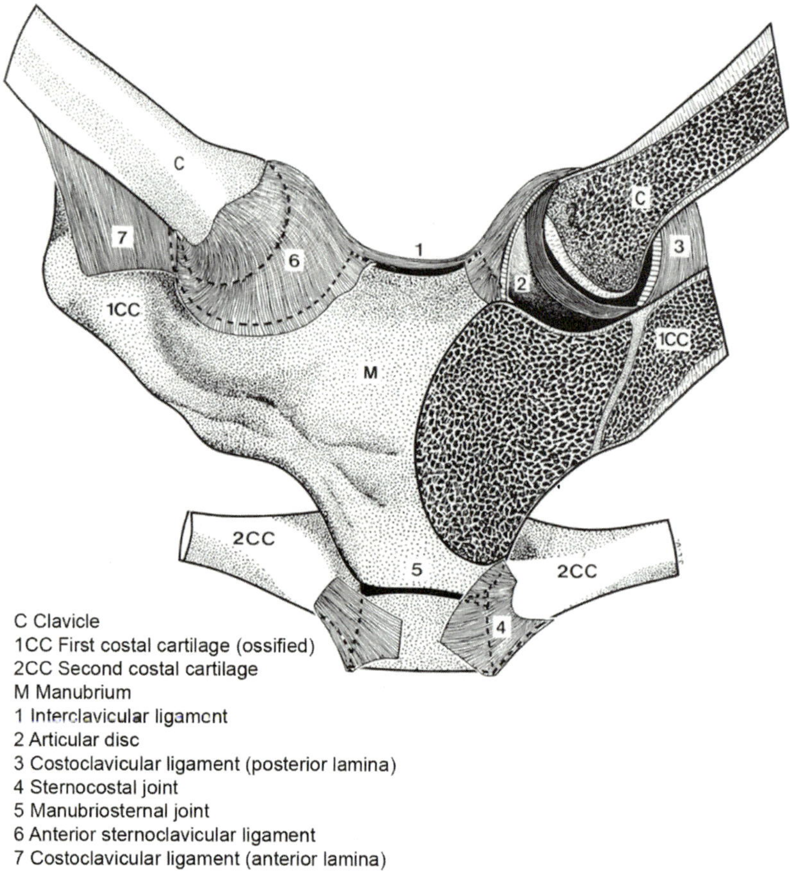

Fig. 1.1 Diagram of the sternoclavicular joint [36]

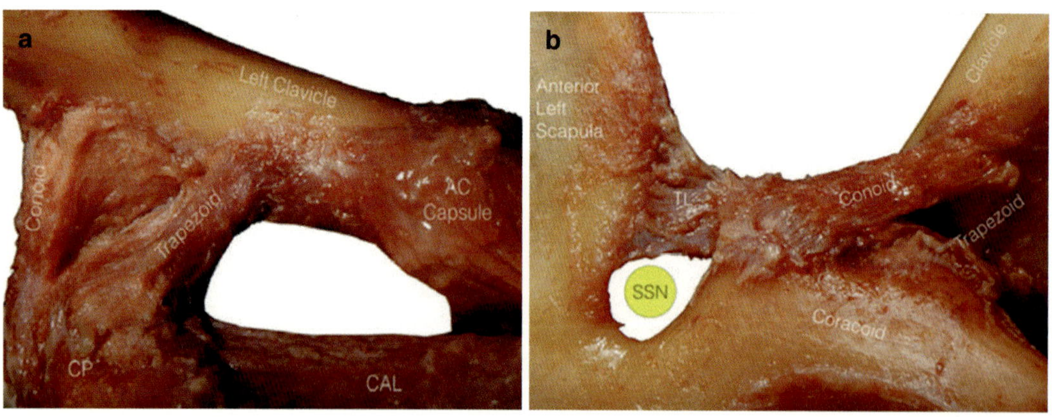

Fig. 1.2 Gross anatomy of the coracoclavicularligaments (**a**) Anteriorview. (**b**) Anteriormedialview. *CP* coracoid process, *TL* transverse ligament, *SSN* suprascapular nerve, *CAL* coracoacromial ligament [37] (Chapter 17, Yon-Sik Yoo)

sis, and 21 mm × 11 mm at the lateral end [4]. The clavicle is stabilized by the acromioclavicular and coracoclavicular (trapezoid and conoid) ligaments (Fig. 1.2). The primary restraint provided by the acromioclavicular ligaments is in the anteroposterior direction. The primary restraint provided by the conoid and trapezoid ligaments is in the craniocaudal direction [5].

The clavicle acts as a strut that supports the arm for activities that are performed away from the body. It also serves as protection for underlying neurovascular structures [6], and potentially as a mechanical advantage for the myofascial sleeve surrounding it [7].

Scapula

The scapula is a flat triangular bone with multiple prominences. It acts as a mobile point of fixation for several of the upper extremity stabilizing muscles. The scapula is curved to articulate over the rib cage. It has a prominent spine posteriorly (Fig. 1.3) to serve as the division between the supraspinatus and infraspinatus fossae. In addition, the coracoid projects anteriorly and is an important landmark in surgical anatomy (sometimes called the "lighthouse of the shoulder") [8]. The conjoined tendon of the coracobrachialis and short head of the biceps take their origin off the coracoid. In addition, the coracoid serves as the insertion site of the pectoralis minor tendon (Fig. 1.4). The coracoclavicular and coracoacromial ligaments also attach to the coracoid. The acromion is one of the more easily palpable prominences of the scapula, and serves as the connection point of the clavicle to the scapula and also serves as the origin of the deltoid muscle. Towards the lateral end of the scapula, the bone flares into the glenoid neck and terminates into the glenoid fossa. The glenoid anatomy can be variable but the version usually ranges between 9.5° of anteversion to 10.5° of retroversion [9]. Mean glenoid inclination is approximately 4° of superior tilt [10]. The same study reported an average glenoid size of 27.8 mm × 37.5 mm in men, and 23.6 mm × 32.6 mm in women.

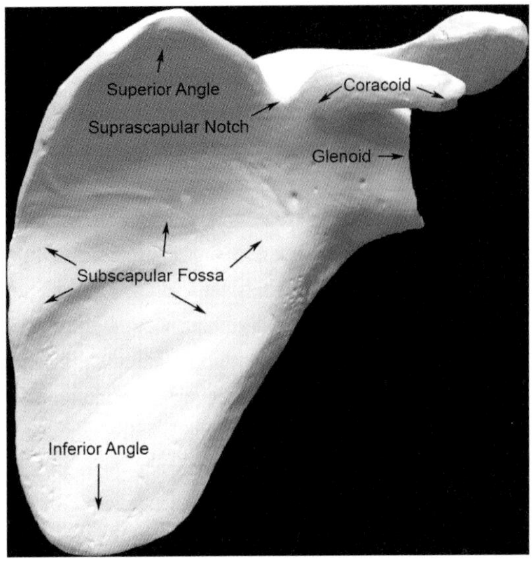

Fig. 1.4 Anterior view of a left scapula

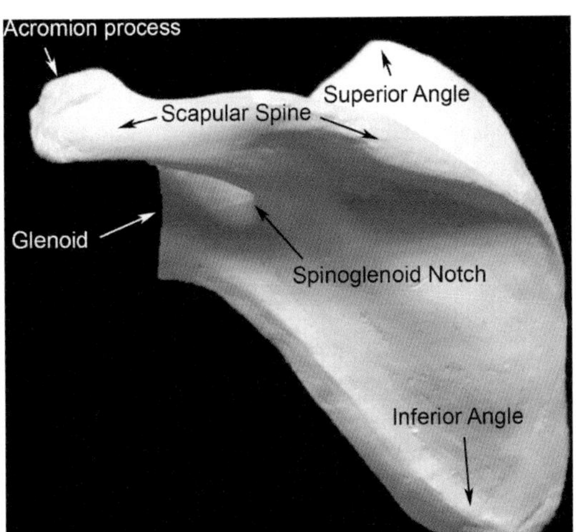

Fig. 1.3 Posterior view of a left scapula

Humerus

The humerus is the extension of the shoulder joint that allows us to position our distal extremity in space. The humeral head is the ovoidproximal end of the humerus that articulates with the glenoid. Its average radius of curvature is 24 mm in the coronal plane, and the average thickness is 19 mm [11]. The average articular surface diameter has been reported as 43 mm [12]. The greater and lesser tuberosities serve as attachment points for the rotator cuff tendons (Fig. 1.5). The subscapularis attaches to the lesser tuberosity. The supraspinatus, infraspinatus, and teres minor attach to the greater tuberosity. The bicipital groove is found between the two tuberosities, and can serve as a landmark during surgery. The retroversion of the proximal humerus can be variable anywhere from 10–50° and is usually quoted as averaging 30° [13].

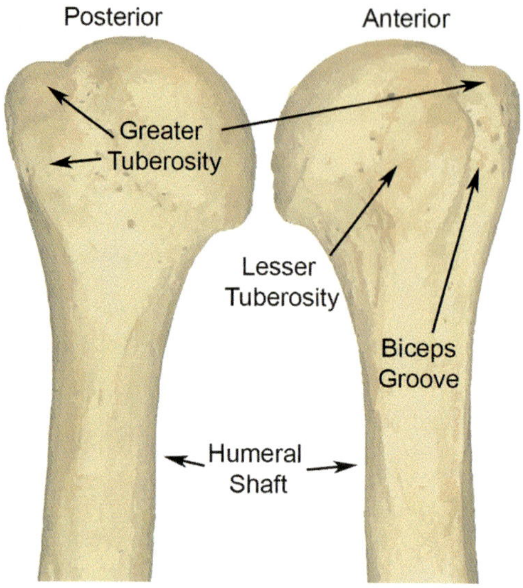

Fig. 1.5 Posterior and anterior views of the proximal humerus demonstrating the tuberosities and the bicipital groove

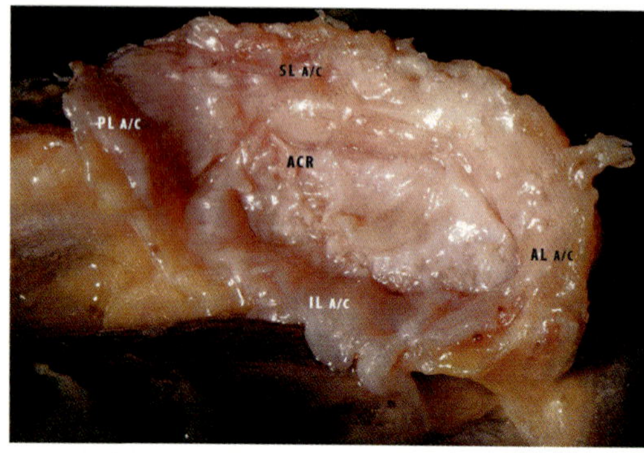

Fig. 1.6 Left shoulder: acromial side of the A/C joint. The entire capsule, detached from the clavicular side, is still attached at the acromial side, making the acromioclavicular ligaments visible (*ACR* acromion, articular side, *AL a/c* anterior acromioclavicular ligament, *IL a/c* inferior acromioclavicular ligament, *PL a/c* posterior acromioclavicular ligament. *SL a/c* superior acromioclavicular ligament) [38]

Sternoclavicular Joint

The sternoclavicular joint is a synovial joint at the superior end of the sternum and the medial aspect of the clavicle [14]. It has been described as both a ball and socket joint and a saddle joint [15]. In addition, the first costal cartilage is at the inferior aspect of the sternoclavicular joint. The sternoclavicular joint serves as the only bony connection of the axial skeleton to the upper extremity. The ligamentous restraints of the joint come from thickenings of the capsule. The primary restraint of the sternoclavicular joint is the posterior sternoclavicular ligament. There is an articular disc that attaches superiorly and inferiorly that lies between the medial end of the clavicle and the sternum [16]. There is also a costoclavicular ligament which connects the medial end of the clavicle to the first rib (Fig. 1.1). This helps restrict superior migration of the clavicle. There is approximately 30–35° of elevation and 35° of flexion and extension [3]. Most of the motion at the sternoclavicular articulation occurs in the first 90° of elevation [17].

Acromioclavicular Joint

Moving laterally, the acromioclavicular (AC) joint is the articulation between the lateral end of the clavicle and the medial end of the acromion. The articular ends of both the clavicle and the acromion are covered with fibrocartilage. In addition to the fibrocartilage, there is an articular disc that is meniscoid in nature and covers mostly the superior portion of the joint [18] (Fig. 1.6). The angle of the joint can be quite variable, and should be considered if any surgical procedure is to be undertaken [19]. Most of the stability in the anterior and posterior direction is provided by the AC ligament. The coracoclavicular (CC) ligaments are composed of the conoid (posteromedial) and the trapezoid (anterolateral) ligaments. These serve to maintain the craniocaudal relationship between the clavicle and the coracoid and provide most of the vertical stability [20].

Glenohumeral Joint

The glenohumeral joint is the "ball in socket" or more appropriately "ball on golf tee" joint that allows a significant amount of mobility to position

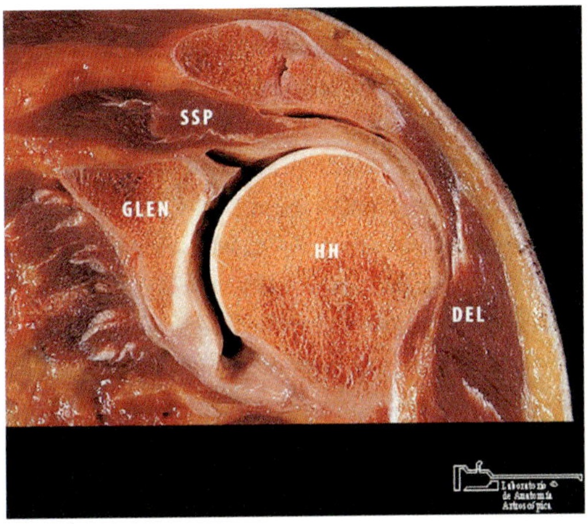

Fig. 1.7 Left shoulder, frontal view (*DEL* deltoid, *GLEN* glenoid, *HH* humeral head, *SSP* supraspinatus) (Digiacomo and Dr. Pau Golanò) [38]

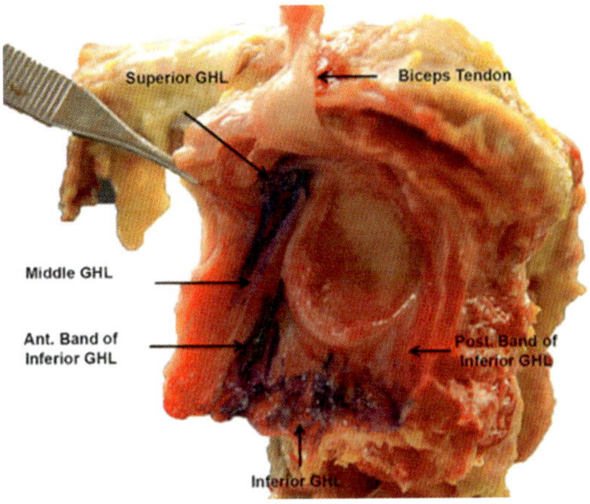

Fig. 1.8 Left cadaveric shoulder demonstrating labrum and intraarticular ligaments [37] (Chapter 9, Apostolakos et al.)

the arm in space (Fig. 1.7). To account for this mobility, there are several static and dynamic restraints to range of motion. Unlike the hip, only a small portion of the humeral articular surface is in contact with the glenoid at any given point [21]. The glenoid labrum surrounds the bony glenoid and is a ring of fibrocartilage that serves to deepen articular surface and provide stability [22]. The labrum also serves as an attachment site for the glenohumeral ligaments, joint capsule, and long head of the biceps tendon [23] (Fig. 1.8).

Any alteration in the structure and morphology of the glenohumeral joint can lead to increased instability. Changes in the articular version can lead to increased instability. Additionally, capsulolabral tears can allow for increased glenohumeral translation. Fractures or recurrent dislocations with bone loss can decrease the effective glenoid articular surface, which can lead to increased instability. The fluid in the shoulder producing an adhesion-cohesion effect can also stabilize the joint [24].

As mentioned previously, the capsule and labrum play a large part in the stability of the joint. There are several named thickenings of the joint capsule that serve as named ligamentous stabilizers of the glenohumeral joint [25] (Fig. 1.8). As static stabilizers, they come into play at the end range of motion in various directions, as the structures are placed on stretch.

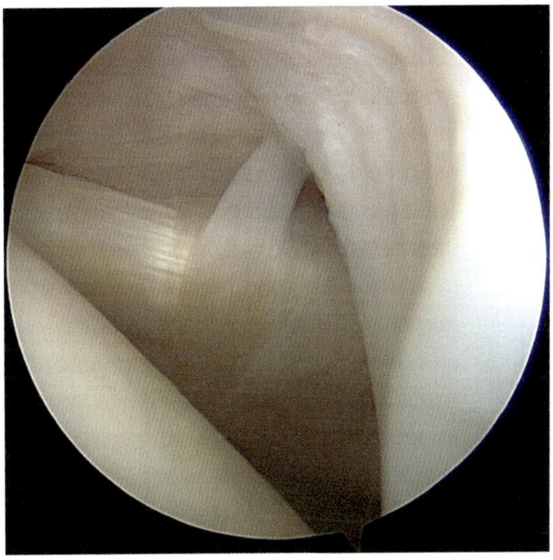

Fig. 1.9 Arthroscopic image of the middle glenohumeral ligament coming off at 90° angle to the subscapularis tendon. Patient is in the beach chair position, image taken from the posterior portal (Nickolas G. Garbis, MD)

The inferior glenohumeral ligament is a hammock like structure at the inferior aspect of the shoulder. It has been described as being composed of three parts: the anterior band (AIGHL), the posterior band (PIGHL) and the axillary pouch (AxIGHL) [26]. When the arm is placed in abduction the ligament tightens and further tightens in external rotation to maintain the humeral head centered in the glenoid. The middle glenohumeral ligament (Fig. 1.9) limits external rotation with the arm at the side. Its anatomy is variable but usually attaches to the upper aspect of the anterior glenoid, runs deep to the subscapularis, and inserts onto the lesser tuberosity. A sublabral foramen is found in 12% of arthroscopies, a cord-like MGHL in 18%, and a Buford complex in 1–2% of arthroscopies [27, 28]. The Buford complex is defined as an absent anterosuperior labrum and a cord like MGHL which originates from the superior labrum. The superior glenohumeral ligament (SGHL) limits inferior translation and external rotation. It also prevents anterior-superior escape of the humeral head. It usually originates from the supraglenoid tubercle anterior to the biceps, but can be variable and has been classified to three different types of origin [29]. The posterior capsule structures are usually thin but can limit posterior translation and can limit adduction across the body. The coracoacromial ligament along with the coracoid and the acromion also serve as static stabilization to prevent superior migration of the humeral head.

The dynamic stabilizers help support the joint through the midrange of motion. These are primarily composed of the rotator cuff and periscapularmuscles. The long head of the biceps may assist in depressing the humeral head, but it's role in shoulder stability is debated [30]. The rotator cuff compresses the humeral head into the glenoid, further enhancing stability [31].

Subacromial Space

The subacromial space contains a bursa that separates the rotator cuff and supraspinatus muscle, from the deltoid and the acromion above it. During arthroscopic approaches, several structures can be assessed from the subacromial space, including the rotator cuff, CA ligament, AC joint, and biceps tendon (Fig. 1.10) The normal acromiohumeral interval on radiographs averages 1.0–1.5 cm [32]. The acromion is often described by the degree of curvature into the subacromial space [33]. Type I is a flat acromion, type II is a curved acromion, and type III is a hooked acromion (Fig. 1.11).

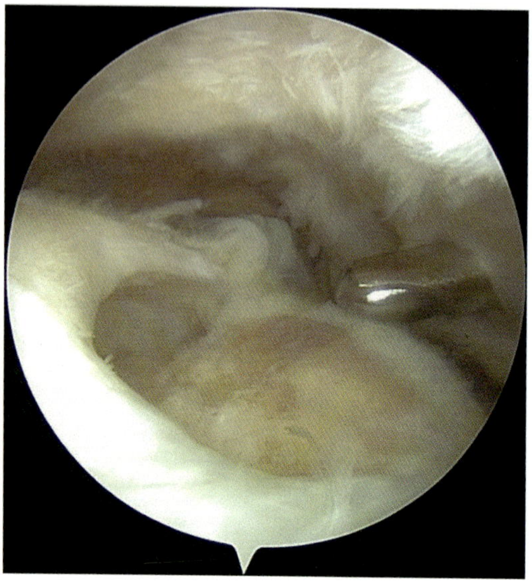

Fig. 1.10 View of the right subacromial space from a posterior portal in beach chair position demonstrating a supraspinatus tear (Nickolas G. Garbis, MD)

Scapulothoracic Bursa

The scapulothoracic articulation consists of several bursae that assist gliding of the scapula over the ribcage. There have been two major and four minor bursae described. The major bursae are the scapulothoracic bursa and the subscapularis bursa. The four minor bursae are not always identifiable and are often secondary to pathologic scapulothoracic articulation (Fig. 1.12).

Muscles

There are several muscles that affect the shoulder, and it's helpful to group them into regions, or to think of them based on their general origin or

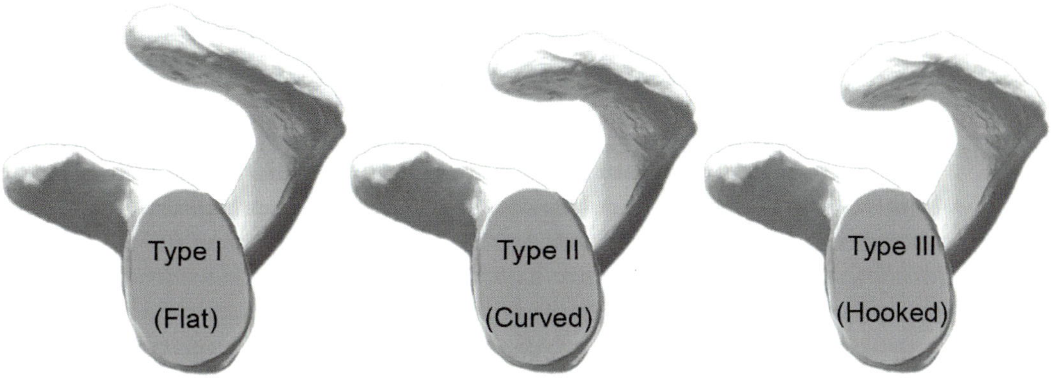

Fig. 1.11 Enface view of the scapula demonstration acromial morphology

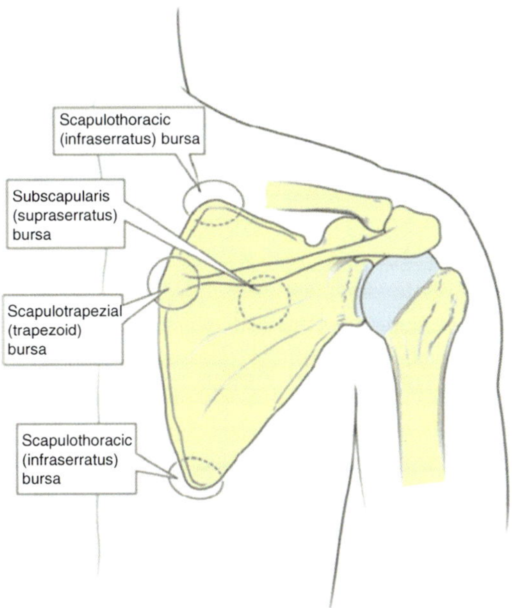

Fig. 1.12 Multiple named bursae around the shoulder, AP view (Hubbard and Poehling p 551,Hubbard JB, Poehling GG. Chapter 46: Scapulothoracic disorders. In: Milano G, Grasso A, editors. Shoulder arthroscopy principles and practice. London: Springer)

insertion. Most of the muscles that act on the shoulder take their origin from either the spinous processes, ribs/chest wall, or the scapula itself. Table 1.1 lists the pertinent muscles about the shoulder girdle. Figures 1.13 and 1.14 demonstrate the anterior and posterior relationships of the rotator cuff muscles and tendons to the shoulder.

Neurovascular Anatomy

The brachial plexus plays a central role in understanding the neuroanatomy about the shoulder girdle. The plexus is composed of nerve roots from C5 to T1, and is responsible for most of the innervation to the upper limb. As the plexus progresses distally, it traditionally is divided into different sections that medical students around the world generated have multiple mnemonics to help remember them. Starting at the roots, they combine to form trunks, divisions, cords, and terminate in branches. One of the more common mnemonics is "Robert Taylor Drinks Cold Beer," or "Rugby Teams Drink Cold Beer" (Fig. 1.13). There are four preclavicular nerve branches which come from the rami and trunks: dorsal scapular nerve, long thoracic nerve, suprascapular nerve, and the nerve to subclavius (Fig. 1.15).

The vascular anatomy about the shoulder usually references the axillary artery and its relationship to the pectoralis minor muscle. The axillary artery is the continuation of the subclavian artery, which comes off of the aorta on the left and the brachiocephalic trunk on the right. The subclavian

Table 1.1 Origins, insertions, innervations, and mechanisms of action of the muscles around the shoulder girdle.

Muscle	Origin	Insertion	Function	Innervation
Pectoralis Minor	Ribs 3–5	Medial aspect of the coracoid	Protracts scapula	Medial pectoral nerve
Pectoralis Major	Sternum, clavicle, ribs	Lateral aspect of the bicipital groove	Adducts and internally rotates arm	Medial and lateral pectoral nerves
Latissimus Dorsi	Spinous processes of thoracolumbar spine and ilium	Medial aspect of the bicipital groove[34]	Extends, adducts, internally rotates humerus	Dorsal scapular nerve
Trapezius	Spinous processes C7–C12	Posterior surface lateral third clavicle, acromion, scapular spine	Rotates scapula	Spinal accessory nerve (cranial nerve XI)
Rhomboid Major	Spinous processes T2–T5	Medial border scapula	Adducts scapula	Dorsal scapular nerve
Rhomboid Minor	Spinous processes C7–T1	Medial aspect of scapular spine	Adducts scapula	Dorsal scapular nerve
Levator Scapulae	Transverse processes C1–C4	Superomedial scapula	Move scapula cephalad and rotate	C3 and C4
Subclavius	First rib	Inferior clavicle	Moves clavicle caudally	Upper trunk brachial plexus
Serratus Anterior	1st–9th ninth ribs	Ventral medial surface of scapula	Holds scapula against chest wall	Long thoracic nerve
Deltoid	Lateral aspect clavicle, acromion, and scapular spine	Deltoid tuberosity of humerus	Abducts arm	Axillary nerve
Teres Major	Inferior scapula	Medial aspect bicipital groove	Adducts, internally rotates, extends arm	Lower subscapular nerve
Subscapularis	Ventral scapula	Lesser tuberosity	Internally rotates arm	Upper and lower subscapular nerves
Supraspinatus	Supraspinous fossa	Greater tuberosity	Abducts and internally rotates arm	Suprascapular nerve
Infraspinatus	Infraspinous fossa	Greater tuberosity	Externally rotates arm	Suprascapular nerve
Teres Minor	Dorsolateral scapula	Greater tuberosity	Externally rotates arm	Axillary nerve
Biceps Brachii	Supraglenoid tubercle (long head) and coracoid (Short head)	Radial tuberosity	Flex and supinate elbow	Musculocutaneous nerve

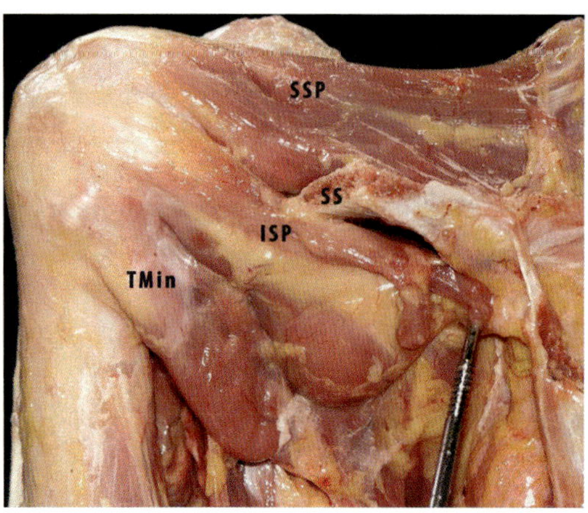

Fig. 1.13 Posterior view of the shoulder demonstrating the rotator cuff musculature. *SSP* supraspinatus, *SS* scapular spine, *ISP* infraspinatus, *Tmin* Teres minor [38]

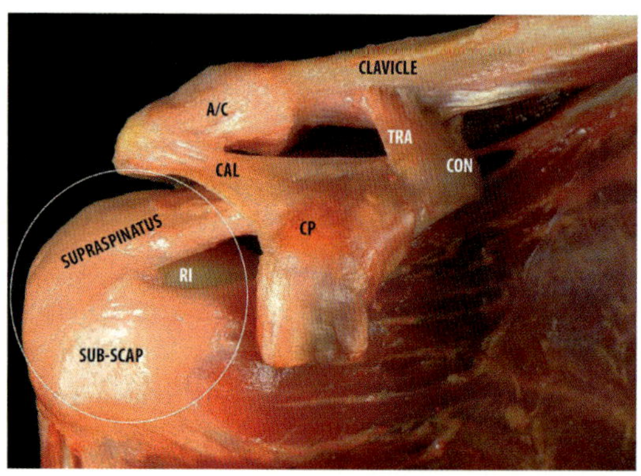

Fig. 1.14 Anterior view of the shoulder demonstrating relationship of subscapularis to the suprapinatus. *RI* rotator interval, *CP* Coracoid process, *A/C* acromioclavicular ligaments, *CAL* coracoacromial ligament, *TRA* trapezoid, *CON* conoid [38]

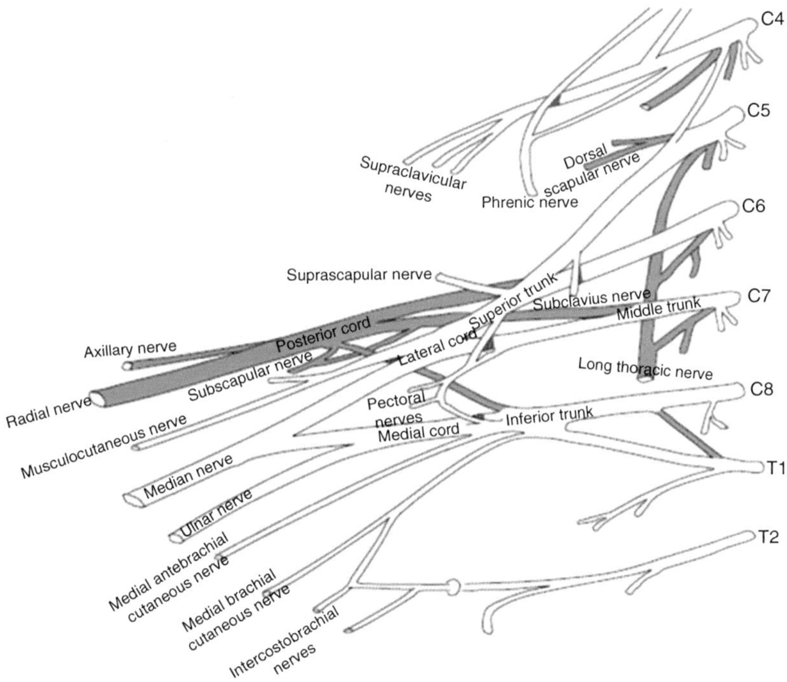

Fig. 1.15 Diagram of the brachial plexus [37], p. 312

artery becomes the axillary artery at the lateral aspect of the first rib. Medial to the pectoralis minor (the first part of the artery), the only branch is the supreme thoracic artery. As the artery passes posterior (deep) to the pectoralis minor (second part), it gives off two branches: the thoracoacromial and lateral thoracic arteries. The thoracoacromial branch divides into four different branches which supply several regions of the shoulder: acromial, clavicular, pectoral, deltoid. Lateral to the pectoralis minor muscle, (third part) it branches off into the subscapular artery, anterior circumflex, and posterior circumflex artery. The vascularity about the shoulder itself contains numerous anastomoses and allows for retrograde filling in case of injury or defect [2, 35].

Shoulder Anatomy

Which bones comprise the shoulder?

A. The humerus and the scapula
B. The humerus, the scapula, and the clavicle
C. The humerus, the scapula, the clavicle and the sternum

Which of the following statements are true for the clavicle

A. It is the first bone in the body which begins to ossifymm in utero
B. The conoid and trapezoid ligaments provide stability in the anteroposterior direction
C. It is formed by both intramembranous and endochondral ossification
D. It is the only long bone that lies horizontally
E. All the above
F. A & C & D
G. A & B & D

Group the bone anatomic regions with the attachments of muscular structures

A. Lesser tuberosity
B. Greater tuberosity
C. Acromion
D. Coracoid
E. Labrum
   1. Subscapularis
   2. Pectoralis minor
   3. Long head of biceps
   4. Supraspinatus
   5. Deltoid

Which is the primary restraint of the sternoclavicular joint
A. Posterior sternoclavicular ligament
B. Anterior sternoclavicular ligament
C. Articular capsule
D. Articular disc

Which of the following statements are correct?
A. The inferior glenohumeral ligament is tight in abduction and external rotation
B. The superior glenohumeral ligament limits inferior translation and external rotation
C. A cord-like MGHL is found in approximately 1 out of 5 patients
D. All the above

Group the types of acromion with their characteristics
A. Type I
B. Type II
C. Type III
   1. Flat acromion
   2. Hooked acromion
   3. Curved acromion

References

1. Baird RN. Anatomy for surgeons volume III: the back and limbs. W. Henry Hollinshead. Third edition. 270 ×185 mm. pp. 878 + viii. Illustrated. 1982. London: Harper and Row. £56.00. Br J Surg. 1983;70(9):570. doi:10.1002/bjs.1800700941.
2. Moore KL, AMR A, Dalley AF. Clinically oriented anatomy. Baltimore: Lippincott Williams & Wilkins; 2010.
3. Rockwood Jr CA, Wirth MA. Disorders of the sternoclavicular joint. In: Rockwood Jr CA, Mattson FA, editors. The shoulder. 2nd ed. Philadelphia: Saunders; 1990. p. 555–609.
4. Galley IJ, Watts AC, Bain GI. The anatomic relationship of the axillary artery and vein to the clavicle: a cadaveric study. J Shoulder Elb Surg. 2009;18(5):e21–5. doi:10.1016/j.jse.2009.01.021.
5. Dawson PA, Adamson GJ, Pink MM, Kornswiet M, Lin S, Shankwiler JA, et al. Relative contribution of acromioclavicular joint capsule and coracoclavicular ligaments to acromioclavicular stability. J Shoulder Elb Surg. 2009;18(2):237–44. doi:10.1016/j.jse.2008.08.003.
6. McKee MD, Wild LM, Schemitsch EH. Midshaft malunions of the clavicle. J Bone Joint Surg Am. 2003;85-a(5):790–7.
7. Abbott LC, Lucas DB. The function of the clavicle; its surgical significance. Ann Surg. 1954; 140(4):583–99.
8. Matsen FA, Rockwood CA. Anterior glenohumeral instability. In: Rockwood CAMF, editor. The shoulder. Philadelphia: WB Saunders; 1990. p. 336–67.
9. Rockwood Jr CA, Matsen III. FA, Wirth MA. Lippitt SB. The shoulder. Philadelphia: Elsevier Health Sciences; 2009.
10. Churchill RS, Brems JJ, Kotschi H. Glenoid size, inclination, and version: an anatomic study. J Shoulder Elb Surg. 2001;10(4):327–32. doi:10.1067/mse.2001.115269.
11. Iannotti JP, Gabriel JP, Schneck SL, Evans BG, Misra S. The normal glenohumeral relationships. An anatomical study of one hundred and forty shoulders. J Bone Joint Surg Am. 1992;74(4):491–500.
12. Boileau P, Walch G. The three-dimensional geometry of the proximal humerus. Implications for surgical technique and prosthetic design. J Bone Joint Surg Br. 1997;79(5):857–65.
13. Pearl ML, Volk AG. Retroversion of the proximal humerus in relationship to prosthetic replacement arthroplasty. J Shoulder Elb Surg. 1995;4(4):286–9.
14. Sewell MD, Al-Hadithy N, Le Leu A, Lambert SM. Instability of the sternoclavicular joint: current concepts in classification, treatment and outcomes. Bone Joint J. 2013;95-B(6):721–31. doi:10.1302/0301-620X.95B6.31064.
15. Renfree KJ, Wright TW. Anatomy and biomechanics of the acromioclavicular and sternoclavicular joints. Clin Sports Med. 2003;22(2):219–37.
16. van Tongel A, MacDonald P, Leiter J, Pouliart N, Peeler J. A cadaveric study of the structural anatomy of the sternoclavicular joint. Clin Anat. 2012;25(7):903–10. doi:10.1002/ca.22021.
17. Inman VT, dec M, Saunders JB, Abbott LC. Observations of the function of the shoulder joint. J Bone Joint Surg Br 1944;26A:1–31.
18. Mall NA, Foley E, Chalmers PN, Cole BJ, Romeo AA, Bach Jr BR. Degenerative joint disease of the acromioclavicular joint: a review. Am J Sports Med. 2013;41(11):2684–92. doi:10.1177/0363546513485359.
19. Nourissat G, Henon A, Debet-Mejean A, Clement P, Dumontier C, Sautet A, et al. Three-dimensional computed tomographic scan of the external third of the clavicle. Arthroscopy. 2007;23(1):29–33. doi:10.1016/j.arthro.2006.08.007.
20. Fukuda K, Craig EV, An KN, Cofield RH, Chao EY. Biomechanical study of the ligamentous system of the acromioclavicular joint. J Bone Joint Surg Am. 1986;68(3):434–40.
21. Soslowsky LJ, Flatow EL, Bigliani LU, Pawluk RJ, Ateshian GA, Mow VC. Quantitation of in situ contact areas at the glenohumeral joint: a biomechanical study. J Orthop Res. 1992;10(4):524–34. doi:10.1002/jor.1100100407.

22. Moseley HF, Övergaard B. The anterior capsular mechanism in recurrent anterior dislocation of the shoulder. J Bone Joint Surg Br. 1962;44-B(4):913–27.
23. Dunham KS, Bencardino JT, Rokito AS. Anatomic variants and pitfalls of the labrum, glenoid cartilage, and glenohumeral ligaments. Magn Reson Imaging Clin N Am. 2012;20(2):213–28. x doi:10.1016/j.mric.2012.01.014.
24. Howell SM, Galinat BJ, Renzi AJ, Marone PJ. Normal and abnormal mechanics of the glenohumeral joint in the horizontal plane. J Bone Joint Surg Am. 1988;70(2):227–32.
25. Steinbeck J, Liljenqvist U, Jerosch J. The anatomy of the glenohumeral ligamentous complex and its contribution to anterior shoulder stability. J Shoulder Elb Surg. 1998;7(2):122–6. doi:10.1016/s1058-2746(98)90221-x.
26. O'Brien SJ, Neves MC, Arnoczky SP, Rozbruck SR, Dicarlo EF, Warren RF, et al. The anatomy and histology of the inferior glenohumeral ligament complex of the shoulder. Am J Sports Med. 1990;18(5):449–56. doi:10.1177/036354659001800501.
27. Ide J, Maeda S, Takagi K. Normal variations of the glenohumeral ligament complex: an anatomic study for arthroscopic Bankart repair. Arthroscopy. 2004;20(2):164–8. doi:10.1016/j.arthro.2003.11.005.
28. Williams MM, Snyder SJ, Buford Jr D. The Buford complex—the "cord-like" middle glenohumeral ligament and absent anterosuperior labrum complex: a normal anatomic capsulolabral variant. Arthroscopy. 1994;10(3):241–7.
29. DePalma AF. Surgery of the shoulder. 3rd ed. Philadelphia: JB Lippincott; 1973.
30. Strauss EJ, Salata MJ, Sershon RA, Garbis N, Provencher MT, Wang VM, et al. Role of the superior labrum after biceps tenodesis in glenohumeral stability. J Shoulder Elb Surg. 2014;23(4):485–91. doi:10.1016/j.jse.2013.07.036.
31. Lippitt SB, Vanderhooft JE, Harris SL, Sidles JA, Harryman 2nd DT, Matsen III FA. Glenohumeral stability from concavity-compression: A quantitative analysis. J Shoulder Elb Surg. 1993;2(1):27–35. doi:10.1016/S1058-2746(09)80134-1.
32. Petersson CJ, Redlund-Johnell I. The subacromial space in normal shoulder radiographs. Acta Orthop Scand. 1984;55(1):57–8.
33. Bigliani LU, Morrison DS, April EW. The morphology of the acromion and its relationship to rotator cuff tears. Orthop Trans. 1986;10:228.
34. Goldberg BA, Elhassan B, Marciniak S, Dunn JH. Surgical anatomy of latissimus dorsi muscle in transfers about the shoulder. Am J Orthop (Belle Mead NJ). 2009;38(3):E64–7.
35. Gerber C, Schneeberger AG, Vinh TS. The arterial vascularization of the humeral head. An anatomical study. J Bone Joint Surg Am. 1990;72(10):1486–94.
36. Guyot J. Atlas of human limb joints. Berlin: Springer; 1990.
37. Bain GI, Itoi E, Di Giacomo G, editors. Normal and pathological anatomy of the shoulder. Heidelberg: Springer; 2015.
38. Di Giacomo G, Pouliart N, Costantini A, De Vita A. Atlas of functional shoulder anatomy. Milan: Springer; 2008.

Surgical Approaches to the Shoulder

2

Nickolas G. Garbis

Deltopectoral Approach

The deltopectoral approach is one of the more common anterior approaches and is useful for a variety of different surgical procedures about the shoulder. As the name suggests, it takes advantage of an internervous plane between the deltoid (axillary nerve) and the pectoralis major (medial and lateral pectoral nerves.) It was described by Henry in 1957 [1]. This approach provides excellent exposure to the anterior shoulder, including the coracoid, subscapularis, anterior humerus, biceps, and glenoid. The deltopectoral approach can also be extended into an anterolateral approach to the humerus in cases of trauma or where more extensile exposure to the humeral shaft is needed.

Operating Room Setup

There are several different positioning methods for the deltopectoral approach to the shoulder. It is usually performed in either the beach chair (semi-sitting) or supine position. It is possible to perform this approach while positioned lateral as well, but the operating surgeon may find it more awkward. In addition to the operating room bed, there are several commercial devices or head holders available to assist with positioning in the beach chair position. These allow for neutral alignment of the cervical spine while also giving more clearance to the posterior shoulder. This access is useful for better clearance with posterior portals in arthroscopic surgery and also assists with dislocation of the humeral head during shoulder arthroplasty procedures (Fig. 2.1).

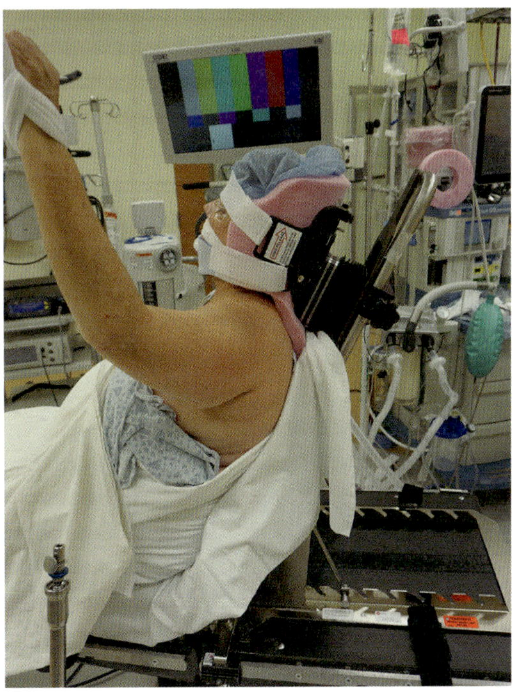

Fig. 2.1 Operating room setup in the beach chair position. Note neutral position of the cervical spine, easy access to the posterior shoulder, and pneumatic arm holder

N.G. Garbis, M.D.
Loyola University Medical Center,
Maywood, IL, USA
e-mail: ngarbis@lumc.edu

G. Huri, N.K. Paschos (eds.), *The Shoulder*, Orthopaedic Study Guide Series,
DOI 10.1007/978-3-319-51979-1_2

How much to elevate the head of the bed is based on surgeon preference. A more seated position (higher angle on the head of the bed) allows for flatter hand positioning during shoulder arthroscopy cases, whereas a more supine angle may allow for easier dislocation of the humeral head during open surgical cases. The beach chair position can be associated with diminished cerebral perfusion [2] but taking precautions such as avoiding hypotensive anesthesia and using compression stockings to improve venous return may help minimize these complications [3]. An arm holder or a padded Mayo stand can also be used to allow for control and positioning of the distal extremity.

Surgical Incision and Dissection

The skin incision for the deltopectoral approach should provide adequate exposure to the deep deltopectoral interval. If an extensile approach is anticipated or may be needed in the future, then an incision along the course of the deltopectoral interval from the coracoid cephalad towards the pecrtoralis insertion on the proximal humerus distally can be easily extended into an anterolateral approach to the humeral shaft (Fig. 2.2). Proximally, the incision can be extended to the clavicle to visualize the entire deltoid origin. Alternately, a more vertical incision from the coracoid into the axillary crease can be used, with subsequent skin flap mobilization to allow exposure to the entire deltopectoral interval. The incision into the axillary crease makes this more difficult to convert to an extensile approach if the humeral shaft needs to be visualized.

Once through the skin, the surgeon can perform superficial dissection through the subcutaneous fat down to the level of the fascia. As a technical point, the fascia of the deltoid is usually more superficial at the cephalad portion of the incision and deeper towards the more caudal end of the incision. At the fascial level, the next step is to develop the interval between the medial aspect of the deltoid and the lateral aspect of the pectoralis major [4] (Fig. 2.3). The interval is easier to identify near the coracoid and towards the clavicle. At this level, the pectoralis and deltoid fiber orientation is easier to distinguish (Fig. 2.4). Distally, the fibers may appear more convergent, and often have interdigitations. This interval can often be identified by looking for the cephalic vein lying in the groove. The vein may be covered in a layer of fat making a longitudinal "fat stripe" parallel to the deltopectoral groove.

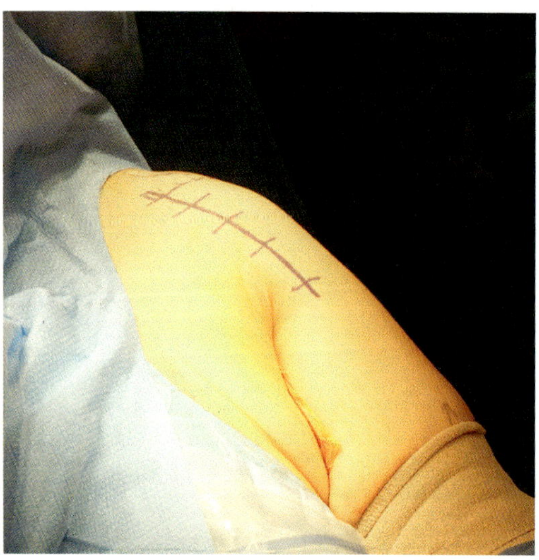

Fig. 2.2 Incision for a deltopectoral approach to the shoulder. Incision is starting at the coracoid and extending towards the pectoralis insertion on the humerus

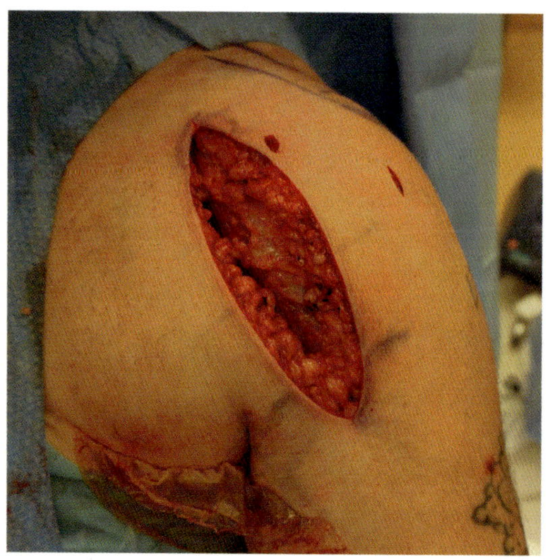

Fig. 2.3 Subcutaneous dissection for the deltopectoral approach

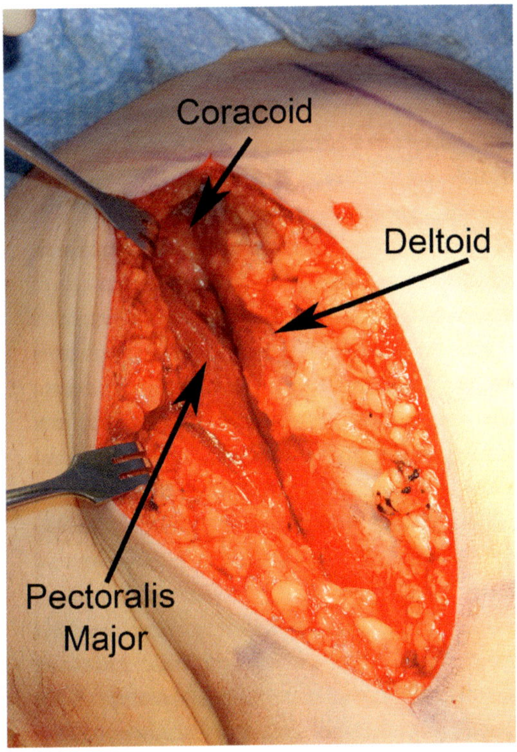

Fig. 2.4 The coracoid is visualized at the superior aspect of the wound. It is easier to distinguish the differing orientation of the pectoralis major and deltoid fibers at this level

Meticulous dissection through this fat stripe and releasing the fascia over the vein proximally and distally will help mobilize the vein and prevent tethering at the proximal and distal ends of the incision. When the vein is difficult to identify, it may be easier to look for it at either the proximal or distal ends of the interval. The vein can also be deep in the interval, and in cases of revision surgery, may be surgically absent or ligated (Fig. 2.5). There are more branch vessels between the deltoid and the vein than between the vein and the pectoralis major [5]. This often makes it easier to dissect and retract the vein laterally with the deltoid. At the proximal aspect of the wound, the vein crosses from medial to lateral, and aggressive deltoid retraction may lacerate the vein. If there appears to be tethering proximally, it may be more protective of the vein to dissect and retract medially with the pectoralis.

Once down in the interval, the pectoralis can be elevated off of the underlying fascia to further accentuate the space between the two muscles. This maneuver will further expose the coracoid and allow the surgeon to identify the conjoined tendon heading distally from the coracoid. The coracoacromial ligament should be visualized at the lateral aspect of the coracoid, heading towards the acromion. Another useful pearl is that the surgeon can often develop the plane between the humeral shaft and the deltoid just laterally to the pectoralis major insertion. This will allow for placement of a distal retractor that can facilitate exposure at the inferior aspect of the approach (Fig. 2.6).

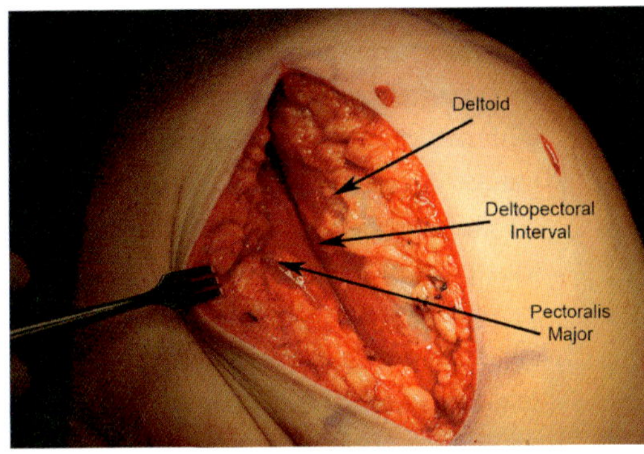

Fig. 2.5 Notice interval between deltoid and pectoralis major. In this patient, the cephalic vein is deep in the interval and not visualized

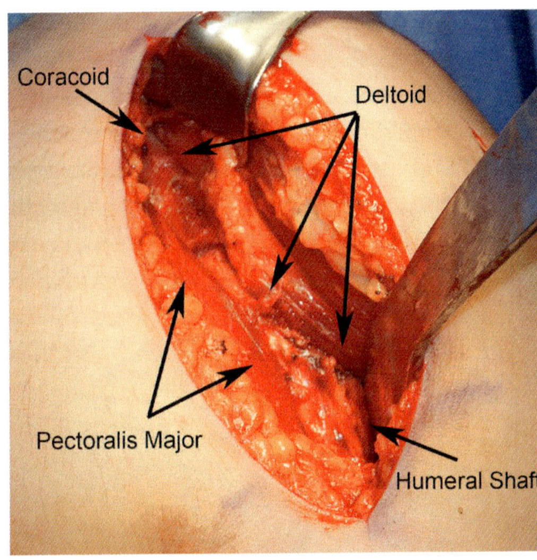

Fig. 2.6 Distal retractor placed around the humeral shaft retracting the deltoid laterally. This exposes the pectoralis insertion. The proximal humerus is still obscured by the overlying deltoid

The clavipectoral fascia can be found lateral to the conjoined tendon and inferior to the coracoacromial ligament. Incision of this fascia will allow easier access to the subcoracoid and subdeltoid spaces. When incising the fascia, take care not to plunge too deep as the subscapularis lies just below the level of the incision. The coracoacromial (CA) ligament should be preserved in cases of anatomic shoulder arthroplasty in order to maintain the integrity of the coracoacromial arch. The incision should also be lateral to the muscle belly of the short head of the biceps instead of following just lateral to the tendon. This will prevent incising into the biceps muscle belly and potentially increase bleeding. This incision of the fascia continues inferiorly until the superior border of the pectoralis insertion on the humerus. Some surgeons will release the upper 1 cm of the pectoralis to allow for greater exposure and easier external rotation. Once the fascia is incised the conjoined tendon is swept medially and the subcoracoid space is developed. The musculocutaneous nerve can sometimes be felt on the posterior aspect of the coracobrachialis approximately 5 cm distal to the coracoid tip, and the axillary nerve can be felt medially at the inferior aspect of the subscapularis (Fig. 2.7). At this point, the subdeltoid space can be identified by developing the plane under the CA ligament. In cases with an intact rotator cuff, the retractor will be in the subacromial space, with the supraspinatus below and the acromion above. In cases where there is a deficient rotator cuff, the humeral head will often be palpable. Once the subdeltoid space is identified proximally and distally, the entire deltoid needs to be mobilized off of the humeral head and underlying bursa. The axillary nerve lies on the deep surface of the deltoid and can be injured if the fascia of the deep deltoid is elevated. When developing this plane, there is a humeral branch from the posterior circumflex vessels that can be a source of brisk bleeding. If seen, this is often at the same level as the axillary nerve and to prevent nerve injury should be coagulated off of the bone of the humerus, not off the deltoid.

Once the deltoid has been completely mobilized, a self-retaining retractor (Kolbel type) can be placed with one blade under the conjoined tendon and one blade under the deltoid muscle. Excessive force on the retractor can injure the musculocutaneous nerve. A deltoid retractor (Browne type) may be useful in exposing more of the proximal humerus during the approach. If there is still restricted access to the proximal humerus, there are some extensile measures that can be performed. One of the problems is that the deltoid can be quite prominent and excessive

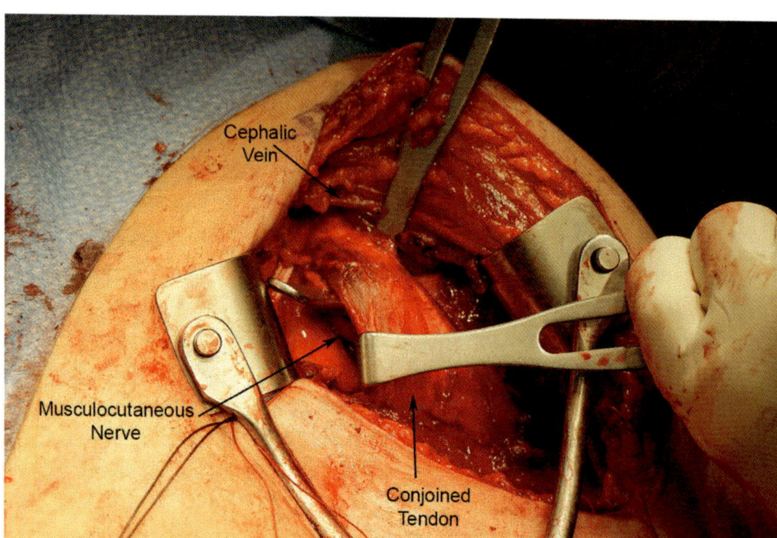

Fig. 2.7 Musculocutaneous nerve seen entering the coracobrachialis when exposing on the medial side of the conjoined tendon. This particular patient is undergoing a pectoralis transfer for subscapularis insufficiency

force is needed to retract it adequately, which can permanently damage the muscle. In his surgical text, Henry observed that "the muscle forms a thick unyielding cowl which gives when pulled aside a grudging revelation of bone and shoulder joint; and that will often be the last successful thing it does" [1]. Removing or reflecting the clavicular origin of the deltoid muscle can improve visualization significantly. Thompson described subperiosteal stripping of the deltoid from the clavicle and acromion with reattachment using cerclage sutures. A Mayo Clinic series of 81 anteromedial approaches to the proximal humerus were studied and found to have excellent results with no deltoid detachments [6]. Redfern et al. [7] described an osteotomy of the anterior cortex of the clavicle to mobilize the anterior deltoid. They reported some minor complications of fracture, fibrous union, and prominent hardware. If more medial or neurovascular exposure is needed, a coracoid osteotomy or conjoined tendon release can be performed as well.

Once the proximal humerus is exposed, the surgeon should take some time to identify key structures. There is sometimes a bursal layer that covers the anterior shoulder structures, and this can be removed to assist with appropriate identification. One of the more useful landmarks to identify is the bicipital groove on the anterior humerus. The long head of the biceps tendon lies within the groove and can be traced up from just above the insertion of the pectoralis major all the way into the rotator interval. As the biceps approaches the rotator interval, it curves medially towards its insertion on the supraglenoid tubercle. The upper border of the subscapularis can be usually felt in the interval. The inferior border of the subscapularis can usually be identified by the presence of the anterior circumflex artery and its two venae comitantes (the "Three Sisters."). If the biceps tendon is elevated out of the groove, the upper border of the latissimus is often visible inserting onto the floor of the bicipital groove. Internal rotation and adduction of the arm will bring the supraspinatus, greater tuberosity, and subacromial bursa into view.

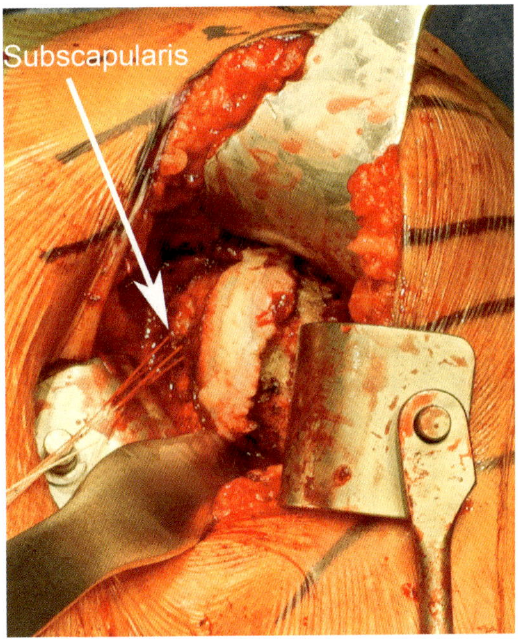

Fig. 2.8 Proximal humerus exposure for an anatomic total shoulder arthroplasty. One blade of the self-retaining retractor is behind the conjoined tendon, and the other behind the deltoid. A Browne retractor is retracting the deltoid superiorly. A blunt Hohmann is protecting the axillary nerve. The subscapularis has been peeled off the lesser tuberosity and tagged for later repair. Notice the proximal humeral osteophytes

Depending on the procedure, the subsequent steps for exposure can be variable. For proximal humerus fracture fixation, the fracture fragments and structures are mobilized and tagged. Procedures needing access into the glenohumeral joint usually involve access through the rotator interval or through the subscapularis (Fig. 2.8). The triangular rotator interval can be excised from the superior border of the subscapularis all the way superior to the leading edge of the supraspinatus. Laterally, the supraspinatus and subscapularis converge near the bicipital groove. Medially, the interval can be developed to the glenoid, and the coracohumeral ligament can often be identified and excised. This can improve subscapularis excursion in cases of internal rotation contracture. If more exposure to the glenohumeral joint is needed, then some sort of access through the subscapularis is necessary.

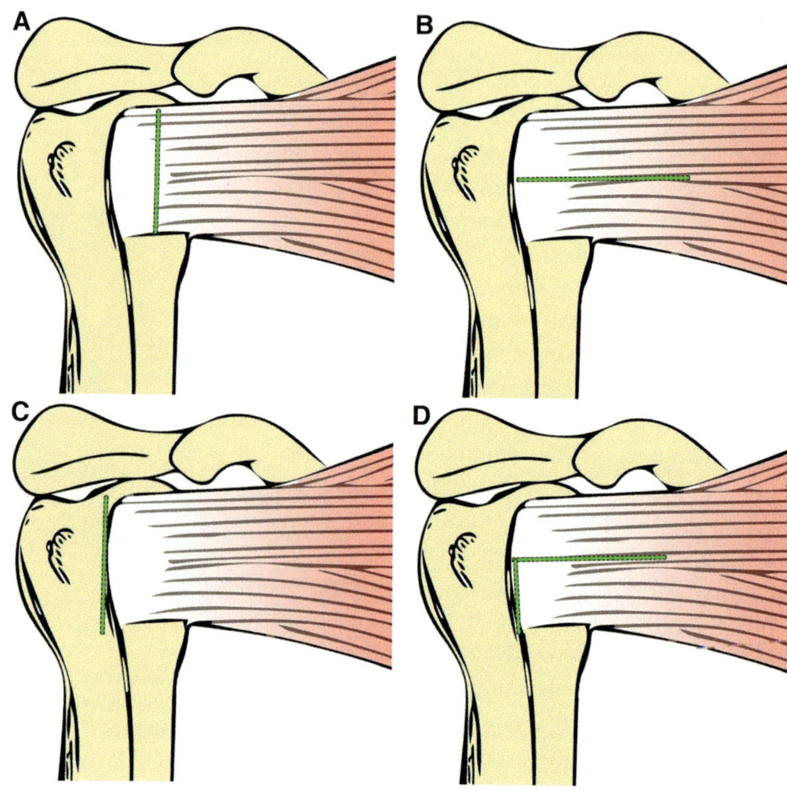

Fig. 2.9 Diagram showing incision lines for subscapularis management. A Subscapularis tenotomy; B: Subscapularis split; C: Subscapularis peel; D: Inferior subscapularis takedown

Management of the subscapularis during anterior shoulder approaches can be controversial [8–12]. Several surgical techniques have been described and the appropriate one can be left at the discretion of the surgeon. These include: subscapularis split (in line with tendon,) L-shaped tenotomy of the inferior half of the subscapularis, vertical tenotomy medial to the lesser tuberosity, subscapularis peel starting from the bicpital groove, and lesser tuberosity osteotomy. Whichever method of subscapularis management is chosen, the surgeon should keep in mind that the capsule and tendon are more intimately related laterally, and become more distinct medially towards the glenoid labrum (Fig. 2.9).

The horizontal subscapularis splitting approach can be useful in reconstruction of shoulder instability, such as Bankart lesions or in cases where a coracoid transfer is performed [13]. The capsule deep to the subscapularis can be opened or released as needed. Recently, there has been more interest in performing reconstructive type procedures such as arthroplasty through a limited subscapularis takedown, such as through the rotator interval [14] or with takedown of the inferior portion of the subscapularis [11]. In cases where significant deformity or osteophytes are present, these minimally invasive approaches should be avoided as this may compromise exposure. The subscapularis tendon can also be tenotomized medial to the lesser tuberosity, allowing a stump of tendon laterally which can be used to secure the cut tendon back to its anatomic position. The repair can be augmented with bony tunnels as well. A variation of this is to perform the subscapularis "peel" where Sharpey's fibers are elevated as one sleeve starting from the bicipital groove moving medially. This method may allow greater flexibility in cases with severe internal rotation contracture. A lesser tuberosity osteotomy is a more recent variation where a fleck of bone is removed with the attached subscapularis, allowing for bone to bone healing. There has been some debate in the literature on the most effective method, with some biomechanical studies showing no difference [15]. Others do show some potential increased tendon integrity at follow up with lesser tuberosity osteotomy [16]. The answer will hopefully become more clear with further research.

Once the subscapularis is reflected, work can be completed inside the glenohumeral joint. For capsular reconstruction, the appropriate anchors can be placed into the glenoid as needed. When a capsular release is necessary, the contracted structures can be released off the glenoid and also off of the neck of the humerus. Care should be taken as the axillary nerve can be intimately related to the inferior capsular structures of the glenohumeral joint. A humeral head cut can be performed in case of arthroplasty to allow access to the glenoid. In cases of shoulder arthroplasty, a complete anterior capsulectomy and inferior capsulotomy may be performed to facilitate exposure. Posterior retractors such as a Fukuda ring retractor or more rigid retractors can be used for final glenoid exposure.

Deltoid Splitting Approach

Deltoid split approaches can be used for a variety of different procedures, including open or "mini-open" rotator cuff repairs, and can be used for proximal humerus fracture fixation or shoulder arthroplasty. The most important consideration in these approaches is the course of the axillary nerve. It is classically described as 5 cm from the lateral edge of the acromion, although several anatomic studies found it can be closer, especially on patients with smaller deltoid muscles [17–19]. A cutaneous incision is made off the anterolateral corner of the acromion, either in the direction of the deltoid fibers or along Langer's lines. The anterolateral corner of the acromion is identified and the deltoid fibers are split in line with the muscle. The acromial attachment of the deltoid can be left intact, or alternately the anterior acromial portion can be elevated subperiosteally and reattached through drill holes or with cerclage sutures. If only a proximal exposure is needed, then the axillary nerve can be palpated on the deep surface of the deltoid, and a stay suture can be placed in the caudal apex of the split to prevent further propagation and a traction injury to the nerve. If more distal exposure is needed, such as for the distal screws of a proximal humerus plate, then the nerve can be exposed. A strip of deltoid around the nerve can be kept and the humerus is exposed below this. This has been described both as an extensile open approach [20] or as a less invasive approach that uses percutaneous incisions for placement of the distal screws [21]. Once the procedure is complete, there should be a meticulous repair of the deltoid muscle.

Approach to the AC Joint

In cases where exposure to the acromioclavicular (AC) joint is required, such as for resection of the distal articular surface [22] or reconstruction of an acromioclavicular joint separation, an isolated to the AC joint can be performed. An important note with any approach to the AC joint is preservation of the thick deltrotrapezial tissue surrounding the AC joint for closure at the end of the case. The skin incision can be in line with the AC joint along Langer's lines or parallel to the

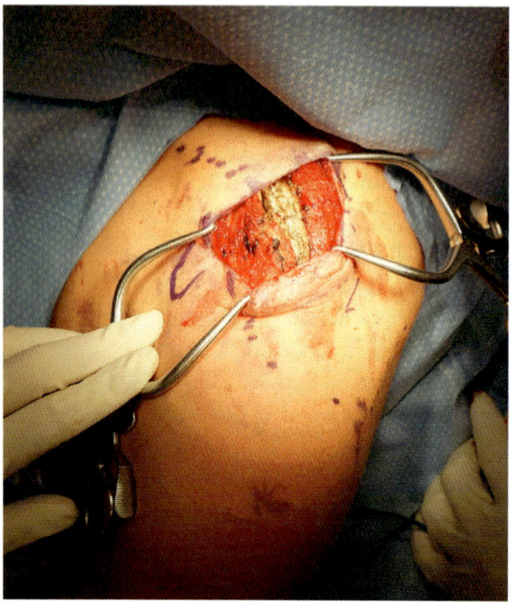

Fig. 2.10 Open approach for reconstruction of an acromioclavicular joint dislocation. The skin incision paralleled Langer's lines and skin flaps were developed to expose medially and laterally. Notice musculoperiostial flaps elevated in line with clavicle

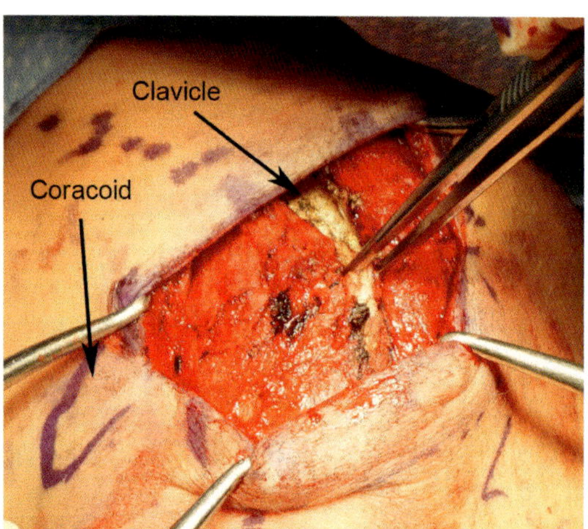

Fig. 2.11 The musculoperiostial flaps should be full thickness to allow for closure at the end of the procedure

clavicle (Fig. 2.10). Once skin and subcutaneous tissue are divided, medial and lateral skin flaps are developed down to the deltotrapezial layer overlying the clavicle. Depending on the procedure and exposure needed, full thickness musculoperiosteral flaps are elevated off the anterior and posterior surfaces of the AC joint. Any resection or reconstructive procedure can be performed and at the end of the case, the anterior and posterior muscle flaps are securely repaired, either to each other or in a tranosseous fashion (Fig. 2.11).

Posterior Approaches to the Shoulder

Occasionally, a deltopectoral or deltoid split approach will not provide the necessary visualization of the posterior shoulder structures or posterior glenoid. Examples where posterior exposure may be needed include: treatment of posterior instability [23–25], glenoid osteotomy [23], oncological surgery, scapular neck fractures, or posterior fracture dislocations. This approach can also be used for open suprascapular nerve decompressions [26]. For scapular fractures, a more extensive Judet approach to the scapular body can be used [27].

For a posterior approach to the shoulder, the patient should be in a prone or lateral decubitus position. All bony landmarks including the spine of the scapula and the posterolateral corner of the acromion should be marked. It may help to feel for the soft spot of the posterior glenohumeral joint and mark where the joint line is estimated. The skin incision can be either horizontal along the scapular spine or in a vertical direction. If a vertical direction is chosen, then it may be centered over the glenohumeral joint or just medial, close to where a posterior arthroscopic portal would typically be made. For more medial work such as nerve decompression, the incision should be shifted more medially. An incision that is too far lateral will make access to the glenohumeral joint difficult. Once through the skin layer, medial and lateral skin flaps should be developed to identify the underlying deltoid. The fibers of the deltoid are in a more horizontal direction. At this point, the deltoid can either be elevated off of the scapular spine, or a deltoid split can be made for a limited approach [28]. The extent of the deltoid split is limited down to the level of the teres minor secondary to the axillary nerve emerging from the quadrilateral space. Once the deltoid is elevated off of the scapular spine or split, the infraspinatus and teres minor can be seen deep to it. These two muscles form an internervous plane between the suprascapular nerve and the axillary nerve. The interval between the two muscles can be developed bluntly and extended laterally towards their insertion on the greater tuberosity. Care should be taken because inferior retractors can damage the axillary nerve and medial retractors can damage the suprascapular nerve. Once between the two muscles, the posterior capsule is identified and incised to give access to the posterior glenohumeral joint.

Judet Approach to Posterior Shoulder

The Judet approach is useful in more complex scapula fractures which require more medial exposure. The skin incision starts along the subcutaneous border of the scapular spine and curves at the superomedial angle of the scapula, following the medial edge to the inferiomedial corner (Fig. 2.12). A large skin flap with all the subcutaneous tissue is elevated off of the underlying musculature. The muscular planes can be developed with a combination of blunt and sharp dissection. The teres minor and major, infraspinatus, upper latissimus, and posterior deltoid should readily be visible. At this point, the posterior deltoid can be taken down in a similar fashion to the method described above. The interval between the infraspinatus and teres minor is identified for approach to the lateral scapular neck and glenohumeral joint. The medial border can be plated from this approach, and any necessary scapular plates can be placed.

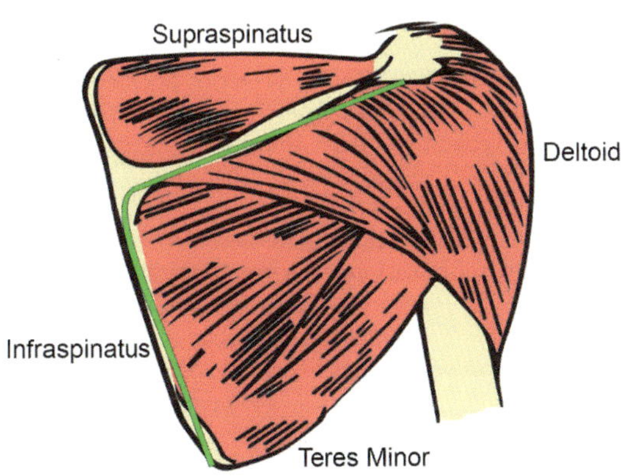

Fig. 2.12 Line signifying skin incision for posterior Judet approach to the scapula. Once through the subcutaneous tissue, the posterior deltoid can be reflected to reveal the insertion of the teres minor and infraspinatus on the proximal humerus

All statements below are correct except:

The deltopectoral approach:

A. Uses the plane between the suprascapular nerve and the axillary nerve
B. It was described by Henry
C. Provides excellent exposure to the anterior shoulder
D. Can be extended into an anterolateral approach to the humerus

All statements below are correct except:

The skin incision for a posterior approach of the shoulder:

A. Can be either horizontal or vertical
B. The vertical incision must be centered over the glenohumeral joint or just medially
C. If medial work such as nerve decompression is needed, the incision should be shifted more medially
D. An incision that is too far medial will make access to the glenohumeral joint difficult

It is important to preserve the thick deltrotrapezial tissue with any approach to the AC joint because

A. If violated the underlying neurovascular bundle can be damaged
B. For closure at the end of the case
C. To use it as a landmark for potential distal excision of the clavicle
D. All the above

References

1. Henry A. Extensile exposure. 2nd ed. Baltimore: Churchill Livingstone; 1957.
2. Papadonikolakis A, Wiesler ER, Olympio MA, Poehling GG. Avoiding catastrophic complications of stroke and death related to shoulder surgery in the sitting position. Arthroscopy. 2008;24(4):481–2. doi:10.1016/j.arthro.2008.02.005.
3. Tauchen AJ, Salazar D, Barton GJ, Francois A, Tonino P, Garbis NG, et al. The effect of compression stockings on cerebral desaturation events in obese patients undergoing shoulder arthroscopy in the beach-chair position. Arthroscopy. 2015;31(12):2352–64. doi:10.1016/j.arthro.2015.06.017.
4. Hoppenfeld S, Buckley R, de Boer P. Surgical exposures in orthopaedics: the anatomic approach. Philadelphia: Wolters Kluwer/Lippincott Williams & Wilkins; 2009.
5. Radkowski CA, Richards RS, Pietrobon R, Moorman III CT. An anatomic study of the cephalic vein in the deltopectoral shoulder approach. Clin Orthop Relat Res. 2006;442:139–42.
6. Gill DR, Cofield RH, Rowland C. The anteromedial approach for shoulder arthroplasty: the importance of the anterior deltoid. J Shoulder Elb Surg. 2004;13(5):532–7. doi:10.1016/S1058274604000850.
7. Redfern TR, Wallace WA, Beddow FH. Clavicular osteotomy in shoulder arthroplasty. Int Orthop. 1989;13(1):61–3. doi:10.1007/bf00266725.
8. Qureshi S, Hsiao A, Klug RA, Lee E, Braman J, Flatow EL. Subscapularis function after total shoulder replacement: results with lesser tuberosity osteotomy. J Shoulder Elb Surg. 2008;17(1):68–72. doi:10.1016/j.jse.2007.04.018.
9. Gadea F, Bouju Y, Berhouet J, Bacle G, Favard L. Deltopectoral approach for shoulder arthroplasty: anatomic basis. Int Orthop. 2015;39(2):215–25. doi:10.1007/s00264-014-2654-x.
10. Van den Berghe GR, Nguyen B, Patil S, D'Lima DD, Mahar A, Pedowitz R, et al. A biomechanical evaluation of three surgical techniques for subscapularis repair. J Shoulder Elb Surg. 2008;17(1):156–61. doi:10.1016/j.jse.2007.04.016.
11. Savoie 3rd FH, Charles R, Casselton J, O'Brien MJ, Hurt III JA. The subscapularis-sparing approach in humeral head replacement. J Shoulder Elb Surg. 2015;24(4):606–12. doi:10.1016/j.jse.2014.07.020.
12. Krishnan SG, Stewart DG, Reineck JR, Lin KC, Buzzell JE, Burkhead WZ. Subscapularis repair after shoulder arthroplasty: biomechanical and clinical validation of a novel technique. J Shoulder Elb Surg. 2009;18(2):184–92. discussion 97-8 doi:10.1016/j.jse.2008.09.009.
13. McFarland EG, Park HB, Chronopoulos E, Kim TK, Wilckens J. Modification of the Subscapularis Splitting Technique for Anterior Shoulder Reconstructions. Tech Should Elbow Surg. 2003;4(1):18–25.
14. Lafosse L, Schnaser E, Haag M, Gobezie R. Primary total shoulder arthroplasty performed entirely thru the rotator interval: technique and minimum two-year outcomes. J Shoulder Elb Surg. 2009;18(6):864–73. doi:10.1016/j.jse.2009.03.017.
15. Van Thiel GS, Wang VM, Wang FC, Nho SJ, Piasecki DP, Bach Jr BR, et al. Biomechanical similarities among subscapularis repairs after shoulder arthroplasty. J Shoulder Elb Surg. 2010;19(5):657–63. doi:10.1016/j.jse.2010.01.014.
16. Buckley T, Miller R, Nicandri G, Lewis R, Voloshin I. Analysis of subscapularis integrity and function after lesser tuberosity osteotomy versus subscapularis tenotomy in total shoulder arthroplasty using ultrasound and validated clinical outcome measures. J Shoulder Elbow Surg. 23(9):1309–17. doi:10.1016/j.jse.2013.12.009.
17. Kontakis GM, Steriopoulos K, Damilakis J, Michalodimitrakis E. The position of the axillary nerve in the deltoid muscle. A cadaveric study. Acta Orthop Scand. 1999;70(1):9–11.
18. Burkhead Jr WZ, Scheinberg RR, Box G. Surgical anatomy of the axillary nerve. J Shoulder Elb Surg. 1992;1(1):31–6. doi:10.1016/S1058-2746(09)80014-1.
19. Kulkarni RR, Nandedkar AN, Mysorekar VR. Position of the axillary nerve in the deltoid muscle. Anat Rec. 1992;232(2):316–7. doi:10.1002/ar.1092320217.
20. Robinson CM, Khan L, Akhtar A, Whittaker R. The extended deltoid-splitting approach to the proximal humerus. J Orthop Trauma. 2007;21(9):657–62. doi:10.1097/BOT.0b013e3180ce833e.
21. Lill H, Hepp P, Rose T, Konig K, Josten C. The angle stable locking-proximal-humerus-plate (LPHP) for proximal humeral fractures using a small anterior-lateral-deltoid-splitting-approach—technique and first results. Zentralbl Chir. 2004;129(1):43–8. doi:10.1055/s-2004-44870.
22. Mumford EB. Acromioclavicular dislocation—a new operative treatment. J Bone Joint Surg. 1941;23:799–802.
23. Rowe CR, Yee LBK. A posterior approach to the shoulder joint. J Bone Joint Surg. 1944;26:580–4.
24. Boyd HB, Sisk TD. Recurrent posterior dislocation of the shoulder. J Bone Joint Surg Am. 1972;54(4):779–86.
25. Hindenach JC. Recurrent posterior dislocation of the shoulder. J Bone Joint Surg Am. 1947;29(3):582–6.
26. Mall NA, Hammond JE, Lenart BA, Enriquez DJ, Twigg SL, Nicholson GP. Suprascapular nerve entrapment isolated to the spinoglenoid notch: surgical technique and results of open decompression. J Shoulder Elb Surg. 2013;22(11):e1–8. doi:10.1016/j.jse.2013.03.009.
27. Obremskey WT, Lyman JR. A modified judet approach to the scapula. J Orthop Trauma. 2004;18(10):696–9.
28. Wirth MA, Butters KP, Rockwood Jr CA. The posterior deltoid-splitting approach to the shoulder. Clin Orthop Relat Res. 1993;296:92–8.

Shoulder Biomechanics

3

Marcheggiani Muccioli Giulio Maria, Lullini Giada, Grassi Alberto, Roberti di Sarsina Tommaso, Raggi Federico, Carbone Giuseppe, and Zaffagnini Stefano

Key Points

The shoulder joint is the most mobile joint in the body; however, it is also the most unstable.

Strength and stability of the joint are highly dependent on both static and dynamic restraints.

The constitutional trait of laxity facilitates extensive motion in multiple planes and may be essential to athletic performance.

The scapulothoracic muscles transfer the potential energy of the trunk to kinetic energy in the shoulder. The scapula is a key link in the kinetic chain between the trunk and the shoulder.

Introduction

The shoulder complex is an association of a number of joints, ligaments and muscles working together to achieve hand positioning in the space. This complex is the most movable of the human body, at the price of a great unstableness [1].

Shoulder complex motion can be described through anatomic coordinate system: internal and external rotations are the movements in the transversal plane and they can be described as the rotation around humerus long axis; abduction and adduction are the movements in the frontal plane; flexion and extension are the movements in the sagittal plane. Moreover glenohumeral joint can translate in anterior-posterior, superior-inferior and medial-lateral directions. Circumduction is generated by combination of elementary movements, described as a complex circle movement, whose trajectory is an irregular cone with the apex centred on glenohumeral joint.

This large range of motion is allowed by a balanced interaction between static and active stabilizers: static stabilizers include bony, cartilaginous, capsular and ligamentous factors; active stabilizers include muscles and neural feedback between capsular and ligamentous structure and muscle.

A slight borderline exists between normal laxity of shoulder complex and pathologic instability.

Laxity, defined as asymptomatic translation of humeral head on the glenoid, may be essential to reach good athletic performance, especially in activities and sports requiring wide motion of the joint. Shoulder instability is defined as an abnormal translation associated with functional deficit and symptoms such as pain and apprehension.

Glenohumeral instability can occur in athletes due to chronic overuse injuries or after acute

M.M.G. Maria, M.D., Ph.D. (✉)
L. Giada, M.D. • G. Alberto, M.D.
R. di S. Tommaso, M.D. • R. Federico, M.D.
C. Giuseppe, M.D. • Z. Stefano, M.D.
Istituto Ortopedico Rizzoli, University of Bologna, Via di Barbiano, 1/10—c/o Lab. Biomeccanicaed Innovazione Tecnologica, 40136 Bologna, Italy
e-mail: marcheggianimuccioli@sportsdoc.it

G. Huri, N.K. Paschos (eds.), *The Shoulder*, Orthopaedic Study Guide Series,
DOI 10.1007/978-3-319-51979-1_3

traumatic event. In any case shoulder instability leads to damage or deficiency of normal shoulder stabilizers, often counterbalanced by neuro-muscolar control. If this mechanism fails, because of acute or chronic worsening, shoulder instability is established.

Static Stabilizers

Static stabilizers include bones, labrum, capsule and the vacuum effect.

Static stabilizers can be divided into bony stabilizers (humeral head and glenoid) and soft tissue stabilizers (glenoid labrum, glenohumeral ligaments and joint capsule, rotator interval, negative intracapsular pressure, adhesion cohesion mechanism and acromio-clavicular joint system) (Fig. 3.1).

Bony Static Stabilizers

The *humeral head* is extremely variable in shape and size: it is retroverted on average 19° (range 9–31°) and inclined on average 41° (range 34–47°); head radius measures 23 mm (range 17–28 mm) and medial and posterior head center offset are on average 7 mm (range 4–12 mm) and 2 mm (range 1–8 mm), respectively [2]. Humeral head is covered by a layer of hyaline articular cartilage; articular surface ending is lined by the anatomic neck, a bony transition from cartilage to capsular attachment and tendinous insertion. Greater and lesser tuberosity, positioned laterally to the anatomic neck, are the insertion point of the rotator cuff tendons and delimit the bicipital groove helping the long head biceps being in place.

The *glenoid* is a shallow socket that holds humeral head; its mean depth is 2.5 mm on

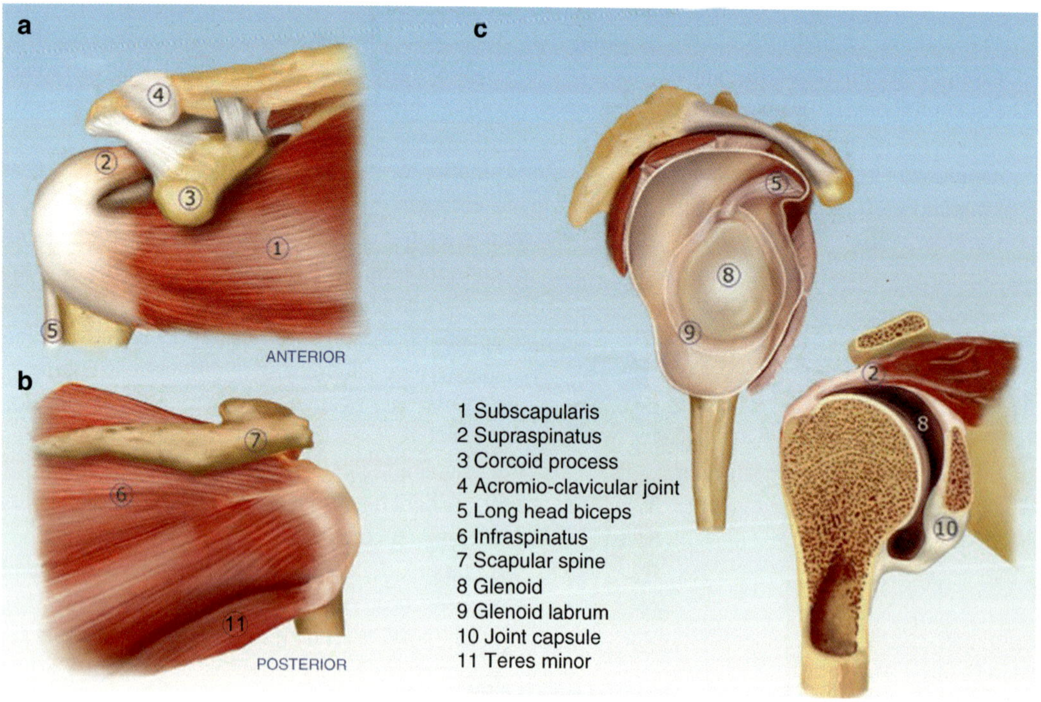

Fig. 3.1 Anatomic representation of the shoulder [(**a**) anterior, (**b**), posterior, (**c**) internal views]. Static bony stabilizers (humeral head and glenoid) and static soft tissue stabilizers (glenoid labrum, glenohumeral ligaments and joint capsule, rotator interval and acromio-clavicular joint system) are surrounded by the dynamic stabilizers of this system: rotator cuff muscles and scapula-thoracic muscles

anteroposterior direction and 9 mm in superior inferior direction. It is retroverted on average 1.23° (range 9.5° of antiversion to 10.5 of retroversion) and inclined superiorly on average 4.2° (range, 7° of inferior inclination to 15.8° of superior inclination) [3]. Friedman and Kessler reported that its bending radius is larger than humeral head radius in 93% of examined joints; the remainders have glenoid and humeral head with the same bending radius [4].

Only 30% of humeral articular surface articulates with glenoid articular surface at any time; [5] the importance of soft tissue static and dynamic restrains in shoulder stability must be noticed. The glenohumeral ratio is the result of the division between the maximum diameter of the glenoid and the maximum diameter of the humeral head. It's different according to considered planes: 0.75 in the sagittal plane and 0.6 in the coronal plane [6].

All changes in bony anatomy could result in shoulder instability.

Most important bony lesions that result in instability occur after traumatic events and involve the anterior-inferior glenoid rim (Bony Bankart lesion) and the postero-lateral aspect of the humeral head (Hill Sachs lesion).

Bony Bankart lesion becomes significant when involves more than 20% of the length of the glenoid and can lead to recurrence despite correct soft tissues repairing; if bony Bankart involves more than 50% of glenoid length, shoulder stability is reduced more than 30% [7]. Bony Bankart lesions are classified according to Bigliani et al. [8]: type I, a displaced avulsion fracture with attached capsule; type II, a medially displaced fragment mal-united to the glenoid rim; type III, an erosion of the glenoid rim lower than 25% (III A) and more than 25% (III B). In any case, if a bone fragment is present, it will be reabsorbed within a year [9]. The PICO method, suggested by Baudi et al. [10], could be used to calculate bony deficiency produced by a bony Bankart lesions: it needs Computed Tomography MultiPlanar Reconstruction of both shoulder and defects is calculated as a ratio between the surface of the damaged glenoid and the surface of not damaged glenoid.

Hill Sachs lesion is the result of an impact fracture occurred after one or more traumatic anterior shoulder dislocation and involves the posterior-lateral articular surface of the humeral head. Smaller Hill Sachs lesions do not influence stability; the level of influence in shoulder instability depends on the lesion's size and its localization. According to the size, Hill Sachs lesions are classified in mild (2 cm × 0.3 cm), moderately severe (4 cm × 0.5 cm) and severe (greater than previous one); [11] according to their orientation Burkhart and De Beer [12] classified them in engaging or not engaging (impact fractures extended at the area of contact between articular surfaces of glenohumeral joint during abduction, external rotation and extension have an higher risk of engagement). Risk of engaging is higher if glenoid surface is reduced. Calandra et al. [13] performed an arthroscopy classification of Hill Sachs lesions in order to recognize three types of defects: Grade I, that doesn't involve subcondral bone; Grade II, that involves subcondral bone; Grade III, that involves subcondral bone widely. Specular lesions occur in posterior traumatic instability: the posterior glenoid rim could be fractured after acute traumatic dislocation or eroded after repeated subluxations (reverse bony Bankart lesion) [14] and the humeral head could be fractured in its anterior articular surface (reverse Hill Sachs lesion or McLaughlin lesion) [15]. Reverse Hill Sachs lesions could be engaging during adduction, flexion and internal rotation if they extends in the zone of contact between articular surface during that motion [16].

It's important to underline, while considering bony stabilizers, the glenoid track concept, defined as the contact area between glenoid and humeral head, originated by the shift of glenoid from the inferomedial to the posterolateral portion of the posterior articular surface of the humeral head when the arm moves in maximum external rotation, extension and abduction. This area's width is 84% of glenoid width, therefore every glenoid articular surface loss (as in Bony Bankart lesion) can influence the width of the glenoid track. The glenoid track influences the risk of engaging of a Hill-Sachs lesion: if the bony loss in the humeral head remains within the glenoid track there is no chance that the Hill-Sachs lesion overrides the glinoid rim. On the other hand, if Hill Sachs lesion extends over the medial margin of the glenoid track risk of engaging rises according to lesion's position [17, 18].

Soft Tissue Static Stabilizers

Soft tissue static stabilizers include glenoid labrum, glenohumeral capsule, glenohumeral ligaments, rotator interval, negative intracapsular pressure and adhesion cohesion mechanism.

The *glenoid labrum* is a triangular section ring around the glenoid rim to which it's connected by fibro-cartilage and fibrous bone. The superior half of glenoid labrum is more movable than inferior half; its superior border blends with the origin of long head of the biceps. Its jobs are to make glenoid socket deeper, to increase contact area and congruity, to generate a suction effect, to function as insertion area for capsular-ligamentous structures and to help muscles to compress humeral head within glenoid. The glenoid labrum acts on the humeral head like a plunger: loss of the glenoid labrum reduces depth of glenoid socket more than 50%, so it reduces stability [19].

There are several kind of labrum lesions and it's very important not to confuse tears with anatomical variants that don't require surgical repair, like sublabral foramen associated with cord-like middle gleno-humeral ligament or meniscoid labrum [20].

The most common injury to the labrumis Bankart lesion, observed in more than 90% of traumatic anterior instability, [21]. It is defined as a detachment of anteroinferior aspect of the labrum and its attached portion of the inferior glenohumeral ligament. Despite of its frequency, it cannot be considered an isolated cause of instability [22]. Green and Christensen [23] classified Bankart lesions in five arthroscopic types: type 1 refers to the entire labrum; type 2 is a simple detachment of labrum with no other significant lesions; type 3 is an intra-parenchymal labrum tear; type 4 and 5 are complex tears with a significant or complete degeneration of the inferior glenohumeral ligament, respectively. This classification also has a prognostic value: type 4 and 5 have a great chance of recurrent instability after arthroscopic Bankart procedure (87%).

Another lesion involving antero-inferior aspect of the labrum is the ALPSA lesion (anterior labroligamentous periosteal sleeve avulsion): the anterior labro-ligamentous complex rolls up in a sleeve-like fashion and becomes displaced medially and inferiorly on the glenoid neck [24]. ALPSA lesions may have a higher risk of re-dislocation than un-displaced Bankart tears, as the normal bumper and capsule stabilizing the front of the shoulder are displaced and the anterior glenoid is deficient of capsule and labrum.

Specular lesions can be described for the posterior aspect of the labrum: reverse Bankart lesion involves the posterior labrum and the posterior band of inferior glenohumeral ligament; [25] POLPSA is the posterior labroligamentous sleeve avulsion, that in chronic conditions could become a Bennett lesion (an extra-articular calcification along the posteroinferior glenoid neck close to the posterior band of the glenohumeral ligament) [26]. Reverse Bankart lesion is quite frequent in athletes, such as rugby players, with a 20% incidence being reported in a study of 142 elite rugby player shoulder arthroscopy [27]. The mechanism of injury could trace back to a direct blow to the anterior and lateral aspect of the shoulder, while the arm is adducted; a rare mechanism of injury is a posterior blow to the arm, while holding a tackle shield [28].

Concerning superior labrum, a very common lesion in throwing overhead athletes is SLAP (superior labrum anterior and posterior) tear. Described for the first time by Snyder et al. [29], SLAP lesion origins during the ending deceleration phase of the throwing, because of a traction force wielded by the long head of biceps on the glenoid labrum. Sneyder classified SLAP tear in four different types: type II and IV are the most significant in determining instability since they involve both labrum and long head of the biceps, resulting in increased total range of motion. Moreover SLAP lesions are common in contact athletes: Funk and Snow have been reported a 35% incidence of SLAP tears, arthroscopically diagnosed, in 51 rugby players shoulders [30].

Capsuloligamentous structures include *joint capsule*, whose mean thickness is 5 mm, and *glenohumeral ligaments* (superior, middle and inferior), described as located thickening of the capsule. These structures received great attention and many cadaveric and clinic studies have tried to clarify their anatomical and biomechanical characteristics and their relationship with dynamic stabilizers.

The constitutional trait of laxity facilitates extensive motion in multiple planes and may be essential to athletic performance. On the other hand, capsular stretching is noted along with a Bankart lesion in up to 28% of patient with recurrent anterior instability [31].

Superior and middle glenohumeral ligaments, together with coracohumeral ligament, long head of the biceps and a thin layer of capsule, help to form rotator interval and they will be treated in detail later.

Inferior glenohumeral ligament, also called inferior glenohumeral ligament complex (IGHLC), is made out of three parts: two thicker bands on anterior and posterior and a thinner recess. During abduction, external rotation and extension IGHLC moves anteriorly, forming a restraint to anterior translation of the humeral head.

During adduction, flexion and internal rotation, IGHLC moves posteriorly, forming a restraint to posterior translation. IGHLC suffers of initial plastic deformation during initial dislocation, but the damage becomes more critical after several episodes [32]. The lesion could more frequently occur at the glenoid insertion (antero-inferior glenoid rim), but also in the middle part or at the humeral insertion [33]. The incidence of humeral avulsion of glenohumeral ligament (HAGL) has been reported as high as 10% [34].

Capsular stretching is often noted along with a Bankart lesion in up to 28% of patients with recurrent anterior instability [31]. Posterior capsular can also be damaged, seeing that recurrent posterior subluxations or luxations produce capsular redundancy and increase joint volume, resulting in posterior instability. Capsular redundancy, both anterior and inferior and posterior, is a very common find in non traumatic multidirectional instability.

The *rotator interval* is a triangular space, with medial base and lateral apex, medially limited by the coracoid, long head of biceps and its groove laterally, superior fibers of subscapularis inferiorly and anterior fibers of supraspinatus superiorly. The rotator interval is composed of coracohumeral ligament (CHL) and superior and middle glenohumeral ligaments deeper, even if middle glenohumeral ligament contribution is relatively variable (different studies reported its absence, in 10–40% of cases). Usually, it is larger in male than in female and becomes smaller with internal rotation. It is an important inferior stabilizers and its insufficiency could be clinically appreciated with sulcus sign. A rotator interval defect could be a little foramen or could reach larger size, significantly influencing inferior stability [35].

A role in shoulder stability is also played by *negative intracapsular pressure* that presupposes the integrity of all structure. Intracapsular pressure is about −42 mmHg H_2O and acts especially when rotator cuff muscles are not contracted and glenohumeral ligaments and capsular structure are not in tension. Loss of intracapsular negative pressure can manifest itself as an augmentation of anterior translation; this factor could be marginal when muscles are contracted and capsuloligamentous structures are in tension, especially in athletes [36].

Furthermore synovial fluid provides to generate *adhesion cohesion mechanism*: when two cartilage wet surfaces, such as the humeral head and glenoid, come into contact with each other and adhesion-cohesion bond is created providing stability to the glenohumeral articulation [37].

The suction effect of the glenoid labrum, the negative intracapsular pressure and the adhesion cohesion mechanism are the three mechanisms providing the *vacuum effect*.

The *acromionclavicular system* (ACS) is composed by a complex of ligaments (conoid, trapezoid and acromioclavicularcapsular ligaments) stabilizing the acromioclavicular joint. The conoid and the trapezoid are attached from the distal clavicula to the coracoid. The ACS help to prevent excessive superior translation of the shoulder. An acromion-clavicular dislocation up to Rockwood type 3 could require surgical repair as these cause pain and functional restrictions [38], with good results even in athletes [39].

Dynamic Stabilizers

Muscles and proprioceptive effects are the dynamic stabilizers.

Rotator cuff muscles act compressing humeral head on the glenoid surface and tightening capsuloligamentous structures, having direct insertion on rotator cuff tendons. The scapular rotators allow the glenoid to modify its orientation in such a way as to follow the humeral head during motion. Long head of biceps and scapulo-thoracic rhythm boost this mechanism.

Propioception

Glenohumeral joint capsule has been shown to havenumerous mechanoreceptors particularly within the anterior and inferior capsule. In abduction and external rotation these mechanoreceptors are most likely activated as the humeral head comes into contact with the capsule sending a signal to the stabilizing muscles of the shoulder providing containment and stability of the humeral head [40]. Moreover, there is a close relationship between glenohumeral ligament and rotator cuff muscles, seeing that muscles contraction act as pre-tensioners or co-tensioners for capsular ligament. Instability could also come from a not coordinated contraction of the rotator cuff; especially in overhead athletes, being the cuff an important decelerator of anterior translation [41].

Rotator Cuff Muscles

The Rotator cuff is composed by four muscles (subscapularis, supraspinatus, infraspinatus and teres minor) originating from the scapula and insert on the humeral head.

Subscapularis origin is on the anterior face of the scapula with insertion on the lesser tuberosity; *supraspinatus* origins in the fossa up to the scapular spine with insertion on the anterior facet of the greater tuberosity; *infraspinatus* origins in the fossa under the spine with insertion on the middle facet of the greater tuberosity; *teres minor* origins from the lateral border of the scapula with insertion on the posterior facet of the greater tuberosity.

The rotator cuff muscles provide significant stability to the shoulder joint, almost hugging the joint to the glenoid. Wuelker et al. [42] showed that a 50% decrease in the rotator cuff muscle forces resulted in nearly a 50% increase in anterior displacement of the humeral head in response to external loading in all glenohumeral joint positions. The sub-scapularis muscle provides anterior stability when the arm is in neutral but less so as the arm comes into abduction [43]. The infraspinatus and teres minor act together to reduce the strain on the antero-inferior glenohumeral ligament in abduction and external rotation [44].

Lesions to rotator cuff can occur after single traumatic event or after degeneration because of overuse, anyway rising of the humeral head occur during abduction and in case of massive lesion, an excessive anterior translation is observed. Degeneration of rotator cuff could occur because of external or internal impingement: external impingement derived from an abnormal contact between coracoacromyal arc and superior surface of the rotator cuff; internal impingement, defined as abnormal contact between rotator cuff joint surface and the posterosuperior glenoid rim, is common in throwing athletes. It could result in tearing of both rotator cuff and labrum. Origin of internal impingement is controversial and can be attributed to anterior micro-instability and tightness of the posterior capsule; others underline the postero-inferior capsular contracture resulting

Part II

Clinical Evaluation

4 History

Edward G. McFarland

The clinical evaluation of the shoulder and accurate diagnosis of shoulder abnormalities are challenging. As in most disciplines of clinical medicine, accurate diagnosis begins with a thorough patient history. Patients often have more than one abnormality contributing to their shoulder symptoms, and the clinician must use all available evidence to make the diagnosis.

The clinician must first determine the patient's chief symptom and how the problem began (Table 4.1). A traumatic injury would lead the clinician to assess for a particular spectrum of disorders such as fracture, rotator cuff tear, dislocation, or acromioclavicular (AC) joint injury. Most shoulder disorders occur insidiously with no trauma. The most common condition that often has no inciting event is a stiff or "frozen" shoulder. Shoulder pain that occurs after activity that is outside the patient's normal routine (e.g., tennis, heavy lifting) typically indicates that the shoulder is inflamed or irritated. In these cases, the most likely diagnoses are rotator cuff syndrome or AC irritation.

If symptoms have followed a shoulder injury, it is important to determine the mechanism of injury. The position of the arm at the time of the trauma, the amount of force applied, and the direction of the force can be important factors in the differential and definitive diagnosis. A patient with an injury that hyperabducts the arm in

Table 4.1 Patient history and possible diagnoses of shoulder abnormalities[a]

Patient history	Possible diagnoses
Trauma	
Arm abducted and externally rotated	Anterior instability; subscapularis tendon tear
Fall onto hyperabducted arm	Luxatio erecta (inferior dislocation)
Fall onto outstretched arm	Proximal humerus fracture; rotator cuff tear; SLAP lesion
Fall onto shoulder	AC separation; fracture; rotator cuff tear; SLAP lesion
Traction injury	SLAP lesion
No trauma	
Insidious onset of pain	Degenerative joint disease; frozen shoulder; tendinitis
Insidious onset of severe pain	Brachial neuritis; shingles
Night pain	Tumor
Weakness without pain	Chronic rotator cuff tear; nerve injury; muscle disease

[a]*Source*: Adapted with permission from *Examination of the Shoulder: The Complete Guide*. New York, NY: Thieme Medical Publishers, Inc.; 2006

AC acromioclavicular, *SLAP* superior labral anterior posterior

E.G. McFarland, M.D.
Division of Shoulder Surgery,
Department of Orthopaedic Surgery,
The Johns Hopkins University,
Baltimore, MD, USA
e-mail: editorialservices@jhmi.edu

G. Huri, N.K. Paschos (eds.), *The Shoulder*, Orthopaedic Study Guide Series,
DOI 10.1007/978-3-319-51979-1_4

external rotation can produce anterior instability but it also can tear the subscapularis tendon, fracture the greater tuberosity, or fracture the glenoid. A fall on an outstretched arm can result in a rotator cuff tear, biceps anchor lesion, or fracture. A fall on a flexed elbow with a posteriorly directed force or a posteriorly directed force from any cause can result in a posterior instability episode. A fall directly on the shoulder (e.g., a fall from a bicycle) typically causes AC injury or clavicle fracture.

Understanding the timing of symptom onset can help narrow the diagnosis. It is common for patients with insidious onset of pain (e.g., from rotator cuff issues) not to move their shoulders because of pain. The shoulder soon becomes stiff, and the patient cannot perform everyday activities such as donning a coat or reaching into the back seat of a car. In such a case, what began as a rotator cuff abnormality becomes a stiff or frozen shoulder. Although both disorders may require treatment, knowing that the stiffness followed an injury or painful condition helps the practitioner decide what to assess during examination and how to create a treatment plan.

Certain activities are strongly associated with particular injuries (Table 4.2). For example, patients who do many push-ups for exercise or in the workplace (such as military or law enforcement officers) commonly present with irritation of the AC joint. Patients who regularly perform bench pressing can present with osteolysis of the distal clavicle. Patients who use heavy weights when bench pressing often tear their pectoralis major tendons. It is helpful for the practitioner to have suspicion for injuries seen in certain sports, especially first-rib stress fractures in overhead athletes, which can present as pleuritic chest pain [1].

Orthopedists are taught to "consider the joint above and below." In the case of the shoulder, the proximal "joint" is the cervical spine, which is often the cause of shoulder and upper extremity pain and weakness [2, 3]. Generally, cervical spine pain radiates down the arm to the hand, often in a dermatomal distribution. Cervical spine conditions cause pain into the trapezius or along the medial border of the scapula (Fig. 4.1) [4]. In patients with trapezius pain, it is important to evaluate the AC joint because it is the only joint in the shoulder where conditions can cause pain into the trapezius.

It is important to ask patients if they have a history of tingling numbness in their upper

Table 4.2 Specific injuries associated with various sports activities[a]

Activity/athlete type	Associated injuries
Adolescent baseball pitchers	Proximal humeral apophysitis ("Little League shoulder")
Archery	Posterior shoulder instability
Bench presses	Pectoralis major tendon tears
Bench presses, dips, push-ups	Osteolysis of the distal clavicle; AC arthritis
Football linemen	Posterior shoulder instability
Golf, rowing	Rib stress fractures
Kayaking	Supraspinatus partial tears; anterior shoulder dislocations
Overhead athletes	SLAP lesions; partial cuff tears; "occult" instability
Trapshooting	Coracoid stress fractures

[a]*Source*: Adapted with permission from *Examination of the Shoulder: The Complete Guide*. New York, NY: Thieme Medical Publishers, Inc.; 2006

AC acromioclavicular, *SLAP* superior labral anterior posterior

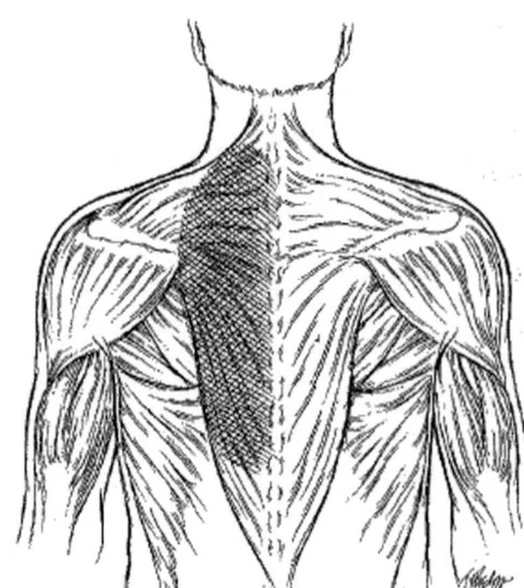

Fig. 4.1 Drawing showing the location of pain along the medial border of the scapula, which is most often caused by cervical spine disease (Reprinted with permission from Examination of The Shoulder: The Complete Guide, Thieme Medical Publishers, Inc., 2006. Figure 1-3, p. 3.)

inpostero-superior instability and a peel-back to the superior labrum and a tearing of the rotator cuff [45].

Long Head of Biceps

Long head of biceps (LHB) is a secondary stabilizer with a predominant role in case of rotator cuff orcapsule-ligamentous deficiency. This tendon, originating from the supraglenoid tubercle and passing through bicipital groove, acts as an anterior stabilizer during internal rotation and as posterior stabilizer during external rotation; during late loading phase of throwing LHB reduces anterior translation, helping to prevent excessive torsion of the glenohumeral joint with a flexing elbow. These concepts can explain why type II or IV Slap lesions are very common in throwing athletes and an hypertrophic tendon is found in patient with insufficient rotator cuff [46].

Scapula-thoracic Muscles

Trapezius, rhomboids, latissimusdorsi, serratus anterior and elevator scapulae belong to scapular rotators. Scapula-thoracic joint is constituted by a sliding surface between anterior face of scapula and thoracic cage. The coordinated movement between the scapula-thoracic joint and the gleno-humeral joint has been defined by Codman as "*scapula-thoracic rhythm*" [5]. The ratio between gleno-humeral and scapula-thoracic joint motion is approximately 2:1, but it's higher during lower degrees and lower at the extreme degrees of motion [47, 48]. The scapula-thoracic muscles transfer the potential energy of the trunk to kinetic energy in the shoulder. The kinetic train is a concept describing the transfer of energy from the trunk to the shoulder and arm. The scapula is a key link in the kinetic chain between the trunk and the shoulder [49].

Any alteration in scapula-thoracic rhythm could predispose to shoulder joint pathology. In particular, in pitchers the weakness of the serratus anterior predispose to development of rotator cuff tendinitis because of an abnormal contact with the coracoacromial arch or nontraumatic shoulder instability [50]. Scapulo-thoracic rhythm recovery by appropriate scapular rotators rehabilitation is essential in younger patient with rotator cuff tendinitis or non traumatic instability.

With progressive instability there will be more proprioceptive loss from the capsule with increased capsular stretch. This proprioceptive disorganization will lead to muscle patterning problems, repeated continued dislocations and subluxations and can progress to bony glenoid wear and affect core stability and the full kinetic chain. It would therefore make sense that early treatment and stabilization would be advantageous based on the principles above.

Conclusion

Glenohumeral joint is a complex articulation with high freedom of motion but innate instability. Many structure are involved in stability maintenance and a balanced and synchronized interplay between passive and dynamic restrains is essential to counteract the forces that could destabilize glenohumeral joint. Damage to one structure is most likely affect other structures and treatment should be directed accordingly. It's interesting to note how different injuries could appear with a similar clinical presentation and how much narrow is the border between anatomical and pathological variants. Only a deep knowledge of anatomy and biomechanical principles could help the surgeon to recognize pathology, choose the best treatment and adapt it according to the anatomy of the patient.

The humeral head

A. Is retroverted with a range 9–31°
B. Is anteverted with a rage of 3–24°
C. Has a radius ranging 5–18 mm
D. Has a radius ranging 17–28 mm
E. A & B
F. A & C
G. A & D
H. B & C
I. B & D

Soft tissue static stabilizers include all the above except:

A. Glenoid labrum
B. Glenohumeral capsule and ligaments
C. Long head of the biceps
D. Rotator interval
E. Negative intracapsular pressure
F. Adhesion cohesion mechanism

The percentage of humeral articular surface that articulates with glenoid articular surface at any time is:

A. 10%
B. 30%
C. 50%
D. 85%

References

1. Rockwood CAJ, Matsen FA. The shoulder. 4th ed. Philadelphia: Saunders-Elsevier; 2009.
2. Robertson DD, Yuan J, Bigliani LU, Flatow EL, Yamaguchi K. Three-dimensional analysis of the proximal part of the humerus: relevance to arthroplasty. J Bone Joint Surg Am. 2000;82-A(11):1594–602.
3. Churchill RS, Brems JJ, Kotschi H. Glenoid size, inclination, and version: an anatomic study. J Shoulder Elb Surg. 2001;10(4):327–32. doi:10.1067/mse.2001.115269.
4. Friedman RJ, An Y, Chokeski R, Kessler L. Anatomic and biomechanical study of glenohumeral contact. J Shoulder Elb Surg. 1994;3:S35.
5. Codman EA. The Shoulder. Boston, MA: Thomas Todd; 1934.
6. Saha AK. Dynamic stability of the glenohumeral joint. Acta Orthop Scand. 1971;42(6):491–505.
7. Piasecki DP, Verma NN, Romeo AA, Levine WN, Bach Jr BR, Provencher MT. Glenoid bone deficiency in recurrent anterior shoulder instability: diagnosis and management. J Am Acad Orthop Surg. 2009;17(8):482–93.
8. Bigliani LU, Newton PM, Steinmann SP, Connor PM, McLlveen SJ. Glenoid rim lesions associated with recurrent anterior dislocation of the shoulder. Am J Sports Med. 1998;26(1):41–5.
9. Nakagawa S, Mizuno N, Hiramatsu K, Tachibana Y, Mae T. Absorption of the bone fragment in shoulders with bony Bankart lesions caused by recurrent anterior dislocations or subluxations: when does it occur? Am J Sports Med. 2013;41(6):1380–6. doi:10.1177/0363546513483087.
10. Baudi P, Righi P, Bolognesi D, Rivetta S, Rossi Urtoler E, Guicciardi N, Carrara M. How to identify and calculate glenoid bone deficit. Chir Organi Mov. 2005;90(2):145–52.
11. Rowe CR, Zarins B, Ciullo JV. Recurrent anterior dislocation of the shoulder after surgical repair. Apparent causes of failure and treatment. J Bone Joint Surg Am. 1984;66(2):159–68.
12. Burkhart SS, De Beer JF. Traumatic glenohumeral bone defects and their relationship to failure of arthroscopic Bankart repairs: significance of the inverted-pear glenoid and the humeral engaging Hill-Sachs lesion. Arthroscopy. 2000;16(7):677–94.
13. Calandra JJ, Baker CL, Uribe J. The incidence of Hill-Sachs lesions in initial anterior shoulder dislocations. Arthroscopy. 1989;5(4):254–7.
14. Fronek J, Warren RF, Bowen M. Posterior subluxation of the glenohumeral joint. J Bone Joint Surg Am. 1989;71(2):205–16.
15. McLaughlin HL. Posterior dislocation of the shoulder. J Bone Joint Surg Am. 1952;24A(3):584–90.
16. Goudie EB, Murray IR, Robinson CM. Instability of the shoulder following seizures. J Bone Joint Surg Br. 2012;94(6):721–8. doi:10.1302/0301-620X.94B6.28259.
17. Di Giacomo G, De Vita A, Costantini A, de Gasperis N, Scarso P. Management of humeral head deficiencies and glenoid track. Curr Rev Muscoskelet Med. 2014;7(1):6–11. doi:10.1007/s12178-013-9194-7.
18. Yamamoto N, Itoi E, Abe H, Minagawa H, Seki N, Shimada Y, Okada K. Contact between the glenoid and the humeral head in abduction, external rotation, and horizontal extension: a new concept of glenoid track. J Shoulder Elb Surg. 2007;16(5):649–56. doi:10.1016/j.jse.2006.12.012.
19. Howell SM, Galinat BJ. The glenoid-labral socket. A constrained articular surface. Clin Orthopaed Relat Res. 1989;243:122–5.
20. Rao AG, Kim TK, Chronopoulos E, McFarland EG. Anatomical variants in the anterosuperior aspect of the glenoid labrum: a statistical analysis of seventy-three cases. J Bone Joint Surg Am. 2003;85-A(4):653–9.
21. Owens BD, Nelson BJ, Duffey ML, Mountcastle SB, Taylor DC, Cameron KL, Campbell S, DeBerardino TM. Pathoanatomy of first-time, traumatic, anterior glenohumeral subluxation events. J Bone Joint Surg Am. 2010;92(7):1605–11. doi:10.2106/JBJS.I.00851.
22. Speer KP, Deng X, Borrero S, Torzilli PA, Altchek DA, Warren RF. Biomechanical evaluation of a simulated Bankart lesion. J Bone Joint Surg Am. 1994;76(12):1819–26.
23. Green MR, Christensen KP. Arthroscopic Bankart procedure: two- to five-year followup with clinical correlation to severity of glenoid labral lesion. Am J Sports Med. 1995;23(3):276–81.

24. Neviaser TJ. The anterior labroligamentous periosteal sleeve avulsion lesion: a cause of anterior instability of the shoulder. Arthroscopy. 1993;9(1):17–21.
25. Kim SH, Ha KI, Park JH, Kim YM, Lee YS, Lee JY, Yoo JC. Arthroscopic posterior labral repair and capsular shift for traumatic unidirectional recurrent posterior subluxation of the shoulder. J Bone Joint Surg Am. 2003;85-A(8):1479–87.
26. Van Tongel A, Karelse A, Berghs B, Verdonk R, De Wilde L. Posterior shoulder instability: current concepts review. Knee Surg Sports Traumatol Arthrosc. 2011;19(9):1547–53. doi:10.1007/s00167-010-1293-z.
27. Badge R, Tambe A, Funk L. Arthroscopic isolated posterior labral repair in rugby players. Int J Shoulder Surg. 2009;3(1):4–7. doi:10.4103/0973-6042.50875.
28. McDonough A, Funk L. Critical reflection of the advanced rehabilitation of an elite rugby league player sustaining a posterior Bankart lesion. Phys Ther Sport. 2013;14(1):60–7. doi:10.1016/j.ptsp.2012.01.002.
29. Snyder SJ, Karzel RP, Del Pizzo W, Ferkel RD, Friedman MJ. SLAP lesions of the shoulder. Arthroscopy. 1990;6(4):274–9.
30. Funk L, Snow M. SLAP tears of the glenoid labrum in contact athletes. Clin J Sport Med. 2007;17(1):1–4. doi:10.1097/JSM.0b013e31802ede87.
31. Rowe CR, Patel D, Southmayd WW. The Bankart procedure: a long-term end-result study. J Bone Joint Surg Am. 1978;60(1):1–16.
32. Robinson CM, Dobson RJ. Anterior instability of the shoulder after trauma. J Bone Joint Surg Am. 2004;86(4):469–79.
33. Bigliani LU, Pollock RG, Soslowsky LJ, Flatow EL, Pawluk RJ, Mow VC. Tensile properties of the inferior glenohumeral ligament. J Orthopaed Res. 1992;10(2):187–97. doi:10.1002/jor.1100100205.
34. Wolf EM, Cheng JC, Dickson K. Humeral avulsion of glenohumeral ligaments as a cause of anterior shoulder instability. Arthroscopy. 1995;11(5):600–7.
35. Jost B, Koch PP, Gerber C. Anatomy and functional aspects of the rotator interval. J Shoulder Elb Surg. 2000;9(4):336–41. doi:10.1067/mse.2000.106746.
36. Kumar VP, Balasubramaniam P. The role of atmospheric pressure in stabilising the shoulder. An experimental study. J Bone Joint Surg Br. 1985;67(5):719–21.
37. Terry GC, Chopp TM. Functional anatomy of the shoulder. J Athl Train. 2000;35(3):248–55.
38. Collins DN (2009) Disorders of the acromioclavicular joint. In: Rockwood CAJ, Matsen FA (eds) The shoulder, vol 1. Saunders-Elsevier, Philadelphia, pp 453–526
39. Marcheggiani Muccioli GM, Manning C, Wright P, Grassi A, Zaffagnini S, Funk L. Acromioclavicular joint reconstruction with the LARS ligament in professional versus non-professional athletes. Knee Surg Sports Traumatol Arthrosc. 2014; doi:10.1007/s00167-014-3231-y.
40. Jerosch J, Thorwesten L, Teigelkotter T. Proprioception of the shoulder joint in young tennis players. Sportverletz Sportschaden. 1997;11(1):1–9. doi:10.1055/s-2007-993356.
41. Lugo R, Kung P, Ma CB. Shoulder biomechanics. Eur J Radiol. 2008;68(1):16–24. doi:10.1016/j.ejrad.2008.02.051.
42. Wuelker N, Korell M, Thren K. Dynamic glenohumeral joint stability. J Shoulder Elb Surg. 1998;7(1):43–52.
43. Turkel SJ, Panio MW, Marshall JL, Girgis FG. Stabilizing mechanisms preventing anterior dislocation of the glenohumeral joint. J Bone Joint Surg Am. 1981;63(8):1208–17.
44. Cain PR, Mutschler TA, Fu FH, Lee SK. Anterior stability of the glenohumeral joint. A dynamic model. Am J Sports Med. 1987;15(2):144–8.
45. Kirchhoff C, Imhoff AB. Posterosuperior and anterosuperior impingement of the shoulder in overhead athletes-evolving concepts. Int Orthop. 2010;34(7):1049–58. doi:10.1007/s00264-010-1038-0.
46. Pagnani MJ, Deng XH, Warren RF, Torzilli PA, O'Brien SJ. Role of the long head of the biceps brachii in glenohumeral stability: a biomechanical study in cadavera. J Bone Joint Surg Br. 1996;5(4):255–62.
47. Halder AM, Itoi E, An KN. Anatomy and biomechanics of the shoulder. Orthop Clin North Am. 2000;31(2):159–76.
48. Poppen NK, Walker PS. Forces at the glenohumeral joint in abduction. Clin Orthop Relat Res. 1978;135:165–70.
49. Kibler WB. The role of the scapula in athletic shoulder function. Am J Sports Med. 1998;26(2):325–37.
50. Glousman R, Jobe F, Tibone J, Moynes D, Antonelli D, Perry J. Dynamic electromyographic analysis of the throwing shoulder with glenohumeral instability. J Bone Joint Surg Am. 1988;70(2):220–6.

extremities. Shoulder conditions rarely are the cause of paresthesias in the upper extremity. Tingling and numbness down the arm should be considered a neurological problem until proven otherwise. The clinician should consider thoracic outlet syndrome or peripheral nerve entrapment such as cubital or carpal tunnel syndromes to be the cause of paresthesia [5]. If a patient has undergone previous surgery involving the cervical spine or shoulder, then the relationship of the symptoms to the timing of the surgery is important to ascertain.

Similarly, painless weakness should be considered a neurological process until proven otherwise. Patients with rotator cuff disorders do not deteriorate suddenly without an injury. Volleyball players often have painless weakness caused by suprascapular nerve entrapment [6, 7]. Bilateral insidious onset of shoulder or upper extremity weakness necessitates a workup for neurological conditions. We recently saw an elderly patient who had insidious onset of bilateral shoulder weakness but no pain. He had undergone reverse total shoulder arthroplasty to treat the weakness, which did not improve after his surgery. Upon examination, we found the weakness to be diffuse in both upper extremities. Neurological workup revealed amyotrophic lateral sclerosis. A careful history and examination would have prevented this unnecessary procedure.

Another factor to consider when making a diagnosis is the patient's age. Rotator cuff conditions typically do not appear before the fourth decade of life [8, 9]. Athletic individuals may have rotator cuff–like symptoms but typically do not have full-thickness rotator cuff tears, so other disorders should be considered. Young athletes who perform repetitive motions such as throwing a baseball may have proximal humerus physeal injuries, whereas athletes with closed physes who perform throwing motions tend to have partial rotator cuff tears or superior labral anterior posterior lesions [10].

Unfortunately, the location of pain in the shoulder does not necessarily indicate the diagnosis (Fig. 4.2). Pain at the AC joint typically is on top of the shoulder and radiates into the trapezius but it also can radiate down the front or back of the shoulder [11]. Pain in the front of the shoulder can indicate many abnormalities, including rotator cuff syndrome, biceps tendon disorders, arthritis, and stiffness of the shoulder. Therefore, some have suggested that pain in the front of the shoulder be called "anterolateral pain syndrome" rather than suggesting it is caused by one particular abnormality [12].

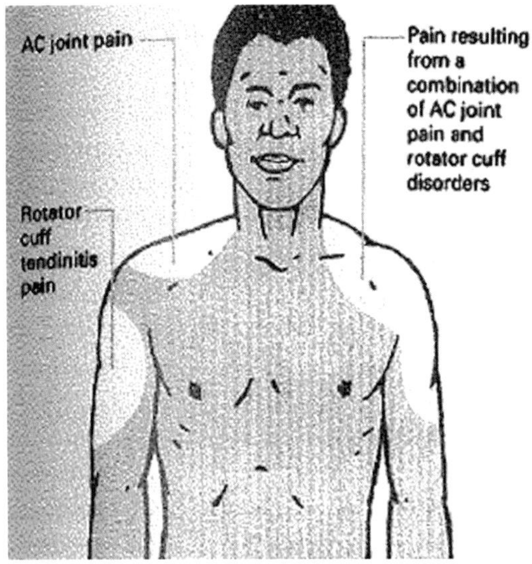

Fig. 4.2 Drawing showing the typical locations of pain from the acromioclavicular joint, the rotator cuff, and both simultaneously (Reprinted with permission from Examination of The Shoulder: The Complete Guide, Thieme Medical Publishers, Inc., 2006. Figure 1-2, p. 3.)

It is important to ascertain the nature of the patient's pain by asking standard questions. The patient's answers indicate the severity of the pain and may also provide warnings that the symptoms are serious in nature [13]. Pain that causes night waking, prevents participation in sports or activities of daily living, is not relieved with ice or heat, is not relieved by nonsteroidal anti-inflammatory drugs, requires increasingly stronger narcotics, or makes the patient miserable may indicate a serious condition such as a malignant tumor or more serious systemic illness. Patients should be asked what activities make their pain worse and what makes their pain better. They should always be asked about gastrointestinal problems, renal disorders, liver conditions, the use of blood thinners, and diabetes before prescribing anti-inflammatory medicines. Patients with stiff shoulders from osteoarthritis or frozen shoulders have the most difficulty with activities of daily living, followed by patients with rotator cuff syndromes (Table 4.3).

Checklists of the symptoms also can be helpful (Table 4.4). The use of checklists will often stimulate the patient to report other symptoms or conditions that might be associated with their more salient symptoms. When using checklists, it is important to note tingling, numbness, and temperature changes because these many indicate nerve involvement or infection.

Table 4.3 Difficulty performing specific activities with various shoulder pathologies[a]

	N	Difficulty with activity (%)[b]							
Disease state		Use back pocket	Wash opposite underarm	Eat with utensil	Comb hair	Use arm at shoulder level	Dress	Use hand overhead	Carry weight[c]
Instability[d]	208	18.0	12.5	9.4	18.5	31.7	13.5	55.1	31.0
External impingement	103	42.6	28.2	17.8	39.4	59.2	35.3	78.4	66.0
Glenohumeral osteoarthritis	99	89.4	78.4	38.3	71.0	79.6	66.3	92.9	73.7
Acromioclavicular joint[e]	78	39.7	33.8	17.3	32.5	47.4	36.4	69.3	62.2
Rotator cuff[f]	376	39.7	34.0	20.1	39.0	61.2	35.8	77.4	58.1
SLAP lesion	19	47.4	47.4	33.3	44.4	52.6	47.4	73.7	38.9

SLAP superior labrum anterior to posterior

[a]*Source*: Adapted with permission from *Examination of the Shoulder: The Complete Guide*. New York, NY: Thieme Medical Publishers, Inc.; 2006

[b]Variable for ability to perform activity from the American Shoulder and Elbow Surgeons score; included here are only those who reported difficulty, with assistance, or not at all

[c]10–15 lb with arm at side using a shoulder and elbow score

[d]Anterior, anterior traumatic, multidirectional, occult, or posterior instability

[e]Acromioclavicular joint arthritis, separation, or osteolysis

[f]Rotator cuff tendinitis, partial tear, or full tear

Table 4.4 Examination history of the shoulder[a]

General Information	Medical information	Symptoms	Injury pattern	Symptom characteristics	Related symptoms
Age	Chronic or acute problem	Pain	Sudden vs. acute onset	Location	Cervical
Dominant arm	Review of systems	Weakness or fatigue	Gradual vs. chronic onset	Character and severity	Peripheral nerve
Participation in sports	Preexisting or recurrent shoulder problem	Instability/subluxation	Traumatic onset	Provocation	Brachial plexus
Level of competition	Other musculoskeletal problems	Stiffness	Recurrent pattern	Duration	Entrapment
		Catching/locking		Paresthesias/referral pattern	
				Effect on sport/other disability	

[a]*Source*: Adapted with permission from *Clinical Examination of the Shoulder*, Vol. 1. New York, NY: Elsevier Science; 2004

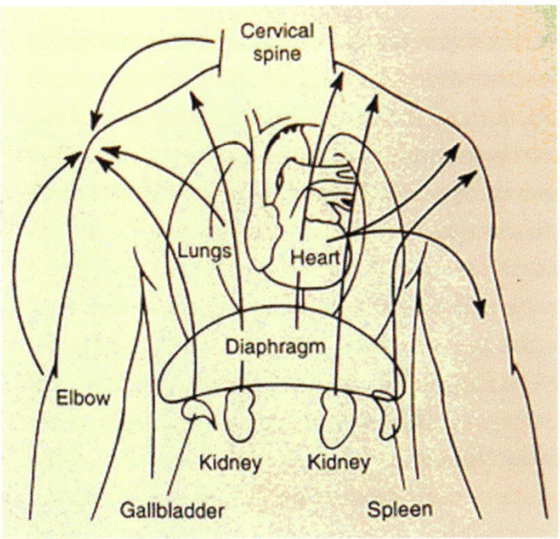

Fig. 4.3 Drawing showing the many possible visceral causes of pain in the upper or lower thorax, which can be mistaken for shoulder pain (Reprinted with permission from Examination of The Shoulder: The Complete Guide, Thieme Medical Publishers, Inc., 2006. Figure 1-6, p. 4.)

Finally, it is important to know the medical history of the patient. For example, a patient with insulin-dependent diabetes who develops insidious onset of pain with no trauma should be considered to have a frozen shoulder until proven otherwise. Patients with a history of oral or intravenous steroid use may have avascular necrosis. Patients with Crohn's disease, psoriasis, or ulcerative colitis might have an underlying immunological cause of pain and arthritis. Patients with a history of cancer should undergo careful examination and early imaging when there is pain in the shoulder area either from trauma or with insidious onset. Patients with abdominal conditions may have pain in the upper or lower thorax (Fig. 4.3). The types of medications the patient is taking and the types of comorbidities the patient has can influence whether the treatment is medical or surgical.

Few shoulder conditions are life-threatening. Therefore, the choice of treatment, be it medical or surgical, involves consideration of many objective and subjective variables. The presence of a lesion on examination or magnetic resonance imaging is not typically an indication for surgery unless it is symptomatic. The axiom, "the lesion is attached to a person," is especially true in shoulder conditions. The type and urgency of treatment are determined by many factors, including the patient's age, occupation, and general health; whether the dominant or nondominant arm is affected; the patient's pain level at rest and at night; what makes the pain worse or better; the effects on exercise, hobbies, or activities of daily living; the ability of medicines to relieve the pain; and the perceived natural history of the condition. Information on all of these factors should be obtained so that an appropriate plan of treatment can be developed for the needs of each patient.

References

1. Wild AT, Begly JP, Garzon-Muvdi J, Desai P, McFarland EG. First-rib stress fracture in a high-school lacrosse player: a case report and short clinical review. Sports Health. 2011;3(6):547–9. doi:10.1177/1941738111416189.
2. Daigneault J, Cooney Jr LM. Shoulder pain in older people. J Am Geriatr Soc. 1998;46(9):1144–51.
3. Lunsford LD, Bissonette DJ, Jannetta PJ, Sheptak PE, Zorub DS. Anterior surgery for cervical disc disease. Part 1: Treatment of lateral cervical disc herniation in 253 cases. J Neurosurg. 1980;53(1):1–11. doi:10.3171/jns.1980.53.1.0001.
4. Hawkins RJ, Bilco T, Bonutti P. Cervical spine and shoulder pain. Clin Orthop. 1990;258:142–6.
5. Muscolino JE. Upper extremity paraesthesia: clinical assessment and reasoning. J Bodyw Mov Ther. 2008;12(3):268–73. doi:10.1016/j.jbmt.2007.07.005.
6. Lajtai G, Wieser K, Ofner M, Raimann G, Aitzetmuller G, Jost B. Electromyography and nerve conduction velocity for the evaluation of the infraspinatus muscle and the suprascapular nerve in professional beach volleyball players. Am J Sports Med. 2012;40(10):2303–8. doi:10.1177/0363546512455395.
7. Sandow MJ, Ilic J. Suprascapular nerve rotator cuff compression syndrome in volleyball players. J Shoulder Elb Surg. 1998;7(5):516–21.
8. Milgrom C, Schaffler M, Gilbert S, Van Holsbeeck M. Rotator-cuff changes in asymptomatic adults. The effect of age, hand dominance and gender. J Bone Joint Surg Br. 1995;77(2):296–8.
9. Sher JS, Uribe JW, Posada A, Murphy BJ, Zlatkin MB. Abnormal findings on magnetic resonance images of asymptomatic shoulders. J Bone Joint Surg Am. 1995;77(1):10–5.
10. Meister K. Injuries to the shoulder in the throwing athlete. Part one: Biomechanics/pathophysiology/classification of injury. Am J Sports Med. 2000;28(2):265–75.

11. Gerber C, Galantay RV, Hersche O. The pattern of pain produced by irritation of the acromioclavicular joint and the subacromial space. J Shoulder Elb Surg. 1998;7(4):352–5.
12. McFarland EG, Maffulli N, Del Buono A, Murrell GAC, Garzon-Muvdi J, Petersen SA. Impingement is not impingement: the case for calling it "Rotator Cuff Disease". Muscles Ligaments Tendons J. 2013;3(3):196–200.
13. McFarland EG, Compton SP, Dawson CA. Guide to good and bad pain for the health/fitness professional. ACSM Health Fitness J. 2003;7(4):11–6.

Physical Evaluation

5

Edward G. McFarland, Kyubo Choi,
Seyedali R. Ghasemi, and Alex Bitzer

Introduction

The evaluation of any joint of the musculoskeletal system should be within the abilities of any health care provider, and the goal of this chapter is to help enable a practitioner of any level of training to perform a competent examination of the shoulder complex. The basic principles of a musculoskeletal evaluation are as follows: (1) expose both shoulders to assess the affected joint; (2) compare both sides; (3) evaluate a joint above (proximal to) and below (distal to) the affected area; (4) always perform a neurovascular examination; and (5) always obtain radiographs in both planes at 90° to each other. By following these simple rules, a clinician can usually make an accurate diagnosis [1].

Basic Principles

Musculoskeletal Evaluation

Shoulder exposure. Once a history has been obtained, the clinician should perform the examination with the patient's shoulders and upper extremities exposed enough to see the posterior thorax, cervical spine, deltoid area, and complete upper extremity (Fig. 5.1). This exposure allows the examiner to evaluate for atrophy of the muscles of the upper extremity and thorax (Fig. 5.2) and to see the interactions of the scapula, thorax, and glenohumeral joint (Fig. 5.3). A "hitch" in the shoulder motion as the patient elevates the arm can indicate various shoulder conditions and is not diagnostic, but it does alert the clinician that the shoulder joint is not moving in a synchronous manner.

Comparison of both sides. The corollary to exposing the shoulders is to compare both sides so that even subtle swelling and atrophy of the affected shoulder and extremity are noted. The ability to see both sides accurately is important not only for the visual examination of the extremity but also for the neurologic and functional examinations.

Consideration of the joints proximal and distal to the affected area. Next, the clinician should evaluate the joints proximal to (above) and distal to (below) the affected area. For a shoulder evaluation, the proximal joint is the neck. The clinician should ask the patient if there is a history of neck problems, surgery of the cervical spine, or neurologic symptoms such as tingling or numbness. The neck should be examined for tenderness and range of motion. Axial compression of the cervical spine can produce radicular symptoms (Spurling sign), but this sign is not positive in many patients with cervical spine nerve irritations [2–4].

E.G. McFarland, M.D. (✉) • K. Choi, M.D.
S.R. Ghasemi, M.D. • A. Bitzer, M.D.
Division of Shoulder Surgery, Department of Orthopaedic Surgery, The Johns Hopkins University, Baltimore, MD, USA
e-mail: editorialservices@jhmi.edu

G. Huri, N.K. Paschos (eds.), *The Shoulder*, Orthopaedic Study Guide Series,
DOI 10.1007/978-3-319-51979-1_5

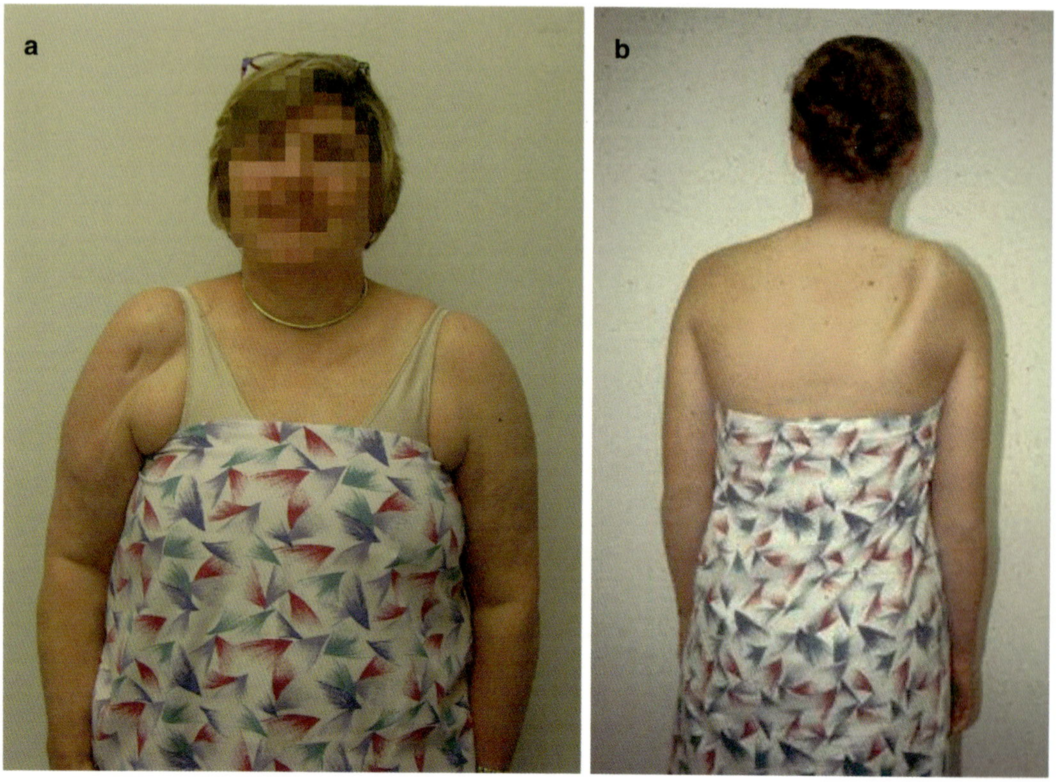

Fig. 5.1 Anterior (**a**) and posterior (**b**) views of a gown designed to allow visualization of the thorax and upper extremity in female patients

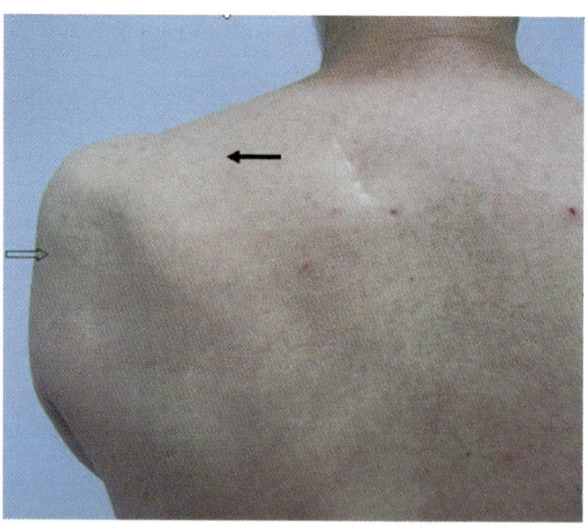

Fig. 5.2 Clinical photograph of patient with atrophy of the supraspinatus muscle (*closed black arrow*) and of the infraspinatus muscle (*open black arrow*). Atrophy of these muscles can be secondary to a neurologic cause or to torn rotator cuff tendons

Neurovascular Examination

One of the most important evaluations when assessing the shoulder joint is the neurovascular examination of the affected upper extremity. A competent neurologic and vascular examination of the upper extremity can rule out or identify the most serious causes of shoulder dysfunction and avoid a missed neurologic or vascular cause of shoulder, arm, or upper extremity pain.

Vascular evaluation. The vascular examination consists of evaluating the color, temperature, and swelling of the extremity and comparing it with the contralateral extremity. This evaluation is particularly important in the patient with acute pain because there may be an occult vascular injury or a deep venous thrombosis (Fig. 5.4). Evaluation of these variables is also important in making the diagnosis of complex regional pain syndrome (Fig. 5.5). Next, the clinician should

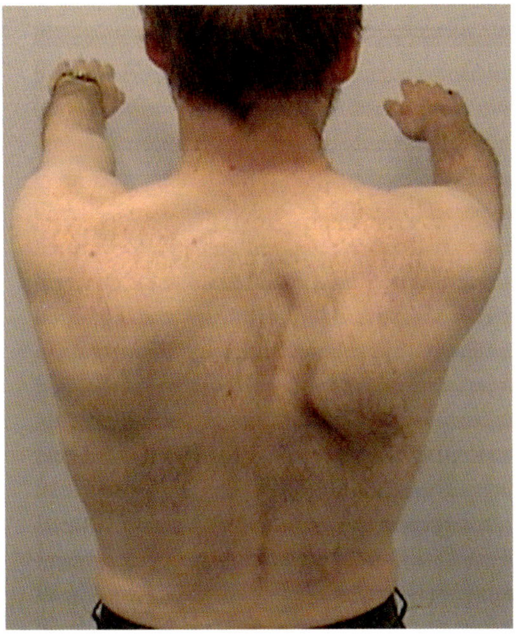

Fig. 5.3 Clinical photograph of patient with scapular winging, which is difficult to detect if the patient is clothed (Reprinted with permission from McFarland EG. General principles of shoulder examination. In: *Examination of the Shoulder: The Complete Guide*. New York: Thieme, 2006:1–14; Figure 25.)

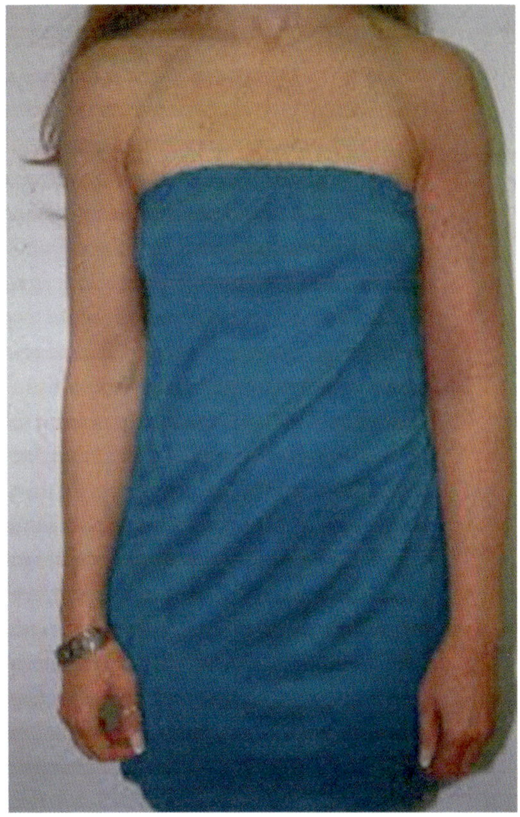

Fig. 5.4 Clinical photograph of a patient with a deep venous thrombosis of the left upper extremity after a clavicle fracture. The diagnosis is more apparent when the two extremities are compared

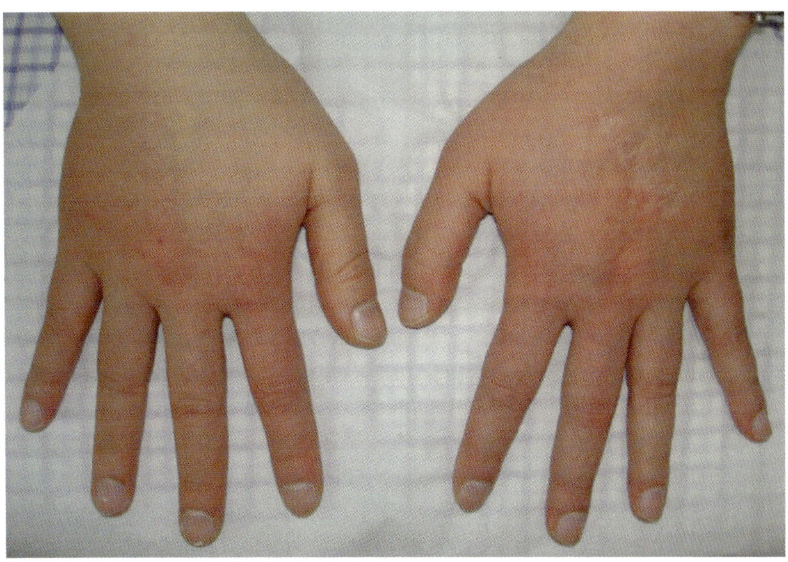

Fig. 5.5 Clinical photograph of a patient with complex regional pain syndrome with classic findings of skin color changes, swelling, and stiffness in the hands

note the presence or absence of a pulse at the wrist, and the capillary refill should be compared with that in the contralateral extremity. Although the scientific literature does not report an absolute value for this criterion, the capillary refill should not be >3 s. Any discrepancy between the two sides might warrant additional investigation with Doppler ultrasonography, plethysmography, or other modalities [5–8].

Sensory evaluation. The sensory examination consists of light touch, deep touch, pain, temperature, position sense, and vibration evaluation. In the office and the emergency department settings, light touch is the modality most frequently used. It usually is unnecessary to test for pain or use the other modalities unless light touch testing is abnormal or there is a clinical suspicion of systemic disease or of higher long-tract lesions that are affecting the nerves.

When assessing light-touch response, it is important to test every dermatome and every peripheral nerve and to compare responses on both sides. The best method is to touch the patient in the same anatomic areas on both upper extremities and ask if the two sides feel the same. A complete sensory examination includes the deltoid (C5 dermatome, axillary nerve), volar side of the thumb (C5–C6 dermatome, median nerve), volar side of the middle finger (C7 dermatome, median nerve), volar side of the little finger (C8 dermatome, ulnar nerve), lateral side of the forearm (C5–C6, lateral antebrachial cutaneous nerve), medial forearm (C7–C8, medial antebrachial cutaneous nerve), medial elbow (T1, medial brachial cutaneous nerve), and dorsal, proximal part of the first web space (C7, radial nerve).

If a patient reports a difference between the two sides, it is often helpful to map out the area of different sensation to delineate the pattern and to determine whether it is dermatomal or a peripheral nerve distribution. Similarly, the use of two-point discrimination in the fingertips can be a valuable guide to the severity of the nerve involvement. Electromyography and nerve conduction testing can be performed in patients for whom the diagnosis is uncertain or for whom more detailed neurologic nerve injury information is needed.

Reflexes and long-tract signs. When examining the patient with upper extremity pain or paresthesias, it is important to evaluate the reflexes. There are only three cervical reflexes: the biceps (C5), the brachioradialis (C6), and the triceps (C7). The reflexes should be noted to be normal, hyporeflexic, or hyperreflexic. In patients with hypotonia, the strength and sensory distribution of the individual nerve root should be evaluated.

In the patient with hyperreflexia, it is important to evaluate for long-tract signs. In the upper extremity, the best sign is the Hoffmann reflex (Fig. 5.6), which is analogous to a Babinski reflex in the lower extremity. A positive Hoffmann reflex indicates an upper motor neuron lesion in the cervical spine or at higher levels in the brain. For a patient with a positive Hoffmann sign, it is important to compare the extremity with the other side; a small percentage of patients will have a bilaterally positive Hoffmann sign, which can be a normal finding. If a patient has a positive Hoffmann sign, consideration also should be given to examining the lower extremity because disease that affects upper motor neurons may also affect those in the lower extremity. An example is cervical spondylopathy (cervical spinal stenosis), which can affect all four extremities.

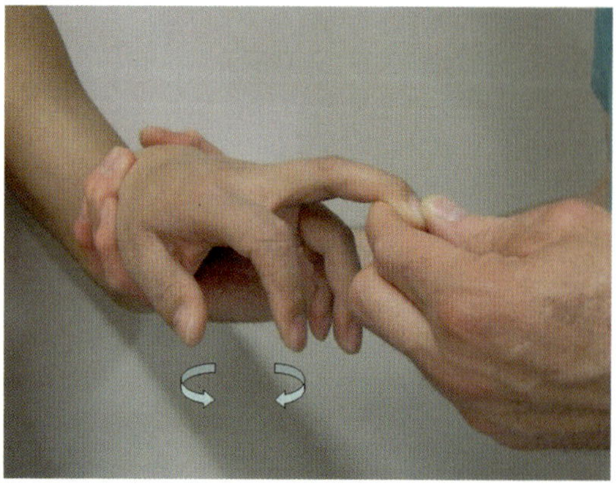

Fig. 5.6 Clinical photograph of how to perform the Hoffmann reflex test. The examiner holds the patient's hand and wrist in a relaxed position and flicks the end of the middle finger

Muscle strength and range of motion. A large portion of the motor strength examination involves determining the range of motion of the shoulder and the joints distal to it. However, testing any of the upper extremity muscles takes some clinical judgment; a patient with acute onset of severe shoulder pain and swelling should be approached differently than an ambulatory patient who has only mild symptoms. For some patients such as those with acute trauma or those who present with very painful shoulders despite an insidious onset, range of motion examination should be deferred until the exact causes of the problem can be determined by radiography or other diagnostic imaging.

In the emergent setting or in patients with severe pain, the goal simply is to determine whether or not the muscle segment is firing. In such situations, it is best to test the extremity in whatever position is comfortable for the patient. Similarly, it is best to test muscles that provide the most information about each cervical level and each peripheral nerve. For the patient with shoulder problems, we recommend asking the patient to contract the muscle to abduct the arm (deltoid, axillary nerve, C5), to flex the elbow (biceps muscle, musculocutaneous nerve, C5–C6), extend the elbow (triceps muscle, radial, C7), abduct the fingers (intrinsic muscles, ulnar nerve, C7–C8), and oppose the tip of the thumb to the tip of the little finger (opponens pollicis, median nerve, C5–C7). Other muscles can be selected as necessary to determine the exact distribution of nerve involvement.

Once it is established that a patient can fire the muscle, it is then recommended that the strength be determined for each muscle group. The first step is to ask the patient to move the extremity against gravity in a full range of motion. A patient's inability to move the extremity through a full range of motion can be the result of various causes such as pain, weakness, contracture, or central nervous system abnormalities. The most commonly used grading system is the manual muscle testing system, which rates muscle action from 0 (no activity) to 5 (normal) (Table 5.1) [9].

Table 5.1 The manual muscle testing system for grading muscle strength

Strength grade	Description
5: Normal	Complete range of motion against gravity with full resistance
4: Good	Complete range of motion against gravity with some resistance
3: Fair	Complete range of motion against gravity
2: Poor	Complete range of motion with gravity eliminated
1: Trace	Evidence of slight contractility; no joint motion
0: None	No evidence of contractility

Originally published in Hoppenfeld S. Physical examination of the shoulder. In: *Physical Examination of the Spine & Extremities*, chapter 1, pp. 1–34. Norwalk (CT): Appleton & Lange, 1976

The neural examination involves having the patient perform full elevation, flex the elbow fully, extend the elbow fully, make a fist, and extend the fingers and wrist. If the patient cannot move the segment against gravity, then the strength rating is graded as a 2. A grade of 4 means that the patient is weak against resistance provided by the examiner but otherwise has full range of motion.

Although there are more sophisticated ways to measure strength such as hand-held dynamometers, we have not found them to be valuable in the routine evaluation of patients. Also, although isokinetic testing via sophisticated machines may be of some value for selected patients, this type of testing usually is not needed except for athletic populations.

For testing shoulder motion specifically, five motions typically are evaluated and recorded as part of the examination: elevation (in flexion or abduction) (Fig. 5.7), external rotation with the arm abducted 90° (Fig. 5.8), internal rotation with the arm abducted 90° (Fig. 5.9), external rotation with the arm at the side (Fig. 5.10), and internal rotation with the arm up the back (Fig. 5.11). Internal rotation can be approximated with the system recommended by Matsen et al. [10], in which the top of the scapula is C7, the

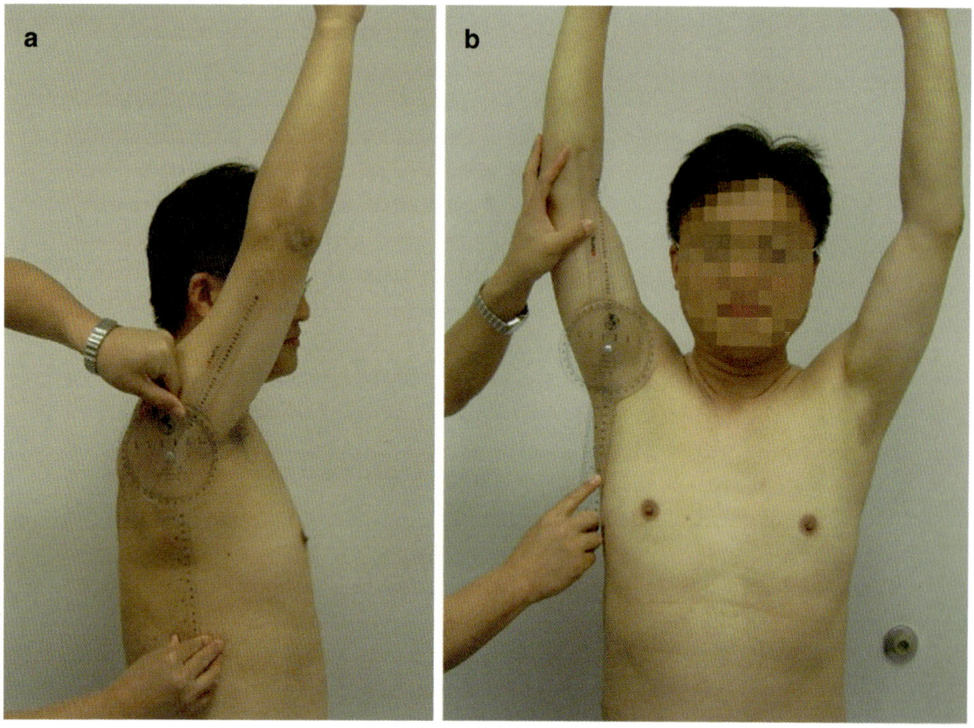

Fig. 5.7 Clinical photograph of the technique for measuring elevation of the arm in flexion (**a**) or abduction (**b**)

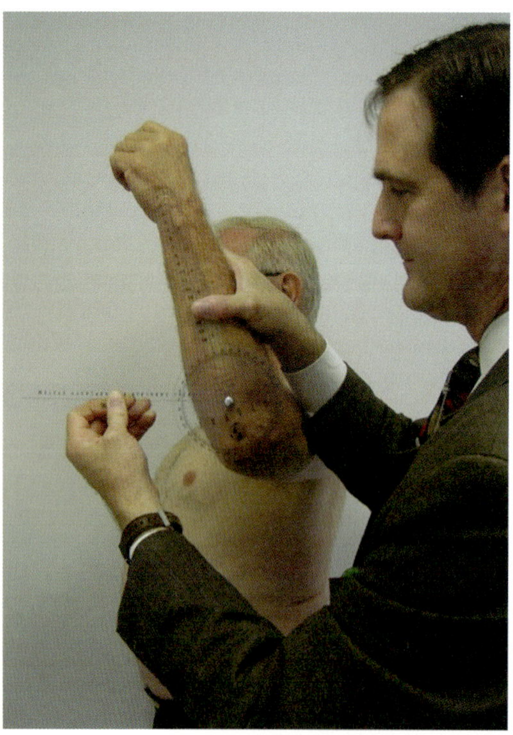

Fig. 5.8 Clinical photograph of the technique for measuring external rotation with the arm in 90° of elevation

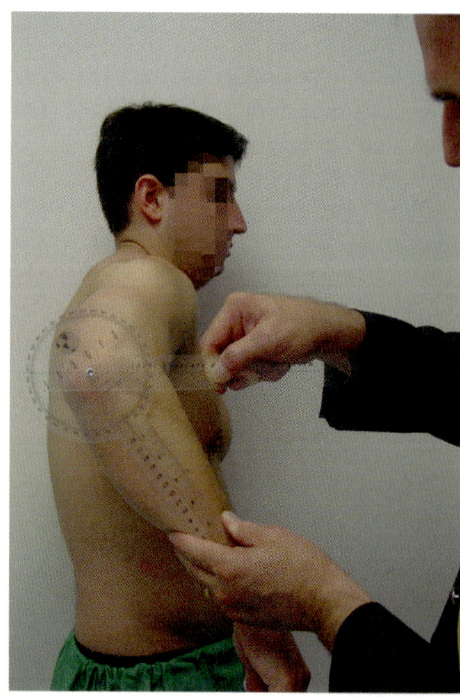

Fig. 5.9 Clinical photograph of the technique for measuring internal rotation with the arm in 90° of elevation (Reprinted with permission from McFarland EG. Shoulder range of motion. In: *Examination of the Shoulder: The Complete Guide*. New York: Thieme, 2006:15–87; Figure 2-23)

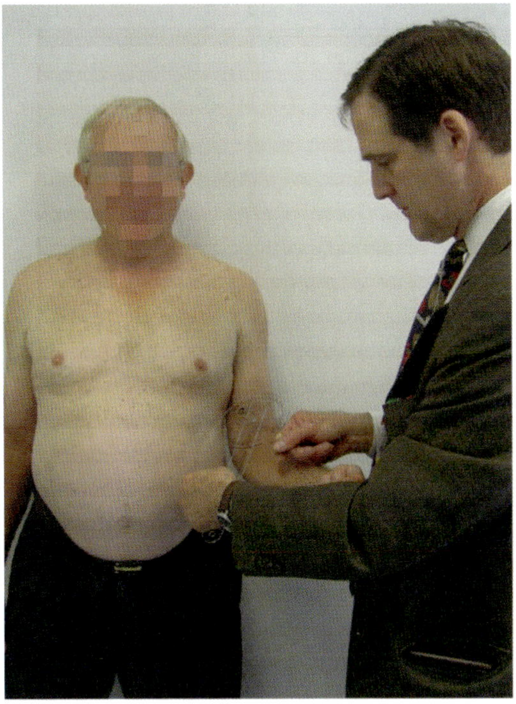

Fig. 5.10 Clinical photograph of the technique of testing external rotation with the arm at the side

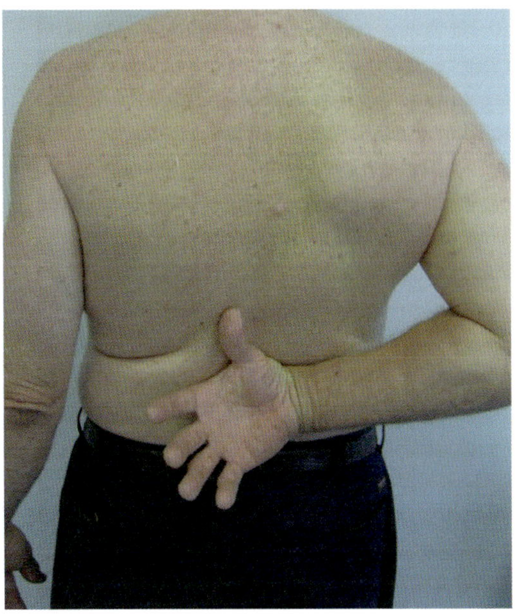

Fig. 5.11 Photograph of measuring internal rotation with the hand up the middle of the back, with the thumb up

midportion of the scapula is T4, the lower border of the scapula is T8, the upper lumbar region is L1, the lumbosacral junction is L5–S1, and the

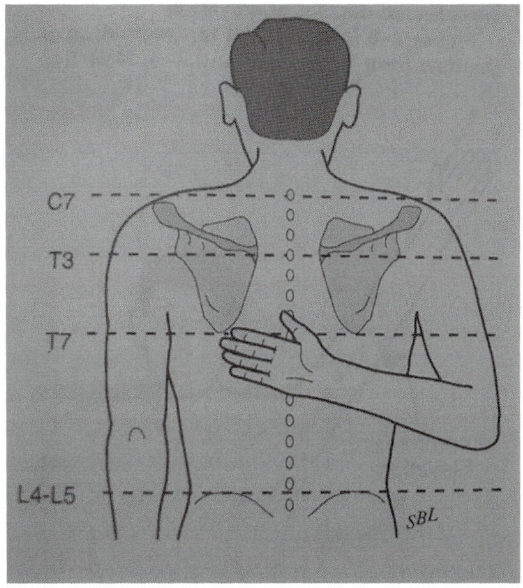

Fig. 5.12 Line drawing of the location of landmarks for internal rotation up the back. (Reprinted with permission from Matsen FA, Lippitt SB, Sidles JA, Harryman DT. Shoulder motion. In: *Practical Evaluation and Management of the Shoulder.* Philadelphia: WB Saunders, 1994:21.)

back pocket and the hip are the last two landmarks (Fig. 5.12). All of these motions in the affected extremity should be compared with those of the opposite extremity.

If a patient has limited range of motion, it is important to try to establish whether the motion the patient obtains actively is as good as the motion obtained passively with assistance from the examiner. When a patient has limited range of motion, the examiner should gently try to make the segment move further with no resistance. If the patient has limited range of motion actively and passively, then the patient may have pain or a mechanical block to movement of the arm. The most common diagnoses that cause loss of active and passive motion are arthritis of any type and frozen or stiff shoulders. For a patient with passive motion that is nearly normal but with restricted active motion, the most common causes are neurological (upper or lower motor neuron) or tears of the tendons of the muscles that control that motion. Patients with limited range of motion should be examined carefully for neurologic causes of the loss of motion unless there are obvious orthopaedic reasons why the motion is limited, such as arthritis or an acute injury.

Tests for Specific Diagnoses

Manual Muscle Testing and Lag Signs

An important part of determining the diagnosis in patients who present with pain and loss of shoulder function is to determine which shoulder muscles function normally and which do not. The shoulder has many "backup systems" that allow it to function with torn tendons or muscles. For example, many clinicians are taught that a patient with a rotator cuff tear cannot lift the arm. In reality, the loss of motion after a rotator cuff tear is most often the result of pain, not a mechanical problem caused by the tear itself.

Two muscles elevate the arm: the deltoid and the supraspinatus muscles. In one study, Colachis and Strohm [11] paralyzed the nerve to the supraspinatus and infraspinatus muscles (the suprascapular nerve). They found that the patients with supraspinatus and infraspinatus muscle paralysis had full range of motion but were weak in abduction and external rotation to strength testing. A similar study found that patients whose axillary nerves (and thus the deltoid muscles) were paralyzed had full range of motion because the supraspinatus was still functioning [12].

The findings of Colachis and Strohm [11] are clinically important because they indicate that patients with very large rotator cuff tears (i.e., the supraspinatus and infraspinatus torn completely from the bone) can have normal shoulder range of motion and little loss of motion in their activities of daily living. However, the most common experience of such patients is weakness when using the arm elevated over shoulder level and when holding objects away from their bodies. As a result, the ability to detect rotator cuff abnormalities depends on the examiner's ability to test specifically the muscles of the rotator cuff and other muscles around the shoulder. Although a detailed description of how to test all muscles of the upper extremity is beyond the scope of this chapter, and excellent texts are available on this subject, several of the techniques used for testing muscle strength are summarized here.

When testing abduction strength of the shoulder, it is impossible to isolate the supraspinatus muscle from the deltoid muscle [13]. The most common position for testing the supraspinatus is with the arm abducted 90°, forward-flexed 30° on the thorax (called the "plane of the scapula" because the scapula is on an angle because of the curve of the thorax), and with the arm in internal rotation (Fig. 5.13). This test can be done with the arm in neutral rotation, internal rotation (called the "empty can" position), or external rotation (called the "full can" position) [14]. When testing the arm for abduction strength, it is important not to cause the patient pain, which is more likely to occur when the arm is tested in the internally rotated position. Some studies have shown that the muscle activity in the supraspinatus is the same whether the arm is tested thumb down, thumb up, or in neutral position [15, 16]. Therefore, we no longer use the empty-can position when testing the supraspinatus because the pain provoked makes the test difficult to interpret.

An important test for determining the strength of abduction is the "drop-arm sign." There are two ways to perform this test. The first is to have the patient elevate the arm fully and then ask him to bring it down slowly to the side (Fig. 5.14). If the patient cannot do this without dropping the arm, the test is considered positive. The second method is to elevate the arm to 90° and ask the patient to hold it in that position. If she cannot do so, and the arm drops to the side, the test is considered positive. This test indicates profound abduction weakness that can be secondary to neurologic causes or a massive tear of the rotator cuff (i.e., the supraspinatus and infraspinatus).

The second important test for determining whether the rotator cuff is torn is testing external rotation strength with the arm at the side (Fig. 5.15). This test is best performed with the elbows at the side, with the examiner pushing the patient's arm into internal rotation against resistance by the patient. If the patient's resistance is weak, it can mean that there is a supraspinatus tendon tear because the supraspinatus muscle is also an external rotator of the shoulder. However, profound weakness in external rotation is indicative of a tear of the infraspinatus tendon or neural injury to that muscle. Rarely will weakness in that muscle be the result of disuse and pain alone.

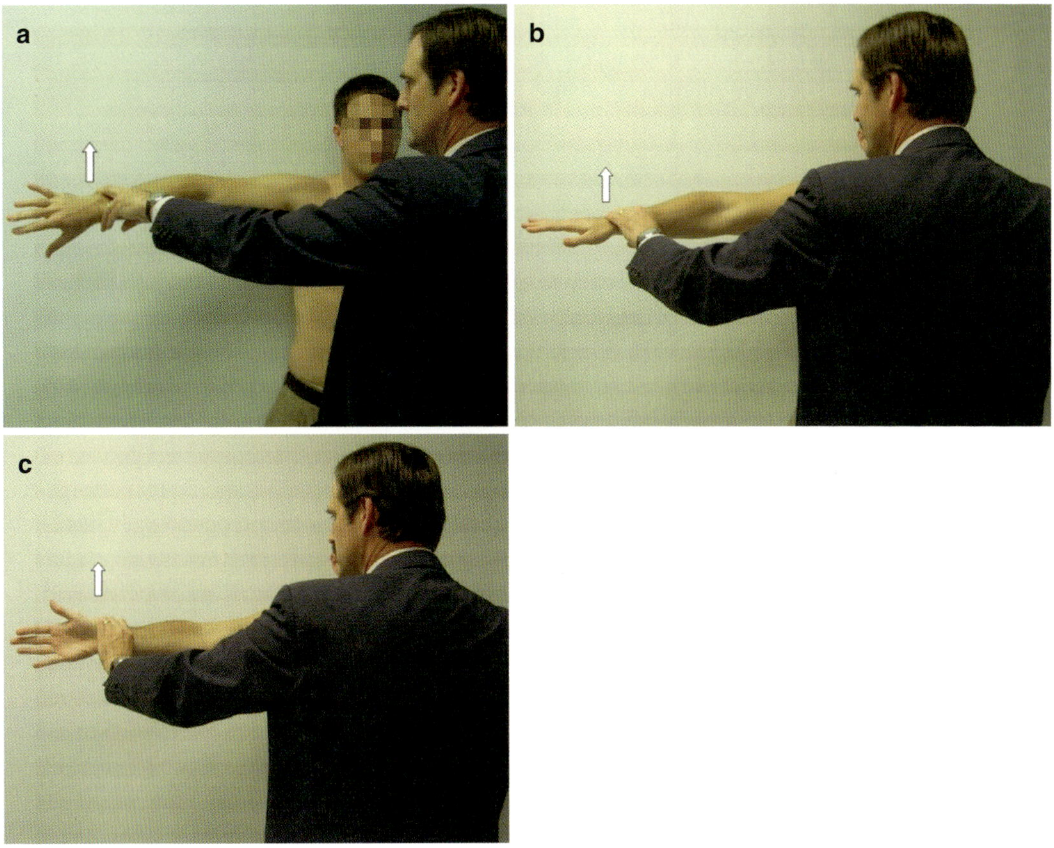

Fig. 5.13 Clinical photographs of testing the strength of abduction with the arm in the plane of the scapula and with the thumb down (known as the "Jobe test" or "empty-can position") (**a**). This test can be performed adequately with the patient's arm in a neutral position (**b**) or with the thumb up (the "full-can position") (**c**)

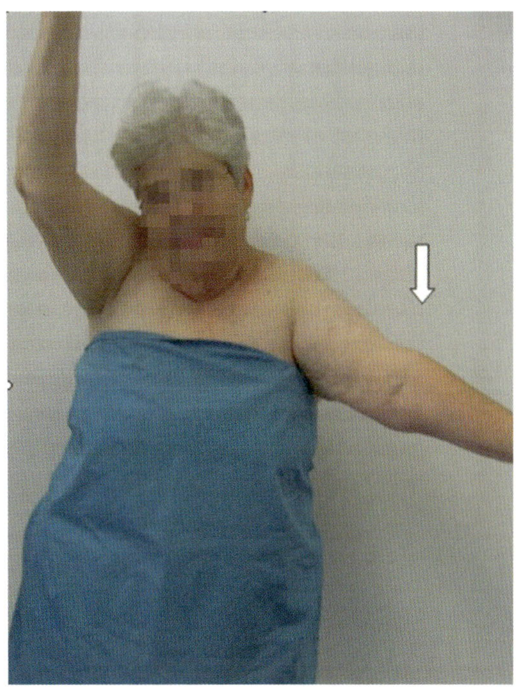

Fig. 5.14 Photograph of a patient with a positive drop-arm sign. The patient cannot hold the arm against gravity (*arrow* shows arm dropping)

Another sign of a large rotator cuff tear or profound neurologic injury to the nerves supplying the rotator cuff is the "external rotation lag sign." In this test, the patient stands with the elbow flexed 90°, and the examiner holds the arm by the elbow (Fig. 5.16). The arm then is maximally externally rotated, and the patient is asked to hold the arm in that position. Inability to hold that position and allowing the arm to rotate internally indicates a complete tear of the supraspinatus and infraspinatus tendons or a severe neurologic deficit to the nerves to those muscles [17].

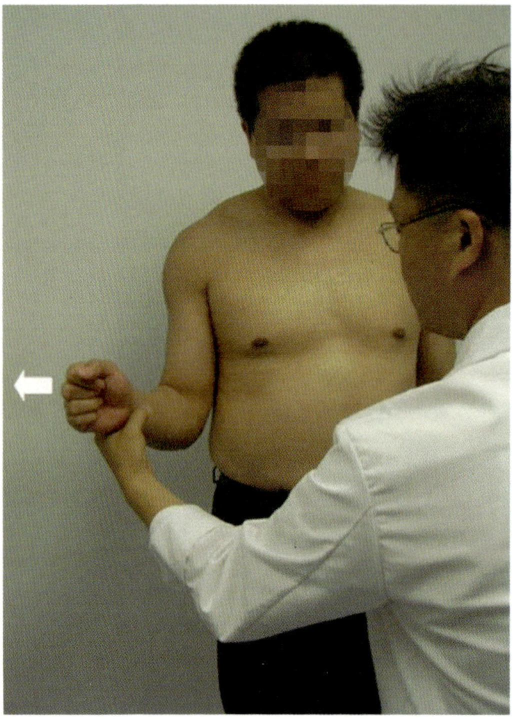

Fig. 5.15 Clinical photograph of the technique of testing the strength of external rotation with the arm at the side

There are three tests for the subscapularis muscle and tendon. The first is the lift-off test, which is performed by asking the patient to rotate the arm internally up the back and then try to lift the hand off the back without extending the elbow [18] (Fig. 5.17). The inability to perform this maneuver is considered a positive test and indicates a complete tear of the subscapularis tendon where it attaches to the lesser tuberosity of the humerus. This test has high accuracy, but it is difficult for patients with a stiff shoulder to perform.

The second test of the subscapularis muscle and tendon is the "subscapularis lag sign" [18]. This test is performed in a manner similar to that for the lift-off test, except that the examiner places the patient's arm just off the low back and asks the patient to hold the position (Fig. 5.18). The inability of the patient to hold the arm away from the body, so that it drops back to the thorax,

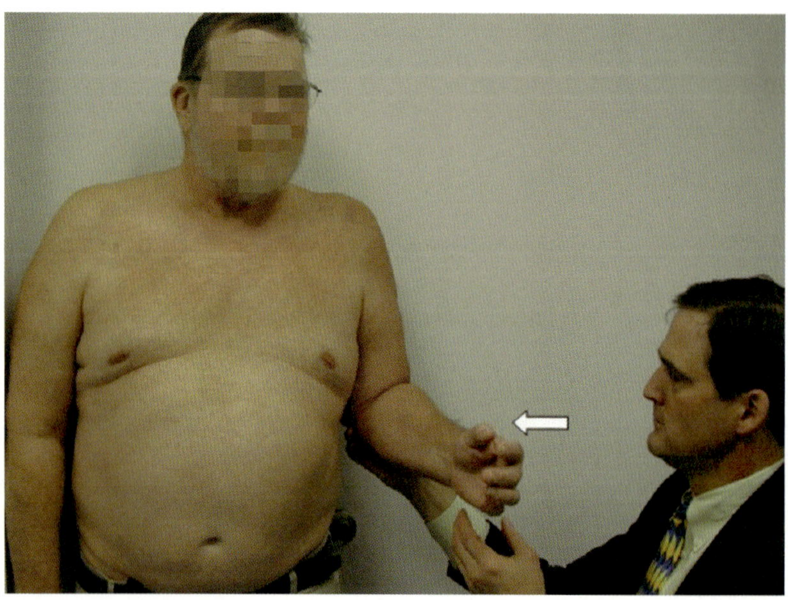

Fig. 5.16 Clinical photograph of the external rotation lag sign, which is positive when the patient cannot hold the arm in maximal external rotation (Reprinted with permission from McFarland EG. Rotator cuff disease and impingement. In: *Examination of the Shoulder: The Complete Guide.* New York: Thieme, 2006:126–161; Figure 4-38.)

is considered a positive test and indicates dysfunction of the subscapularis muscle or tendon.

The third test is the "belly press test." In this test, the patient is asked to place his or her hand on the abdomen, and the examiner brings the elbow forward (Fig. 5.19). The patient is then asked to hold that position. If the elbow falls back so that the wrist flexes, the test is considered to be positive and it indicates subscapularis muscle or tendon dysfunction [18].

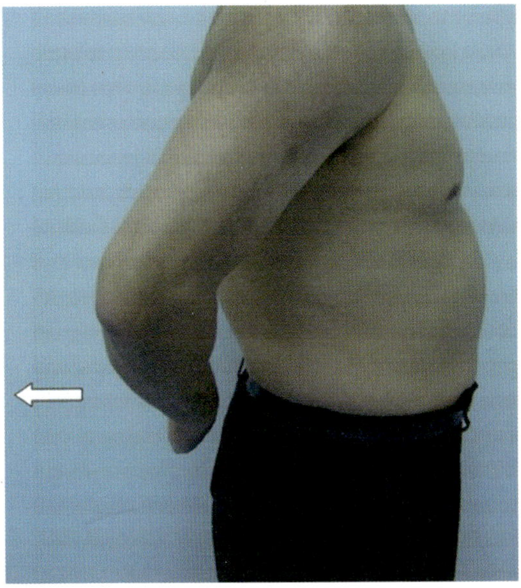

Fig. 5.17 Clinical photograph of the lift-off test

Rotator Cuff Disease

Until recently, it was assumed that the reason the rotator cuff tendons became frayed (partial-thickness tears) and eventually tore completely (full-thickness

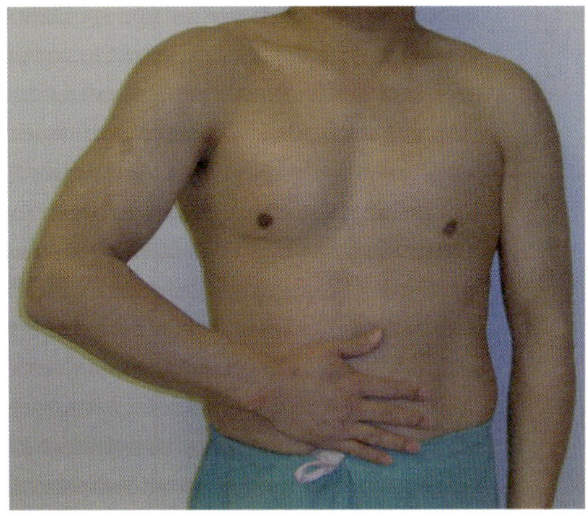

Fig. 5.19 Clinical photograph of the "belly press" test. A positive test is when the wrist flexes with the arm in this position as the patient pushes against the abdomen

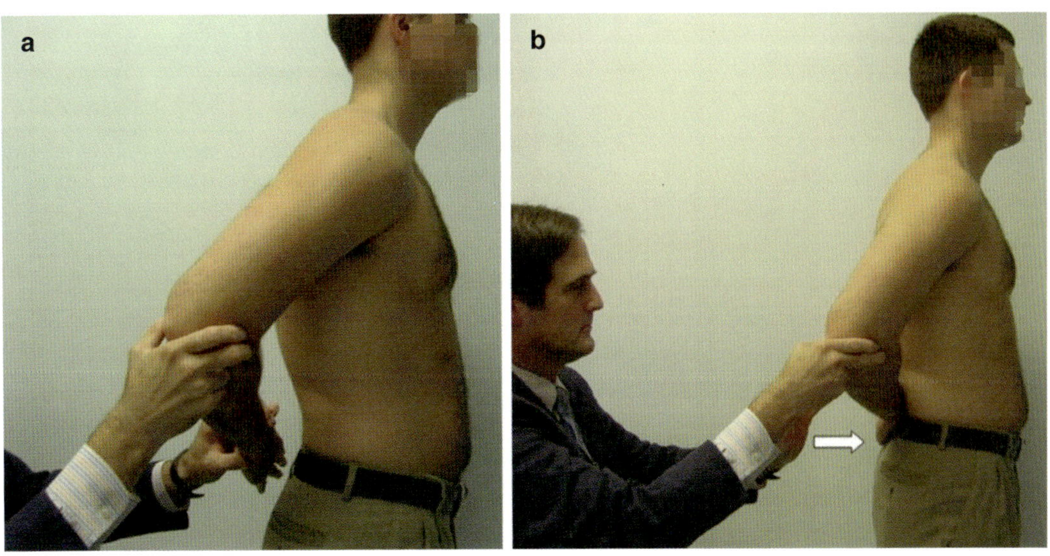

Fig. 5.18 Clinical photographs of the subscapularis lag sign. The arm is lifted off the lower back, and the patient is asked to hold it in that position (**a**). If the arm falls toward the back (**b**), then this is a positive test

tears) was because the tendons rubbed against or "impinged" on the acromion or coracoacromial ligament (called "outlet impingement"), the superior glenoid (called "internal impingement"), or the coracoid (called "coracoid impingement") [19].

Although impingement of the tendons on other structures has been the prevailing theory for the past 50 years, new evidence suggests that rotator cuff tendons wear and eventually tear secondary to senescence alone. Therefore, it has been suggested that the gradual wear and tearing of rotator cuff tendons be called "rotator cuff disease" and not "impingement" [19, 20].

Impingement signs. Two impingement signs have been described for the physical examination for rotator cuff disease. The classic impingement sign, described by Neer in 1972 [21], consists of forward-elevating the arm in flexion (Fig. 5.20) while stabilizing the scapula. A positive test is when the patient reports pain radiating into the deltoid region with this maneuver. Although this test can be helpful when making the diagnosis of rotator cuff abnormality, it also can be positive for almost any shoulder condition, including shoulder stiffness (frozen shoulder), glenohumeral arthritis, acromioclavicular (AC) arthritis, and labral lesions [22, 23]. Therefore, a positive Neer sign when used alone is not specific for any one disease entity, and it must be interpreted with caution.

The second impingement sign for rotator cuff disease is the Kennedy-Hawkins sign [24, 25]. This test is performed by the examiner flexing the patient's shoulder in front of the body to approximately 90° and then internally rotating the shoulder (Fig. 5.21). A test is considered positive if the patient reports pain in the deltoid area or pain that radiates down the arm. Like the Neer impingement sign, this test is not specific for any one shoulder condition. In addition, this test can be especially painful in patients with a stiff or arthritic shoulder, so in those patients it must be performed with caution. Although the Kennedy-

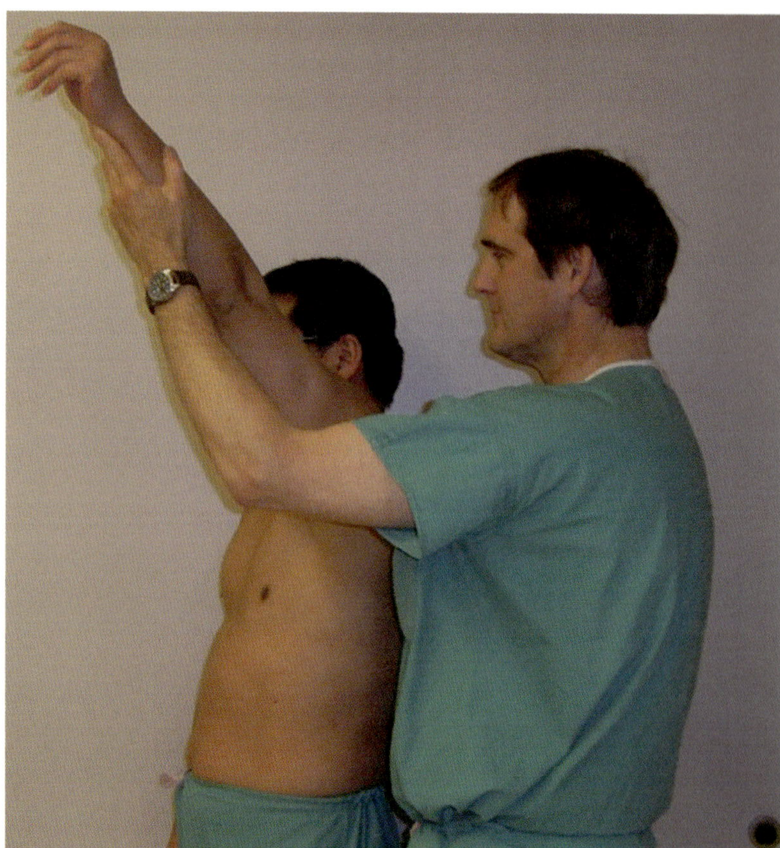

Fig. 5.20 Clinical photograph of the Neer impingement sign test. A positive test is pain in the deltoid region with elevation of the arm

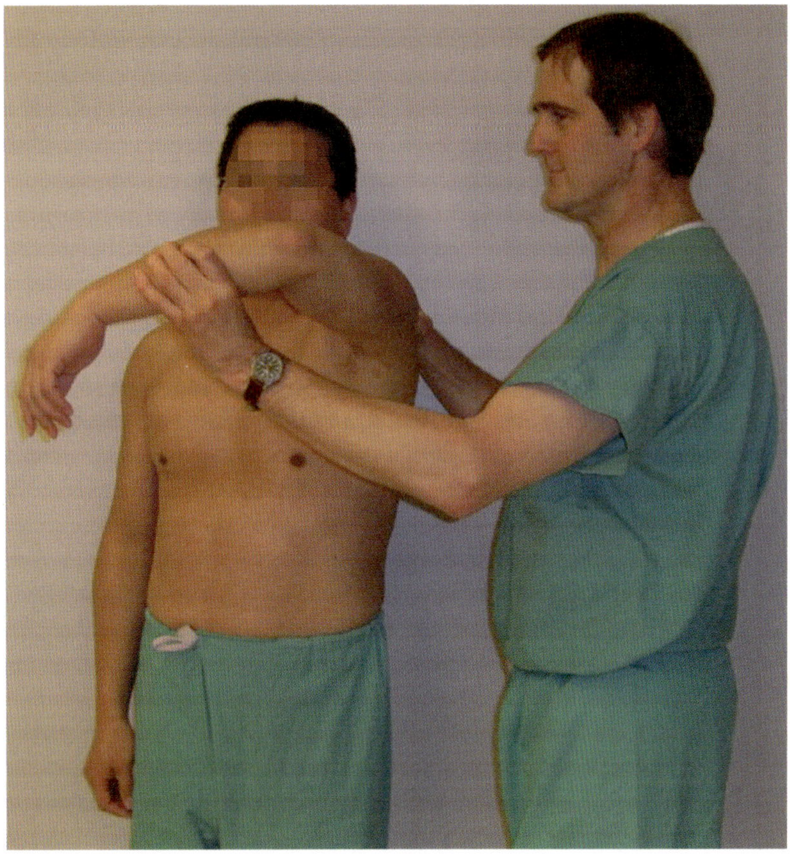

Fig. 5.21 Clinical photograph of the Kennedy-Hawkins impingement sign test. A positive test is pain into the deltoid region with the arm in flexion and internal rotation

Hawkins sign has been shown to be more sensitive than the Neer test for rotator cuff abnormality of any type, Park et al. [23] found that the Neer sign was only nearly equal in sensitivity and specificity to the Kennedy-Hawkins sign. Therefore, this sign should be considered in the context of the entire shoulder examination.

Painful arc sign. The last sign considered important in making the diagnosis of symptomatic rotator cuff disease is the "painful arc" [23, 26]. This test is performed by having the patient fully elevate both arms. In some patients with symptomatic rotator cuff tears, the patient will report pain when the arms are between approximately 70° and 120° of elevation [27]. Although this test is most commonly positive when the rotator cuff is inflamed or torn, it can be positive in patients with arthritis, a stiff or frozen shoulder, or other conditions.

Putting it all together. The evaluation of the patient with a painful shoulder takes a thorough approach and attention to the basic details of the axioms mentioned above. Inspection is necessary to determine if there is atrophy of the muscles, and a neurologic evaluation is necessary to rule out more proximal causes of the dysfunction. Range-of-motion testing will indicate if the patient is stiff but it will not define the cause of the stiffness. Strength testing not only indicates which muscles and tendons work but it reveals possible tendon tears or underlying neural causes of the condition.

Using these tests in combination increases the chance that a diagnosis can be made accurately. For example, if a patient is >60 years old, has weakness in abduction, and has a positive impingement sign (Neer or Kennedy-Hawkins sign), there is a >98% chance that he or she has a rotator cuff tear [28]. One study found that patients with a positive drop-arm sign, weakness in external rotation, and a painful arc had a 91% chance of having a rotator cuff tear [23]. However, it should be remembered that weakness is a neurologic symptom first and an orthopaedic symptom second; in other words, it cannot be assumed that the weakness is the result of rotator cuff abnormality without confirmation via conventional radiography, arthrography, ultrasonography, or magnetic resonance imaging.

Acromioclavicular Joint Abnormalities

The first diagnostic test for an AC joint abnormality is visually to assess the AC joint and compare it with the contralateral joint. The second diagnostic test is palpation directly on the joint itself. Although the AC joint is arthritic by MRI criteria in >90% of people who are >30 years old [29], these changes are not important unless the patient can localize the pain to the AC joint. We frequently ask patients to perform what we call the "one-finger test," asking them to point only one finger at the spot that hurts (Fig. 5.22). Patients with AC arthritis typically point directly at the AC joint, whereas patients with rotator cuff abnormality point to the deltoid area or front of the shoulder (Fig. 5.23).

Other tests described for the AC joint include the cross-arm adduction stress test, the arm extension test, and the active compression test (all described elsewhere) [30, 31]. These secondary tests can help confirm the diagnosis in symptomatic AC joint conditions. When multiple tests are positive, these tests have increased clinical utility (Table 5.2). When there is a question about the

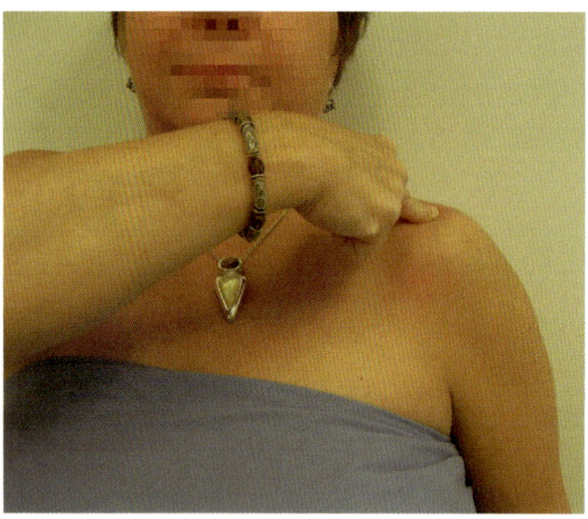

Fig. 5.22 Clinical photograph of the one-finger test, in which the patient places one finger on the spot in the shoulder that hurts the most

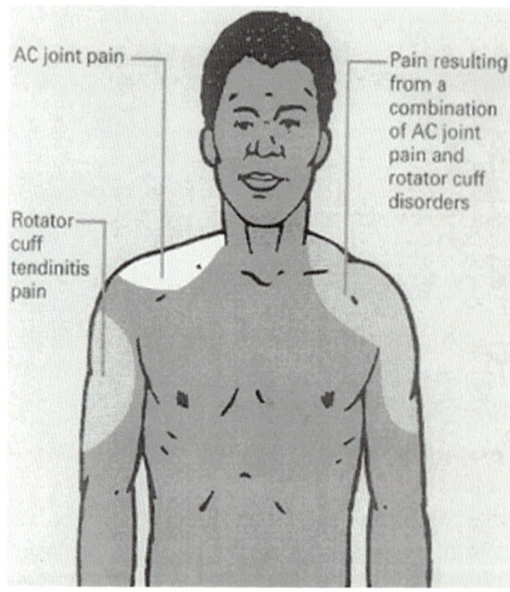

Fig. 5.23 Artist's sketch of pain in the shoulder joint area, in the acromioclavicular joint area, and in a combination of both areas (Reprinted with permission from McFarland EG. General principles of shoulder examination. In: Examination of the Shoulder: The Complete Guide. New York: Thieme, 2006:1–14)

Table 5.2 Clinical usefulness of three physical examination tests[a] for acromioclavicular joint abnormality

	Sensitivity		Specificity		PPV		NPV		Overall Accuracy	
Positive results	%	No.	%	No.	%	No.	%	No.	%	No.
In all 3 tests	25	4 of 16	97	290 of 299	31	4 of 13	96	290 of 302	93	294 of 315
In any 2 tests	81	13 of 16	89	266 of 299	28	13 of 46	99	266 of 269	89	279 of 315
In 1 test	100	16 of 16	74	221 of 299	17	16 of 94	100	221 of 221	75	237 of 315

PPV positive predictive value, *NPV* negative predictive value

Originally published in Chronopoulos E, Kim TK, Park HB, Ashenbrenner D, McFarland EG. Diagnostic value of physical tests for isolated chronic acromioclavicular lesions. *Am J Sports Med.* 2004;32:655–661

[a]The 3 tests analyzed were the cross-body adduction stress test, the acromioclavicular-resisted extension test, and the active compression test

diagnosis, an injection of local anesthetic into the AC joint is considered diagnostic.

Shoulder Instability

Shoulder instability, which is abnormal movement of the humeral head on the glenoid, can be classified by magnitude and direction. In terms of magnitude, a subluxation is defined as the humeral head moving too far on the glenoid but reducing spontaneously, and a dislocation is defined as the humeral head locking outside the confines of the glenoid. A subluxation typically is characterized by pain and limited motion for a few days or weeks. A dislocation presents with acute pain and loss of motion secondary to the humeral head being out of the socket. Patients with dislocations may have nerve or artery damage, rotator cuff tears, or fractures, so a complete neurologic evaluation as described above is also necessary in these patients. After the shoulder is reduced, the patient may have pain and loss of range of motion for several weeks, but a careful neurovascular examination can still be accomplished.

Shoulder instability can also be classified by direction. Anterior instability is defined as the humeral head coming anterior to the glenoid, and posterior instability is defined as the reverse. True inferior instability is quite rare, although increased inferior laxity (as shown by a high-grade sulcus sign) is common, especially in adolescent athletes.

Anterior instability. The arm position that produces anterior glenohumeral or shoulder instability is abduction over the shoulder level and external rotation. It can sometimes be caused by an anterior pull on the arm (as by a ski rope) or a blow to the back of the shoulder.

The classic test for anterior instability is the anterior apprehension test [32], which is performed by the clinician carefully abducting and externally rotating the patient's arm until he or she feels apprehensive that the shoulder might subluxate or dislocate (Fig. 5.24). This test is highly sensitive and accurate if the patient feels a sense of impending subluxation and is apprehensive. Some clinicians have suggested that pain alone with this test might indicate anterior shoulder instability [32–34]. However, several studies

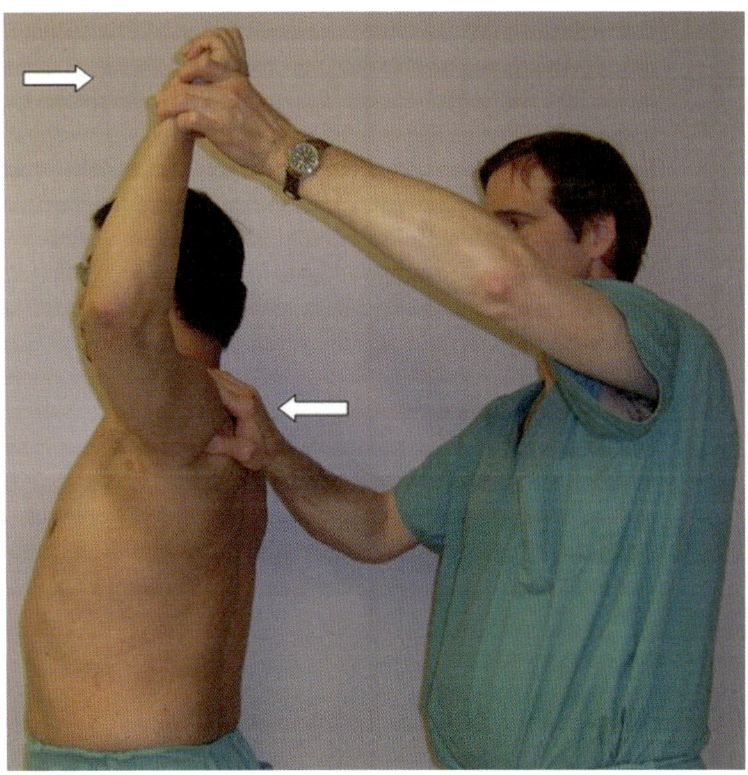

Fig. 5.24 Clinical photograph of the anterior apprehension sign test. The test is positive if the patient expresses concern that the shoulder may subluxate or dislocate with the arm in abduction and external rotation

have shown that if pain is used as the criterion for a positive test, the anterior apprehension test is neither sensitive nor accurate [35, 36].

Posterior instability. Posterior instability of the shoulder is much less common than anterior glenohumeral instability. The most common mechanism for posterior instability is an axial load along the arm when it is flexed in front of the body. It is seen in patients who fall on the arm in front of them with the elbow flexed. If the patient sustains a subluxation, there may be pain and no deformity. If the shoulder is dislocated posteriorly, the patient's arm will be locked in a flexed and internally rotated position. Nearly any motion of the shoulder will be painful until the shoulder is reduced.

The classic test for posterior instability has been called the "posterior apprehension sign" [37]. In this examination, the arm is forward-flexed and internally rotated while the clinician applies a posterior force to the shoulder (Fig. 5.25). This maneuver should make the patient apprehensive that the shoulder might dislocate. Unfortunately, this test is not very accurate and is not positive in most patients [38]. Several other tests for posterior shoulder instability have been described, but those tests are difficult to perform and their accuracy is in question. One test that might be useful is a posterior drawer sign, in which the examiner subluxes the patient's shoulder posteriorly with the patient in the supine position. If the patient states that the subluxation reproduces not only the symptoms of instability but also the direction of the instability, then it can be diagnostic for posterior instability [39].

Inferior instability. As indicated above, true inferior instability is rare, although increased inferior laxity is common in young, athletic individuals, especially swimmers, gymnasts, and baseball pitchers. Inferior laxity is measured via a sulcus sign, which is the gap produced when the arm is pulled inferiorly by the examiner (Fig. 5.26). This test is graded from I to III on the basis of the distance of the gap between the humeral head and the acromion:

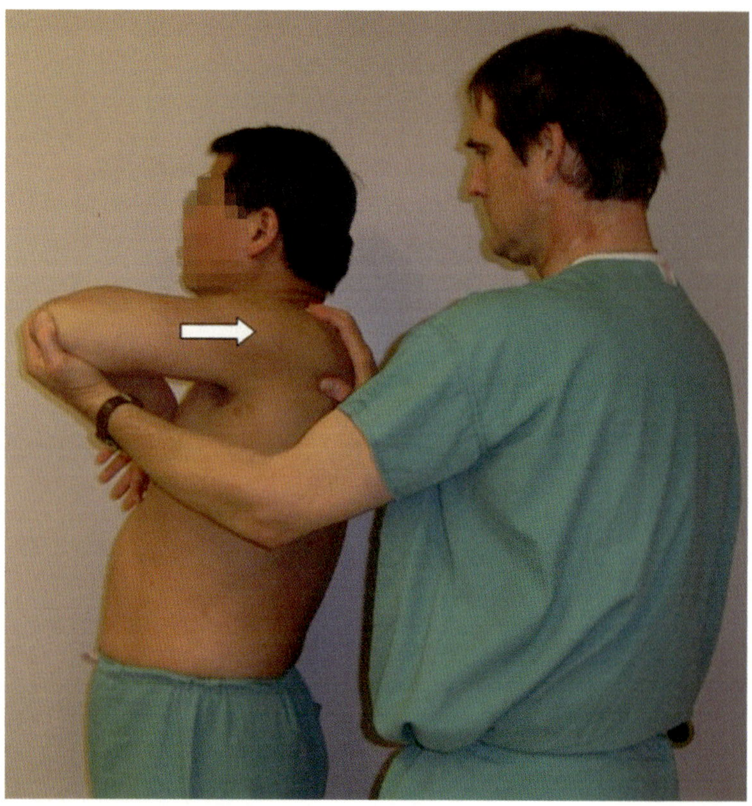

Fig. 5.25 Clinical photograph of the posterior apprehension sign test. A test is positive if the patient feels the shoulder may subluxate or dislocate with a posteriorly directed force with the arm in flexion and internal rotation

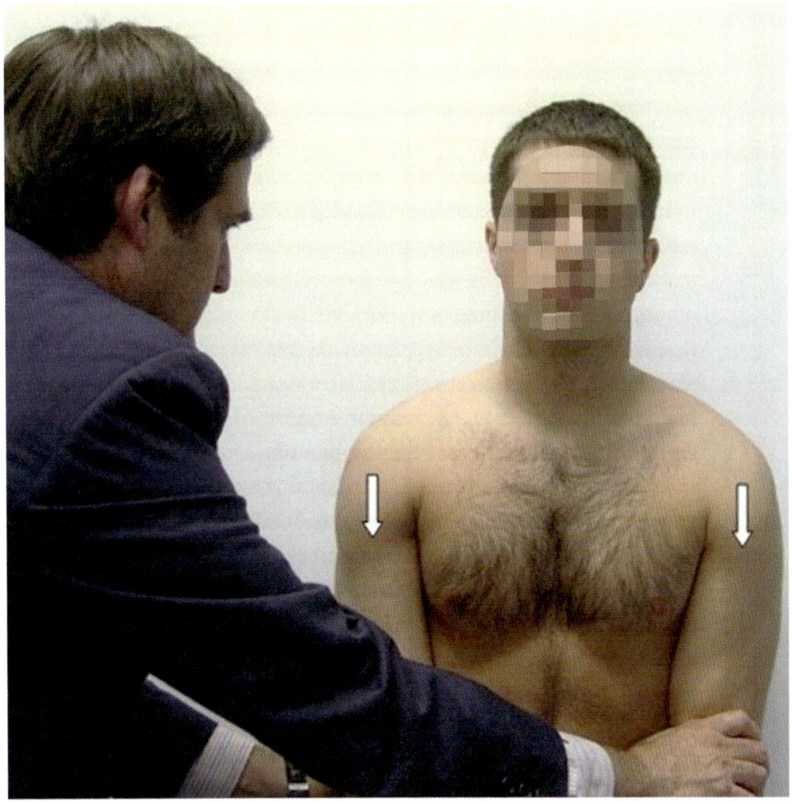

Fig. 5.26 Clinical photograph of the sulcus sign test. This test is a measure of shoulder laxity

grade I, 0.5–1.0 cm; grade II, 1.0–2.0 cm; and grade III, >2 cm [40]. This test has been used inappropriately to make the diagnosis of inferior instability, and it reflects the looseness of the shoulder joint. Unless the patient states during sulcus testing that it reproduces a sense of instability, it reflects only general ligamentous laxity and should not be interpreted to mean the shoulder is unstable inferiorly [41].

Labral Lesions

Tears of the glenoid labrum are difficult to diagnose on physical examination. Although many tests have been described, the most accurate way to make the diagnosis is with arthroscopy of the shoulder [42]. Even when multiple tests are used during the physical examination, the accuracy of those tests does not increase [43]. It has been suggested that a painful click in the shoulder might represent a labrum tear [31, 44], but one study [45] found that the incidence of a click in patients with a superior labrum lesion was the same as that in patients with no labrum tears. Patients who are suspected of having a labrum tear should undergo magnetic resonance arthrography, and consultation with an orthopedic surgeon should be considered.

Biceps Tendon Pain

Many clinicians have observed that the biceps tendon is a source of pain in some patients in whom the tendon eventually ruptures and the pain dissipates. Typically, the pain in such patients radiates down the front of the shoulder into the biceps tendon. Unfortunately, the tests described for eliciting biceps tendon pain are difficult to study because it is rare for the biceps tendon to be inflamed, partially torn, or even unstable without the presence of coexisting rotator cuff disease [46]. Therefore, when a test for the biceps tendon is performed during the physical examination, it is possible that the pain comes from the rotator cuff tear, the biceps tendon, or both.

Similarly, palpation of the biceps tendon is difficult because the tendon is difficult to isolate, especially in larger patients. The best technique for palpating the biceps tendon is for the clinician to rotate the patient's arm externally approximately 20–30°, then flex and extend the elbow while trying to feel the tendon move under the finger, which should be approximately 4–5 cm below the anterior acromion (Fig. 5.27). One study suggested that palpation of the biceps tendon is neither sensitive nor specific for biceps tendon abnormalities, and that pain in the region of the biceps in the anterior shoulder cannot be presumed to be secondary to biceps tendon abnormality alone [46].

Other physical examination tests for the biceps tendon are also not very helpful in making the diagnosis. In our experience, the Yergason test, which is pain in the biceps area with resisted forearm supination, is rarely positive. Parentis et al. [47] found this test to be unhelpful in the diagnosis of biceps tendon pathologies.

Another examination test is the Speed test [48, 49]. This test is performed by having the patient forward-flex the arm to 90° and hold it in a slightly horizontal extended position (Fig. 5.28). The examiner applies a force toward the floor as the patient resists that motion, and a positive test is pain into the biceps area in the anterior shoulder. Despite its widespread use and acceptance, studies have been unable to substantiate its clinical usefulness. One study found that it was neither sensitive nor specific for biceps tendon pathology [46].

Thoracic Outlet Syndrome

One of the more difficult conditions to diagnose accurately is thoracic outlet syndrome (TOS), which is caused by compression of the nerves of the brachial plexus or the vascular bundle in the arm between the first rib, the middle scalene muscle, and the clavicle (see Chap. 8 for details).

Three forms of TOS have been postulated, representing a spectrum of disorders: vascular, neurogenic, and "disputed" or "common" [50]. The vascular form is characterized by compression of the major blood vessels (subclavian artery or vein) as they course beneath the clavicle. In the neurogenic form, the brachial plexus is com-

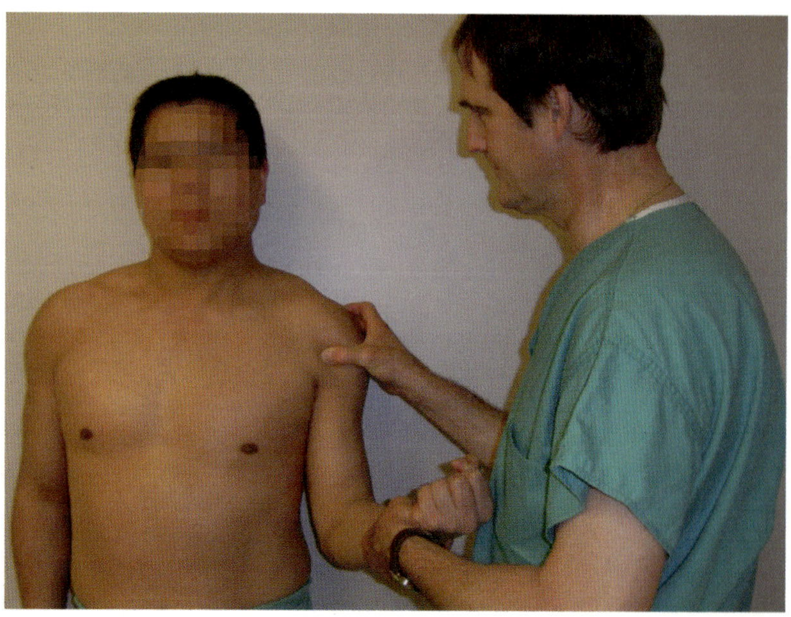

Fig. 5.27 Palpation of the biceps tendon is performed by externally rotating the arm and flexing and extending the elbow

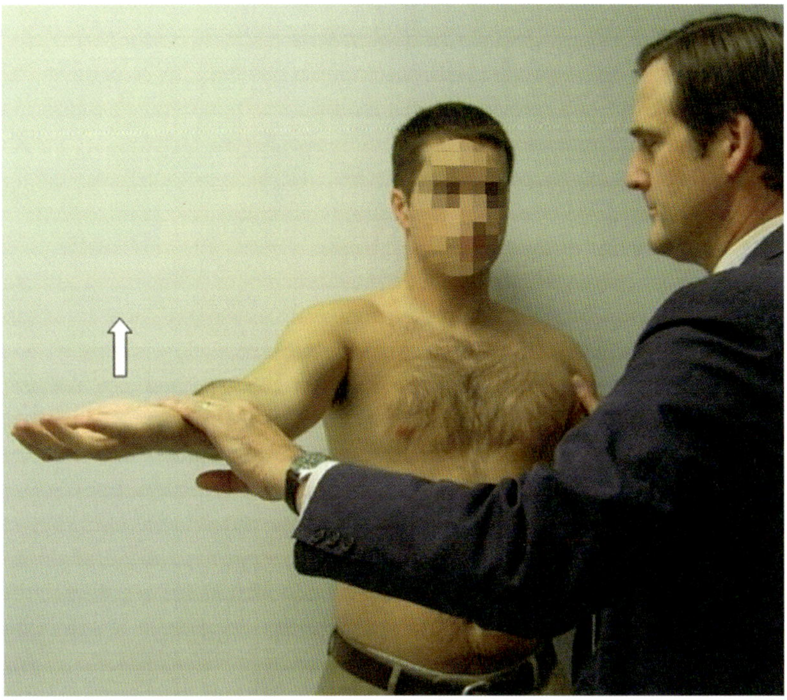

Fig. 5.28 The Speed test is performed by resisting elevation of the arm in this position. A positive test is when the patient reports pain in the anterior shoulder. This test is not accurate for biceps tendon pathology

pressed beneath the scalene muscles or in the costoclavicular space. In the disputed or common form, there is no physical evidence of nerve compression but the patient has pain suggestive of compression of the brachial plexus [50, 51]. As in patients with multiple lesions in the glenohumeral joint, patients with TOS may have one or more forms of the syndrome, and they may concomitantly have other peripheral nerve compressions (such as carpal tunnel syndrome and cubital tunnel syndrome) that can obfuscate the diagnosis [52].

TOS is difficult to diagnose accurately, primarily because the disputed form has no one specific history or physical examination finding that confirms the diagnosis. The vascular form is characterized by symptoms one would expect from intermittent vascular occlusion: color or temperature changes in the extremity, swelling, and paresthesias from nerve ischemia. The neurogenic form is characterized by pain, atrophy, weakness, and paresthesias. The common type is characterized by pain and weakness but it typically does not involve atrophy or vascular changes. The physical findings in TOS can be nonspecific, and as a result it has often been said to be a diagnosis of exclusion [50, 53].

The dilemma for the clinician diagnosing a patient with possible TOS is that there is no one accepted standard that can verify the diagnosis, no one physical examination for TOS that has independent validity, and no radiologic or serologic test that can confirm the diagnosis. Several studies have found that no single ancillary diagnostic tool such as angiography or electromyography can predict the disease or the results of treatment [53–55]. With the caveat that additional study is required to determine the clinical usefulness of these tests during physical examination for TOS, we review below some of the tests described for making the diagnosis.

The Adson test [56], as described in 1947, is an example of the difficulties with the examination for TOS. This test is performed by having the patient elevate the chin and turn it to the affected side while the clinician palpates the pulse (Fig. 5.29). If the person has diminution or loss of the radial pulse with this maneuver, then the patient most likely has TOS. A variation of this test was described by Rayan and Jensen [57], in

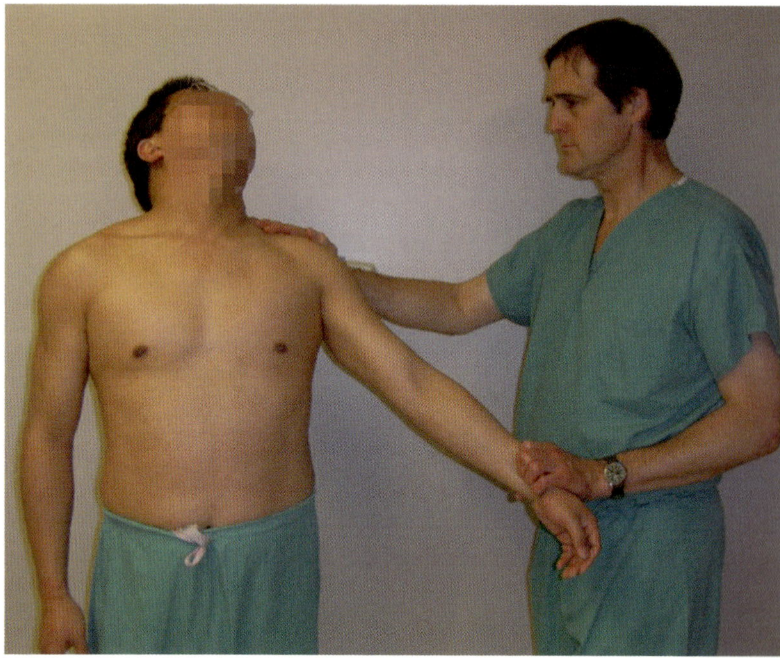

Fig. 5.29 Clinical photograph of the Adson test for thoracic outlet syndrome. A positive test is reproduction of symptoms of pain, paresthesias, or vascular changes in the extremity

which the patient is asked to rotate the head toward the examiner and inhale deeply.

Unfortunately, subsequent study has shown that loss of a pulse with this maneuver is physiological and normal [55]. In a plethysmographic study of the upper extremities of healthy volunteers, Gergoudis et al. [58] found that 53% of the symptom-free volunteers lost a pulse when performing the Adson test. Similarly, Rayan and Jensen [57] studied both extremities of asymptomatic individuals with the Adson test. They found that 13.5% of the extremities had a positive Adson test for loss of a pulse and that only 2% of the extremities experienced paresthesias with this maneuver.

The costoclavicular maneuver was first described by Falconer and Weddell [59] in 1943. With arms at the side, the patient is asked to bring the shoulders back, depress the shoulders, and stick out the chest in an exaggerated military position. The patient is asked to hold this position for at least 1 min. The test is considered positive test if there is diminution of the radial pulse or if the patient develops paresthesias. Rayan and Jensen [57] studied this test in healthy, asymptomatic volunteers and found that 48% had a positive vascular response and 10% had a positive neurologic response with paresthesias.

The hyperabduction test was first described by Wright [60] in 1945. His rationale for this test was the observation that people who sleep with their hands over their heads can produce symptoms of paresthesias or vascular compromise. In the hyperabduction test, the arm is elevated >90° with the elbows extended or flexed <45°. The patient is then asked to hold that position for 1 min. The test is considered positive if there is diminution or loss of the pulse or the presence of paresthesias. Rayan and Jensen [57] studied this test in healthy volunteers and found that a positive vascular response was seen in 57% of volunteers and that paresthesias were reported in 16.5%.

Other provocative tests include direct digital compression of the brachial plexus in the anterior cervical triangle, also known as the supraclavicular fossa, or inferior to the clavicle in the infraclavicular fossa (Fig. 5.30). These tests are collectively known as "compression tests." The rationale behind such tests is that they compress the brachial plexus similarly to a Phalen test for median nerve compression at the wrist. Roos [55] suggested that compression by the examiner's thumb for 30 s indicates that the brachial plexus may be the source

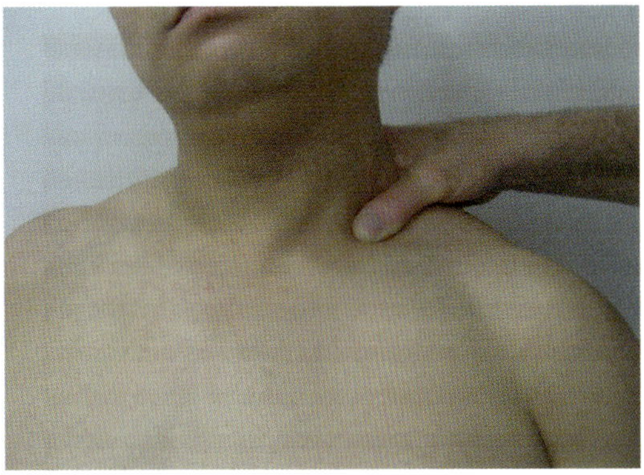

Fig. 5.30 Clinical photograph of the anterior cervical triangle palpation test. This test is analogous to the Phalen test at the wrist

of the patient's symptoms. Novak et al. [61] studied a cohort of patients with suspected TOS and found that, with a positive abduction test as described above and a reproduction of symptoms with downward pressure on the arms, all patients had pain, numbness, or paresthesias within 30 s.

Novak et al. [61] reported on the use of the Tinel maneuver at the supraclavicular or infraclavicular fossa to reproduce symptoms of TOS. They found that a positive Tinel maneuver in this area supports a diagnosis of TOS. Gillard et al. [53] studied 48 patients suspected of having TOS and found that a Tinel sign had a sensitivity of 46% and a specificity of 56% for the diagnosis of TOS.

Another test for TOS is the Roos test [55], in which the patient places both arms in 90° of abduction and external rotation, with the elbows bent. The patient then opens and closes the hands slowly for 3 min. A positive test is when the patient reports reproduction of the symptoms of pain and paresthesias (Fig. 5.31). Several investigators [52, 55, 62] have emphasized that TOS is a clinical diagnosis based on a consideration of the constellation of evidence, including the patient's symptoms and physical examination. Roos [55] suggested that a combination of pain with percussion of the supraclavicular or infraclavicular area, thumb compression of these two areas, weakness to manual muscle testing, hypesthesia to touch and pinprick, and a positive Roos test are the best findings for supporting the diagnosis. However, these observations were not studied statistically and therefore must be considered level-V evidence [63–65].

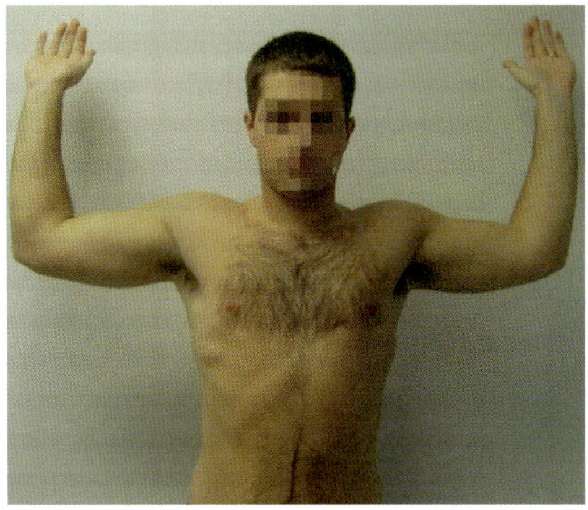

Fig. 5.31 Clinical photograph of the Roos test. A positive test is reproduction of symptoms of pain, paresthesias, or vascular changes in the extremity

Gillard et al. [53] conducted the only study that evaluated the physical examination tests for a cohort of patients who had symptoms of TOS (Table 5.3). They found that the highest sensitivity was for the Wright test when a positive test was considered the reproduction of symptoms. The most specific test was the hyperabduction test for abolition of the pulse (90%). If the patient had more than one positive test, then the specificity increased, but the sensitivity did not. There was no analysis of the relationship of these tests to successful medical or surgical treatment of the condition.

In summary, the diagnosis of TOS on the basis of physical examination alone is difficult, and the clinician must consider carefully all other conditions that might cause similar symptoms in the upper extremity. Studies of the physical examination are hampered by the lack of a standard by which to determine the diagnosis of TOS. Therefore, the physical examination for this condition can contribute toward making the diagnosis but often ancillary diagnostic techniques, such as magnetic resonance angiography or regular angiography, may be necessary. Additional study of the relationship of the physical findings to the diagnosis of TOS and to the results of treatment is warranted.

Table 5.3 Diagnostic usefulness of provocative tests for thoracic outlet syndrome based on final diagnosis

Provocative tests	No.	Sensitivity (%)	Specificity (%)	PPV (%)	NPV (%)
Adson[a]	46	79	76	85	72
Hyperabduction (pulse abolition)[a]	31	52	90	92	47
Hyperabduction (symptom reproduction)	46	84	40	74	55
Wright (pulse abolition)	47	70	53	72	50
Wright (symptom reproduction)	47	90	29	69	63
Roos	48	84	30	68	50
Tinel	42	46	56	63	39

NPP negative predictive value, *PPV* positive predictive value
Originally published in Gillard J, Perez-Cousin M, Hachulla E, Remy J, Hurtevent JF, Vinckier L, Thevenon A, Duquesnoy B. Diagnosing thoracic outlet syndrome: contribution of provocative tests, ultrasonography, electrophysiology, and helical computed tomography in 48 patients. Joint Bone Spine 2001;68:416–424 .
[a]Maneuver was significantly ($p < 0.05$) associated with the diagnosis

The basic principles of a musculoskeletal evaluation are
A. Expose both shoulders to assess the affected joint
B. Compare both sides
C. Evaluate a joint above and below
D. Obtain radiographs in both planes at 90° to each other
E. All of the above

Match sensory examination and area
A. C5
B. C6
C. C7
D. C8
E. T1

1. Deltoid area
2. Volar side of the middle finger
3. Medial elbow
4. Volar side of the little finger
5. Volar side of the thumb

What are the muscles that elevate the arm?
A. Deltoid
B. Infraspinatus
C. Subscapularis
D. Supraspinatus
E. All of the above
F. A & B
G. A & C

What are the tests for the subscapularis muscle?
A. Lift-off test
B. "Subscapularis lag sign"
C. "Belly press test"
D. Kennedy-Hawkins sign
E. All of the above
F. A & B & C
G. A & B & D

References

1. McFarland EG. General principles of shoulder examination. In: Kim TK, Park HB, El Rassi G, Gill H, Keyurapan E, editors. Examination of the shoulder: the complete guide. New York: Thieme; 2006. p. 1–14.
2. Malanga GA, Landes P, Nadler SF. Provocative tests in cervical spine examination: historical basis and scientific analyses. Pain Physician. 2003;6(2):199–205.
3. Uchihara T, Furukawa T, Tsukagoshi H. Compression of brachial plexus as a diagnostic test of cervical cord lesion. Spine. 1994;19(19):2170–3.
4. Viikari-Juntura E, Porras M, Laasonen EM. Validity of clinical tests in the diagnosis of root compression in cervical disc disease. Spine. 1989;14(3):253–7.
5. Challoner AVJ, Ramsay CA. A photoelectric plethysmograph for the measurement of cutaneous blood flow. Phys Med Biol. 1974;19(3):317–28.
6. Cooke ED, Steinberg MD, Pearson RM, Fleming CE, Toms SL, Elusade JA. Reflex sympathetic dystrophy and repetitive strain injury: temperature and microcirculatory changes following mild cold stress. J R Soc Med. 1993;86(12):690–3.
7. LeFlore JL, Engle WD. Capillary refill time is an unreliable indicator of cardiovascular status in term neonates. Adv Neonatal Care. 2005;5(3):147–54.

8. Lima AP, Beelen P, Bakker J. Use of a peripheral perfusion index derived from the pulse oximetry signal as a noninvasive indicator of perfusion. Crit Care Med. 2002;30(6):1210–3.
9. Hoppenfeld S. Physical examination of the shoulder. In: Hoppenfeld S, editor. Physical examination of the spine and extremities. Norwalk (CT): Appleton & Lange; 1976. p. 1–34.
10. Matsen III FA, Lippitt SB, Sidles JA, Harryman II DT. Shoulder motion. In: Practical evaluation and management of the shoulder. Philadelphia: W.B. Saunders; 1994. p. 19–58.
11. Colachis Jr SC, Strohm BR. Effect of suprascapular and axillary nerve blocks on muscle force in upper extremity. Arch Phys Med Rehabil. 1971;52(1):22–9.
12. Colachis Jr SC, Strohm BR, Brechner VL. Effects of axillary nerve block on muscle force in the upper extremity. Arch Phys Med Rehabil. 1969;50(11):647–54.
13. Kuhlman JR, Iannotti JP, Kelly MJ, Riegler FX, Gevaert ML, Ergin TM. Isokinetic and isometric measurement of strength of external rotation and abduction of the shoulder. J Bone Joint Surg Am. 1992;74(9):1320–33.
14. McFarland EG. Strength testing. In: Kim TK, Park HB, El Rassi G, Gill H, Keyurapan E, editors. Examination of the shoulder: the complete guide. New York: Thieme; 2006. p. 88–125.
15. Kelly BT, Kadrmas WR, Speer KP. The manual muscle examination for rotator cuff strength. An electromyographic investigation. Am J Sports Med. 1996; 24(5):581–8.
16. Malanga GA, Jenp YN, Growney ES, An KN. EMG analysis of shoulder positioning in testing and strengthening the supraspinatus. Med Sci Sports Exerc. 1996;28(6):661–4.
17. Hertel R, Ballmer FT, Lambert SM, Gerber C. Lag signs in the diagnosis of rotator cuff rupture. J Shoulder Elbow Surg. 1996;5(4):307–13.
18. Gerber C, Krushell RJ (1991) Isolated rupture of the tendon of the subscapularis muscle. Clinical features in 16 cases. J Bone Joint Surg Br 73(3):389-394
19. McFarland EG, Selhi HS, Keyurapan E. Clinical evaluation of impingement: what to do and what works. Instr Course Lect. 2006;55:3–16.
20. Uhthoff HK, Sano H. Pathology of failure of the rotator cuff tendon. Orthop Clin North Am. 1997;28(1):31–41.
21. Neer II CS. Anterior acromioplasty for the chronic impingement syndrome in the shoulder: a preliminary report. J Bone Joint Surg Am. 1972;54(1):41–50. doi:10.2106/JBJS.8706.cl.
22. Neer II CS. Impingement lesions. Clin Orthop. 1983; 173:70–7. doi:10.1097/00003086-198303000-00010.
23. Park HB, Yokota A, Gill HS, El Rassi G, McFarland EG. Diagnostic accuracy of clinical tests for the different degrees of subacromial impingement syndrome. J Bone Joint Surg Am. 2005;87(7):1446–55. doi:10.2106/JBJS.D.02335.
24. Hawkins RJ, Hobeika PE. Impingement syndrome in the athletic shoulder. Clin Sports Med. 1983;2(2): 391–405.
25. Hawkins RJ, Kennedy JC. Impingement syndrome in athletes. Am J Sports Med. 1980;8(3):151–7. discussion 157-158 doi:10.1177/036354658000800302.
26. Kessel L, Watson M. The painful arc syndrome. Clinical classification as a guide to management. J Bone Joint Surg Br. 1977;59(2):166–72.
27. Neer II CS, Welsh RP. The shoulder in sports. Orthop Clin North Am. 1977;8(3):583–91.
28. Murrell GAC, Walton JR. Diagnosis of rotator cuff tears. Lancet. 2001;357(9258):769–70.
29. Stein BES, Wiater JM, Pfaff HC, Bigliani LU, Levine WN. Detection of acromioclavicular joint pathology in asymptomatic shoulders with magnetic resonance imaging. J Shoulder Elbow Surg. 2001;10(3):204–8.
30. Chronopoulos E, Kim TK, Park HB, Ashenbrenner D, McFarland EG. Diagnostic value of physical tests for isolated chronic acromioclavicular lesions. Am J Sports Med. 2004;32(3):655–61. doi:10.1177/0363546503261723.
31. O'Brien SJ, Pagnani MJ, Fealy S, McGlynn SR, Wilson JB. The active compression test: a new and effective test for diagnosing labral tears and acromioclavicular joint abnormality. Am J Sports Med. 1998;26(5):610–3.
32. Rowe CR, Zarins B. Recurrent transient subluxation of the shoulder. J Bone Joint Surg Am. 1981;63(6):863–72. doi:10.1097/00003086-198710000-00003.
33. Jobe FW, Giangarra CE, Kvitne RS, Glousman RE. Anterior capsulolabral reconstruction of the shoulder in athletes in overhand sports. Am J Sports Med. 1991;19(5):428–34.
34. Jobe FW, Kvitne RS, Giangarra CE (1989) Shoulder pain in the overhand or throwing athlete. The relationship of anterior instability and rotator cuff impingement [published erratum appears in Orthop Rev 1989 Dec;18(12):1268]. Orthop Rev 18:963-975
35. Lo IKY, Nonweiler B, Woolfrey M, Litchfield R, Kirkley A. An evaluation of the apprehension, relocation, and surprise tests for anterior shoulder instability. Am J Sports Med. 2004;32(2):301–7.
36. Speer KP, Hannafin JA, Altchek DW, Warren RF. An evaluation of the shoulder relocation test. Am J Sports Med. 1994;22(2):177–83.
37. Kessel L. Posterior dislocation of the shoulder. In: Clinical disorders of the shoulder. New York: Churchill Livingstone; 1982. p. 150–65.
38. McFarland EG. Instability and laxity. In: Kim TK, Park HB, El Rassi G, Gill H, Keyurapan E, editors. Examination of the shoulder: the complete guide. New York: Thieme; 2006. p. 162–212.
39. Gerber C, Ganz R. Clinical assessment of instability of the shoulder With special reference to anterior and posterior drawer tests. J Bone Joint Surg Br. 1984; 66(4):551–6.
40. Silliman JF, Hawkins RJ (1993) Classification and physical diagnosis of instability of the shoulder. Clin Orthop 291:7-19
41. McFarland EG, Kim TK, Park HB, Neira CA, Gutierrez MI. The effect of variation in definition on the diagnosis of multidirectional instability of the shoulder. J Bone Joint Surg Am. 2003;85(11): 2138–44.

42. Andrews JR, Carson Jr WG, McLeod WD. Glenoid labrum tears related to the long head of the biceps. Am J Sports Med. 1985;13(5):337–41. doi:10.1177/036354658501300508.
43. Kim TK, Queale WS, Cosgarea AJ, McFarland EG. Clinical features of the different types of SLAP lesions. An analysis of one hundred and thirty-nine cases. J Bone Joint Surg Am. 2003;85(1):66–71.
44. Kibler WB. Specificity and sensitivity of the anterior slide test in throwing athletes with superior glenoid labral tears. Arthroscopy. 1995;11(3):296–300.
45. McFarland EG, Kim TK, Savino RM. Clinical assessment of three common tests for superior labral anterior-posterior lesions. Am J Sports Med. 2002; 30(6):810–5.
46. Gill HS, El Rassi G, Bahk MS, Castillo RC, McFarland EG. Physical examination for partial tears of the biceps tendon. Am J Sports Med. 2007;35(8):1334–40. doi:10.1177/0363546507300058.
47. Parentis MA, Mohr KJ, Elattrache NS. Disorders of the superior labrum: review and treatment guidelines. Clin Orthop. 2002;400:77–87.
48. Bennett WF. Specificity of the Speed's test: arthroscopic technique for evaluating the biceps tendon at the level of the bicipital groove. Arthroscopy. 1998;14(8):789–96.
49. Crenshaw AH, Kilgore WE. Surgical treatment of bicipital tenosynovitis. J Bone Joint Surg Am. 1966;48(8):1496–502.
50. Huang JH, Zager EL. Thoracic outlet syndrome. Neurosurgery. 2004;55(4):897–902.
51. Landry GJ, Moneta GL, Taylor LM, Jr., Edwards JM, Porter JM (2001) Long-term functional outcome of neurogenic thoracic outlet syndrome in surgically and conservatively treated patients. J Vasc Surg. 33(2): 312–7; disc 317–9
52. Brantigan CO, Roos DB. Diagnosing thoracic outlet syndrome. Hand Clin. 2004;20(1):27–36.
53. Gillard J, Perez-Cousin M, Hachulla E, Remy J, Hurtevent JF, Vinckier L, Thevenon A, Duquesnoy B (2001) Diagnosing thoracic outlet syndrome: contribution of provocative tests, ultrasonography, electrophysiology, and helical computed tomography in 48 patients. Joint Bone Spine. 68(5):416–4.
54. Passero S, Paradiso C, Giannini F, Cioni R, Burgalassi L, Battistini N. Diagnosis of thoracic outlet syndrome. Relative value of electrophysiological studies. Acta Neurol Scand. 1994;90(3):179–85.
55. Roos DB (1976) Congenital anomalies associated with thoracic outlet syndrome. Anatomy, symptoms, diagnosis, and treatment. Am J Surg 132(6):771–8.
56. Adson AW. Surgical treatment for symptoms produced by cervical ribs and the scalenus anticus muscle. Surg Gynecol Obstet. 1947;85(6):687–700.
57. Rayan GM, Jensen C (1995) Thoracic outlet syndrome: provocative examination maneuvers in a typical population. J Shoulder Elbow Surg. 4(2):113–7.
58. Gergoudis R, Barnes RW. Thoracic outlet arterial compression: prevalence in normal persons. Angiology. 1980;31(8):538–41.
59. Falconer MA, Weddell G. Costoclavicular compression of the subclavian artery and vein. Lancet. 1943;242(6270):539–44.
60. Wright IS (1945) The neurovascular syndrome produced by hyperabduction of the arms. The immediate changes produced in 150 normal controls, and the effects on some persons of prolonged hyperabduction of the arms, as in sleeping, and in certain occupations. Am Heart J 29(1):1–19.
61. Novak CB, MacKinnon SE, Patterson GA. Evaluation of patients with thoracic outlet syndrome. J Hand Surg. 1993;18A(2):292–9.
62. Leffert RD, Perlmutter GS. Thoracic outlet syndrome. Results of 282 transaxillary first rib resections. Clin Orthop. 1999;368:66–79.
63. Sackett DL (1997) Evidence-based medicine and treatment choices. Lancet 349 9051:570
64. Sackett DL. Evidence-based medicine. Spine. 1998; 23(10):1085–6.
65. Wright JG, Swiontkowski MF, Heckman JD. Introducing levels of evidence to the journal. J Bone Joint Surg Am. 2003;85(1):1–3.

6 Assessing Outcomes

Jacob Joseph and Edward G. McFarland

Introduction

The first shoulder surgeon to advocate for following patients who have had shoulder surgery was Ernest Amory Codman [1]. His belief in the need for analyzing clinical results was a clarion call for the health profession that has only recently gained acceptance. There is increasing emphasis on reporting patient outcomes after shoulder surgery for clinical, economic, and political reasons. Since the 1990s, governing bodies for surgeons have prioritized the ability to objectively and independently produce evidence of treatment efficacy and patient satisfaction [2].

Unfortunately, the science of measuring patient satisfaction and outcomes has not progressed rapidly. There are many outcome measures for the whole body, the upper extremity, and the shoulder specifically, but many of them have not been validated, are impractical to use, do not have established minimally important differences, lack statistical rigor, and are used inappropriately [2, 3]. For example, although satisfaction with surgery has been typically measured with a Likert scale (with categories of very unsatisfied, unsatisfied, neutral, satisfied, and very satisfied), the scale is not parametric and has not been validated for many shoulder disorders. An analog scale for patient satisfaction after treatment has not been validated for any shoulder disorder, yet both analog scales and the Likert scale are reported widely across shoulder studies.

There is a practical side to reporting patient outcomes, which may serve to increase our knowledge and allow comparison of treatments [4]. This chapter reviews the various issues regarding outcome measures, which determine their validity and usefulness. The strengths and limitations of each shoulder outcome measure will be explained, and this chapter should serve as a guide for practitioners and scientists alike.

Patient-Reported Outcome Measures

Patient-reported outcomes are defined as the assessment of any aspect of a patient's health state reported directly by the patient. By definition, patient-reported outcomes are subjective information, which is used to create standards for these indirect measures [3]. This subjective information may be augmented with objective data such as quantification of range of motion and strength. Patient-reported health-related quality of life (HRQoL) is now viewed as a primary outcome of surgical treatment. Patient-reported

J. Joseph, B.A. • E.G. McFarland, M.D. (✉)
Division of Shoulder Surgery,
The Department of Orthopaedic Surgery,
The Johns Hopkins University,
10753 Falls Road, Suite 215, Lutherville,
MD 21093, USA
e-mail: editorialservices@jhmi.edu

G. Huri, N.K. Paschos (eds.), *The Shoulder*, Orthopaedic Study Guide Series,
DOI 10.1007/978-3-319-51979-1_6

outcomes and HRQoL measures are often combined into questionnaires as patient-reported outcome measures (PROMs). PROMs have been used widely in research studies and clinical trials. PROMs are also useful in clinical care for screening, monitoring care, and promoting patient-centered care [5]. PROMs have been used in orthopaedic surgery for many years and for various joints and conditions. PROMs have been designed with different levels of specificity by domain or system (e.g., general health, extremity, or joint) and disease condition (Table 6.1).

This chapter discusses the primary general health PROMs used in research and screening, along with upper extremity–specific, shoulder-specific, and disease-specific PROMs. General health PROMs capture the overall health of the individual and encompass physical, mental, and social health. These PROMs also include domains relating to quality of life [6]. General health PROMs are sensitive to various health issues simultaneously and therefore are often unable to distinguish problems with high specificity.

Upper extremity PROMs typically encapsulate the whole arm from mid-clavicle to the fingers. They can capture information from multiple areas of the arm simultaneously, which may provide a good sense of how the extremity functions. However, these PROMs do this at the expense of more specific information about a single joint, which may be the joint of interest [7].

Shoulder-specific PROMs focus on the glenohumeral, acromioclavicular, sternoclavicular, and scapulothoracic joints. Upper extremity– and shoulder-specific PROMs often include domains related to pain, motion, function, and use of the arm for activities of daily living (ADLs). Specific information about the domains of each PROM are outlined below. The final group of PROMs are disease-specific measures. They are designed to assess a single state or condition and are the narrowest outcome measures. Disease-specific PROMs use questionnaires that gather information related to a specific diagnosis or treatment option. They assess pain, function, and ability to perform ADLs [7].

PROMs should have optimally established psychometric validity of their material. This means that a questionnaire asks the appropriate questions and an individual can answer the

Table 6.1 Validity and joint specificity of patient-reported outcome measures

Outcome measure	Validation[a]	Shoulder conditions
American Shoulder and Elbow Surgeons (ASES) score	Yes	General shoulder
Constant-Murley score	Yes	Rotator cuff repair, shoulder arthroplasty, adhesive capsulitis, proximal humeral fractures
Simple Shoulder Test	Yes	General shoulder
Disabilities of the Arm, Shoulder, and Hand (DASH) score	Yes	General upper extremity
Oxford Shoulder Score	Yes	General shoulder except instability
UCLA Shoulder Score	No	General shoulder
University of Pennsylvania Score	Yes	General shoulder
Rowe Score for Instability	Yes	Bankart repair
L'Insalata Shoulder Rating Questionnaire	Yes	General shoulder
Single Assessment Numeric Evaluation (SANE) score	No	General shoulder
Shoulder Pain and Disability Index	Yes	Shoulder pain
Western Ontario Osteoarthritis of the Shoulder (WOOS) Index	Yes	Osteoarthritis
Western Ontario Shoulder Instability (WOSI) Index	Yes	Instability
Western Ontario Rotator Cuff (WORC) Index	Yes	Rotator cuff tears
Rotator Cuff Quality-of-Life Score	Yes	Rotator cuff tears

[a]"Yes" indicates that a published study has established the construct validity, reliability, and responsiveness of the patient-reported outcome measure

questions appropriately [4]. This method is essential to establishing the accuracy and quality of a PROM's ability to capture information. The following three measures of validity are important to understand when considering the accurate use of any PROM: construct validity, test-retest reliability, and responsiveness. Construct validity is the ability of a PROM to effectively measure the concept it was designed to assess. For example, a shoulder-specific PROM should be able to capture information pertinent to the function of the shoulder such as pain, motion, and ease of use for ADLs. Such a measure would ask about when pain occurs and what activities can be performed with what level of comfort [8].

Test-retest reliability is the ability of the measure to produce the same results at similar time points. Test-retest reliability is gauged by having a subject complete a PROM and then repeat it 5–30 days later. Test-retest reliability is typically reported as a correlation of the two results [8].

Responsiveness is the PROM's ability to detect meaningful changes over time. This is measured by correlating the scores on the survey with clinical factors of interest to the researcher or clinician. For example, if a patient experiences more pain over time or a decrease in function and difficulty with ADLs, then a PROM should capture the changes over time, and it should create a sense of whether the changes are enough to create change in the patient's performance or expectations [8].

Some commonly used PROMs have not been psychometrically validated nor designed with a validation method. Many PROMs were developed and introduced before the medical community became aware of the standards of psychometric validation [6].

Although PROMs can be used to measure the effects of intervention, there are multiple concepts to consider when interpreting changes in scores over time. Although a patient's outcome score may change, it may not represent a true clinical change in state. Therefore, it is important to realize that changes in scores that are statistically significant may not be clinically important to the patient or provider. The concept of the minimally clinically important difference (MCID) is that the difference in score represents a meaningful clinical change in the patient's state. This value will vary from PROM to PROM. It also may vary for different diagnoses using the same PROM. For example, for a given PROM, a MCID for the results of the treatment of rotator cuff disease will be different than for the treatment of arthritis of the shoulder. Therefore, although the MCID might be published for a PROM, it is imperative to know what conditions that MCID represents. For some PROMs, the MCID has never been determined nor published, so the use of MCID should be interpreted with caution [9].

There are multiple methods for establishing MCIDs, and there is little consensus regarding the most appropriate method to be used in orthopedics. It is often difficult for studies to define MCID appropriately because of lack of consensus, which may be a reason few MCID values are defined [9].

Outcome measures may be limited by what is called a "floor" or "ceiling" effect. This is the limitation of the PROM to detect changes above or below a certain threshold. A floor or ceiling effect also can occur when the patient approaches the minimum or maximum score at baseline. Further changes cannot be measured as the score approaches the limit at the bottom or top of the scale. This is often an issue with young, healthy patients who may score highly on an outcome measure at baseline. This makes assessing the benefit of the intervention difficult because postoperative improvement cannot be captured [10].

Reviews of the literature have described 39 published PROMs of the shoulder or PROMs used in studies of interventions in shoulder conditions [11]. There is little consensus or consistency regarding the choice of PROM in studies [2, 11]. Often, PROMs are used that are inappropriate for a particular study design or patient population, potentially leading to invalid conclusions about treatment [2]. Various health states can be assessed by PROMs, ranging from general health, health of the upper extremity, health of the shoulder, and disease type. This chapter provides a synopsis of the most common PROMs currently used in shoulder research.

General Health Measures

36-Item Short-Form Health Survey (SF-36)

Developed by the RAND Corporation, the SF-36 is commonly used in shoulder research. The SF-36 has two main domains of measurement: (1) physical health and (2) emotional or mental health. The survey is scored on a 100-point scale with 0 being the worst result and 100 being the best result. The SF-36 has been extensively psychometrically validated for construct validity, reliability, and responsiveness [6, 12].

EQ-5D

The EQ-5D is a general health questionnaire developed by the EuroQol Group. It is administered as two parts: the EQ-5D descriptive system, and the EQ visual analog scale (VAS). It contains five questions regarding mobility, self-care, ADLs (work and leisure), pain, and mental health factors such as anxiety and depression. The VAS is a 100-mm grading scale that represents overall health on that day. The questionnaire can be scored as a representation of a health profile rather than a numeric sore. The profile is a representation of the patient's health state. The responses to the questionnaire can be represented as a code, with each question's numerical value combined, thus creating 243 possible combinations representing health status. This code can be combined with population-specific data from EuroQol to generate a normalized 100-point score [13].

Upper Extremity–Specific Outcome Measure

The Disabilities of the Arm, Shoulder, and Hand (DASH) score was developed by the American Academy of Orthopaedic Surgeons to measure single or multiple joints within the upper extremity [14]. It has three main domains: physical, symptoms, and social function of the arm. All questions on the DASH are in the form of a 5-point Likert scale. The DASH has high levels of construct validity, reliability, and responsiveness. The MCID of the DASH for shoulder-related issues is 12 points. The DASH also shows high consistency with other shoulder-related PROMs when used for studying shoulder treatments and conditions [4, 15–22].

Shoulder-Specific Outcome Measures

Constant-Murley Score

The Constant-Murley score was originally presented as a thesis project in 1987. The score was not validated at the time of its presentation [23–25]. Subsequent studies have been performed to validate its use after total shoulder arthroplasty, rotator cuff repair, adhesive capsulitis, and treatment of proximal humerus fractures [26–32]. It has not been validated for other shoulder conditions. The Constant-Murley score has been used to assess many shoulder-specific conditions for which it has not been strictly validated. However, it is currently the most reported outcome score for shoulder-related pathology in the literature [11]. The 100-point scale consists of three domains: pain, range of motion, and ADLs. The MCID of the score is version-dependent. The Constant-Murley score has been modified many times since its introduction [24, 25].

American Shoulder and Elbow Surgeons (ASES) Score

The ASES score was developed in 1994 by the American Shoulder and Elbow Surgeons [33]. It is one of the most common shoulder-related PROMs [11]. The questionnaire consists of a physician-determined domain and a self-assessment domain. The self-assessment portion comprises three domains: pain, instability, and ADLs. Pain and instability are rated on a 5-point ordinal scale. ADLs comprise ten questions and are rated on a 4-point ordinal scale. This score is converted to a 100-point scale [34–36]. The MCIDs are 12–17 points for rotator cuff pathology, 10 points for open or arthroscopic Bankart repair, and 6.4 points for instability.

University of California Los Angeles (UCLA) Shoulder Score

The UCLA Shoulder Score was first described in 1981. It was one of the first PROMs for the shoulder and, similarly to the Constant-Murley score, it was not validated at first introduction [37]. It was designed for use in shoulder arthroplasty and later used for other shoulder conditions. The UCLA Shoulder Score contains five domains: pain, function, forward flexion, forward flexion strength, and overall satisfaction. The maximum score is 35 points. Comparison studies with other shoulder PROMs have reported low consistency with the UCLA Shoulder Score [37].

Simple Shoulder Test (SST)

The SST is a questionnaire composed of 12 yes/no questions about pain and function of the shoulder. The questionnaire did not originally include a scoring method. A later study established a scoring method for the SST in which "yes" responses are 1 point and "no" responses are 0 points. The score is summed to a maximum of 12 points. The SST has shown to be valid, reliable, and responsive. It correlates moderately with other shoulder PROMs [15, 38].

Single Assessment Numeric Evaluation (SANE)

The SANE was designed as a simple, 1-question assessment tool. The score is the answer to the question, "How would you rate your shoulder today as a percentage of normal (0% to 100% scale, with 100% being normal)?" It has not undergone formal psychometric validation. One study showed that it correlated well with ASES and SST scores for Bankart repair surgery. It has gained popularity because of its ease of administration and data collection, but it needs further study to be used as a standalone PROM and may not be appropriate for use in all scenarios [39].

Oxford Shoulder Score

The Oxford Shoulder Score was developed at Oxford University in 1996. The questionnaire was designed to assess patient outcomes after surgery (with the exception of surgery for instability, for which a separate measure was developed) [40]. It consists of 12 questions graded on a 5-point ordinal scale. Each question is weighted differently so that the maximum score is 48 points. The questionnaire has moderate validity and high reliability. No MCID has been determined [15, 41].

Disease-Specific Outcome Measures

Western Ontario Osteoarthritis of the Shoulder (WOOS) Index

The WOOS Index was developed by the University of Western Ontario in 2001 as a primary PROM for clinical trials. This PROM is specific only to patients with symptomatic primary osteoarthritis of the shoulder. The WOOS Index is a 19-item questionnaire that includes four domains: sport, recreation, and work; pain; lifestyle function; and emotional function. Each item uses a 100-mm VAS. The VAS scores from each question are summed to a final score ranging from 0 to 1900 points, with a higher raw score equating with worse function. The score can also be presented as a percentage of the maximum score, with a higher score representing better function for simpler interpretation. The MCID has not been established [42].

Western Ontario Rotator Cuff (WORC) Index

The WORC Index was developed in 2003 as a PROM specific to primary rotator cuff tears. It assesses five domains: pain and physical symptoms, sports and recreation, work function, social function, and emotional function. It consists of 21 questions using a 100-mm VAS. The VAS scores from all questions are summed to produce a final score ranging from 0 to 2100, with a higher raw score representing worse function. The score can also be presented as a percentage of the maximum score, with a higher score representing better function for simpler interpretation [43]. The MCID for the questionnaire is 245 points (or 11.7% of the total score).

Western Ontario Shoulder Instability Index (WOSI)

The WOSI was developed in 1998 as a PROM specific to shoulder instability. The WOSI consists of five domains: physical symptoms, work, ADLs, emotions, and sport and recreation. It includes 21 questions using a 100-mm VAS. The VAS scores from all questions are summed to produce a final score ranging from 0 to 2100. The score can also be presented as a percentage of the maximum score, with a higher score representing better function for simpler interpretation [43]. The MCID is 225 points (or 11% of total score).

Rotator Cuff Quality-Of-Life Score

The Rotator Cuff Quality-of-Life score was developed in 2000 as a rotator cuff pathology–specific PROM [44]. It assesses five domains: symptoms and physical issues, sport and recreation, work, ADLs, and social and emotional issues. It is scored on a 100-point scale, with higher number representing better function. The MCID has not been defined [45].

Questions

What are the measures of validity for accurate use of any patient-reported outcome measures?

A. Construct validity
B. Test-retest reliability
C. Availability
D. Cost
E. Responsiveness
F. A & B & D
G. A & B & E
H. All the above

Disabilities of the Arm, Shoulder, and Hand (DASH) Score

A. Has two domains and the score for a completely normal patient is 0
B. Has three domains and the score for a completely normal patient is 0
C. Has two domains and the score for a completely normal patient is 100
D. Has three domains and the score for a completely normal patient is 100

What are the most commonly used scores in the orthopedic community for shoulder assessment?

A. DASH, ASES, UCLA Shoulder Score
B. DASH, SF-36, Oxford Shoulder Score
C. SANE, Oxford Shoulder Score, UCLA Shoulder Score
D. SST, ASES, Oxford Shoulder Score

References

1. Brand RA. Ernest Amory Codman, MD, 1869–1940. Clin Orthop. 2009;467(11):2763–5. doi:10.1007/s11999-009-1047-8.
2. Harvie P, Pollard TC, Chennagiri RJ, Carr AJ. The use of outcome scores in surgery of the shoulder. J Bone Joint Surg Br. 2005;87(2):151–4.
3. US Food and Drug Administration. Guidance for industry patient-reported outcome measures: use in medical product development to support labeling claims. 2016. http://google2.fda.gov/search?q=cache:iFPFRPkPORMJ:www.fda.gov/downloads/drugs/guidancecomplianceregulatoryinformation/guidances/ucm193282.pdf+Guidance+for+Industry+Patient-Reported+Outcome+Measures:+Use+in+Medical+Product+Development+to+Support+Labeling+Claims&client=FDAgov&site=FDAgov&lr=&proxystylesheet=FDAgov&output=xml:no_dtd&ie=UTF-8&access=p&oe=UTF-8. Accessed 11 Feb 2016.
4. Desai AS, Dramis A, Hearnden AJ. Critical appraisal of subjective outcome measures used in the assessment of shoulder disability. Ann R Coll Surg Engl. 2010;92(1):9–13. doi:10.1308/003588410x12518836440522.
5. Gonçalves Bradley DC, Gibbons C, Ricci-Cabello I, Bobrovitz NJH, Gibbons EJ, Kotzeva A, Alonso J, Fitzpatrick R, Bower P, van der Wees PJ, Rajmil L, Roberts NW, Taylor RS, Greenhalgh J, Porter I, Valderas JM. Routine provision of information on patient-reported outcome measures to healthcare providers and patients in clinical practice. Cochrane Database Syst Rev. 2015;4:CD011589. doi:10.1002/14651858.CD011589.
6. Kosinski M, Keller SD, Hatoum HT, Kong SX, Ware Jr JE. The SF-36 Health Survey as a generic outcome measure in clinical trials of patients with osteoarthritis and rheumatoid arthritis: tests of data quality, scaling assumptions and score reliability. Med Care. 1999;37(5 Suppl):MS10–22.
7. Wright RW, Baumgarten KM. Shoulder outcomes measures. J Am Acad Orthop Surg. 2010;18(7):436–44.
8. Davidson M, Keating J. Patient-reported outcome measures (PROMs): how should I interpret reports of measurement properties? A practical guide for clinicians and researchers who are not biostatisticians.

Br J Sports Med. 2014;48(9):792–6. doi:10.1136/bjsports-2012-091704.
9. Tashjian RZ, Deloach J, Green A, Porucznik CA, Powell AP. Minimal clinically important differences in ASES and simple shoulder test scores after non-operative treatment of rotator cuff disease. J Bone Joint Surg Am. 2010;92(2):296–303. doi:10.2106/jbjs.h.01296.
10. Bot SD, Terwee CB, van der Windt DA, Bouter LM, Dekker J, de Vet HC. Clinimetric evaluation of shoulder disability questionnaires: a systematic review of the literature. Ann Rheum Dis. 2004;63(4):335–41.
11. Gartsman GM, Morris BJ, Unger RZ, Laughlin MS, Elkousy HA, Edwards TB. Characteristics of clinical shoulder research over the last decade: a review of shoulder articles in the Journal of Bone & Joint Surgery from 2004 to 2014. J Bone Joint Surg Am. 2015;97(5):e26. doi:10.2106/jbjs.n.00831.
12. Ware Jr JE, Sherbourne CD. The MOS 36-item short-form health survey (SF-36). I. Conceptual framework and item selection. Med Care. 1992;30(6):473–81.
13. Brooks R. EuroQol: the current state of play. Health Policy. 1996;37(1):53–72.
14. Hudak PL, Amadio PC, Bombardier C. Development of an upper extremity outcome measure: the DASH (disabilities of the arm, shoulder and hand) [corrected]. The Upper Extremity Collaborative Group (UECG). Am J Ind Med. 1996;29(6):602–8. doi:10.1002/(sici)1097-0274(199606)29:6<602::aid-ajim4>3.0.co;2-l.
15. Angst F, Schwyzer HK, Aeschlimann A, Simmen BR, Goldhahn J. Measures of adult shoulder function: Disabilities of the Arm, Shoulder, and Hand Questionnaire (DASH) and its short version (QuickDASH), Shoulder Pain and Disability Index (SPADI), American Shoulder and Elbow Surgeons (ASES) Society standardized shoulder assessment form, Constant (Murley) Score (CS), Simple Shoulder Test (SST), Oxford Shoulder Score (OSS), Shoulder Disability Questionnaire (SDQ), and Western Ontario Shoulder Instability Index (WOSI). Arthritis Care Res. 2011;63(Suppl 11):S174–88. doi:10.1002/acr.20630.
16. Beaton DE, Katz JN, Fossel AH, Wright JG, Tarasuk V, Bombardier C. Measuring the whole or the parts? Validity, reliability, and responsiveness of the disabilities of the arm, shoulder and hand outcome measure in different regions of the upper extremity. J Hand Ther. 2001;14(2):128–46.
17. Hunsaker FG, Cioffi DA, Amadio PC, Wright JG, Caughlin B. The American academy of orthopaedic surgeons outcomes instruments: normative values from the general population. J Bone Joint Surg Am. 2002;84-A(2):208–15.
18. Jester A, Harth A, Germann G. Measuring levels of upper-extremity disability in employed adults using the DASH Questionnaire. J Hand Surg Am. 2005;30(5):1074 e1071–10. doi:10.1016/j.jhsa.2005.04.009.
19. MacDermid JC, Solomon P, Prkachin K. The shoulder pain and disability index demonstrates factor, construct and longitudinal validity. BMC Musculoskelet Disord. 2006;7:12. doi:10.1186/1471-2474-7-12.
20. McConnell S, Beaton DE, Bombardier C. The DASH outcome measure: a user's manual. Toronto, ON: Institute for Work and Health; 1999.
21. Schmitt JS, Di Fabio RP. Reliable change and minimum important difference (MID) proportions facilitated group responsiveness comparisons using individual threshold criteria. J Clin Epidemiol. 2004;57(10):1008–18. doi:10.1016/j.jclinepi.2004.02.007.
22. Veehof MM, Sleegers EJ, van Veldhoven NH, Schuurman AH, van Meeteren NL. Psychometric qualities of the Dutch language version of the Disabilities of the Arm, Shoulder, and Hand questionnaire (DASH-DLV). J Hand Ther. 2002;15(4):347–54.
23. Constant CR Age related recovery of shoulder function after injury. MCh Thesis, University College, Cork, 1986.
24. Constant CR, Gerber C, Emery RJ, Sojbjerg JO, Gohlke F, Boileau P. A review of the Constant score: modifications and guidelines for its use. J Shoulder Elb Surg. 2008;17(2):355–61. doi:10.1016/j.jse.2007.06.022.
25. Constant CR, Murley AHG. A clinical method of functional assessment of the shoulder. Clin Orthop. 1987;214:160–4.
26. Bankes MJ, Crossman JE, Emery RJ. A standard method of shoulder strength measurement for the Constant score with a spring balance. J Shoulder Elb Surg. 1998;7(2):116–21.
27. Brinker MR, Cuomo JS, Popham GJ, O'Connor DP, Barrack RL. An examination of bias in shoulder scoring instruments among healthy collegiate and recreational athletes. J Shoulder Elb Surg. 2002;11(5):463–9.
28. Conboy VB, Morris RW, Kiss J, Carr AJ. An evaluation of the Constant-Murley shoulder assessment. J Bone Joint Surg Br. 1996;78(2):229–32.
29. Fialka C, Oberleitner G, Stampfl P, Brannath W, Hexel M, Vecsei V. Modification of the Constant-Murley shoulder score-introduction of the individual relative Constant score Individual shoulder assessment. Injury. 2005;36(10):1159–65. doi:10.1016/j.injury.2004.12.023.
30. Katolik LI, Romeo AA, Cole BJ, Verma NN, Hayden JK, Bach BR. Normalization of the Constant score. J Shoulder Elb Surg. 2005;14(3):279–85. doi:10.1016/j.jse.2004.10.009.
31. Othman A, Taylor G. Is the constant score reliable in assessing patients with frozen shoulder? 60 shoulders scored 3 years after manipulation under anaesthesia. Acta Orthop Scand. 2004;75(1):114–6. doi:10.1080/00016470410001708230.
32. Walton MJ, Walton JC, Honorez LA, Harding VF, Wallace WA. A comparison of methods for shoulder strength assessment and analysis of Constant score change in patients aged over fifty years in the United Kingdom. J Shoulder Elb Surg. 2007;16(3):285–9. doi:10.1016/j.jse.2006.08.002.

33. Richards RR, An KN, Bigliani LU, Friedman RJ, Gartsman GM, Gristina AG, Iannotti JP, Mow VC, Sidles JA, Zuckerman JD. A standardized method for the assessment of shoulder function. J Shoulder Elb Surg. 1994;3(6):347–52. doi:10.1016/s1058-2746(09)80019-0.
34. Michener LA, Leggin BG. A review of self-report scales for the assessment of functional limitation and disability of the shoulder. J Hand Ther. 2001;14(2):68–76.
35. Michener LA, McClure PW, Sennett BJ. American shoulder and elbow surgeons standardized shoulder assessment form, patient self-report section: reliability, validity, and responsiveness. J Shoulder Elb Surg. 2002;11(6):587–94. doi:10.1067/mse.2002.127096.
36. Sallay PI, Reed L. The measurement of normative American Shoulder and Elbow Surgeons scores. J Shoulder Elb Surg. 2003;12(6):622–7. doi:10.1016/s105827460300209x.
37. Amstutz HC, Sew Hoy AL, Clarke IC. UCLA anatomic total shoulder arthroplasty. Clin Orthop. 1981;155:7–20.
38. Lippitt SB, Harryman II DT, Matsen III FA. A practical tool for evaluating function: the simple shoulder test. In: Matsen III FA, Fu FH, Hawkins RJ, editors. The shoulder: a balance of mobility and stability. Rosemont, IL: American Academy of Orthopaedic Surgeons; 1993. p. 501–18.
39. Williams GN, Gangel TJ, Arciero RA, Uhorchak JM, Taylor DC. Comparison of the single assessment numeric evaluation method and two shoulder rating scales. Outcomes measures after shoulder surgery. Am J Sports Med. 1999;27(2):214–21.
40. Dawson J, Fitzpatrick R, Carr A, Murray D. Questionnaire on the perceptions of patients about total hip replacement. J Bone Joint Surg Br. 1996;78(2):185–90.
41. Baker P, Nanda R, Goodchild L, Finn P, Rangan A. A comparison of the Constant and Oxford shoulder scores in patients with conservatively treated proximal humeral fractures. J Shoulder Elb Surg. 2008;17(1):37–41. doi:10.1016/j.jse.2007.04.019.
42. Lo IKY, Griffin S, Kirkley A. The development of a disease-specific quality of life measurement tool for osteoarthritis of the shoulder: The Western Ontario Osteoarthritis of the Shoulder (WOOS) index. Osteoarthr Cartil. 2001;9(8):771–8. doi:10.1053/joca.2001.0474.
43. Kirkley A, Alvarez C, Griffin S. The development and evaluation of a disease-specific quality-of-life questionnaire for disorders of the rotator cuff: the Western Ontario Rotator Cuff iIndex. Clin J Sport Med. 2003;13(2):84–92.
44. Hollinshead RM, Mohtadi NG, Vande Guchte RA, Wadey VM. Two 6-year follow-up studies of large and massive rotator cuff tears: comparison of outcome measures. J Shoulder Elb Surg. 2000;9(5):373–81. doi:10.1067/mse.2000.108389.
45. Mohtadi NG, Hollinshead RM, Sasyniuk TM, Fletcher JA, Chan DS, Li FX. A randomized clinical trial comparing open to arthroscopic acromioplasty with mini-open rotator cuff repair for full-thickness rotator cuff tears: disease-specific quality of life outcome at an average 2-year follow-up. Am J Sports Med. 2008;36(6):1043–51. doi:10.1177/0363546508314409.

Part III

Investigations

Three-Dimensional Visualization in Clinical Shoulder Practice

7

Young Lae Moon

Introduction

Recent advances in medical imaging have enabled the use of surgical simulations for diagnosis, surgery planning, and education purposes. Improved and enhanced medical imaging techniques allow high-definition imaging and three-dimensional (3D) visualization, thus leading to a better understanding of surgical and educational needs.

There has been long-standing interest in developing techniques for 3D medical imaging. During the past decade, several commercial solutions have been offered for 3D visualization. As a result, we are witnessing the development of next-generation medical instruments that utilize 3D imaging technology.

Physicians performing medical interventions have been reluctant to accept this novel emerging technology. However, patients may actually benefit from using cutting-edge sophisticated technology. One technique that is widely used in next-generation imaging devices is modeling-assisted 3D imaging of anatomical structures.

Computer-aided design (CAD)-based modeling has recently been subject to significant technological improvement [1]. These modeling techniques are becoming increasingly popular in the field of medical modeling, because medical applications necessitate relatively detailed and reliable modeling as well as processing massive medical data.

The data for modeling anatomical structures are collected using computerized tomography (CT), magnetic resonance imaging (MRI), and optical microscopy, to name a few. The acquired images are analyzed for deducing the human articular structure and kinetics as well as for simulating and designing structures such as artificial joints. Technologies such as CAD, computer-aided manufacturing (CAM), rapid prototyping (RP), and solid freeform fabrication (SFF) are used for designing artificial structures.

The human field of view is stereoscopic. Therefore, given the acquired two-dimensional (2D) images, it is necessary to perform stereoscopic reconstruction mimicking a surgeon's field of view. 3D imaging has been proposed to alleviate the need for such stereoscopic reconstruction. By enhancing 3D visualization, 3D imaging can significantly shorten the time required for surgeons to make correct decisions in complex situations.

Y.L. Moon, M.D.
3D Medical Application Work Group, IEEE-SA, Milano, Italy

3D Printing Work Group, ISO-TC 261, Berlin, Germany

American Shoulder and Elbow Surgeons, San Diego, CA, USA

Orthopaedic Department, Chosun University Medical Research Center, Chosun University Hospital, Gwangju, South Korea
e-mail: ylm2103@gmail.com

G. Huri, N.K. Paschos (eds.), *The Shoulder*, Orthopaedic Study Guide Series,
DOI 10.1007/978-3-319-51979-1_7

Using 3D imaging data it has become possible to simulate a variety of medical procedures and scenarios, such as virtual endoscopy, surgical planning, and real-time interaction. This article describes the principles and recent applications of state-of-the-art shoulder imaging techniques, with a special focus on medical 3D reconstruction techniques.

Segmentation

3D models of human body organs can be generated by 3D reconstruction of serial sectional images of these organs, acquired using CT and MRI [2].

Tomography refers to continuous imaging of structures separated by a 1–3 mm gap. The CT and MRI techniques differ in some aspects. The apparatus of CT involves the device for producing X-rays that is connected to a computer. CT amounts to irradiating the body parts of interest using highly specialized X-rays for obtaining segmented images of different body tissues. As the projected X-rays exit the body, the computer evaluates the amount of X-ray radiation absorbed by the body. Since different body organs (e.g., bone, muscle, and liver) have different densities, the projected X-rays will be absorbed by different organs depending on the organ density, and computer software will account for these differences when generating images. On the other hand, MRI addresses the magnetic property of the analyzed substance and images are calculated based on the difference between magnetic properties of different body tissues. In addition, MRI is more advantageous than CT owing to its higher resolution.

The two imaging technologies have their unique strengths and weaknesses. In the case of CT, bone is clearly identifiable; therefore, bone- or joint-related abnormalities can be addressed. In the case of MRI, cartilage, muscle, and nerves are clearly identifiable, as well as the bone, making MRI more effective (Fig. 7.1) [3, 4]. Considering these characteristics of the two techniques, in practice a combination of CT and MRI is often used [5–7].

After acquiring serial 2D images, the area of interest in these 2D images should be segmented. In the image segmentation procedure, an image is divided into homogeneous structures of the same region or similar nature by defining the boundaries of transitional edges. To generate 3D images, an outline of structures captured by 2D images needs to be provided. This process is known as 'segmentation' [8]. Several methods have been developed for achieving precise segmentation; these methods include thresholding, region growing, dynamic region growing, 3D livewire, morphology operation, Boolean operation, edit masks, multiple edit masks, and 3D edit masks.

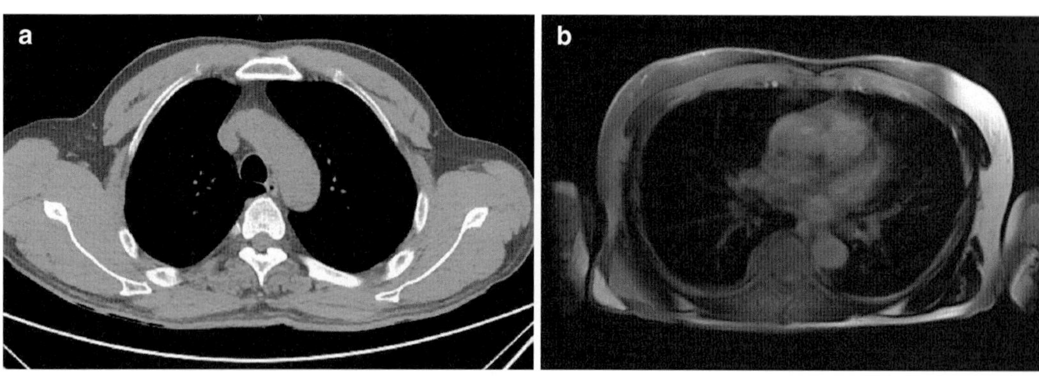

Fig. 7.1 Comparison of (**a**) CT and (**b**) MR images of the thoracic region. In the CT image, bones and airways are clearly seen. In the MR image, the boundaries of muscles and organs are more clearly seen compared with the CT image

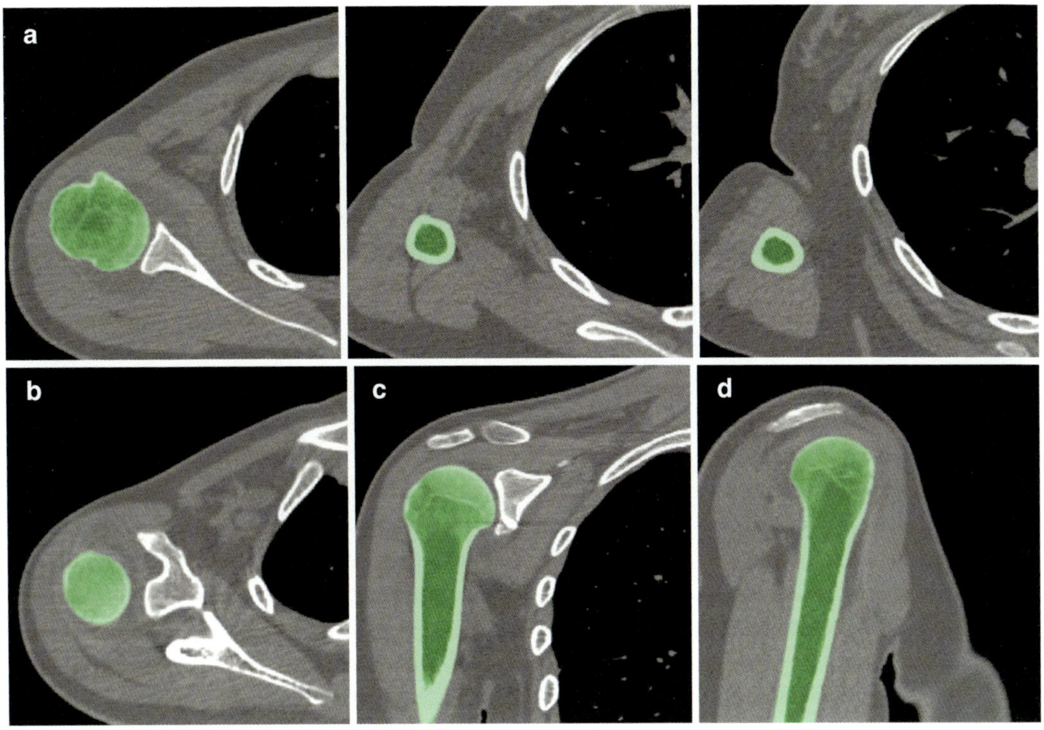

Fig. 7.2 Segmentation of the humerus for the CT image in Fig. 7.1. (**a**) The humerus is serially segmented into horizontal-plane images. (**b**) Axial-plane images. (**c**) Coronal-plane images. (**d**) sagittal-plane images

3D models are generated by stacking serial 2D images; therefore, segmentation is performed on a collection of consecutive 2D images. Usually, segmentation is performed on horizontal-plane images; however, in some cases segmentation is performed on coronal- or sagittal-plane images that are obtained by stacking horizontal-plane images and then cutting in the coronal or sagittal plane (Fig. 7.2).

When MRI is used for segmentation of images, e.g., for 3D imaging of the subscapularis muscle, axial-, coronal-, and sagittal-plane 2D images of the subscapularis muscle outline are marked for segmentation (Fig. 7.3).

Segmentation in medical imaging is generally considered a challenging problem, because many structures have similar densities with respect to imaging. In addition, sampling artifacts, noise, and low contrast may blur the contours of anatomical structures. To address this problem, a variety of algorithms have been developed for automating the process of segmentation, including edge detection, region growing, thresholding, morphological operation, watershed segmentation, edit mask, and manual operation (Fig. 7.4) [9, 10]. Owing to the nature of the problem of segmentation, most of these algorithms are specific to a particular problem and thus are not generalizable to other problems. However, some anatomical structures, such as some fine muscles and ligaments, cannot be segmented automatically, because the contours of neighboring structures are not clearly identifiable in 2D images [11].

Commercial software for medical imaging provides high-quality segmentation [12–14]. Commercial software packages are equipped with many functions for performing optimal segmentation, including semiautomatic segmentation.

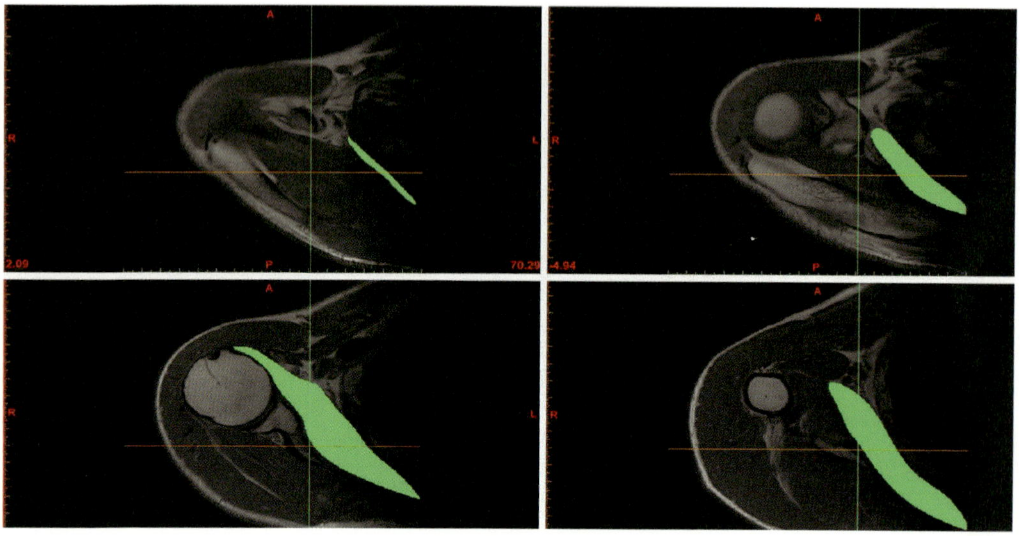

Fig. 7.3 *Green*: schematic of the surface of the subscapularis muscle border in a transverse section. *Green*-colored schematic surface of the subscapularis muscle in the transverse section can be seen here. Drawing the outline of the subscapularis muscle in the transverse section

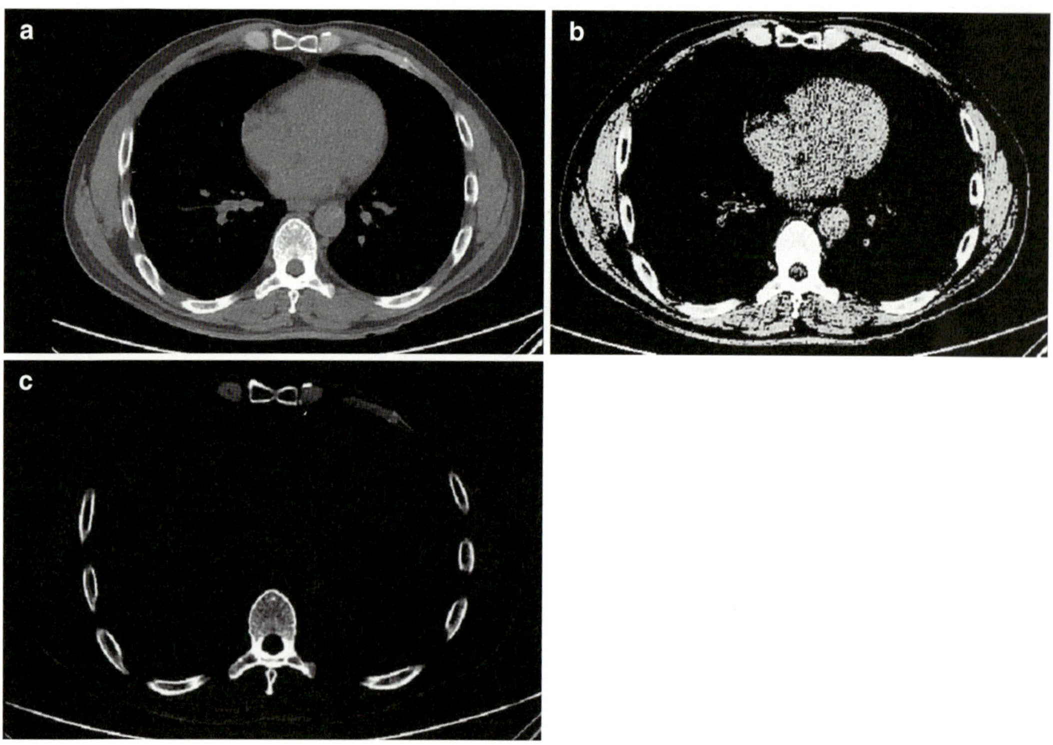

Fig. 7.4 Image segmentation. (**a**) The original image. (**b**) Detection of edges. (**c**) The image morphology

3D Reconstruction

A 3D model with laminating 2D slices can be rendered in two ways, depending on the region of interest (ROI): (1) surface rendering, which visualizes only the surface of the imaged structure and (2) volume rendering, which allows visualizing the inner compartments (Fig. 7.5) [2].

3D models are generated by stacking serial segmented images. Volume 3D models are generated as follows: the segmented images are simultaneously expanded onto the next set of images for building several small-volume models, referred to as the volume reconstruction. Next, all small-volume models are combined to yield a full-scale 3D model. A surface model is extracted from this full-scale 3D model, and the resulting surface model is referred to as the surface reconstruction (Fig. 7.6) [15]. Usually, the volume and surface reconstructions are performed using the

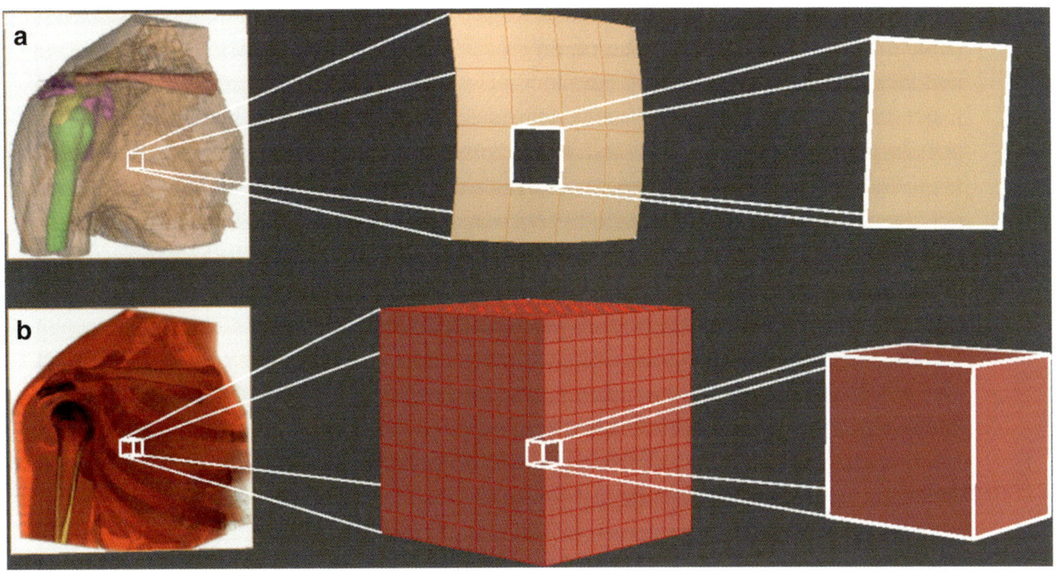

Fig. 7.5 Surface and volume reconstructions. (**a**) Surface reconstruction, with outer surface visualization. (**b**) Volume reconstruction, with inner and outer visualization

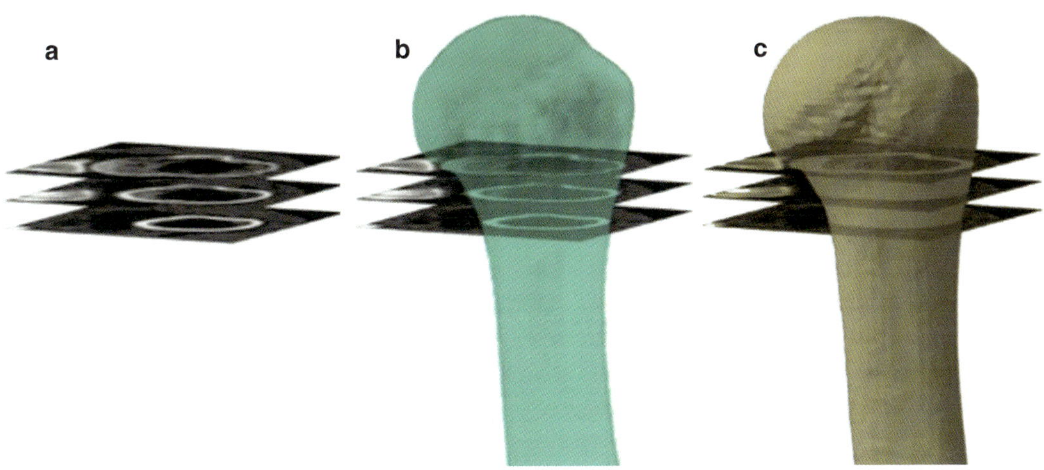

Fig. 7.6 The 3D reconstruction procedure. (**a**) A stack of images. (**b**) Several 3D small-volume models built from the images in (**a**). (**c**) A 3D model of the bone surface extracted from the 3D small-volume models in (**b**)

same reconstruction software. The resulting surface model consists of the original stacked contours and numerous triangular surfaces between the contours [16].

Such 3D reconstruction can be performed using specialized medical software or in-house software [17], but in some cases, non-specialized software may be used for surface reconstruction, not requiring specific programming implementation (Fig. 7.7) [18–20].

Volume and surface 3D models require different file formats that depend on the utilized software, making data exchange difficult. Therefore, a surface model, comprised of stacked contours and polygons between the contours, should be converted to the drawing exchange format (DXF) or a different popular format. In some cases, 3D models are converted to a non-uniform rational B-spline (NURBS) surface.

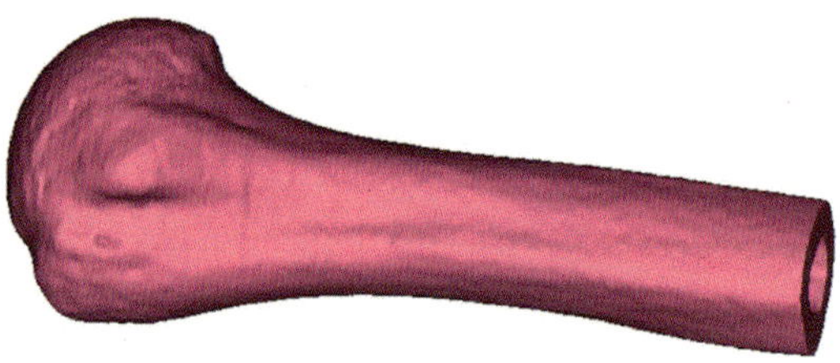

Fig. 7.7 A 3D model of a humerus. After volume reconstruction, the surface was extracted using commercial reconstruction software

As described above, subscapularis images can be segmented using 3D reconstruction software, to obtain a 3D reconstruction (Fig. 7.8).

3D Texture Mapping

Both CT and MRI generate grayscale images; however, each anatomical structure has its own coloration that is dictated by its composition. Therefore, 3D texture mapping is used to generate 3D models with realistic coloration. The technique of 3D texture mapping involves coating 3D models with realistic organ textures (Fig. 7.9). Today, realistic textures of different organs can be acquired from cadavers or surgery rooms. Such 3D texturing yields more realistic models [17, 21]. This technique enhances visualization of relatively fine details of organs/structures.

Kinematic Imaging

In the field of human body modeling, rigging and animation are popular techniques for simulating motion in 3D. These techniques are also important for acquiring 2D medical images, surgery planning, and simulations [22].

3D imaging-based models are used in Finite Element Analysis (FEA), implant design, and RP

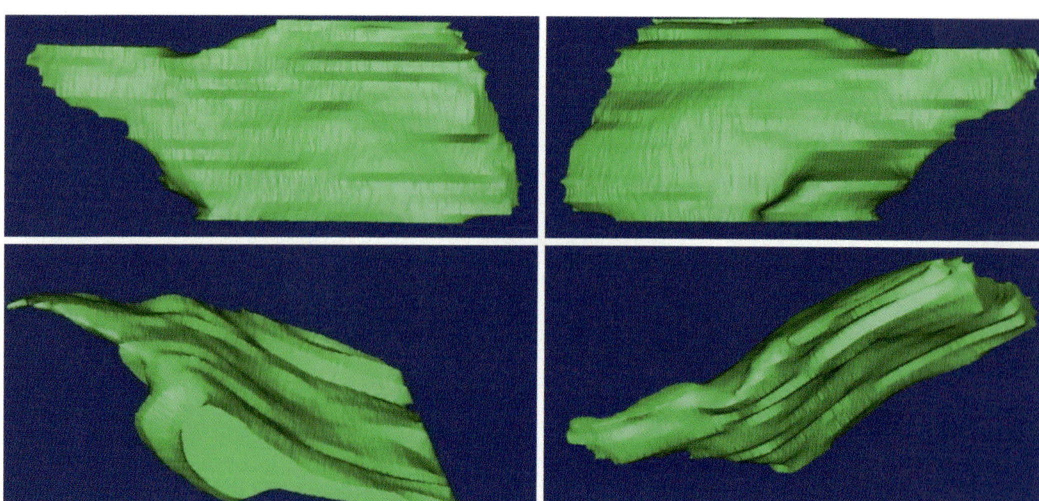

Fig. 7.8 A 3D reconstruction of the subscapularis muscle in Fig. 7.3

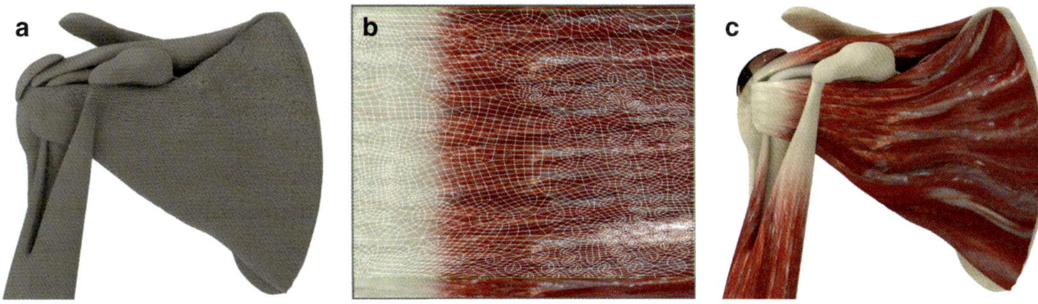

Fig. 7.9 Texture mapping. (**a**) A 3D model of a surface before texture mapping. (**b**) Texture source and mapping coordinates. (**c**) The 3D model of the same surface after texture mapping

fabrication. These procedures involve cutting specific areas, fitting the matter properties to the model, and moving the model. These models are used in computer-assisted surgery, surgery planning, and diagnosis.

Shoulder kinematics can be studied using CT or MRI of various shoulder positions. Information about the shoulder spatial relationships and moment arms is necessary for virtual shoulder surgeries. This kinematic information can be acquired using measurements from 3D reconstructed shoulder models and CAD software [23–25].

In addition to CT and MRI, electromagnetic devices for capturing 3D motion are also used for detecting shoulder movements [26, 27]. Four-dimensional (4D) CT is also used, providing adequate and novel assessment of biomechanics, both before and after surgical repair [28]. 4D kinematic MRI datasets allow us to view an anatomical structure from any viewing perspective in real time [29].

The scapula moves as follows [30]. As the scapula is protracted or retracted, its internal side slides over the thoracic cage. During this motion, the sternoclavicular joint becomes the axis of rotation. This mechanism allows, e.g., to hold a book using both scapulae. If the scapulae are elevated or depressed, the humerus and the clavicle, the bones that connect to the scapulae, will be elevated or depressed as well. This type of motion occurs when the shoulder moves up and down. During this motion, the scapula makes a dangerous joint; the scapula-sternoclavicular joint connecting to the thoracic cage. The scapula will not move until the humerus turns by 90°. However, when the humerus turns by more than 90°, the humerus will touch the coracoid process of the scapula, forcing the scapula to slide and move together with the humerus. At this stage, an accurate description of the extent by which the scapulae and the clavicles are twisted is required for producing realistic movement.

Surgical Simulations

In the twenty-first century, developments in the field of 3D medical imaging resulted in cutting-edge technologies such as virtual endoscopes and surgical simulations, opening new vistas [31]. Specifically, these developments suggest a possibility to use high-speed communication networks in a variety of interesting applications. In many medical applications, simulating the treatment plan prior to performing the actual treatment has become an acceptable practice.

Interactive virtual reality-based simulations require several components, such as a virtual camera, a surgical equipment model, a reference patient model, and texturing and rendering (Fig. 7.10) [32]. Each component must have the same display and material properties as its real analogue. For example, in the case of a camera, for displaying a screen similar to the one that is used during actual surgeries, the virtual camera should have the same optical angle as a real endoscope view (Fig. 7.11).

A controller is required for the user to be able to execute penetration and cutting procedures on a 3D human body model. Controller devices such as the mouse, joystick, haptic devices, and blue

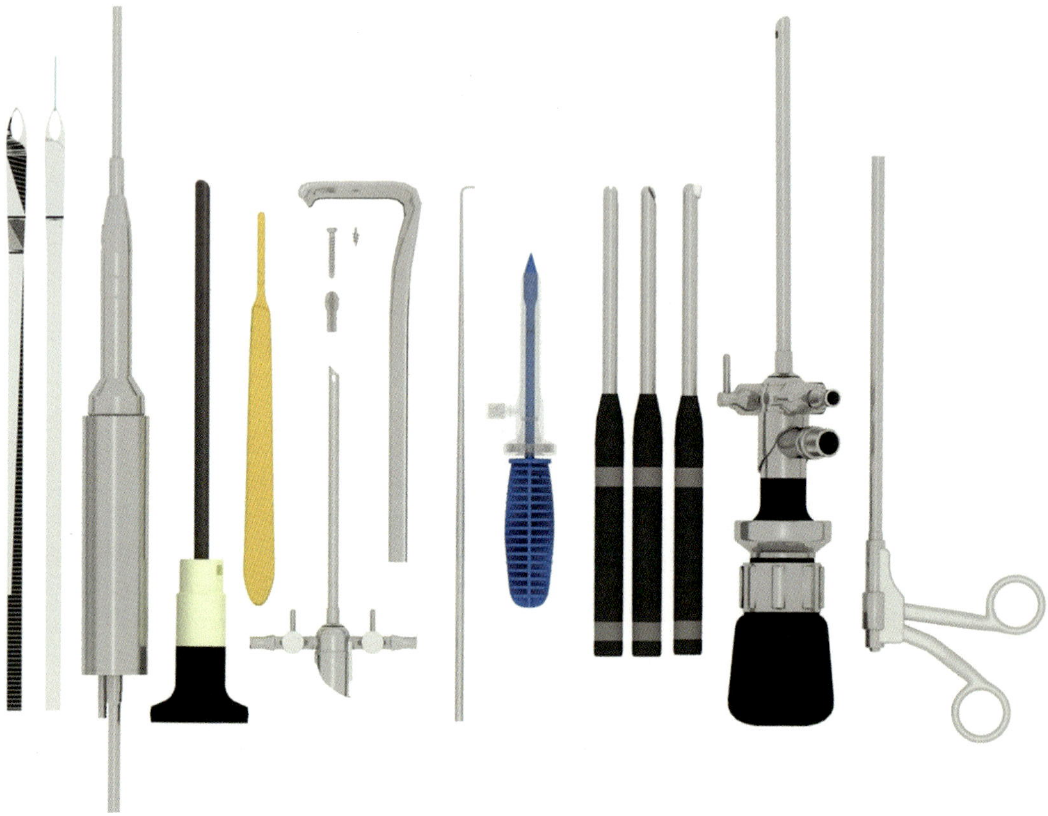

Fig. 7.10 A collection of modeled tools

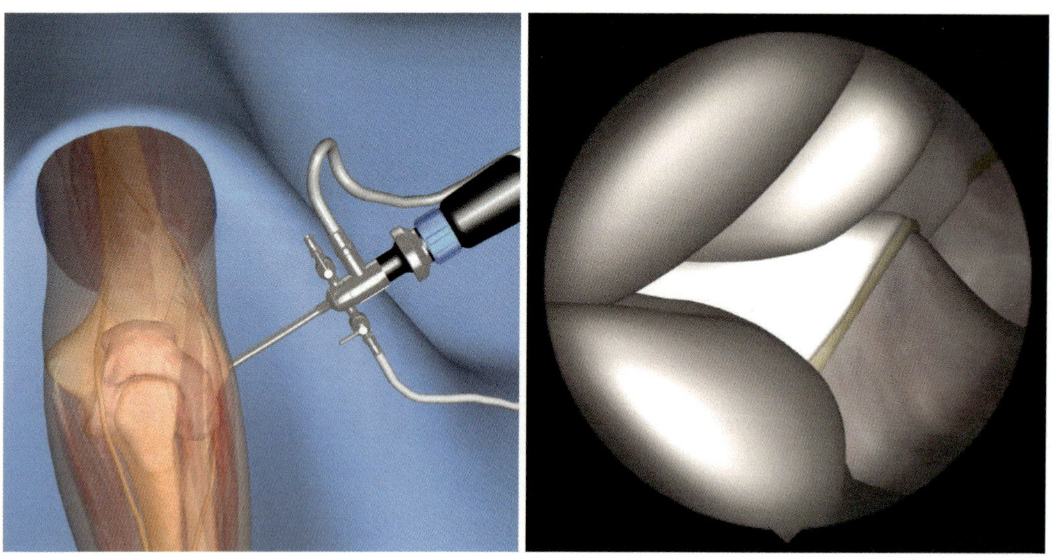

Fig. 7.11 The process of surgery, showing inside of the shoulder joint by virtual endoscopy

tooth systems are often used. Arthroscopy simulators are often designed using these principles and components. Although instruments and 3D human body models based on real models are used, the performance significantly differs from that of real arthroscopic intervention. This difference arises because real arthroscopy magnifies distorted images tenfold to retain the optic angle over 120°, compared with arthroscopy simulators that do not achieve such magnification.

Soft tissues often possess elaborate nonlinear material characteristics that make these tissues soft and compliant to small strains. Therefore, to capture these material characteristics, constraint-based finite-element algorithms are used for efficiently simulating nonlinear incompliant materials for interactive simulation applications [33].

Surgeries that use computer navigation can minimize problems that are likely to occur during surgeries, and can help increase the surgery accuracy. After the information about a patient is supplied to the navigation device, a computer uses this information and provides the surgeon with real-time information required for the surgery. A surgeon can perform a more accurate surgery because the surgeon can utilize this real-time feedback to determine the progress of the surgery.

When a patient needs total shoulder arthroplasty, the symptoms and the indication are the same, whether or not the surgeon plans to use a navigation device. For experienced surgeons, navigation is not necessary. However, total shoulder arthroplasty with fracture or total shoulder arthroplasty revision surgery can present with abnormal anatomical findings. In these cases, navigation can be of use to experienced surgeons, because even they can be confused during this type of surgery [34].

The principle of navigation is as follows. A 3D digital mock-up is obtained based on the CT images of a patient. After that, a prosthesis mock-up, equipped with navigation, is adjusted according to the acquired images. A virtual mock-up is thus obtained. Then, the obtained virtual mock-up is used for simulating the process of surgery before the actual surgery, and is used for analyzing the patient's status in real time during a real surgery [35].

A surgery that uses computer navigation proceeds as follows. First, the patient's shoulder joint is exposed and an optical marker is attached to the upper part of the humerus. At the lower part of the humerus dotting is performed for navigation, for recognizing the entire bone shape. The marker is also applied to the scapula. In the glenoid cavity, a tunnel is drilled at the center. After that, the tunnel is dilated and penetrated to insert a temporary instrument using cement. During this procedure, navigation identifies whether the dilator dilates and penetrates properly as planned before the surgery, using the dilator with the marker attached. Usually, the marker is not attached to the instrument when inserting the instrument into the dilated tunnel. After the instrument is inserted, proper joint stability is ensured before inserting the final implant. The surgery is completed after the implant is inserted and the wound is closed.

The use of navigation in total shoulder arthroplasty is advantageous owing to the higher accuracy of surgery that is achieved by providing real-time intraoperative information regarding the anatomical position. However, an additional incision is required for using a fixation pin, and a fracture can be created on the pinned side when fixating the pin. This procedure becomes especially undesirable if a natural infection or an active infection exists around the artificial joint. In addition, the time spending and cost associated with these surgeries are to expansive, and surgeons performing this surgery with the computer aided training system. Furthermore, computer-related errors and navigation errors due to tracker loosening can occur. Therefore, additional research and longitudinal studies are needed for determining the correlation between the clinical outcomes and errors. On the other hand, automated navigation can be advantageous or disadvantageous, depending on the user, as demonstrated by the example of automated car navigation. Finally, computer-assisted surgery is likely to becoming one of the standard tool in the future medical practice.

3D Printing

Broadly defined, 3D printing is a technology for fabricating 3D objects by stacking evenly spaced slices of a source object [1]. This technology is used for creating realistic objects. Medical applications can be easily envisioned, e.g., 3D printing of body parts, medical instruments, and surgery tools. Today, customized medical instruments, reflecting the individual patient needs and characteristics, can be fabricated using 3D printing, while mass production can hardly meet these needs. Patients differ in their injuries, their needs for replacement body parts, and their disability and diseases. Therefore, it is difficult if not impossible to practically meet these individual needs using the existing manufacturing systems for mass production. By utilizing 3D printing, customized treatments can become more economical and easier to achieve.

A concept similar to that of 3D printing is computer numerical control (CNC), with 3D printing being a CNC-category application. CNC utilizes shaving down to create a model; on the other hand, in 3D printing a model is created by stacking up slices. Thus, the difference between these two methods is that 3D printing does not require additional tools and is advantageous for creating inner shapes in spaces that might be inaccessible to tools.

Many methods have been developed for 3D printing. On a large scale, extrusion, wire, granular, laminate, and light polymerizing are used. On a smaller scale, fused filament fabrication (FFF), fused deposition modeling (FDM), plastic jet printing (PJP), and smooth curvature printing (SCP) are used. Wire techniques include electron beam freeform fabrication (EBF3). Granular techniques include direct metal laser sintering (DMLS), laser-aided direct metal tooling (DMT), electron beam melting (EBM), selective heat sintering (SHS), selective laser sintering (SLS), color jet printing (CJP), and plaster-based 3D printing (PP). Laminate techniques include laminated object manufacturing (LOM). Light polymerized techniques include stereolithography apparatus (SLA), digital light processing (DLP), photopolymer jetting (Polyjet), and multi jet modeling (MJM) [1].

In today's medical market, extrusion is the most widely used technique. This technique can be easily explained as a syringe and glue gun. In this technique, the same material is melted and extruded at the same point and by the same amount for gradually stacking, to obtain a model. In each step of this process, an extruder accepts a certain amount of material, melts it, and then extrudes it. The extruded material stacks to obtain a model. In addition, material can be extended in various ways, and the thicknesses of individual layers can be controlled. The granular method uses a larger beam to partially melt the powder that is evenly spread. Using this method, it is possible to create more detailed models (compared with those created using the extrusion method); however, the associated cost is much higher.

Medical instruments are fabricated using 3D printing with an important advantage of meeting specific patients' needs. For example, using 3D printing it is in principle possible to fabricate customized implants for total shoulder arthroplasty. With improving material properties, these applications are likely to extend to additional organs/body parts.

Conclusion

Advances in CT, MRI, and other imaging modalities have led to new applications and possibilities in the field of shoulder imaging. Among these, 3D imaging bears the promise to become very useful in clinical and basic research fields. This technology can help the clinician to more effectively and faster detect the pathology and reach the optimal decision. In addition, 3D imaging opens new vistas for advanced medical applications, and thus is likely to become a powerful instrument for clinicians and students alike.

Questions

In the process of Volume 3D models generation please place the steps in the correct order

A. Extraction of a surface model (surface reconstruction)
B. The segmented images are simultaneously expanded onto the next set of images
C. Small-volume models are combined to yield a full-scale 3D model
D. Building several small-volume models (volume reconstruction).

Four-dimensional (4D) CT is a valuable tool for:

A. Providing adequate and novel assessment of biomechanics
B. Providing a more accurate imaging than 3D models

C. Detecting abnormalities not seen with 3D reconstruction
D. All the above

All the following statements for 3D printing are correct except:
A. Extrusion is the most widely used technique
B. On a large scale, extrusion, granular, plastic jet printing, and light polymerizing are used
C. The associated cost is extremely high
D. The granular method creates more detailed models compared to the extrusion method

References

1. Jakus AE, Rutz AL, Shah RN. Advancing the field of 3D biomaterial printing. Biomed Mater. 2016;11(1):014102.
2. Lin Q, et al. Immersive virtual reality for visualization of abdominal CT. Proc SPIE Int Soc Opt Eng. 2013;8673:10.1117/12.2008050.
3. Torkzad MR, et al. Comparison between MRI and CT in prediction of peritoneal carcinomatosis index (PCI) in patients undergoing cytoreductive surgery in relation to the experience of the radiologist. J Surg Oncol. 2015;111(6):746–51.
4. Zhong BS, et al. CT and MRI findings in patients with autoimmune pancreatitis. Zhejiang Da Xue Xue Bao Yi Xue Ban. 2014;43(1):94–100.
5. Kim YN, et al. A proposal for combined MRI and PET/CT interpretation criteria for preoperative nodal staging in non-small-cell lung cancer. Eur Radiol. 2012;22(7):1537–46.
6. Donati OF, et al. Combined cardiac CT and MRI for the comprehensive workup of hemodynamically relevant coronary stenoses. Am J Roentgenol. 2010;194(4):920–6.
7. Lee YS, et al. Anatomical evaluation of CT-MRI combined femoral model. Biomed Eng Online. 2008;7:6.
8. Arezoomand S, et al. A 3D active model framework for segmentation of proximal femur in MR images. Int J Comput Assist Radiol Surg. 2015;10(1):55–66.
9. Grau V, et al. Improved watershed transform for medical image segmentation using prior information. IEEE Trans Med Imaging. 2004;23(4):447–58.
10. Yang Z, et al. Automatic bone segmentation and bone-cartilage interface extraction for the shoulder joint from magnetic resonance images. Phys Med Biol. 2015;60(4):1441–59.
11. Chaoui J, et al. Recognition-based segmentation and registration method for image guided shoulder surgery. Conf Proc IEEE Eng Med Biol Soc. 2011;2011:6212–5.
12. Wu Y, et al. Creation of a female and male segmentation dataset based on Chinese Visible Human (CVH). Comput Med Imaging Graph. 2012;36(4):336–42.
13. Huang YX, et al. Three-dimensional reconstruction of the superior mediastinum from Chinese Visible Human Female. Surg Radiol Anat. 2010;32(7):693–8.
14. Shin DS, et al. Outlining of the detailed structures in sectioned images from Visible Korean. Surg Radiol Anat. 2012;34(3):235–47.
15. Shin DS, Park JS, Chung MS. Three types of the serial segmented images suitable for surface reconstruction. Anat Cell Biol. 2012;45(2):128–35.
16. Shin DS, et al. Accessible and informative sectioned images and surface models of a cadaver head. J Craniofac Surg. 2012;23(4):1176–80.
17. Cho SW, et al. Three-dimensional templating arthroplasty of the humeral head. Surg Radiol Anat. 2013;35:685–8.
18. Shin DS, et al. Three-dimensional surface models of detailed lumbosacral structures reconstructed from the Visible Korean. Ann Anat. 2011;193(1):64–70.
19. Shin DS, et al. Surface model of the gastrointestinal tract constructed from the Visible Korean. Clin Anat. 2009;22(5):601–9.
20. Shin DS, et al. Advanced surface reconstruction technique to build detailed surface models of the liver and neighboring structures from the Visible Korean Human. J Korean Med Sci. 2009;24(3):375–83.
21. Shin DS, et al. Surface models of the male urogenital organs built from the Visible Korean using popular software. Anat Cell Biol. 2011;44(2):151–9.
22. Ferre R, et al. Differentiation of fibroadenomas and pure mucinous carcinomas on dynamic contrast-enhanced MRI of the breast using volume segmentation for kinetic analysis: a feasibility study. Am J Roentgenol. 2016;206(2):253–8.
23. Cabezas AF, et al. Kinematic impact of size on the existing glenohumeral joint in patients undergoing reverse shoulder arthroplasty. Clin Biomech (Bristol, Avon). 2014;29(6):622–8.
24. von Eisenhart-Rothe R, et al. Simultaneous 3D assessment of glenohumeral shape, humeral head centering, and scapular positioning in atraumatic shoulder instability: a magnetic resonance-based in vivo analysis. Am J Sports Med. 2010;38(2):375–82.
25. Van Hoof T, et al. 3D computerized model for measuring strain and displacement of the brachial plexus following placement of reverse shoulder prosthesis. Anat Rec (Hoboken). 2008;291(9):1173–85.
26. Kwon YW, et al. Kinematic analysis of dynamic shoulder motion in patients with reverse total shoulder arthroplasty. J Shoulder Elb Surg. 2012;21(9):1184–90.
27. Raiss P, et al. Range of motion of shoulder and elbow in activities of daily life in 3D motion analysis. Z Orthop Unfall. 2007;145(4):493–8.

28. Shores JT, Demehri S, Chhabra A. Kinematic "4 Dimensional" CT imaging in the assessment of wrist biomechanics before and after surgical repair. Eplasty. 2013;13:e9.
29. Schulz H, et al. Real-time interactive viewing of 4D kinematic MR joint studies. Med Image Comput Comput Assist Interv. 2005;8(Pt 1):467–73.
30. Kijima T, et al. In vivo 3-dimensional analysis of scapular and glenohumeral kinematics: comparison of symptomatic or asymptomatic shoulders with rotator cuff tears and healthy shoulders. J Shoulder Elb Surg. 2015;24(11):1817–26.
31. Stefanidis D, et al. Research priorities in surgical simulation for the 21st century. Am J Surg. 2012;203(1): 49–53.
32. Rose AS, et al. Multi-material 3D models for temporal bone surgical simulation. Ann Otol Rhinol Laryngol. 2015;124(7):528–36.
33. Tang W, Wan TR. Constraint-based soft tissue simulation for virtual surgical training. IEEE Trans Biomed Eng. 2014;61(11):2698–706.
34. Verborgt O, et al. Computer navigation and patient-specific instrumentation in shoulder arthroplasty. Sports Med Arthrosc. 2014;22(4):e42–9.
35. Sadoghi P, et al. Benefit of intraoperative navigation on glenoid component positioning during total shoulder arthroplasty. Arch Orthop Trauma Surg. 2015; 135(1):41–7.

Part IV

Shoulder Trauma

Clavicle Fractures

8

Filippo Familiari, Gazi Huri, Olimpio Galasso, Giorgio Gasparini, and Mahmut Nedim Doral

The clavicle is one of the most commonly fractured bones. It accounts for 2.6–4% of all adult fractures and approximately 35% of injuries to the shoulder girdle [1]. Fractures can involve the midshaft (approximately 70%), lateral-end (28%), and/or medial-end (2–3%) of the clavicle and are typically caused by a fall on an outstretched arm or by a direct blow on the shoulder. Midshaft fractures occur most frequently in young and active adults, whereas lateral and medial fractures are more frequent in elderly patients [2].

In children, clavicle fractures account for 10–15% of all fractures. Fractures involving the midshaft are most common (approximately 90%) and most clavicle fractures in childhood can be treated conservatively because of their excellent remodeling capabilities [3].

Anatomy

The clavicle is the sole bone structure connecting the trunk to the shoulder and arm, and it is the only bone of the shoulder girdle that forms a synovial joint with the trunk [4]. The superior aspect of the clavicle is subcutaneous over its course, with only the thin platysma providing muscular coverage to the inner two thirds of the bone. The supraclavicular nerves, which provide sensation to skin in that area, are located just deep to the platysma muscle layer. The clavicle appears almost straight when viewed from the front; however, when viewed from above, the clavicle appears as an S-shaped double curve that is concave ventrally in the outer half and convex ventrally in the medial half. The cross section of the clavicle differs in shape along its length: it is flat along the outer third and prismatic along the inner third. The flat part is most compatible with pull from muscles and ligaments, whereas the tubular part is consistent with axial pressure or pull. The junction between the two cross sections is a weak spot particularly with axial loading [4], and it may be one of the reasons why fractures occur so commonly at the middle third.

The clavicle articulates with the sternum through the sternoclavicular (SC) joint, which has little articular contact but strong ligamentous attachments. The medial-end of the clavicle is firmly attached against the first rib by the intra-articular SC joint cartilage, the oblique fibers of the costoclavicular ligaments, and the subclavius muscle, as described by De Palma [5]. The scapula and clavicle are bound securely by both the AC and coracoclavicular (CC) ligaments [6]. The tubular part of the clavicle offers protection for the important neurovascular structures that pass

F. Familiari, M.D. (✉) • O. Galasso, M.D.
G. Gasparini, M.D.
Department of Orthopaedic and Trauma Surgery, Magna Græcia University, Catanzaro, Italy
e-mail: filippofamiliari@gmail.com

G. Huri, M.D. • M.N. Doral, M.D.
Department of Orthopaedics and Traumatology, Hacettepe University, Ankara, Turkey

G. Huri, N.K. Paschos (eds.), *The Shoulder*, Orthopaedic Study Guide Series,
DOI 10.1007/978-3-319-51979-1_8

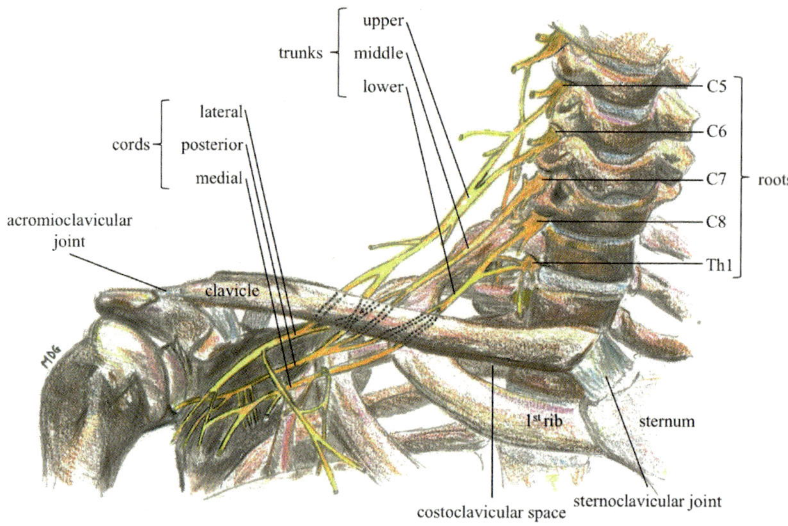

Fig. 8.1 Schematic representation of the brachial plexus and its relations to the clavicle. Courtesy of Marco De Gori, MD

beneath the medial third of the clavicle. The space between the clavicle and the first rib has been called the costoclavicular space. The brachial plexus, when crosses beneath the clavicle, consists of three main cords (Fig. 8.1). Of these, two are anterior: the lateral cord originates from the 5th, 6th, and 7th cervical roots and forms the musculocutaneous nerve and a branch of the median nerve; the medial cord originates from the 8ht cervical and 1st thoracic roots and forms another branch of the median nerve, the ulnar nerve, and the medial cutaneous nerve of the forearm. The posterior cord of the plexus originates from C5 to T1 roots and forms the axillary and radial nerves. The internal jugular is adjacent to the SC joint and the subclavian vessels are in proximity to the medial third of the clavicle. Consequently, vessels (especially the subclavian and axillary vessels) and nerves (especially the ulnar nerve) are potentially subject to injury, pressure, or irritation [7]. The clavicle also appears to be unique as a long bone because it has only a periosteal blood supply and no intramedullary or nutrient arterial blood supply.

The clavicle acts as a bony framework for muscle origin and insertion. The trapezius muscle inserts into the posterior border of the lateral third of the clavicle, while the deltoid muscle originates from the anterior border of the lateral third of the clavicle. The clavicular head of the sternocleidomastoid muscle originates from the superior surface of medial third of the clavicle. The clavicular head of the pectoralis major muscle originates from the anterior edge of the clavicle. The subclavius muscle after arising from the first rib anteriorly at the costochondral junction, it proceeds obliquely and posteriorly into a groove on the undersurface of the clavicle into the middle of the posterior surface of clavicle. It extends in both later and medial parts of clavicle.

Epidemiology

The annual incidence of clavicular fractures is estimated to be between 29 and 64 per 100,000 population per year [1, 8, 9]. The first, largest peak incidence is in males <30 years of age; these fractures tend to be of the shaft, sustained when a direct force is applied during sports activity [10]. The second, smaller peak of incidence occurs in elderly patients (>80 years of age), with a slight female predominance [2]. These fractures tend to be lateral and medial-end of the clavicle and related to osteoporosis, sustained during low-energy trauma, often in the domestic environment. Most shaft fractures are displaced, whereas the majority of lateral-end fractures are undisplaced [1].

Classification

Allman [11] proposed a classification based on the anatomic location of the fracture (group I, fractures of the middle third; group II, fractures of the lateral third; group III, fractures of the medial third). Neer [12] classified fractures of the lateral third of the clavicle according to whether they were undisplaced (type I) or displaced (type II). Displaced lateral-end fractures were then subclassified according to the integrity of the coronoid and trapezoid ligaments: type-IIA, the ligaments remain intact; type-IIB, the CC ligaments are partially or completely detached [12]. Craig then further modified Neer type II lateral clavicle fractures to differentiate between ligamentous injury patterns in the lateral third and include intra-articular and paediatric fractures [13].

The Edinburgh classification has been proposed by Robinson and it has been used to subclassify shaft fractures according to displacement and degree of comminution [1] (Fig. 8.2). Anatomically, fractures are divided into medial (type I), middle (type II), and lateral (type III) thirds. Each of these types is then subdivided based on fracture displacement: fracture displacement of <100% characterizes subgroup A, whereas fractures displaced by >100% account for subgroup B. Type I (medial) and type III (lateral) fractures are further subdivided based on articular involvement: subgroup 1, no articular involvement; subgroup 2, inter-articular extension. Moreover, type II (middle) fractures are subcategorized by the degree of fracture comminution: subgroup 1, simple or wedge-type fractures; subgroup 2, comminuted or segmental fractures. This classification system has been shown to have acceptable levels of interobserver and intraobserver variation.

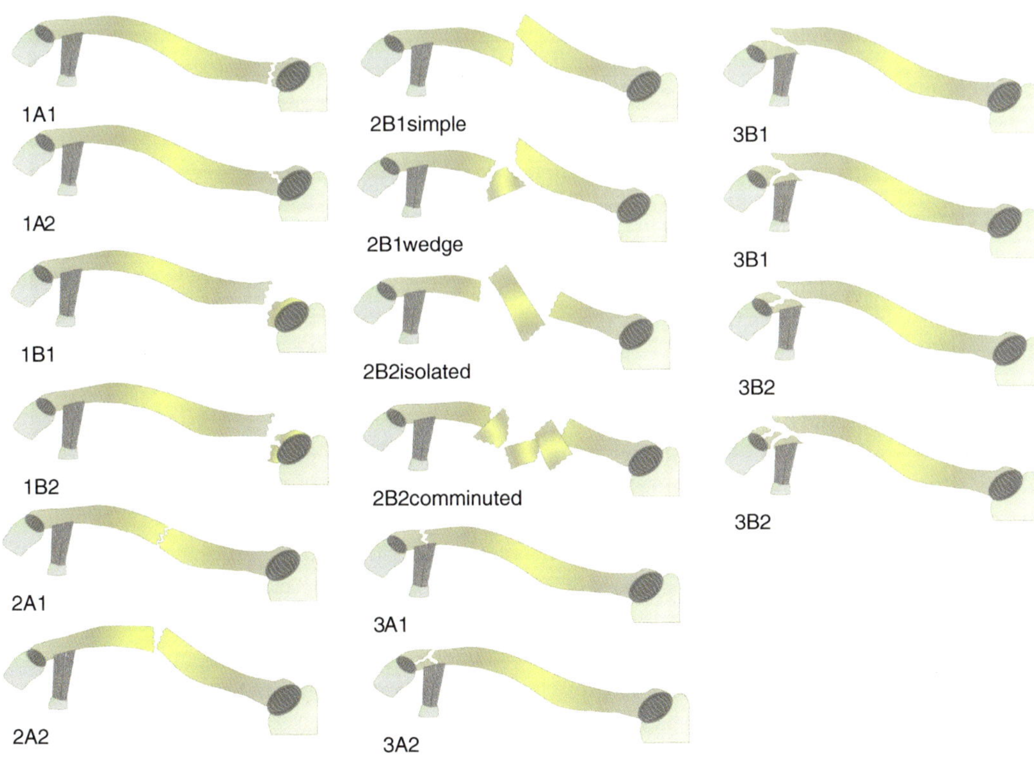

Fig. 8.2 The Edinburgh classification of clavicle fractures. (adapted from: Robinson CM. Fractures of the clavicle in the adult. Epidemiology and classification. J Bone Joint Surg Br. 1998;80:477)

Clinical and Radiographic Assessment

A detailed history should be obtained, focusing on standard demographic information and the mechanism of injury. A clavicle fracture which results from a simple fall is unlikely to be associated with other significant injuries. However, fractures occurring in the context of a high-energy trauma should prompt a thorough search for concomitant injuries. Posterior displacement of a medial-end fracture can cause compression of the mediastinum and major vessels, requiring urgent operative intervention, but this is very rare [14–16]. The majority of fractures result from direct force to the point of the shoulder, although fractures can also result from a traction injury [17]. If the clavicle fractures with minimal force, the possibility of pathologic fractures secondary to metabolic processes and tumours must be considered.

Clavicular fractures typically produce an obvious painful deformity, with tenderness localized over the site of the fracture (Fig. 8.3). There is often downward displacement of the lateral fragment under the weight of the shoulder and elevation of the medial fragment from the unopposed pull of the sternocleidomastoid muscle [13]. A droopy, shortened, and medially-driven shoulder has been described as shoulder "ptosis" [1, 18]. With severely angulated or comminuted fractures, fragments may "button-hole" subcutaneously through the platysma muscle. Despite the superficial position of the clavicle, open fractures producing skin necrosis are uncommon [1].

A thorough physical examination should be performed to exclude co-existing injuries, particularly as a result of high-energy trauma. Because the clavicle is in close proximity to the brachial plexus and subclavian vessels, associated neurovascular injury may occur (3%) [2]. The risk of neurovascular injury increases with high-energy trauma and marked fracture displacement or comminution. A blood pressure discrepancy between the two upper extremities is suggestive of vascular injury. Duplex scanning or arteriography should be undertaken if the diagnosis is suspected.

The radiographic diagnosis is usually made on the basis of a single anteroposterior (AP) view. A

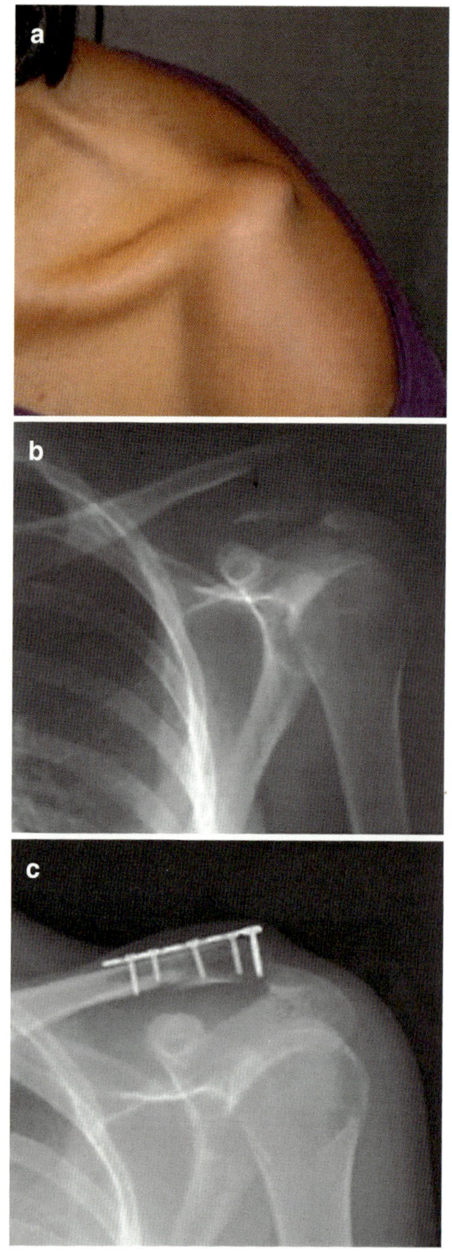

Fig. 8.3 (**a**) Clinical photograph of a displaced left distal clavicle fracture in a 21-year-old woman who fell onto her left shoulder. (**b**) Preoperative AP radiograph demonstrating fracture displacement with no residual cortical contact between the bone ends. (**c**) AP radiograph obtained 3 months postoperatively (the patient was treated with a distal radius 2.4-mm locking plate and simultaneous coracoclavicular stabilization using suture) demonstrating fracture healing. (Reprinted with permission from Banerjee R, Waterman B, Padalecki J, Robertson W. Management of distal clavicle fractures. J Am Acad Orthop Surg. 2011;19(7):392–401)

true AP view of the clavicle and a 30° cephalic tilt view should be obtained to allow biplanar assessment of the bony deformity. Computed tomography with three-dimensional reconstructions may be helpful in special situations, such as the evaluation of medial clavicular physeal fractures or SC fracture-dislocations. Stress radiographs are occasionally used to assess the integrity of the CC ligaments in association with lateral-end fractures [19]. A careful clinical and radiographic survey is also needed to exclude an associated chest injury, such as a pneumothorax or hemothorax [20], which occurs in 3% of patients and is almost always associated with multiple ipsilateral rib fractures. Evidence of an ipsilateral shoulder injury should also be specifically sought on the initial trauma series radiographs.

Treatment

Mid-Shaft Fractures

There is general agreement that undisplaced fractures should be treated nonoperatively. Fractures of the middle third of the clavicle usually proceed to bony union uneventfully without the need for surgery. Studies have reported that significant risk factors for nonunion include older age, female sex, fracture displacement (with shortening of 2 cm or more), and fracture comminution [21]. In most studies, the rate of nonunion when patients were treated nonoperatively has been <1% [19, 22–25]. However, these studies included fractures in children, which nearly always unite. The standard of care is initial immobilization in either a sling or figure-of-8 bandage, with immobilization discontinued when the level of pain allows. More recent studies have demonstrated higher rates of nonunion and poorer functional outcomes after nonoperative treatment, while the results of primary operative reduction and fixation have improved considerably [26–28]. Currently, there is considerable debate about whether acute displaced fractures should be treated operatively or nonoperatively.

Plate fixation provides immediate rigid stabilization and pain relief and facilitates early mobilization. Most commonly, the plate is implanted on the superior aspect of the clavicle; biomechanical studies have shown this to be advantageous, especially in the presence of inferior cortical comminution [29]. Superior plating techniques have greater load to failure and bending failure stiffness than anterior-inferior plating [30]. Despite the biomechanical advantages, the superior approach is associated with a greater risk of injury to the underlying neurovascular structures during fracture manipulation and drilling. In addition, plate prominence with the superior approach may require hardware removal in symptomatic patients. Currently, the implants most commonly used are either dynamic compression or locking plates. Reconstruction plates have fallen into disfavor, since they are susceptible to deformation at the fracture site, leading to malunion. Site specific precontoured locking plates have become increasingly popular and may be less prominent after healing, leading to lower rates of hardware removal after union [29].

Intramedullary nailing is another option in the surgical treatment of clavicle fractures. Intramedullary repair of midshaft clavicle fractures with a titanium elastic nail can be safe and minimally invasive [31]; however, implant related complications can include medial perforations, lateral penetrations, nail breakage, and hardware irritations, as described by Frigg et al. [32]. There is biomechanical evidence to suggest that plate fixation provides a stronger construct than intramedullary fixation [33]. A variety of devices, including Knowles pins, Hagie pins, Rockwood pins, and minimally invasive titanium nails, have been used [34]. Two methods of implant insertion have been described: antegrade, through an anteromedial entry point in the medial fragment, and retrograde, through a posterolateral entry portal in the lateral fragment [2]. More studies are needed to fully define the role of intramedullary nail fixation in clavicular fractures.

Lateral Third Fractures

According to Neer classification [12], nonsurgical management is the treatment of choice for type I fractures, and the protocol is similar to that of shaft fractures. In type II fractures, deforming forces, such as the weight of the arm and muscular attachments, lead to inferior and medial displacement of the distal fragment via its ligamentous attachments. These fracture patterns are associated with delayed union and nonunion. Type III fractures extend into the articular surface of the AC joint with no ligamentous injury and are generally stable. Although several retrospective studies have reported high rates of nonunion after nonsurgical treatment of displaced lateral-third fractures, a study showed a low incidence of nonunion after nonsurgical treatment, whereas high complication rates have been reported with surgical fixation [21, 35]. Because most of these injuries occur in middle-aged and elderly patients, nonunion is often tolerated, with few patients requiring delayed surgical intervention [21, 35]. In the small number of patients in whom substantial arthritis of the AC joint develops, resection of the lateral segment may result in a functional shoulder [2]. Treatment options for type II fractures include CC screws, hook-plate fixation, locking plates, Kirschner wire fixation, and suture techniques. Intra-articular fractures (type III) carry an increased risk of late AC osteoarthritis, which may require further treatment. Type III fractures are generally adequately managed nonsurgically, although open reduction and internal fixation (ORIF) may be indicated if a large fragment resulting in significant articular step-off is present.

Medial Third Fractures

Medial third clavicle fractures are rare, and most are extra-articular and minimally displaced [1]. Stability depends on the integrity of the costoclavicular ligaments. If the ligaments are ruptured, the lateral fragment displaces anteriorly and may overlap the medial fragment. These fractures are usually managed nonsurgically, unless fracture displacement produces mediastinal compromise. In such circumstances, an emergent attempt at closed reduction should be made, with open reduction performed next if that is unsuccessful. If surgical stabilization of this fracture is required, a thoracic surgeon should be available. A variety of internal fixation techniques, including use of the modified Balser plate and use of polyester fiber suture or other strong braided interosseous sutures, have been described [36]. However, supporting evidence is limited for each technique, and there is a lack of consensus regarding the optimal treatment of fractures that require surgical treatment.

Complications

The main intraoperative complication in clavicular fracture fixation is injury to the subclavian artery or vein from drill penetration or at the time of fracture mobilization. As with any other failed osteosynthesis, postoperative wound complications, scar dysesthesia, infection, fixation failure, nonunion, and malunion may occur and eventually require revision surgery.

Nonunion

Recent studies have suggested that adults suffering from a displaced fracture have a higher rate of nonunion (up to 15%) [1, 19, 21, 23, 24, 37–41]. The risk factors associated with nonunion include increasing age, female sex, fracture displacement, and comminution [1, 21].

Shaft nonunions in active individuals are usually symptomatic, causing pain [24, 38, 42–44] and a clicking sensation during motion [24, 38]. Clinical and radiographic signs of nonunion include mobility or pain on stressing of the fracture and an absence of bridging callus on radiographs [21, 45]. CT scans may be helpful by demonstrating whether bridging callus is present across the fracture site. A number of operative techniques have been described to treat shaft nonunions [38, 42, 43, 46, 47]. Plate fixation permits early mobilization of the shoulder while providing secure fixation, with a predictably high rate of union and a low risk of complications [42, 48, 49]. A variety of implants have been used, including reconstruction, wave, dynamic compression, and low-contact dynamic compression plates. Supplementary autologous bone-grafting (from the iliac crest, fibula, or medial femoral condyle) is commonly used and may shorten the time to union [2]. Intramedullary fixation and external fixation have been used only in small series.

A nonunion rate of 11.5% after nonoperative treatment of lateral-end fractures has been reported [21]. The independent risk factors for this complication include age and displacement of the fracture [2, 21]. The symptoms of nonunion in this area include pain and loss of shoulder function. The treatment options for an established symptomatic nonunion include excision of the lateral end of the clavicle, or fracture fixation with or without bone graft. Excision is usually preferred if the lateral fragment is small and the CC ligaments are intact, whereas fixation is used when there is a larger fragment, with good bone stock. The results of treatment have been assessed only in small studies mainly focusing on the treatment of midshaft nonunions.

Malunion

All displaced fractures that are treated nonoperatively heal with some degree of malunion due to angulation and/or shortening [50], but often with few or no symptoms [51]. However, some authors have reported that shortening of >15 mm is associated with shoulder discomfort and dysfunction [23, 39, 41]. Others have suggested that permanent shortening has no clinical relevance [52, 53]. Corrective osteotomy (with or without) adjuvant autologous bone-grafting and plate fixation can improve function in patients in whom symptomatic malunion has produced neurovascular problems or cosmetic deformity [2]. Since many clavicular malunions are asymptomatic, careful patient selection and counseling before surgery is recommended.

Neurological Complications

Nerve compression can be caused acutely by displacement of the fracture fragments, or it can be caused by chronic malunion or nonunion [54, 55]. Brachial plexus palsy may also occur as a complication of operative treatment with use of intramedullary fixation [56]. The exact prevalence is poorly defined and the clinical tests for these syndromes are nonspecific. Consequently, the diagnosis should be made only if the patient has a suggestive clinical history with supportive evidence on electrophysiological testing, arteriography or venography, and specialized imaging. The treatment should be directed toward correction of the malunion or nonunion.

Refracture

Refracture can occur after both nonoperative and operative treatment, with risk factors including epilepsy and alcohol abuse and an early return to contact sports [57]. Reinjury after operative treatment may cause breakage of the fixation device, or fracture around the implant, whereas a reinjury after implant removal may produce further fracture at the site of the previous injury. Nonunion is relatively common after refracture, and internal fixation is often required.

Osteoarthritis of the Acromioclavicular Joint

This complication occurs most frequently following an intra-articular fracture and the major symptom is activity-related pain. Physical examination reveals local swelling and tenderness, with a positive active compression test as described by O'Brien et al. [58]. Plain radiographs may reveal signs of osteoarthritis. Symptomatic osteoarthritis of the AC joint should be treated with either arthroscopic or open excision of the lateral fragment [12, 59]. In cases where there is concomitant ligamentous instability, the Weaver-Dunn CC ligament transfer procedure [60] should be performed to restore stability to the lateral end of the clavicle.

Questions

1. Which of the following is not a risk factor for non-union in clavicle fractures?
   A. Male sex
   B. Older age
   C. Communition
   D. Lateral third fractures
   E. <1 cm displacement
   A

2. A patient who is injured in a car accident referred to your hospital's ER. You recognize in his examination and on radiological evaluation that the patient has a displaced lateral third clavicle fracture. You suspect from injury to the CC ligaments. Which of the following is the most appropriate type of fracture according to Allman classification with Neer modification?
   A. Group 1
   B. Group 2 type I
   C. Group 2 type II
   D. Group2 type III
   E. Group 3
   C

3. What is the most appropriate management of a displaced non-union of midshaft clavicle?
   A. Sling
   B. Closed reduction + percutaneous pinning
   C. Open reduction + intramedullary nailing
   D. Weaver Dunn procedure
   E. Open reduction + plate fixation
   E

What is new?

A new double endobutton technique is described for unstable distal clavicle fractures by two researches from New York University Hospital for Joint Diseases. This technique seems successful to achieve a high rate of union and does not need any removal of hardware after healing. A larger case group is needed to improve the reliability of the study.

Closed-Loop Double Endobutton Technique for Repair of Unstable Distal Clavicle Fractures, The Orthopaedic Journal of Sports Medicine, 2016 July, Struhl S, Wolfson TS.

References

1. Robinson CM. Fractures of the clavicle in the adult. Epidemiology and classification. J Bone Joint Surg Br. 1998;80(3):476–84.
2. Khan LA, Bradnock TJ, Scott C, Robinson CM. Fractures of the clavicle. J Bone Joint Surg Am. 2009;91(2):447–60.
3. Kubiak R, Slongo T. Operative treatment of clavicle fractures in children: a review of 21 years. J Pediatr Orthop. 2002;22(6):736–9.
4. Ljunggren AE. Clavicular function. Acta Orthop Scand. 1979;50:261–8.
5. De Palma A. Surgery of the shoulder. 3rd ed. Philadelphia: JB Lippincott; 1983.
6. Fukuda K, Craig EV, An KN, Cofield RH, Chao EY. Biomechanical study of the ligamentous system of the acromioclavicular joint. J Bone Joint Surg Am. 1986 Mar;68(3):434–40.
7. Berkheiser EJ. Old united clavicular fractures in the adult. Surg Gynecol Obstet. 1937;64:1064–72.
8. Nordqvist A, Petersson C. The incidence of fractures of the clavicle. Clin Orthop Relat Res. 1994;300:127–32.
9. Nowak J, Mallmin H, Larsson S. The aetiology and epidemiology of clavicular fractures. A prospective study during a two-year period in Uppsala, Sweden. Injury. 2000;31:353–8.
10. Stanley D, Trowbridge EA, Norris SH. The mechanism of clavicular fracture. A clinical and biomechanical analysis. J Bone Joint Surg Br. 1988;70:461–4.
11. Allman Jr FL. Fractures and ligamentous injuries of the clavicle and its articulation. J Bone Joint Surg Am. 1967;49:774–84.
12. Neer II CS. Fractures of the distal third of the clavicle. Clin Orthop Relat Res. 1968;58:43–50.
13. Craig EV. Fractures of the clavicle. In: Rockwood Jr CA, Matsen 3rd FA, editors. The shoulder. Philadelphia: WB Saunders; 1990. p. 367–412.
14. Eskola A. Sternoclavicular dislocation. A plea for open treatment. Acta Orthop Scand. 1986;57:227–8.
15. Hanby CK, Pasque CB, Sullivan JA. Medial clavicle physis fracture with posterior displacement and vascular compromise: the value of three-dimensional computed tomography and duplex ultrasound. Orthopedics. 2003;26:81–4.
16. Jougon JB, Lepront DJ, Dromer CE. Posterior dislocation of the sternoclavicular joint leading to mediastinal compression. Ann Thorac Surg. 1996;61:711–3.

17. McKee MD. Clavicle fractures. In: Bucholz RW, Court-Brown CM, Heckman JD, Tornet P, editors. Rockwood and Green's fractures in adults. 7th ed. Oxford: Lippincott Williams and Wilkins; 2009. p. 1106–43.
18. Hertel R, Hempfing A, Stiehler M, Leunig M. Predictors of humeral head ischemia after intracapsular fracture of the proximal humerus. J Shoulder Elb Surg. 2004;13(4):427–33.
19. Rowe CR. An atlas of anatomy and treatment of midclavicular fractures. Clin Orthop Relat Res. 1968;58:29–42.
20. Dugdale TW, Fulkerson JP. Pneumothorax complicating a closed fracture of the clavicle. A case report. Clin Orthop Relat Res. 1987;221:212–4.
21. Robinson CM, Court-Brown CM, McQueen MM, Wakefield AE. Estimating the risk of nonunion following nonoperative treatment of a clavicular fracture. J Bone Joint Surg Am. 2004;86(7):1359–65.
22. Andersen K, Jensen PO, Lauritzen J. Treatment of clavicular fractures. Figure of- eight bandage versus a simple sling. Acta Orthop Scand. 1987;58:71–4.
23. Eskola A, Vainionpää S, Myllynen P, Pätiälä H, Rokkanen P. Outcome of clavicular fracture in 89 patients. Arch Orthop Trauma Surg. 1986;105:337–8.
24. Neer II CS. Nonunion of the clavicle. J Am Med Assoc. 1960;172:1006–11.
25. Sankarankutty M, Turner BW. Fractures of the clavicle. Injury. 1975;7:101–6.
26. Canadian Orthopaedic Trauma Society. Nonoperative treatment compared with plate fixation of displaced midshaft clavicular fractures. A multicenter, randomized clinical trial. J Bone Joint Surg Am. 2007;89:1–10.
27. McKee MD, Wild LM, Schemitsch EH. Midshaft malunions of the clavicle. J Bone Joint Surg Am. 2003;85:790–7.
28. McKee MD, Pedersen EM, Jones C, Stephen DJ, Kreder HJ, Schemitsch EH, Wild LM, Potter J. Deficits following nonoperative treatment of displaced midshaft clavicular fractures. J Bone Joint Surg Am. 2006;88:35–40.
29. Iannotti MR, Crosby LA, Stafford P, Grayson G, Goulet R. Effects of plate location and selection on the stability of midshaft clavicle osteotomies: a biomechanical study. J Shoulder Elb Surg. 2002;11(5):457–62.
30. Robertson C, Celestre P, Mahar A, Schwartz A. Reconstruction plates for stabilization of mid-shaft clavicle fractures: differences between nonlocked and locked plates in two different positions. J Shoulder Elb Surg. 2009;18(2):204–9.
31. Mueller M, Rangger C, Striepens N, Burger C. Minimally invasive intramedullary nailing of midshaft clavicular fractures using titanium elastic nails. J Trauma. 2008;64(6):1528–34.
32. Frigg A, Rillmann P, Perren T, Gerber M, Ryf C. Intramedullary nailing of clavicular midshaft fractures with the titanium elastic nail: problems and complications. Am J Sports Med. 2009;37(2):352–9.
33. Golish SR, Oliviero JA, Francke EI, Miller MD. A biomechanical study of plate versus intramedullary devices for midshaft clavicle fixation. J Orthop Surg. 2008;3:28.
34. Jubel A, Andermahr J, Schiffer G, Tsironis K, Rehm KE. Elastic stable intramedullary nailing of midclavicular fractures with a titanium nail. Clin Orthop Relat Res. 2003;408:279–85.
35. Robinson CM, Cairns DA. Primary nonoperative treatment of displaced lateral fractures of the clavicle. J Bone Joint Surg Am. 2004;86(4):778–82.
36. Franck WM, Siassi RM, Hennig FF. Treatment of posterior epiphyseal disruption of the medial clavicle with a modified Balser plate. J Trauma. 2003;55(5):966–8.
37. Zenni Jr EJ, Krieg JK, Rosen MJ. Open reduction and internal fixation of clavicular fractures. J Bone Joint Surg Am. 1981;63:147–51.
38. Wilkins RM, Johnston RM. Ununited fractures of the clavicle. J Bone Joint Surg Am. 1983;65:773–8.
39. Wick M, Müller EJ, Kollig E, Muhr G. Midshaft fractures of the clavicle with a shortening of more than 2 cm predispose to nonunion. Arch Orthop Trauma Surg. 2001;121:207–11.
40. Davids PH, Luitse JS, Strating RP, van der Hart CP. Operative treatment for delayed union and nonunion of midshaft clavicular fractures: AO reconstruction plate fixation and early mobilization. J Trauma. 1996;40:985–6.
41. Hill JM, McGuire MH, Crosby LA. Closed treatment of displaced middle-third fractures of the clavicle gives poor results. J Bone Joint Surg Br. 1997;79:537–9.
42. Jupiter JB, Leffert RD. Non-union of the clavicle. Associated complications and surgical management. J Bone Joint Surg Am. 1987;69:753–60.
43. Der Tavitian J, Davison JN, Dias JJ. Clavicular fracture non-union surgical outcome and complications. Injury. 2002;33:135–43.
44. Johnson Jr EW, Collins HR. Nonunion of the clavicle. Arch Surg. 1963;87:963–6.
45. Nowak J, Holgersson M, Larsson S. Can we predict long-term sequelae after fractures of the clavicle based on initial findings? A prospective study with nine to ten years of follow-up. J Shoulder Elb Surg. 2004;13:479–86.
46. Rosenberg N, Neumann L, Wallace AW. Functional outcome of surgical treatment of symptomatic nonunion and malunion of midshaft clavicle fractures. J Shoulder Elb Surg. 2007;16:510–3.
47. Khan SA, Shamshery P, Gupta V, Trikha V, Varshney MK, Kumar A. Locking compression plate in long standing clavicular nonunions with poor bone stock. J Trauma. 2008;64:439–41.
48. Marti RK, Nolte PA, Kerkhoffs GM, Besselaar PP, Schaap GR. Operative treatment of mid-shaft clavicular non-union. Int Orthop. 2003;27:131–5.
49. Nowak J, Rahme H, Holgersson M, Lindsjö U, Larsson S. A prospective comparison between external fixation and plates for treatment of midshaft nonunions of the clavicle. Ann Chir Gynaecol. 2001;90:280–5.
50. Edelson JG. The bony anatomy of clavicular malunions. J Shoulder Elb Surg. 2003;12:173–8.

51. McKee MD, Wild LM, Schemitsch EH. Midshaft malunions of the clavicle. Surgical technique. J Bone Joint Surg Am. 2004;86(Suppl 1):37–43.
52. Nordqvist A, Redlund-Johnell I, von Scheele A, Petersson CJ. Shortening of clavicle after fracture. Incidence and clinical significance, a 5-year follow-up of 85 patients. Acta Orthop Scand. 1997;68:349–51.
53. Oroko PK, Buchan M, Winkler A, Kelly IG. Does shortening matter after clavicular fractures? Bull Hosp Jt Dis. 1999;58:6–8.
54. Barbier O, Malghem J, Delaere O, Vande Berg B, Rombouts JJ. Injury to the brachial plexus by a fragment of bone after fracture of the clavicle. J Bone Joint Surg Br. 1997;79:534–6.
55. Chen CE, Liu HC. Delayed brachial plexus neurapraxia complicating malunion of the clavicle. Am J Orthop. 2000;29:321–2.
56. Ring D, Holovacs T. Brachial plexus palsy after intramedullary fixation of a clavicular fracture. A report of three cases. J Bone Joint Surg Am. 2005;87:1834–7.
57. Flinkkilä T, Ristiniemi J, Lakovaara M, Hyvönen P, Leppilahti J. Hook-plate fixation of unstable lateral clavicle fractures: a report on 63 patients. Acta Orthop. 2006;77:644–9.
58. O'Brien SJ, Pagnani MJ, Fealy S, McGlynn SR, Wilson JB. The active compression test: a new and effective test for diagnosing labral tears and acromioclavicular joint abnormality. Am J Sports Med. 1998;26:610–3.
59. Petersson CJ. Resection of the lateral end of the clavicle. A 3 to 30-year follow-up. Acta Orthop Scand. 1983;54:904–7.
60. Weaver JK, Dunn HK. Treatment of acromioclavicular injuries, especially complete acromioclavicular separation. J Bone Joint Surg Am. 1972;54:1187–94.

Proximal Humerus Fractures

9

Cem Zeki Esenyel

Introduction

Proximal humeral fractures are the third most common fragility fracture and it account for 5–9% of all fractures [1, 2]. Proximal humerus fractures have a dual age distribution occurs either young people following high energy trauma or in those older than 50 years with low velocity injuries like simple fall [3]. In the elderly population, most of these fractures are related to osteoporosis [1, 3]. They have a bimodal age distribution. Proximal humeral fractures are the third most common fracture in elderly patients and pose an important socioeconomic problem [4]. More than 70% of the patients with these fractures are older than 60 years of age, and 80% are women [3, 5]. Complex three- and four part fractures account for >50% of cases in patients older than 60 years [6].

Fifty one percent of all humeral fractures are displaced fractures [7]. Because conservative management of displaced or unstable proximal humeral fractures often results malunion and poor functional outcome, surgical treatment is recommended [1, 7]. The treatment of choice remains a matter of controversy. There is no single method to impose itself as the gold standard of treatment [1].

Commonly utilized techniques include percutaneous fixation, open reduction with locking plate fixation (ORIF), intramedullary nailing (IMN), hemiarthroplasty (HA), and reverse shoulder arthroplasty (RSA) [6].

Anatomy

The proximal humerus includes the humeral head, greater tuberosity, lesser tuberosity, and the humeral shaft [8]. In the sagittal plane, the humeral head is retroverted an average of 30° relative to humeral shaft [8]. In the coronal plane, it is angled 130–150° cephalad relative to the diaphysis. Fracture through anatomic neck can result in significant vascular compromise to humeral head leading to avascular necrosis.

Because of their musculotendinous rotator cuff attachments, the greater and lesser tuberosities are deformed during the fracture. The supraspinatus muscle, the infraspinatus muscle, and the teres minor muscle attaches to the greater tuberosity [3, 9]. These three muscles yield a posteromedially directed deforming force. During the surgical neck fracture, these muscles can remain intact and causes typically varus and external rotation deformity [8].

Anterior and posterior humeral circumflex arteries supply humeral head vascularity [8]. The

C.Z. Esenyel, M.D.
Department of Orthopaedic Surgery,
Giresun University Medical Faculty,
Giresun, Turkey
e-mail: esenyel@yahoo.com

G. Huri, N.K. Paschos (eds.), *The Shoulder*, Orthopaedic Study Guide Series,
DOI 10.1007/978-3-319-51979-1_9

anterior humeral circumflex artery is the most important blood supply to the proximal humerus. The posterior humeral circumflex artery and muscular attachments of the proximal humerus are secondary important source of blood supplies. However, more recently, it was suggested that the contribution of the proximal humeral circumflex artery was more important than the anterior humeral circumflex artery [8, 9]. Sixty four percent of humeral head perfusion arises from the posterior humeral circumflex artery. The anterior humeral circumflex artery only contributes 36% of humeral head perfusion [9].

The axillary nerve is the most frequently injured nerve in proximal humeral fractures, and the suprascapular nerve is the second most commonly injured [8].

Clinical Evaluation

History and Physical

The most common mechanism is a fall from standing in an elderly, osteoporotic woman [8]. Other causes are high-energy traumas such as fall from height, motor vehicle crashes, seizures, and electric shocks. If a fracture of the proximal humerus in a young person occurs with a low energy, pathological fracture should be considered [2, 8].

Associated injuries of the shoulder girdle, upper extremity, and cervical spine should be considered [8].

The shoulder is usually swollen and ecchymotic. Physical examination may be limited in the acute fracture setting because of pain and swelling. The skin should be inspected for associated lesion, ecchymosis, and prior surgical scars [8]. The area of bruising is most commonly seen in the chest as well as the arm distal to the deltoid muscle. Gross deformity may indicate glenohumeral dislocation.

Neurovascular examination should be done, with particular attention to axillary nerve. Acute neurovascular compromise may need for emergent surgical intervention [8]. Distal pulses should be evaluated and compared to the contralateral side. Differences in distal pulses may be an indication for arteriogram.

Radiographic examination should be limited to a trauma series, which does not require the patient to move the arm.

1. True Anteroposterior Radiograph
   It is taken perpendicular to the glenohumeral joint by angling the beam 40 degrees away from midline to account for scapulothoracic and glenoid version.
2. The lateral or scapular-Y view
3. A velpeau axillary view
   This view is critical to confirm location of the humeral head.
   These views allow for adequate evaluation of fracture anatomy, comminution, and fragment displacement.
   Computed tomography (CT) has been shown to improve the accuracy of fracture classification. It is also very beneficial for surgical planning.
   Magnetic resonance imaging (MRI) rarely indicated in the acute setting. If underlying bony pathology or malignancy is suspected, it becomes a useful tool.

Classification

A lot of classifications have been described, including the Kocher, Codman, and Jakob and Ganz systems.

Codman's Classification

In 1934, Codman described the segment theory for the classification of proximal humeral fractures [10]. In this classification, there are four main segments (shaft, head, greater tuberosity, and lesser tuberosity), and it has twelve basic patterns 3).

Disadvantages:

- Distinction between anatomic and surgical neck fractures is not made.
- It does not include fracture displacement

AO Classification

The AO classification for proximal humerus fractures was initially described by Muller in 1988 [11]. This AO/OTA classification distinguishes three basic fracture types:

A. extra-articular, unifocal
B. extra-articular, bifocal
C. articular

This clasification has also a total of 27 subtypes.

Neer Classification

Neer classification is the most widely used classification [12]. In this classification, the proximal humerus is divided into four parts: the greater tuberosity, the lesser tuberosity, the articular segment (head), and the humeral shaft. The classification based on displacement of one or more of these four main segment. The fracture is thought displaced if there is 1 cm of displacement or 45° of angulation. However, if the greater tuberosity is displaced more than 0.5 cm it is accepted as a displaced fracture [3].

It has six group:

I. minimal displacement
II. displaced anatomic neck fracture
III. displaced surgical neck fracture
IV. displaced greater tuberosity fracture
V. displaced lesser tuberosity
VI. fracture-dislocation

Displaced number of main segments indicates one, two, three or four-part fractures.

The varus and valgus fractures are different from each other [13]. The varus fracture may present as an impaction or distraction (disruption) type. Valgus fractures may be impacted in straight lateral or posterolateral direction [13]. It is assumed that the periosteum leading medially to the humeral head is intact and that the vessels passing through the periosteum are also intact. Because of this survival of the humeral head segment is protected [13].

Hertl et al. [14] identified he morphologic risk factors for humeral head ischemia. The most relevant predictors of ischemia are the length of the dorsomedial metaphyseal extension, the integrity of the medial hinge, and the basic fracture type determined with the binary description system. Disruption of the medial hinge is a critical factor for fractures with medial metaphyseal extensions below 8 mm, and distruption of the medial hinge with displacement of >2 mm. Displacement-induced stripping of the periosteum (and vessels) might distinguish between perfusion and ischemia in this specific subgroup.

Treatment

Approximately 20% of proximal humeral fractures require surgical intervention; most are 3- to 4- part fractures [24]. Fracture treatment depends on the type of fracture, the degree of fragment displacement and fracture stability [2].

Nonoperative Treatment

Nondisplaced or minimally displaced fractures can be treated conservatively. Two weeks of sling immobilization is suggested. Then passive range of motion should be started. Patients should be controlled with serial radiographs of the proximal humerus weekly until ensure fracture stability [1, 3].

Outcomes for nonoperative management of the minimally displaced fractures in elderly patients are good to excellent. Valgus impacted fractures could also be treated conservatively with a good to excellent outcomes. Patients with valgus impacted fractures regained approximately 80% of the abduction and flexion strength compared with the contralateral extremity [15]. Court-Brown et al reported positive results in displaced 2 part fractures treated nonoperatively. They compared to nonoperative and operative management, and found that surgery did not improve outcome in elderly patients [16].

In elderly, low demand patients, or those with significant medical comorbidities, even more complex fractures may be treated without surgery.

Complications of Non-operative Treatment

- Delayed union or nonunion (7%)
- Malunion
- Osteonecrosis of the humeral head (6.5%)
- Axillary nerve lesions (30%)
- Loss of reduction

Surgical Treatment

Severely displaced fractures warrant surgical management [3]. Surgical management options are guided by bone quality, fracture pattern, degree of comminution, and age and activity level of patients [3].

Surgical options include closed reduction and percutaneous pinning, transosseous suture fixation, open reduction and internal fixation with plate, haemiarthroplasty, or revers shoulder arthroplasty [3].

In osteoporotic elderly patients, bone quality is poor, which makes screw purchase and fixation less secure. Also, healing capacity in osteoporosis is decreased. Failure of implant fixation is increased [3].

Surgical treatment requires anatomic reduction and stable fixation.

Percutaneous Pinning

Closed reduction and percutaneous pinning with Kirschner (K) wires is a minimally invasive technique (Fig. 9.1) [17]. This offers advantages over open techniques that limit the exposure, minimizing surgical trauma and reducing the risk of osteonecrosis [7]. Theoretically, it limits iatrogenic vascular damage, postoperative pain, operative time, and blood loss as well as improving cosmesis [7, 17]. However, the procedure requires advanced skill, minimal fracture comminution, and a cooperative patient. It has disadvantages such as migration of K wires (33%), need for implant removal, reduced primary fixation stability, or risk of neurovascular damage [7].

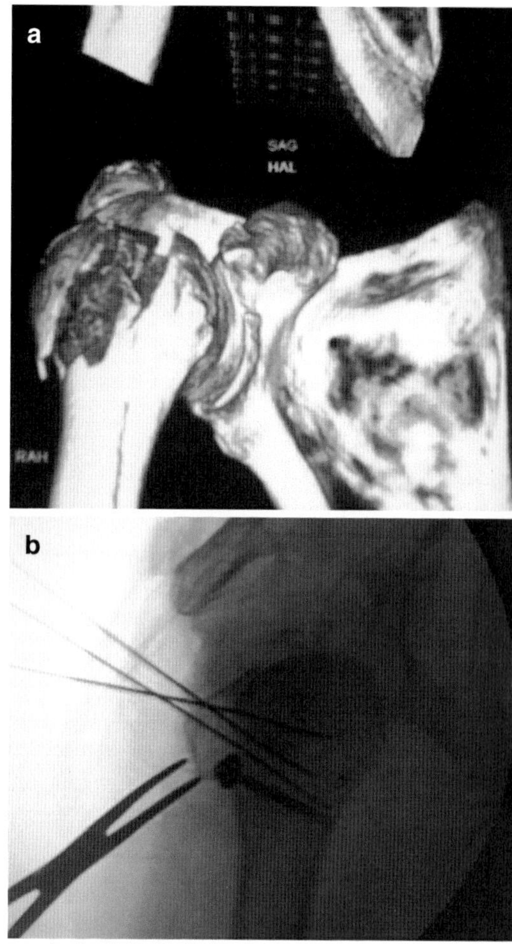

Fig. 9.1 Closed reduction and percutaneous pinning with Kirschner (K) wires is a minimally invasive technique for the treatment of proximal humeral fracture (**a**): fracture of the proximal humerus is seen; (**b**): The humeral fracture was treated by closed reduction and percutaneous osteosynthesis with Kirschner wires

Necessities for percutaneous pinning:

- Good bone quality.
- Lack of communication in the proximal humeral metaphysis at the medial aspect of the anatomic neck.
- Acceptable stability should be obtained.
- Indications:
- Two-parts proximal humeral fractures ideally surgical neck.

- Three-or four part fractures with adequate bone stock.
- All valgus impacted 3-part and 4- part fractures.
- In elderly patient, the goal is rather to provide a painless range of motion.
- Although percutaneous fixation has demonstrated good midterm results, avascular necrosis rates are high [6].

Plating

Conventional plate osteosynthesis of proximal humeral fractures has been associated with a high complication rate [3]. The initial results showed that up to 100% of an implant failure rate was reported with osteoporotic bone. Initial plates were bulky, associated with the unacceptable infection rate and the high rate fixation failure in elderly osteoporotic patients [1].

Locking plate provide more stable osteosynthesis, significantly greater holding power of the humeral head, and leading to lower rates of implant failure or loss of fixation, thus allowing earlier mobilization [1].

Locking plates are different from the conventional plates, because of:

- Locking plates function as a locked internal fixator and do not need to be compressed for stability, allowing preservation of periosteal vascularity.
- They provide greater angular stability and better screw anchorage in osteoporotic bone [1].
- Locking plates provide better torsional fatigue resistance and stiffness than the blade plates. Accurate fracture reduction and correct screw placement in the humeral head should be check fluoroscopically in both anteroposterior and lateral planes with rotation of the humeral head. Primary screw perforation, implant related impingement, implant position and inadequate fracture reduction should be avoided [1]. Locking plates fail catastrophically as a complete "monoblock" by pulling out of the humeral head as shaft, because of osteoporosis of the humeral head [1].

Less invasive plating has been described for reduction and fixation of the proximal fractures the aim of this is minimal soft tissue dissection. The anterolateral acromial approach to the proximal humerus is used (Fig. 9.2). In this approach, the plane of the avascular anterior deltoid raphe is used. The axillary nerve should then be found and protected (Fig. 9.3) [18]. The fracture is reduced and plate is applied the lateral aspect of the fracture proximal humerus (Fig. 9.4). The aim is to apply the plate without dissection of the critical blood supply of the humeral head. Second incision is made distal to the humeral shaft. AVN rates are significantly lower (range from 0 to 2.6%) with minimally invasive deltoid splitting approach [19, 20].
Indications:

- Two, three and four pout-fractures with tuberosity on head fragment displacement.
- Risk factors for the early failure of the locking compression plate in osteoporotic proximal humeral fractures are:
- Malreduction
- Loss of medial support

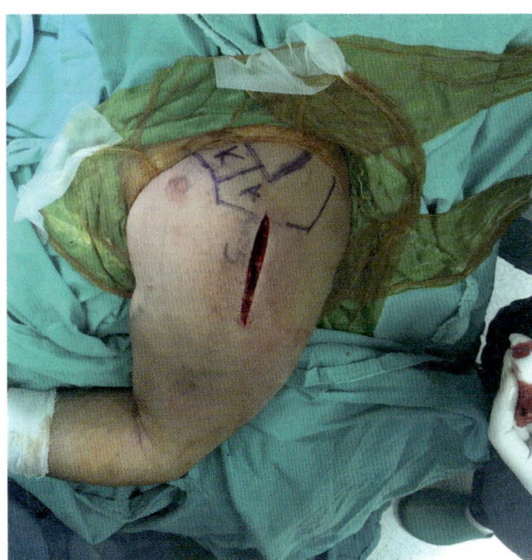

Fig. 9.2 Anterolateral or lateral transdeltoid approach to proximal humerus fractures can be used for various treatments of proximal humeral fractures. Incision is started from the tip of acromion down the lateral aspect of humerus

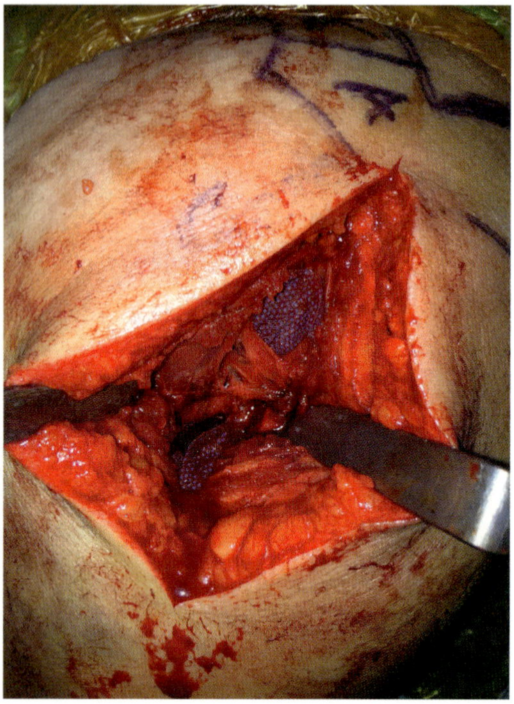

Fig. 9.3 Deltoid is splitted in the line of skin incision and axillary nerve is explored and secured under vision

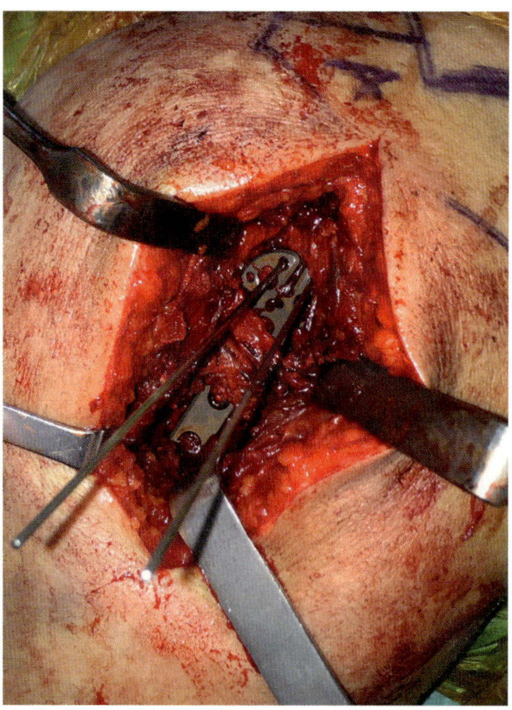

Fig. 9.4 The fracture is reduced and a plate is then slided beneath this nerve on the lateral surface of humerus

- Negligence of tension band sutures on the tuberosities [21].
- Aim for anatomical locking plate fixation:
- An anatomic on slightly impacted stable reduction is important
- A minimum of five equally distributed divergent fixed-angle plate screws should be placed in the humeral head.
- At least one superiorly directed oblique locked screw in the inferomedial region of the proximal fragment should be applied in order to achieve more stable medial column support.
- Screws in the humeral head should be left at least 5-10 mm below the subcortical bone to increase the stability.
- Factors for affecting the final outcome:
- Varus angulation of the humeral head is associated with a significantly worse clinical outcome.
- Patients age
- The length of the intact metaphysical segment attached to the articular fragment.
- Metaphysical segment length is less than 2 mm is associated with developing avascular necrosis.
- Smoking
- Osteoporosis
- Medical and psychiatric co-morbidities.

(The above are associated with an increased risk of nonunion.)

- Metaphysical communication on a fracture line extension distally.
- The medial side is defection and medial support is last.
- Complications [22]:
- The complication and reoperation rates of locked proximal humerus plating remain high [1, 3, 6].
- Avascular necrosis (4.5–16%).
- Screw cut-out (11.6%). Screw penetration is commonly due to varus deformation of the fragments. To prevent such complication, support of the medial column is advocated [21, 22].
- Re-operation (13.7–15.8%) [6].
- Intraoperative screw perforation of the humeral head (14%).

- Varus malunion (16.3%)
- Intraarticular screw perforation (7.5%)
- Subacromial impingement (4.8%)
- Infection (3.5%)
- Nonunion (3.4%)
- Miscellaneous complications (2.5%)

Although a vascular necrosis is initiated by fracture pattern itself, extensive soft tissue dissection may further put humeral head vascularity endanger. It is important that soft tissue stripping should be avoided during the surgery. Alignment and fracture reduction should be done with palpation and checked with fluoroscopically without soft tissue stripping.

Traditionally, the deltopectoral approach is mainstay for surgical treatment of proximal humerus fractures (Fig. 9.5) [17]. This approach allows for good access to the glenohumeral joint. However, this is suboptimal for the treatment of proximal humerus fractures, especially with locking plates and screws [17]. This anterior approach provides limited access to the lateral and posterior portion of the humerus.

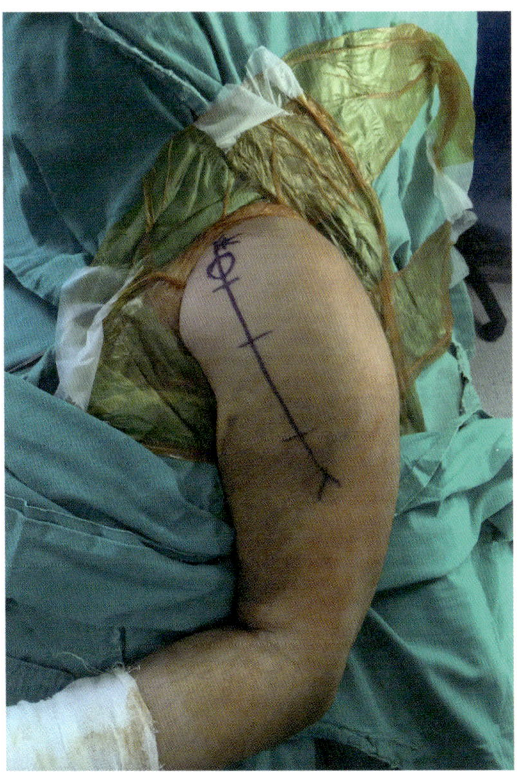

Fig. 9.5 The (*anterior*) deltopectoral approach can be used for almost any proximal humeral fracture treatment and is often the preferred approach

External Fixation

External fixation has been done to minimize the risk of infection and to protect humeral vascularity. External fixators are especially used in polytrauma patients. This can be applied in supine position.

External fixation should be reserved for open fractures and constable polytrauma patients.

Intramedullary Nailing

Indication:

- Three and four part fractures with metaphyseal comminution or diaphyseal involvement but only minor displacement of the tuberosities.
- Intramedullary nails demonstrate higher stiffness values, thus generating greater primary stability than extra-medullary load carries [1]. Intramedullary nails are load-sharing devices and these have been reported to provide clinical outcomes comparable to locking plates, with less soft tissue dissection and a possibly improved complication profile [1, 6]. Intramedullary nails can be excellent solution in complex cases of proximal humeral fractures with concomitant shaft fractures [1].
- Application of intramedullary nails for from part fractures is technically difficult [6].
- Complication associated with intramedullary nail [6]:
- Loss of reduction
- Malunion. It is associated with poor outcome
- Avascular necrosis. The incidence of avascular necrosis is between 3.7% and 11%.
- Reoperation rate with intramedullary nail is remains rather high (30%) and mostly due to screw penetration [1, 6]
- Values deformity

- Humeral head collapse (range between 20% and 37%)
- Great tuberosity displacement
- Producing an additional fracture through the entry point of the nail. This iatrogenic complication reported in up to 17,9% of cases [23, 24, 25].

Age is important for a good result more than 65 years of age have a worse functional result. This may be due to osteoporosis which causes reduce implant guy.

The nail should be inserted at least 5 mm below the subchondral bone of the humeral head and proximal screw length fluoroscopically verified. A more medial articular entry point may cause less damage to the rotator cuff. The medial aspect of the rotator cuff has more vascularity [6]. Despite meticulous repair, rotator cuff symptoms can persist.

Primary Hemiarthroplasty

Primary hemiarthroplasty may a choice for complex fractures of the proximal humerus, where adequate reduction and fixation cannot be achieved.

Indication:

- Four part fractures,
- Osteoporotic three-part fracture, fracture dislocation
- A short (< 8m) metaphyseal head extension
- Disruption of the medial periosteal hinge
- A shell-like head fragment
- Non-reconstructable head split
- Humeral head impression fractures

If there is not glenoid cartilage damage, hemiarthroplasty is usually preferred to total shoulder arthroplasty [3].

The important surgical principles when performing a hemiarthroplasty for the proximal humeral fractures include the following:

- The use of a deltopectoral approach
- Restoration of humeral length
- Restoration of humeral retroversion
- Secure fixation of the tuberosities to the prosthesis, to the shaft and to one another.

The poor prognostic factors are associated with:

- the old age
- the delay between injury and surgery. Surgery within one week of injury is associated with improved outcomes.
- preoperative neurologic deficit
- history of cigarette smoking
- Excessive alcohol consumption
- Female sex
- Tuberosity malposition and non-healing. Tuberosity position of more than 5mm above or more than 10mm below the prosthetic head is associated with poor results.
- Improper humeral stem position
- *Operative technique:*
- The patient is placed in the beach chair position with the back of the table elevated approximately 30–45°. The patients are placed at the edge of the operating table. Medial border of the scapula should be free from the table. All bony prominence should be well padded.
- These kinds of surgeries are performed under interscalene block anesthesia or general anesthesia exposure. If there is a documented neurological injury interscalene block is contraindicated.
- Antibiotics should be used for prophylaxis.

Surgical approach is planned to contribute minimal additional trauma to the soft tissues and vascular structures in the area of the proximal humerus.

A deltopectoral incision is made beginning at the level superior to the coracoid and passing to a point directly anterior to the deltoid insertion. The cephalic vein is dissected laterally. During the operation, the axillary nerve must be identified and protected. Continuity of the axillary nerve can be verified using the Tug Test [26]. 1 cm of the superior border of the pectoralis major tendon is released (Fig. 9.6). The tuberosities the found and heavy non-absorbable sutures are placed through the tendinous part rotator cuffs to fix the tuberosities later (Fig. 9.7a, b).

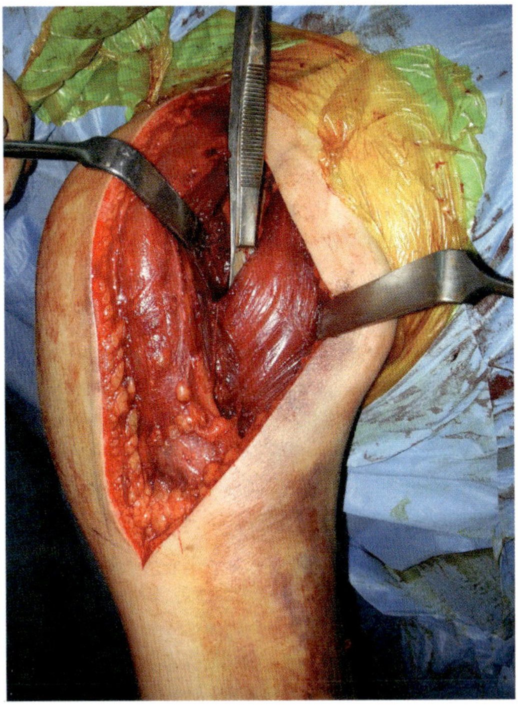

Fig. 9.6 One cm of the superior border of the pectoralis major tendon is released to increase the exposure and external rotation

The humeral head is removed and all cancellous bone in the humeral head is harvested and used for bone grafting of the tuberosities prior to fixation (Fig. 9.8a, b).

Adequate positioning of the prosthesis both in terms of height and version is critical towards the success of the procedure and in reestablishing relatively normal anatomy for the patient postoperatively. The positioning is important to reestablish the normal resting length of the deltoid muscle.

Options for determining adequate height for the prosthesis:

- The upper margin of the pectoralis major insertion site constitutes a reliable land mark to restore humeral head height, and is typically 56 mm from the superior aspect of the greater tuberosity [27]. The humeral head must be places just superior to the greater tuberosity in this location and by reducing the greater tuberosity to the shaft.
- Tension on the biceps has been recommended as a guide for the prosthetic height but is less reliable.

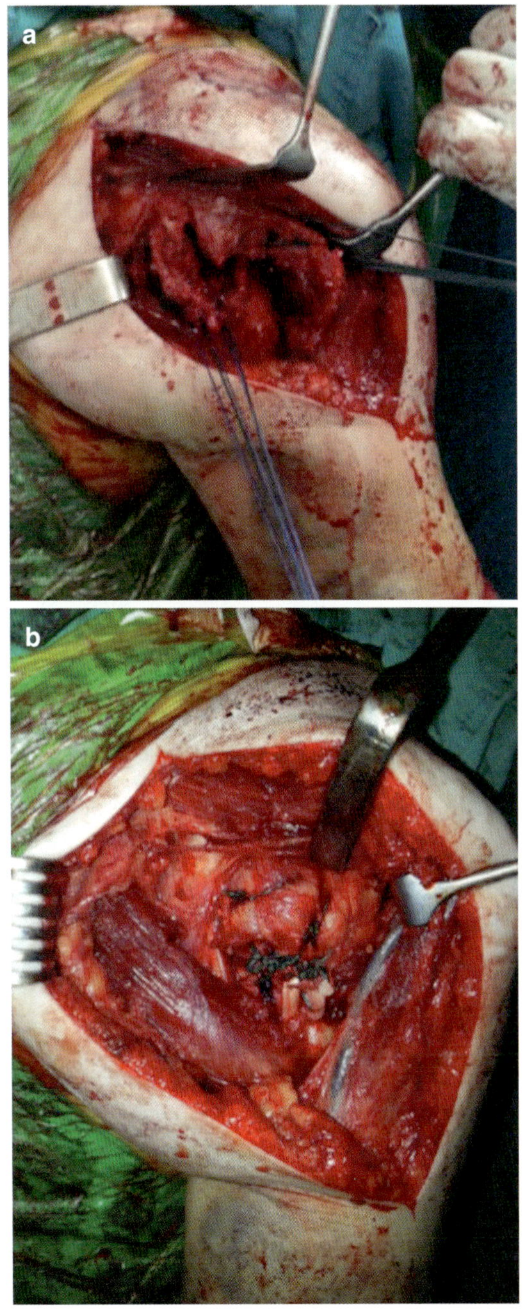

Fig. 9.7 The tuberosities the found and heavy non-absorbable sutures are placed through the tendinous part rotator cuffs (**a**) to fix the tuberosities later (**b**)

- Preoperative templating relative to the contralateral arm with jigs can be utilized for determining length.

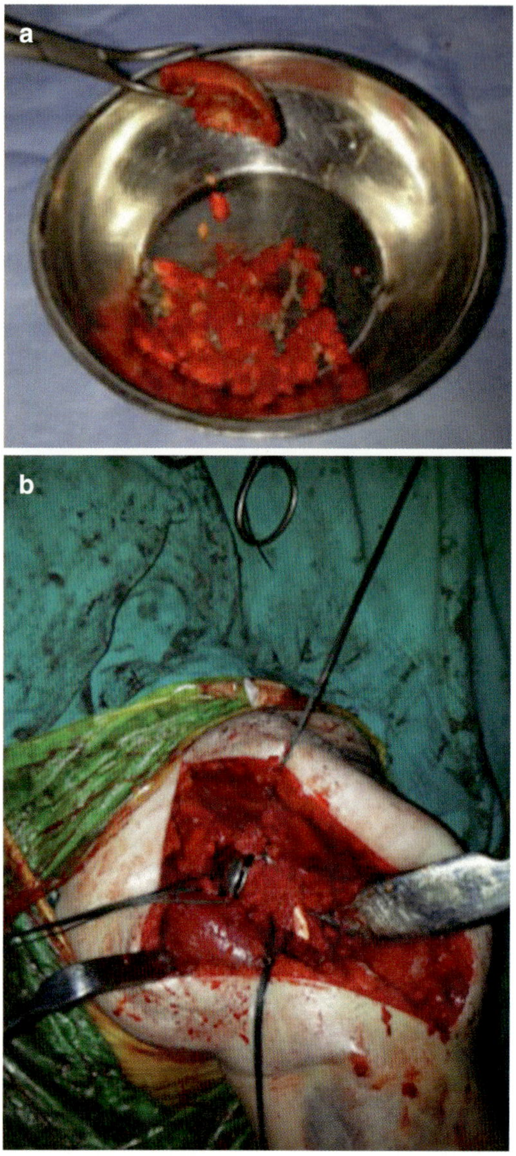

Fig. 9.8 All cancellous bone in the humeral head is harvested (**a**), used for bone grafting and put around the proximal part of the prosthesis and under the tuberosities to accelerate the healing of tuberosities (**b**)

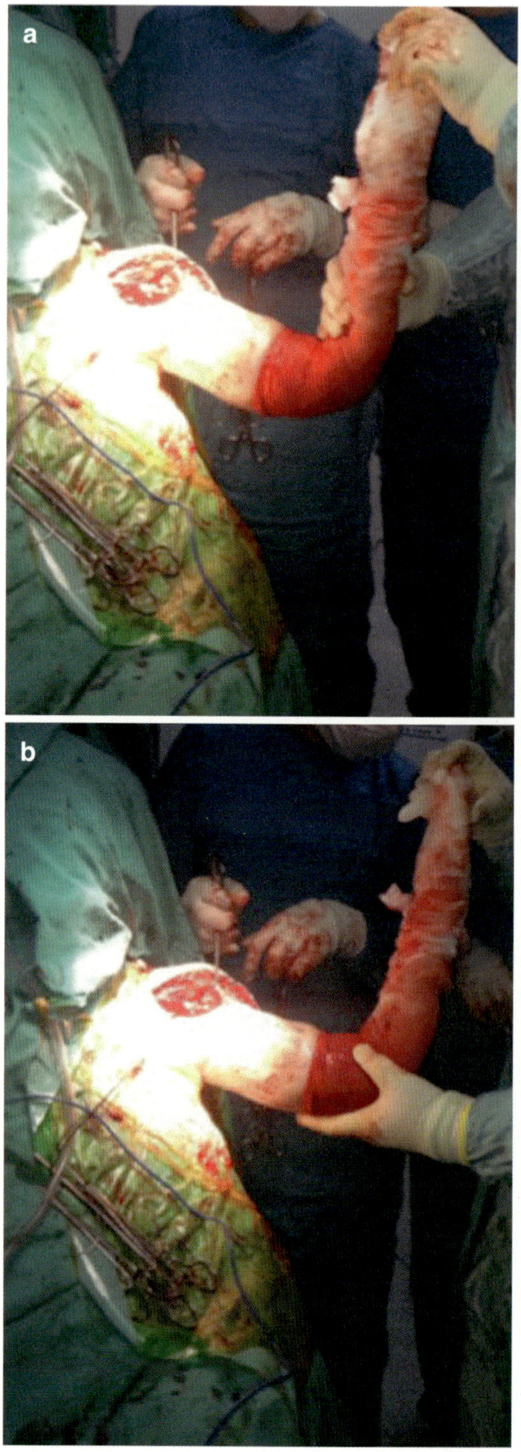

Fig. 9.9 During the operation, the arm is kept parallel to the floor with the elbow at 90 degree of flexion. A gentle traction is applied to the arm (a). Then the arm is turned to 20 degree of external rotation (b). In this position the humeral head of the prosthesis is turned towards the glenoid. At this position, land marks for humeral version and humeral heights are done with cautery

- During the operation, the arm is kept parallel to the floor with the elbow at 90 degree of flexion. A gentle traction is applied to the arm. Then the arm is turned to 20 degree of external rotation. In this position the humeral head of the prosthesis is turned towards the glenoid. At this position, land marks for humeral version and humeral heights are done with cautery (Fig. 9.9a, b).

Too low placement of the prosthesis will result in inferior subluxation of the humeral head relative to the glenoid. This will cause weakness in elevation. Too high placement of the prosthesis will lead to overstuffing of the joint superior subluxation, pain and stiffness.

Anatomic version of the humeral head should be kept between 20° and 40° of retroversion. Less version of approximately 20° is recommended, which places less tension on the greater tuberosity fragment during internal rotation and benefit healing. The posterior fin should generally be located just posterior to the bicipital groove. Because the stabilizing effect typically afforded by the tuberosities, which has been lost due to fractures, the humeral stem is generally cemented in place to avoid subsidence and malrotation.

Tuberosity Fixation

The success of the tuberosity healing is directly releated to the adequate reduction and fixation of the tuberosities during the surgery. Tuberosity healing is a major challenge and greater tuberosity pull off remains the most common complication of this surgery [5, 28]. The tuberosities must heal to each other and to the shaft as well as to the ingrowth material of the humeral prosthesis. The tuberosities are fixed to each other, to the prosthesis and to the shaft of the humerus with non-absorbable number 5 sutures. The bone graft is inserted between the prosthesis and the tuberosities to assist with healing [5]. Anatomic healing of the tuberosities significantly improves patients' satisfaction. Non-unions of the tuberosities are associated with lower results [5]. Because of that, fluoroscopic control should be done before fixation of the tuberosities (Fig. 9.10).

A randomized controlled study found significantly superior outcomes related to pain and quality of life for hemiarthroplasty compared with nonoperative treatment [29].

Complications of primary hemiarthroplasty

I. Intraoperative complications

- Component malpositioning
- Iatrogenic fracture
- Axillary nerve injury

II. Early postoperative complications

- Tuberosity pull-off (23%)
- Glenohumeral stiffness (5%)

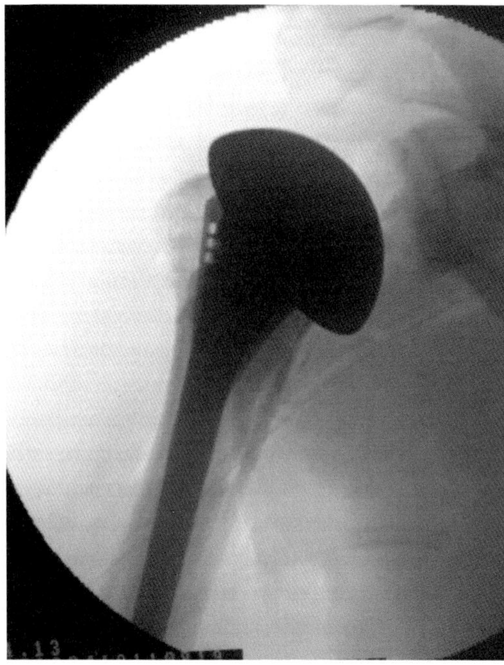

Fig. 9.10 Fluoroscopic control of the tuberosities positions should be done before fixation

- Instability (15%)
- Infection (6%)

III. Late complications

- Tuberosity absorption (7%)
- Tuberosity non-union (17%)
- Rotator Cuff dysfunction (25%)
- Glenoid erosion on arthrosis (35%)
- Loosening (3%)
- Periprosthetic fracture (2%)
- Heterotopic ossification (30%)

The "unhappy triad" involves prosthesis with excessive height and retroversion and the greater tuberosity is positioned too low.

Reverse Shoulder Arthroplasty

Reverse shoulder arthroplasty is indicated in elderly patients with pre-existing or anticipated rotator cuff deficiency and represents a salvage procedure for failed first-line treatment [5]. This prosthesis is generally not recommended in younger patients and it's use has most often been reported in patients around the age of 70.

Complications of reverse shoulder arthroplasty

- Scapular notching
  - It is the most frequent complication for reverse shoulder arthroplasty.
  - It causes polyethylene wear, synovitis (polyethylene disease), and glenoidal bone loss with potential loosening of the glenoid component.
- Acromial insaficiency

Conclusion

Treatment of proximal humeral fractures still remains a matter of controversy. Especially in osteoporotic bones, a lot of fixation techniques have been described.

The patient and fracture characteristics are very important while deciding the type of the surgical technique.

Questions

1. Which of the following is not an advantage of deltopectoral approach comparing with minimal invasice deltoid splitting approach?
   A. Lower AVN risk
   B. Lower axillary nerve injury risk
   C. Better deltoid function postoperatively
   D. Easier surgical technique
      A. Minimal invasive deltoid splitting approach has a lower risk for AVN of humeral head. Axillary nerve injury and better deltoid function postoperatively is associated with deltopectoral approach

2. What is the best treatment option for an elderly patient with 4-part fracture of the humeral head with no significant glenoid and rotator cuff injury ?
   A. Plate fixation
   B. K-wire fixation
   C. Arthroscopically assisted open fixation
   D. Hemiarthroplasty
   E. Reverse shoulder arthroplasty
      D. Even hemiarthroplasty is the first choice in multiple part humeral head fractures, new studies with reverse shoulder arthroplasty in patients with 3-4 part fracture of humeral head is promising.

3. Which one of the stated below is an inappropriate fixation technique for OR+IF with locking plate?
   A. Five divergent screw placed in humeral head
   B. Superiorly directed oblique screw below the proximal fragment
   C. Screws in the humeral head must pass both cortexes to increase the stability
   D. Medial column stabilization is important to avoid implant failure.
      C.

References

1. Karataglis D, Stavridis SI, Petsatodis G, Papadopoulos P, Christodoulou A. New trends in fixation of proximal humeral fractures: a review. Injury. 2011;42(4):330–8. doi:10.1016/j.injury.2010.10.016.
2. Rabi S, Evaniew N, Sprague SA, Bhandari M, Slobogean GP. Operative vs non-operative management of displaced proximal humeral fractures in the elderly: a systematic review and meta-analysis of randomized controlled trials. World J Orthop. 2015;6(10):838–46.
3. Banik II R, Mondal S. Evaluation of internal fixation with locking proximal humerus plate in osteoporotic proximal humeral fractures. IOSR-JDMS. 2015;14(1):12–9.
4. Helmy N, Hintermann B. New trends in the treatment of proximal humerus fractures. Clin Orthop Relat Res. 2006;442:100–8.
5. Maier D, Jaeger M, Izadpanah K, Strohm PC, Suedkamp NP. Proximal humeral fracture treatment in adult. J Bone Joint Surg Am. 2014;96(3):251–61.
6. Wong J, Newman JM, Gruson KI. Outcomes of intramedullary nailing for acute proximal humerus fractures: a systematic review. J Orthop Traumatol. 2016;17(2):113–22.
7. Calvo E, de Miguel I, de la Cruz JJ, López-Martín N. Percutaneous fixation of displaced proximal humeral fractures: Indications based on the correlation between clinical and radiographic results. J Shoulder Elb Surg. 2007;16(6):774–81.
8. Khmelnitskaya E, Lamont LE, Taylor SA, Lorich DG, Dines DM, Dines JS. Evaluation and management of proximal humerus fractures. Adv Orthop. 2012;2012:861598.
9. Hettrich CM, Boraiah S, Dyke JP, Neviaser A, Helfet AD, Lorich DG. Quantitative assessment of the vascularity of the proximal part of the humerus. J Bone Joint Surg Am. 2010;92(4):943–8.
10. Codman EA. The shoulder, rupture of the supraspinatus tendon and other lesions in or about the subacromial bursa. Boston: Thomas Tood Company; 1934.
11. Muller M, Perren S, Allgower M. Appendix A: the comprehensive classification of fracture of long bones. In: Allgower M, editor. Manual of internal fixation: techniques recommended by the AO-ASIF Group. Berlin: Springer; 1991. p. 118–25.

12. Neer II CS. Four-segment classification of proximal humerus fractures: purpose and reliable use. J Shoulder Elb Surg. 2002;11(4):389–400.
13. Resch H, Beck E, Bayley I. Reconstruction of the valgus-impacted humeral head fracture. J Shoulder Elb Surg. 1995;4(2):73–80.
14. Hertel R, Hempfing A, Stiehler M, Leunig M. Predictors of humeral head ischemia after intracapsular fracture of the proximal humerus. J Shoulder Elb Surg. 2004;13:427–33.
15. Court-Brown CM, Garg A, McQueen MM. The translated two-part fracture of the proximal humerus. Epidemiology and outcome in the older patient. J Bone Joint Surg Br. 2001;83(6):799–804.
16. Court-Brown CM, Cattermole H, McQueen MM. Impacted valgus fractures (B1.1) of the proximal humerus. J Bone Joint Surg Br. 2002;84(4):504–8.
17. Esenyel CZ, Yesiltepe Y, Bulbul M, Bagriacik A, Kara AN. Treatment of proximal humeral fractures with open reduction and internal fixation with Kirschner wires. Acta Orthop Traumatol Turc. 2001;35:10–5.
18. Esenyel CZ, Dedeoglu S, Imren Y, Kahraman S, Cakar M, Ozturk K. Relationship between axillary nerve and percutaneously inserted proximal humeral locking plate: a cadaver study. Acta Orthop Traumatol Turc. 2014;48(5):553–7.
19. Gardner MJ, Boraiah S, Helfet DL, Lorich DG. The anterolateral acromial approach for fractures of the proximal humerus. J Orthop Trauma. 2008;22(2):132–7.
20. Hertel R. Fractures of the proximal humerus in osteoporotic bone. Osteoporos Int. 2005;16(Suppl 2):S65–72.
21. Kralinger F, Unger S, Wambacher M, Smekal V, Schmoelz W. The medial periosteal hinge, a key structure in fractures of the proximal humerus: a biomechanical cadaver study of its mechanical properties. J Bone Joint Surg Br. 2009;91(7):973–6.
22. Burke NG, Kennedy J, Cousins G, Fitzpatrick D, Mullett H. Locking plate fixation with and without inferomedial screws for proximal humeral fractures: a biomechanical study. J Orthop Surg (Hong Kong). 2014;22(2):190–4.
23. Agel J, Jones CB, Sanzone AG, Camuso M, Henley MB. Treatment of proximal humeral fractures with Polarus nail fixation. J Shoulder Elb Surg. 2004;13(2):191–5.
24. Gradl G, Dietze A, Arndt D, Beck M, Gierer P, Börsch T, Mittlmeier T. Angular and sliding stable antegrade nailing (Targon PH) for the treatment of proximal humeral fractures. Arch Orthop Trauma Surg. 2007;127(10):937–44.
25. Popescu D, Fernandez-Valencia JA, Rios M, Cuñé J, Domingo A, Prat S. Internal fixation of proximal humerus fractures using the T2-proximal humeral nail. Arch Orthop Trauma Surg. 2009;129(9):1239–44.
26. Flatowel BLU. Location and protecting the axillary nerve in the shoulder surgery; Tug test. Orthop Rev. 1992;21:503–5.
27. Murachovsky J, Ikemoto RY, Nascimento LG, Milani C, Warner JJ. Pectoralis major tendon reference (PMT): a new method for accurate restoration of humeral length with hemiarthroplasty for fracture. J Shoulder Elb Surg. 2006;15(6):675–8.
28. Boileau P, Krishnan SG, Tinsi L, Walch G, Coste JS, Molé D. Tuberosity malposition and migration: Reasons for poor outcomes after hemiarthroplasty for displaced fractures of the proximal humerus. J Shoulder Elb Surg. 2002;11(5):401–12.
29. Olerud P, Ahrengart L, Ponzer S, Saving J, Tidermark J. Hemiarthroplasty versus nonoperative treatment of displaced 4-part proximal humeral fractures in elderly patients: a randomized controlled trial. J Shoulder Elb Surg. 2011;20(7):1025–33.

Reverse Shoulder Arthroplasty for 3-Part and 4-Part Proximal Humerus Fractures

10

E. Boyer, G. Menu, R. Saadnia, F. Loisel, J. Uhring, A. Adam, S. Rochet, P. Clappaz, E. Baudouin, T. Lascar, and L. Obert

Introduction

Four-part fractures of the proximal humerus in patients between 60 and 70 years of age should theoretically be treated by hemiarthroplasty (HA). In this age group, use of reverse shoulder arthroplasty (RSA) implants is contraindicated and fracture fixation is not always feasible, either because of compromised humeral head vascularity (varus, extensive comminution, very osteoporotic bone) [1, 2] or because of a complex fracture pattern (varus, associated dislocation, low head volume). However, because the functional outcomes of HA for these fractures are correlated to implant height and anatomical reduction of the tuberosities [5–7], less and less surgeons are using this technique. For the same type of fracture, the results are more predictable with an RSA implant; this has contributed to a marked increase in the number of RSA procedures performed on patients between 60 and 70 years of age. We report the first serie of locked stem of implant in trauma (hemi and reverse).

Materials and Methods

The first part of the study consisted of an assessment of a fracture-specific stem with diaphyseal locking (Humelock™, FX Solutions, Viriat, France) on 11 cadavers (22 shoulders) (Fig. 10.1). The goals of the cadaver study were, to determine whether the diaphyseal locking mechanism was mechanically reliable, determine whether the implant was safe for the vascular and nerve structures, and verify the data generated by Murachowsky [3] and Torrens [4] regarding the distance between the upper margin of the pectoralis major tendon and the top of the humeral head.

To set the stem height, we decided to directly lock the chosen stem; this allowed us to focus our time on the aspect we felt was most important: the fixation of the tuberosities. After locating the upper margin of the clavicular head of the pectoralis major, the stem was locked in a trial position that placed the head 5.5 cm from the pectoral

E. Boyer • G. Menu • R. Saadnia • F. Loisel
J. Uhring • A. Adam • S. Rochet • L. Obert (✉)
Orthopedic, Traumatology, and Hand Surgery Unit, Research Unit: Nano Medicine, CHRU Besancon, University of Bourgogne—Franche Comte, Bd Fleming, 25030 Besancon, France
e-mail: laurentobert@yahoo.fr

P. Clappaz
Clinique Convert, Bourg-en-Bresse, 62 Avenue de Jasseron, 01000 Bourg-en-Bresse, France

E. Baudouin
Centre Hospitalier de Chambéry, Place Lucien Biset, 73000 Chambéry, France

T. Lascar
Centre Hospitalier Princesse-Grace, 1 Avenue Pasteur, 98012 Monaco, France

G. Huri, N.K. Paschos (eds.), *The Shoulder*, Orthopaedic Study Guide Series,
DOI 10.1007/978-3-319-51979-1_10

landmark. A K-wire was used to lock the distal end of the stem temporarily; this enabled carrying out primary tuberosity reduction using trial heads and check the configuration on fluoroscopy with the arm in neutral position, internal rotation and external rotation (Figs. 10.2 and 10.3).

Patients were recruited for the prospective clinical study conducted between 2009 and 2011. Patients of each center were reviewed prospectively by an independent assessor. Ninety-three patients have been treated by locked stem, 49 with hemiarthroplasty and 44 with reversed. The clinical review consisted of measuring the shoulder range of motion and calculating the Constant score and QuickDASH. The radiological review consisted of an analysis of the position and consolidation of the tuberosities around the implant; these elements were analysed according to looped suture use.

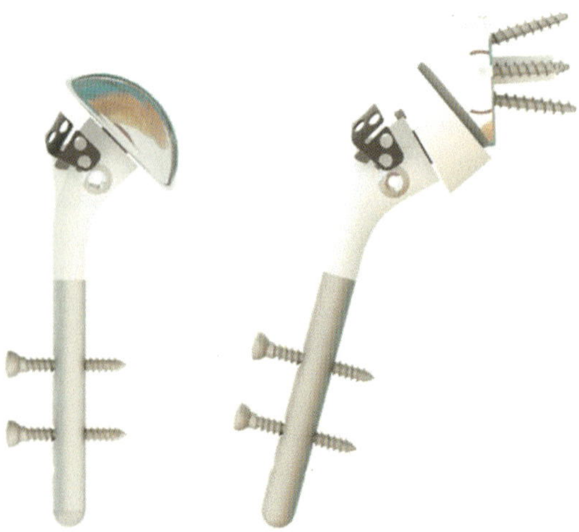

Fig. 10.1 New generation of hemi and reverse arthrosplasty with a locked and uncemented stem but which can be cemented. The stem is reversible allowing to use the platform as hemi or reversed prostheses (reprinted with permission from FX Solutions)

This study also allowed us to assess tuberosity reattachment using specially-designed suture loops (Smartloop®, FX Solutions), aiming to generate a reliable and reproducible construct, independent of fracture type. We also evaluated the mechanical advantage of adding a cage (Offset Modular System®, OMS, FX Solutions) below the head. This optional cage was developed to make it easier to position and fix the tuberosities as a function of the remaining tuberosity volume and to provide a recess where cancellous autograft taken from the patient's humeral head can be added against the prosthesis. The shoulder was immobilized in an internal rotation cast or sling for 4 weeks with no passive or active mobilization during this time-period.

Results

In the cadaver study, the distance between the top of the humeral head and the pectoralis major was 5.8 cm ± 5 mm, which is consistent with published data. This finding validated the height adjustment gauge developed for this implant. All

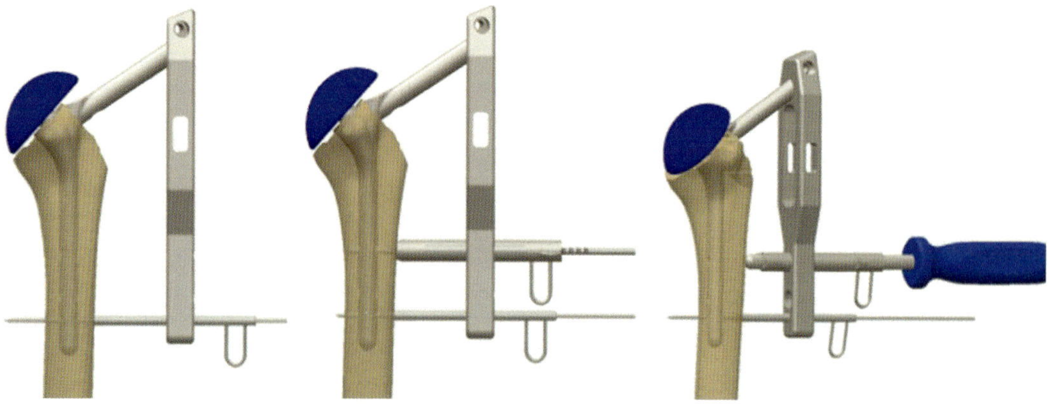

Fig. 10.2 The stem is permanently fitted at the correct height then the prosthesis is secured to the bone using a pin (Fig. 10.2 reprinted with permission from FX Solutions)

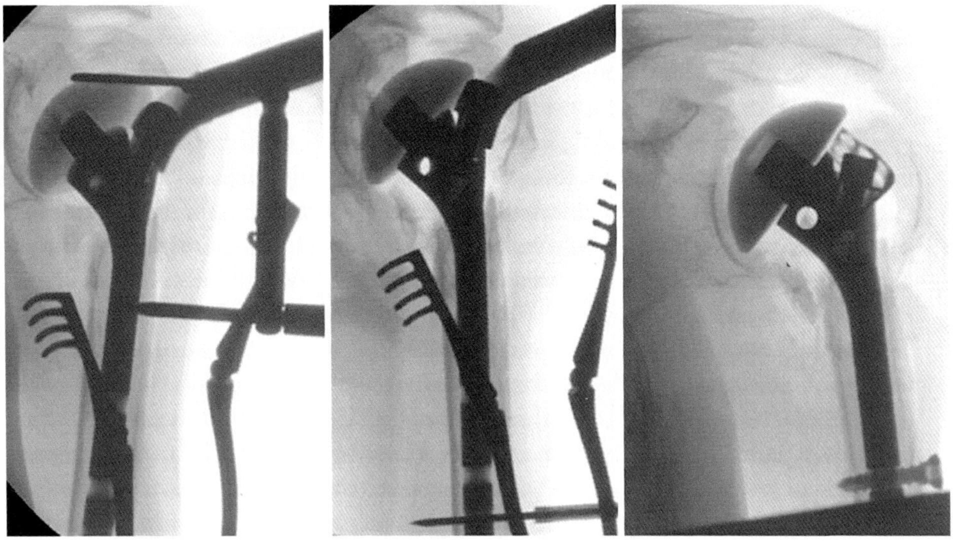

Fig. 10.3 The surgeon can apply tuberosities and assess they anatomical reduction finally locking is completed

stems could be solidly locked using the distal dual-locking instrumentation. The mechanical advantage of using the OMS to help positioning the tuberosities was evident in the cadaver study. The cage walls were further refined based on our findings to improve the biological exchanges around the implant.

The clinical study enrolled ninety-three 3 & 4 part patients with 93 fractures which have been treated by locked stem, 49 with hemiarthroplasty (mean age 67yo (50–90)) and 44 with reversed (mean age: 76.8 (59–90)). Five senior surgeons at four different hospitals performed the surgical procedures. The patients were operated at a mean of 7.1 days [1–17] after the fracture event by delto pectoral approach in 91% of cases. Immobilisation in internal rotation for 1 month was proposed in case of hemiathroplasty and a sling for 3 weeks in case of reverse prosthesis.

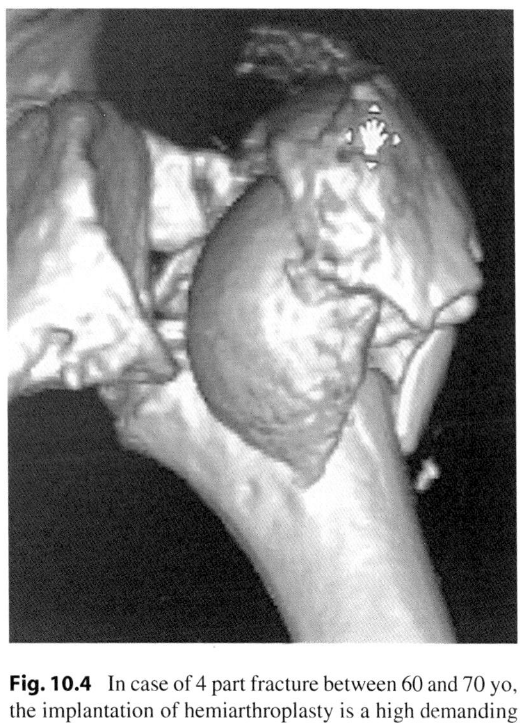

Fig. 10.4 In case of 4 part fracture between 60 and 70 yo, the implantation of hemiarthroplasty is a high demanding procedure

In the group of hemiarthroplasties, active flexion reached 99° (25°–160°), active abduction 89° (35°–160°) and active external rotation 27.5° (0°–55°). Constant score with ponderation reached 72.3 (31.5–120) and QDash 30.2 (4.5–68.1) with a mean FU of 18 months (12–96) (Figs. 10.4 and 10.5).

In the group of reversed prosthesis, active flexion reached 98.5° (30°–160°), active abduction 89.5° (10°–150°) and active external rotation 18° (0°–50°). Constant score with ponderation reached 79 (36.4–109.4) and QDash 36.5 (2.27–70.4) with a mean FU of 16 months [12–34] (Figs. 10.6, 10.7 and 10.8). No complications

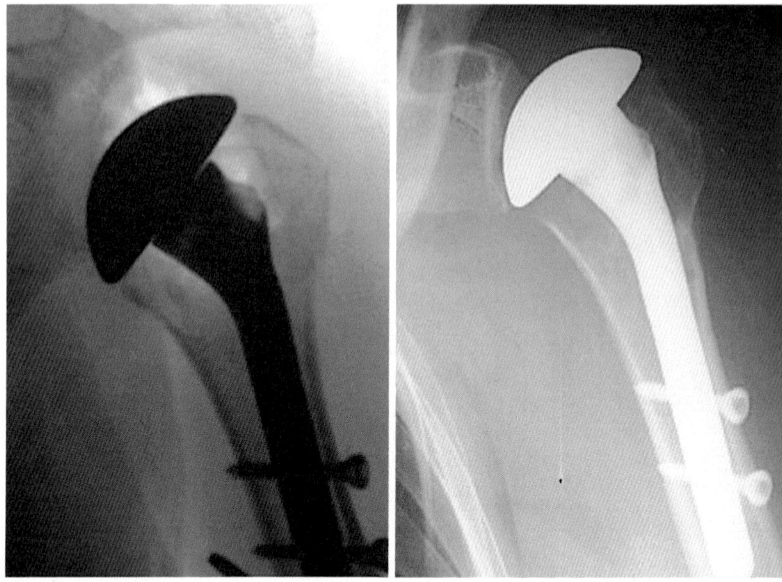

Fig. 10.5 Osteosuture of tuberosities and peroperative X-ray control are mandatory in order to achieve bone union at the right place

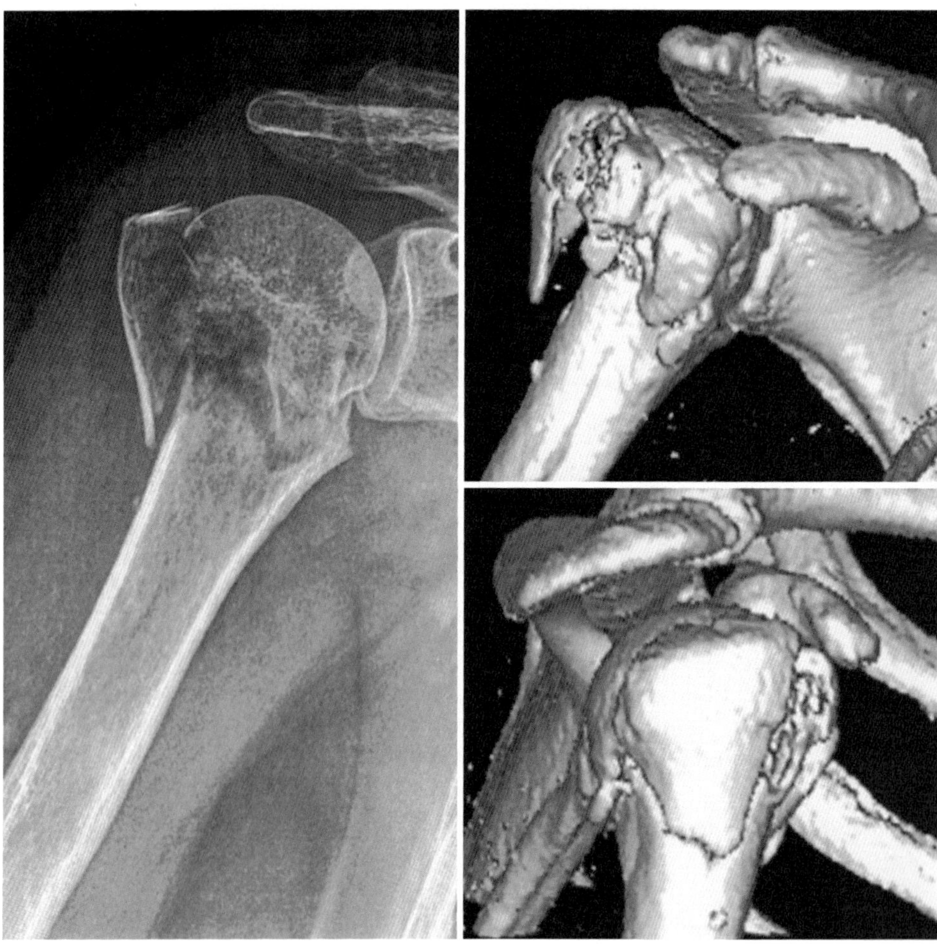

Fig. 10.6 In case of 4 part fracture after 70 yo, the implantation of reversed prosthesis provide more predictible functionnal results

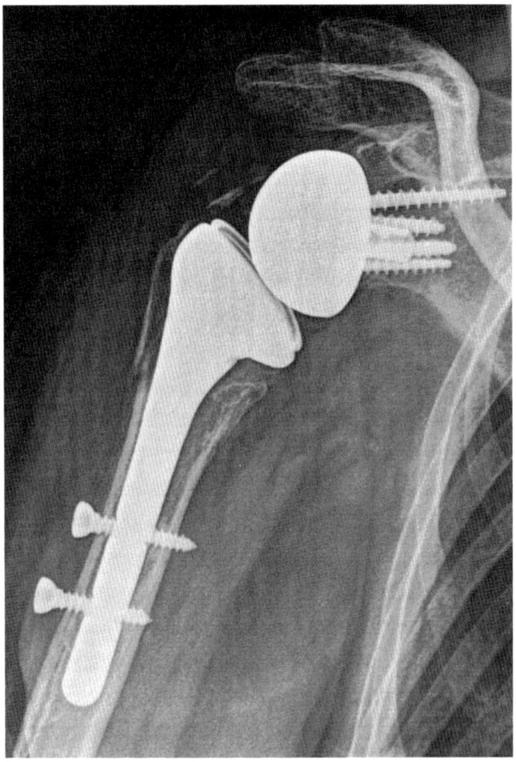

Fig. 10.7 Reinsertion of tuberosities is mandatory to reach better results even in case of reversed prosthesis

related to stem locking were observed. 28 complications occurred, 15 in the "hemi group" and 12 in the "reverse group". Complications are described in the Table 10.1.

Two of these rotator cuff cases required RSA conversion, which was easy to perform because no cement had been used initially. In the reverse group and at this follow-up only 1 case of notch (grade 1) was pointed (Fig. 10.9).

Discussion

Hemiarthroplasty

Consolidation of the lesser tuberosity and retroversion of the humeral stem are difficult to evaluate reliably. CT scanning would have provided a more accurate assessment, but also would have exposed the patient to more radiation. It was not possible to determine whether humeral length had been restored because X-rays of the entire humerus were not taken.

The number of patients in this study, as well as their ages and genders, were comparable to other published studies. The effect of age on tuberosity consolidation, and in parallel, the functional outcomes, has been demonstrated by several authors. Reuther [5] found that the tuberosity union rate was 61.5% in patients under 60 years of age, but only 26.5% in those over 80 years of age. Grönhagen [6] showed that the Constant–Murley score was significantly better in patients under 60 years of age. Boileau [7] found that tuberosity migration was significantly correlated to being over 75. In the current study, no differences were observed between patients over and under 60 years of age. Comorbidities also impact the functional outcomes. Kabir [8] found that the Constant-Murley score decreased from 41 to 27 when patients have three or more comorbidities.

Many studies have shown that women have worse functional outcomes and joint range of motion [7, 9, 10]. This can be explained by poor bone quality and increased risk of tuberosity nonunion. However, we found no differences in the outcomes between genders in the current study.

We did not find the time before surgery to have any impact on clinical outcomes. Mighell [11] reported that functional outcomes were significantly better when patients were operated within 2 weeks of the fracture event; this concept was not supported by Fallatah's study [12]. The deltopectoral approach used in this study is the same approach used in most published studies. A significant correlation between stem height and consolidation of the tuberosities in their anatomical position has been found [7]. A reliable reference for appropriate stem height is the distance between the apex of the humeral head and the superior margin of the pectoralis major tendon [3]. This distance can be measured only when using the deltopectoral approach. Better clinical outcomes have been found when the height is set using the distance between the apex of the humeral head and the superior margin of the pectoralis major tendon [13, 14]. In our opinion,

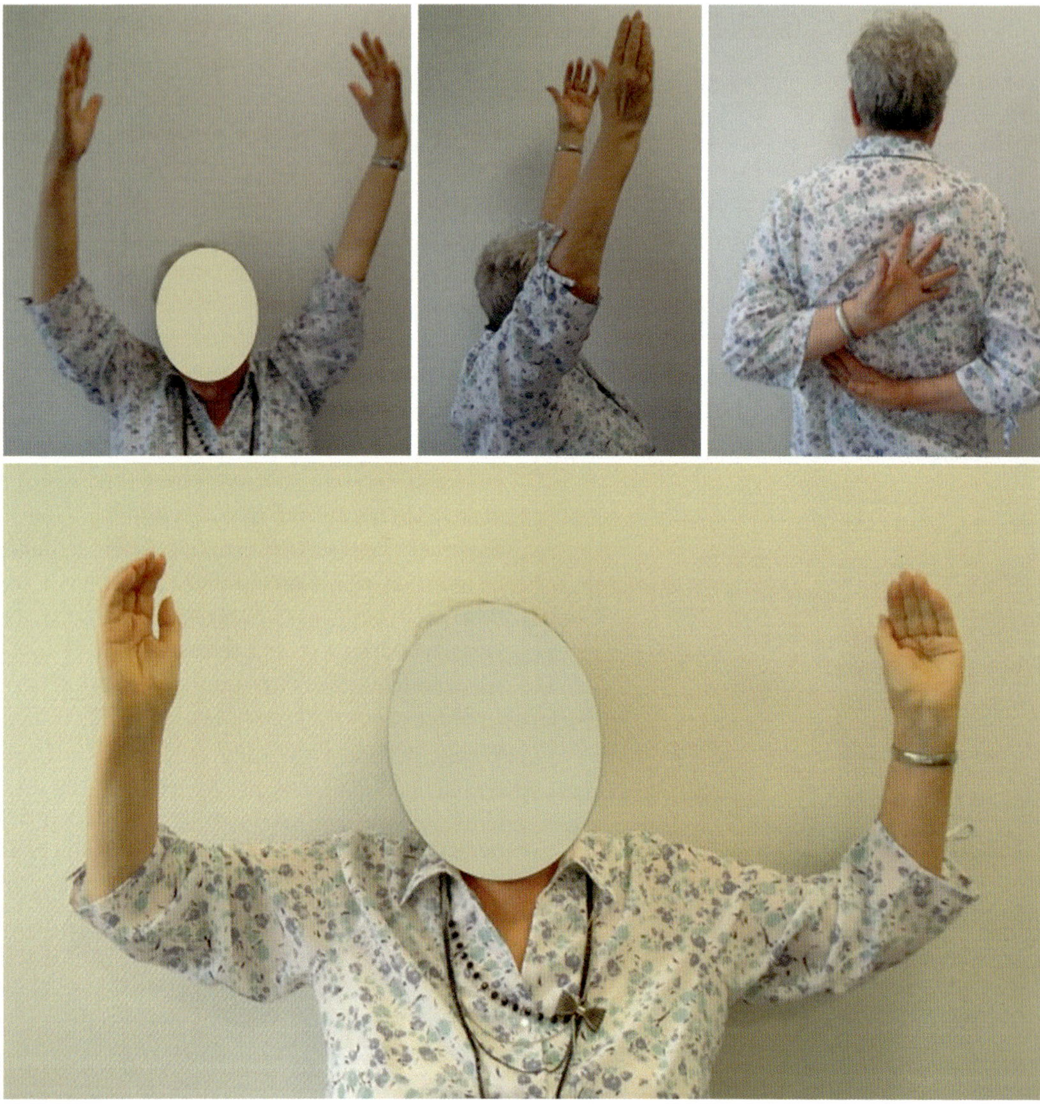

Fig. 10.8 Functional results are otain in 2 to 3 months

Table 10.1 Complications in subgroups

Complications	Hemi arthroplasty	Reverse prosthesis
Capsulitis	8	4
Phlebitis of upper limb		2
Axilary palsy		1
Lysis of great tuberositie	1	3
Infection		1
Problem with locking	2 (screw removal)	1
Secondary Cuff rupture	3	
Lymphoedema	1	

bone grafting is essential because it increases the primary stability of the tuberosities and adds a biological element to the healing process. We believe that the HA results are more predictable when the tuberosities are stabilized by transosseous sutures placed around the implant's metaphysis, which is filled with autograft.

Some authors have shown that tuberosity consolidation is not significantly affected by the use of bone graft [5, 15]. However, several teams have shown that tuberosity consolidation is critical to achieving good functional outcomes [5, 7,

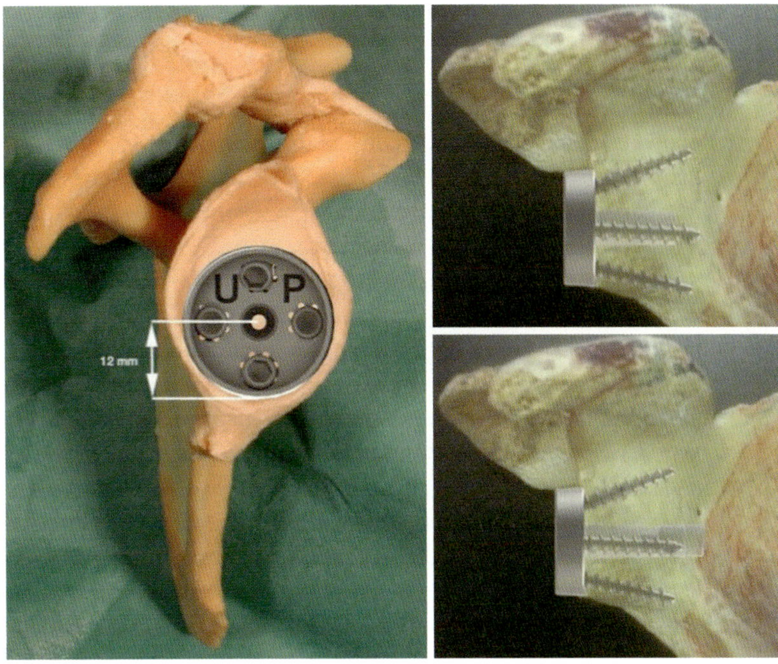

Fig. 10.9 With the smallest base plate of the market and a low implantation on the glenoid bone, the FX reverse prosthesis allow to diminish the notch

15–18]. Complications related to tuberosity consolidation are the main cause of functional catastrophy.

The nonunion rate in the current study (11.5%) falls within the range (0% to 17%) reported in other studies [7, 9]. Transosseous tuberosity suturing must be performed meticulously. Anatomical reduction of the tuberosities is an essential prerequisite for good functional outcomes. The malunion rate in the current study (23.7%) falls within the range (0–39%) reported in other studies [7, 9].

More recent studies found a tuberosity nonunion or malpositioning rate of 40–66% [19–21]. The transosseous sutures are as important as the implant's design and height for ensuring that the tuberosities heal in the correct position. Krishnan [22] and Boileau [23] have recently reported tuberosity nonunion rates of 21 and 13%, respectively, when a fracture-specific stem was used. This reinforced our research on implant that effectively treats humeral fractures involving the head and tuberosities.

The intraoperative complication rate in this study was low. The published rate is under 2%. Boileau [10] reported one case of axillary artery damage (1.6% complication rate). Brandao reported one periprosthetic humeral fracture (1.5% rate).

All the patients in this study underwent postoperative immobilization for 1 month using a shoulder immobilizer with the arm internally rotated. This position is controversial. Some authors recommend immobilization in neutral position or external rotation to reduce tension on the lesser trochanter, as this is a source of migration [7, 24]. However, this position is difficult to maintain during sleep.

Although Robinson [25] has shown that the Constant score levels out starting at the sixth postoperative month; very few studies have more than 2 years' follow-up. An analysis of published results shows a wide variation in the resulting shoulder range of motion (ROM). The mean forward flexion ranges from a low of 53.5° [26] to a high of 149° [17]. The Constant–Murley score ranges from a low of 42 points [6] to a high of 73.6 points [18]. The overall Constant–Murley score of 45.9 in this study falls within this range.

The condition of the rotator cuff directly affects the functional results of HA for fracture. Impaired functional outcomes due to reduced subacromial space has been demonstrated in many studies [6, 9, 11] and can reach 52% [6].

At the latest review, the functional outcomes were significantly altered when the subacromial space was less than 7 mm. In this study, it can be attributed to secondary rotator cuff damage in all cases. No damage to the rotator cuff was identified intraoperatively. One cause of postoperative rotator cuff damage is excessive humeral length. According to Boileau [7], length of more than 10 mm had two effects:

- Rotator cuff damage (less subacromial space) due to excessive tension on the supraspinatus muscle
- Tuberosity migration due to lack of union with the humeral shaft

Humerus length could not be determined in the current study because X-rays of the entire humerus were not taken.

Mighell [11] found a smaller subacromial space in 20.8% of patients. This radiological finding is systematically associated with impaired functional outcomes. Shah [27] counters these results and finds no significant difference between patients who have reduced subacromial space and those who have not.

No infections were identified in this study but with short follow up. The published rate of deep infection after HA for fracture is 1.6% [10]. For all etiologies combined, the prevalence of infection of anatomical shoulder implants is 2% according to Pelegri [28]. *Staphylococci* and *Propionibacterium acnes* are the most commonly found microorganisms (23–40%). The infectious prognosis is relatively good: the infection is resolved in 71% cases when all treatments are considered altogether.

Ectopic bone formation identified on X-rays is generally not considered as a complication. Grönhagen has reported ectopic bone formation in 54% of cases [6]. The impact of this abnormal radiological finding on functional outcomes is controversial. Grönhagen [6] and Goldman [9] found no changes in the functional outcomes in patients with ectopic ossification. Kjaergaard-Andersen [29] described three stages of ectopic ossification in a series of 26 out of 58 arthroplasty cases. In stage III, the bone bridges the humerus and acromion. The functional outcome is negatively affected only after ossification reaches stage III.

Reversed Prosthesis

The epidemiological variables are comparable to the published series. The mean age was 77 years (range, 72–86 years). The proportion of female patients varied from 70% for Klein et al. [39] to 100% for Hubert et al. [40]. The mean follow-up reported in the literature is 33 months (range, 10–86 months).

The superolateral and deltopectoral approaches can be used in reversed arthroplasty with fracture. In previous studies, the superolateral approach remains the most widely used. Bufquin et al. [41] found no differences in the results for these two approaches. For Sirveaux et al. [42], the superolateral approach is preferable because it results in fewer dislocations. However, this approach presents the disadvantage of weakening the deltoid muscle, the main motor of the prosthesis, whereas in a fracture situation the subscapular tendon does not need to be resected. Osteosuture of the tuberosities should be attempted whenever possible. Bufquin et al. [41] and Gallinet et al. [26] showed that this reinsertion was possible and effective in restoring rotation. The literature does not report criteria for defining anatomic union of the tuberosities in reversed prostheses. In another study, Gallinet et al. [43] showed significant improvement of the Constant score and throughout range of movement when anatomic union of the tuberosities was observed. Cuff et al. [44] nuanced these observations, considering that reinsertion of the tuberosities and their union significantly influences external rotation but not the functional scores.

Of the 12 series reported in the literature, the functional range of motion reached 118.6° (range, 97–139°) for anterior elevation, 107.4° (range, 80–128°) for abduction, and 16° (range,

8–27°) for external rotation with the elbow against the body. The mean crude Constant score varied from 44 points for Bufquin et al. [41] to 67.9 points for Klein et al. [39].

Intraoperative fractures are exceptional but they aggravate the prognosis. Bufquin et al. [41] reported fractures of the glenoid (2.3% of the complications). In these symposium series, we found no acromion or spine of scapula fractures. Dislocation is one of the most stressful complications for the patient. The risk of recurrence is even higher when the first episode occurs early. Its rate has been reported to be 16.6% in recent injuries [45]. The factors of instability described in the literature are the approach and most particularly the deltopectoral approach, which may be related to an increased risk of dislocation compared to the superolateral approach [46], because of the antero-inferior capsular release (more frequently used in scheduled surgery); a humeral length defect and therefore deltoid tension [47]; fat degeneration of the subscapularis muscle [48]; and finally, use of a small-diameter glenoid sphere (36 mm) [49].

Neurological lesions are not rare. The distinction between post-traumatic and iatrogenic neurological impairment remains subject to a preoperative examination that is often difficult. In the literature, the axillary nerve is the most frequently injured. The neurological lesion rate was 12.5% for Bufquin et al. [41].

The infection rate in series of reversed prostheses with fractures was 10% for Klein et al. [39]. The series of the 2006 SOFCOT symposium found 5.1% infections in scheduled surgery [49]. Pelegri et al. [28] found 3% infections all indications combined, with an 80% healing rate.

The rate of a notch on the lower side of the neck of scapula varies from 0% for Cuff et al. and Valenti et al. [44, 50] to 96% for Werner et al. [51]. This is a specific radiological anomaly of the reversed prosthesis but the analysis of this phenomenon can be delicate because it depends on the quality of the x-ray. Most frequently, the notch is partially hidden by the glenoid sphere when the patient is positioned too frontal. The use of a horizontal or slightly ascending ray coupled with radioscopy makes it possible to assess the presence of a notch. This scapular notch generally appears in the 1st year after surgery. In the 2006 SOFCOT series [49], the notch rate was 48% at 1 year of follow-up. These changes remain difficult to assess because it varies from case to case. Lévigne et al. [52] found a tendency towards progression of the notch over time. This notion of aggravation over time was also observed by Cazeneuve and Cristofari [53] and may stem from two related phenomena: mechanical impingement between the medial edge of the humeral cup and the lower edge of the neck of scapula and an osteolytic reaction to the polyethylene particles released in the joint capsule. The notch's clinical and radiological consequences continue to be debated in the literature. According to Lévigne et al. [52], the presence of a notch has no significant incidence on the Constant-Murley score or joint range of movement. On the other hand, it is associated with a significant decrease in strength. The 2006 SOFCOT symposium series [49] showed that the presence of a notch was significantly correlated with lower anterior elevation and less strength. For Sirveaux et al. [54], presence of a stage 3 or 4 notch is significantly associated with a lower Constant-Murley score. Even in cases of fracture, prevention of the notch seems logical to improve the longevity of reversed prostheses. The means to reduce its incidence are well known: low implantation of the glenoid insert flush with the lower edge of the glenoid [51], positioning the glenoid insert with at least 10% downward inclination, polyethylene cup depth as low as possible to preserve satisfactory stability, lateralization of the glenoid implant pulling away the humerus from the neck of scapula [55], and reduction (verticalization) of the neck-shaft angle of the humeral implant [56].

Conclusion

This is a relatively short-term study, but optimization of a fracture-specific implant leads to more predictable results if the tuberosities are reduced, they will heal. In case of hemi arthroplasty, the predictable results with this implant can be explained by the ease of setting the stem height, the ability to lock the stem in place without cement, the use of suture loops for transosseous fixation and the stabilization of the horseshoe-shaped graft in the metaphyseal area. In the hands of an experienced surgeon who makes use of fluoroscopy, the results of HA can be improved without having to perform RSA on every fracture cases. At shoulder level, the removal of a cemented stem remains a highly demanding procedure with sometimes bad functional results and high level of complications. This series is the first one of locked stem without significant complications. Locked stem remains a new but logical tool in trauma.

Questions

Select the unique problems related to massive rotator cuff arthritis/total shoulder arthroplasty:

A. Suturing of co-existing RC tears in arthroplasty is not effective due to poor RC tissue quality
B. Glenohumeral joint congruity is distorted.
C. A superior migration of the humeral head is seen
D. Persistent pain is the most common reason for failure of total shoulder arthroplasty with patient with massive RC tears while range of motion is typically restored and component integration is normal
E. During arm elevation rotation is partially replaced with translation at the GH joint that leads to early wear and loosening

Why Dr Grammont's work is considered key for the evolution of reverse shoulder arthroplasty?

A. He developed the concept of the glenoid being convex, whereas the humeral side being concave, so that this system would be inherently stable
B. He proposed lateralization of the acromion. With the hypothesis that a more lateral position of the acromion to the joint's center of rotation would create an increase in the abductor component of the deltoid
C. He proposed medialization of the COR of the prosthesis with the conception of a possible "nonanatomic" solution
D. A central screw to fix the glenosphere to the scapula
E. A & B & C
F. A & B & D

Which of the following statements are correct (select all that apply:)

A. With medialized implants, the center of rotation is placed at the glenoid component–bone interface which results in less shear stress
B. Lateralized implants can result in increased force at the glenoid bone–implant interface encroachment on the glenoid
C. Lateralized implants can result in laxity of the remaining cuff
D. Medialized implants result in lower risk of scapular notching

Factors that can increase range of motion of a reverse shoulder are all the above except:

A. Lateral offset of the implant
B. Inferior positioning of the glenoid
C. Inferior glenoid tilt
D. superior positioning with inferior tilting of the glenosphere

All the above can be considered indications for reverse arthroplasty except:

A. Rotator cuff tear arthropathy
B. Osteoarthritis with severe glenoid bone loss
C. Glenoid osteoporosis
D. Dislocation arthropathy
E. Failed proximal humeral head replacement

References

1. Seggl W, Weiglein A. Die arterielle Blutversorgung des Oberarmkopfes und ihre prognostische Bedeutung bei Luxationen, Frakturen und Luxationsfrakturen des Oberarmkopfes. Vienna: Blackwell-MZV; 1991.
2. Gerber C, Schneeberger AG, Vinh TS. The arterial vascularization of the humeral head. An anatomical study. J Bone Joint Surg Am. 1990;72(10):1486–94.
3. Murachovsky J, Ikemoto RY, Nascimento LGP, Fujiki EN, Milani C, Warner JJP. Pectoralis major tendon reference (PMT): a new method for accurate restoration of humeral length with hemiarthroplasty for fracture. J Shoulder Elb Surg. 2006;15(6):675–8.

4. Torrens C, Corrales M, Melendo E, Solano A, Rodríguez-Baeza A, Cáceres E. The pectoralis major tendon as a reference for restoring humeral length and retroversion with hemiarthroplasty for fracture. J Shoulder Elb Surg. 2008;17(6):947–50.
5. Reuther F, Mühlhäusler B, Wahl D, Nijs S. Functional outcome of shoulder hemiarthroplasty for fractures: a multicentre analysis. Injury. 2010;41(6):606–12.
6. Grönhagen CM, Abbaszadegan H, Révay SA, Adolphson PY. Medium-term results after primary hemiarthroplasty for comminuted proximal humerus fractures: a study of 46 patients followed up for an average of 4.4 years. J Shoulder Elb Surg. 2007;16(6):766–73.
7. Boileau P, Krishnan SG, Tinsi L, Walch G, Coste JS, Molé D. Tuberosity malposition and migration: reasons for poor outcomes after hemiarthroplasty for displaced fractures of the proximal humerus. J Shoulder Elb Surg. 2002;11(5):401–12.
8. Kabir K, Burger C, Fischer P, Weber O, Florczyk A, Goost H, et al. Health status as an important outcome factor after hemiarthroplasty. J Shoulder Elb Surg. 2009;18(1):75–82.
9. Goldman RT, Koval KJ, Cuomo F, Gallagher MA, Zuckerman JD. Functional outcome after humeral head replacement for acute three- and four-part proximal humeral fractures. J Shoulder Elb Surg. 1995;4(2):81–6.
10. Boileau P, Winter M, Cikes A, Han Y, Carles M, Walch G, et al. Can surgeons predict what makes a good hemiarthroplasty for fracture? J Shoulder Elb Surg. 2013;22(11):1495–506.
11. Mighell MA, Kolm GP, Collinge CA, Frankle MA. Outcomes of hemiarthroplasty for fractures of the proximal humerus. J Shoulder Elb Surg. 2003;12(6):569–77.
12. Fallatah S, Dervin GF, Brunet JA, Conway AF, Hrushowy H. Functional outcome after proximal humeral fractures treated with hemiarthroplasty. Can J Surg. 2008;51(5):361–5.
13. Greiner SH, Kääb MJ, Kröning I, Scheibel M, Perka C. Reconstruction of humeral length and centering of the prosthetic head in hemiarthroplasty for proximal humeral fractures. J Shoulder Elb Surg. 2008;17(5):709–14.
14. Lascar T, Rocher S, Vidil A, Hery J-Y, Juvanspan M, Bellumore Y, et al. Intérêt d'une prothèse anatomique dédiée au traitement des fractures céphalo-tubérositaires. Présentation des solutions techniques pour améliorer la consolidation des tubérosités et analyses radiologiques et cliniques des résultats. Rev Chir Orthopédique Traumatol. 2012;98(4, Supplement):S68–72.
15. Kralinger F, Schwaiger R, Wambacher M, Farrell E, Menth-Chiari W, Lajtai G, et al. Outcome after primary hemiarthroplasty for fracture of the head of the humerus A retrospective multicentre study of 167 patients. J Bone Joint Surg Br. 2004;86(2):217–9.
16. Antuña SA, Sperling JW, Cofield RH. Shoulder hemiarthroplasty for acute fractures of the proximal humerus: a minimum five-year followup. J Shoulder Elb Surg. 2008;17(2):202–9.
17. Kontakis GM, Tosounidis TI, Christoforakis Z, Hadjipavlou AG. Early management of complex proximal humeral fractures using the Aequalis fracture prosthesis. A two- to five-year followup report. J Bone Joint Surg Br. 2009;91(10):1335–40.
18. Esen E, Doğramacı Y, Gültekin S, Deveci MA, Suluova F, Kanatlı U, et al. Factors affecting results of patients with humeral proximal end fractures undergoing primary hemiarthroplasty: a retrospective study in 42 patients. Injury. 2009;40(12):1336–41.
19. Jacquot N, Kempf J-F, Favard L, Le Huec J-C, Molé D, Walch G, et al. 247 Résultats d'une prothèse d'épaule spécifiquement dessinée pour les fractures de l'extrémité supérieure de l'humérus. Rev Chir Orthop Réparatrice Appar Mot. 2004;90(6, Supplement 1): 145.
20. Boileau P, Walch G, Krishnan SG. Tuberosity osteosynthesis and hemiarthroplasty for four-part fractures of the proximal humerus. Tech Shoulder Elb Surg. 2000;1(2):96–109.
21. Reuther F, Müller S, Wahl D. Management of humeral head fractures with a trauma shoulder prosthesis: correlation between joint function and healing of the tuberosities. Acta Orthop Belg. 2007;73(2):179–87.
22. Krishnan SG, Reineck JR, Bennion PD, Feher L, Burkhead WZ. Shoulder arthroplasty for fracture: does a fracture-specific stem make a difference? Clin Orthop Relat Res. 2011;469(12):3317–23.
23. Boileau P, Pennington SD, Alami G. Proximal humeral fractures in younger patients: fixation techniques and arthroplasty. J Shoulder Elb Surg. 2011;20(2 Suppl):S47–60.
24. Krishnan SG, Pennington SD, Burkhead WZ, Boileau P. Shoulder arthroplasty for fracture: restoration of the « gothic arch ». Tech Shoulder Elb Surg. 2005;6(2):57–66.
25. Robinson CM, Page RS, Hill RM, Sanders DL, Wakefield AE. Primary hemiarthroplasty for treatment of proximal humeral fractures. J Bone Joint Surg. 2003;85(7):1215–23.
26. Gallinet D, Clappaz P, Garbuio P, Tropet Y, Obert L. Three or four parts complex proximal humerus fractures: hemiarthroplasty versus reverse prosthesis: a comparative study of 40 cases. Orthop Traumatol Surg Res. 2009;95(1):48–55.
27. Shah N, Iqbal HJ, Brookes-Fazakerley S, Sinopidis C. Shoulder hemiarthroplasty for the treatment of three and four part fractures of the proximal humerus using Comprehensive® Fracture stem. Int Orthop. 2011;35(6):861–7.
28. Pelegri C, Jacquot N, Coste J-S, Boileau P. Infection des prothèses d'épaule : spécificité et prise en charge: Infection in shoulder prostheses: specificities and management. In: Boileau P, Walch G, éditeurs. Prothèses d'épaule État actuel [Internet]. Paris: Elsevier Masson; 2008. p. 382–390.
29. Kjaersgaard-Andersen P, Frich LH, Søjbjerg JO, Sneppen O. Heterotopic bone formation follow-

ing total shoulder arthroplasty. J Arthroplasty. 1989;4(2):99–104.
30. Prakash U, McGurty DW, Dent JA. Hemiarthroplasty for severe fractures of the proximal humerus. J Shoulder Elb Surg. 2002;11(5):428–30.
31. Christoforakis JJ, Kontakis GM, Katonis PG, Maris T, Voloudaki A, Prassopoulos P, et al. Relevance of the restoration of humeral length and retroversion in hemiarthroplasty for humeral head fractures. Acta Orthop Belg. 2003;69(3):226–32.
32. Loew M, Heitkemper S, Parsch D, Schneider S, Rickert M. Influence of the design of the prosthesis on the outcome after hemiarthroplasty of the shoulder in displaced fractures of the head of the humerus. J Bone Joint Surg Br. 2006;88(3):345–50.
33. Padua R, Bondì R, Ceccarelli E, Campi A, Padua L. Health-related quality of life and subjective outcome after shoulder replacement for proximal humeral fractures. J Shoulder Elb Surg. 2008;17(2):261–4.
34. Castricini R, Benedetto M, Pirani P, Panfoli N, Pace N. Shoulder hemiarthroplasty for fractures of the proximal humerus. Musculoskelet Surg. 2011;95(S1):49–54.
35. Liu J, Li S, Cai Z, Lou L, Wu X, Zhu Y, et al. Outcomes, and factors affecting outcomes, following shoulder hemiarthroplasty for proximal humeral fracture repair. J Orthop Sci. 2011;16(5):565–72.
36. Padua R, Padua L, Galluzzo M, Ceccarelli E, Alviti F, Castagna A. Position of shoulder arthroplasty and clinical outcome in proximal humerus fractures. Musculoskelet Surg. 2011;95(S1):S55–8.
37. Fucentese SF, Sutter R, Wolfensperger F, Jost B, Gerber C. Large metaphyseal volume hemiprostheses for complex fractures of the proximal humerus. J Shoulder Elb Surg. 2014;23(3):427–33.
38. Brandão BL, Amaral MVG, Cohen M, Correia RG de M, CHG A, Monteiro MT, et al. Treatment of complex acute proximal humerus fractures using hemiarthroplasty. Rev Bras Orthop Engl Ed. 2013;48(1):29–35.
39. Klein M, Juschka M, Hinkenjann B, Scherger B, Ostermann PA. Treatment of comminuted fractures of the proximal humerus in elderly patients with the Delta III reverse shoulder prosthesis. J Orthop Trauma. 2008;22(10):698–704.
40. Hubert L, Lahogue J-F, Hersan A, Gournay A, Massin P. 116 Prothèse inversée Delta® en traumatologie de l'épaule : résultats préliminaires. Rev Chir Orthop Réparatrice Appar Mot. 2004;90(6, Supplement 1):83.
41. Bufquin T, Hersan A, Hubert L, Massin P. Reverse shoulder arthroplasty for the treatment of three-and four-part fractures of the proximal humerus in the elderly a prospective review of 43 cases with a short-term follow-up. J Bone Joint Surg Br. 2007;89(4):516–20.
42. Sirveaux F, Navez G, Favard L, Boileau P, Walch G, Mole D. Reverse prosthesis for acute proximal humerus fracture, the multicentric study. In: Walch G, Boileau P, Mole D, editors. Reverse shoulder arthroplasty: clinical results, complications, revisions. Montpellier, France: Sauramps Medical; 2006. p. 73–80.
43. Gallinet D, Adam A, Gasse N, Rochet S, Obert L. Improvement in shoulder rotation in complex shoulder fractures treated by reverse shoulder arthroplasty. J Shoulder Elb Surg. 2013;22(1):38–44.
44. Cuff DJ, Pupello DR. Comparison of hemiarthroplasty and reverse shoulder arthroplasty for the treatment of proximal humeral fractures in elderly patients. J Bone Joint Surg Am. 2013;95(22):2050–5.
45. Van Seymortier P, Stoffelen D, Fortems Y, Reynders P. The reverse shoulder prosthesis (Delta III) in acute shoulder fractures: technical considerations with respect to stability. Acta Orthop Belg. 2006;72(4):474–7.
46. Molé D, Wein F, Dézaly C, Valenti P, Sirveaux F. Surgical technique: the anterosuperior approach for reverse shoulder arthroplasty. Clin Orthop Relat Res. 2011;469(9):2461–8.
47. Walch G, Nové-Josserand L. Instabilité de la prothèse totale inversée de l'épaule: Instability of the reverse shoulder prosthesis. In: Boileau P, Walch G, éditeurs. Prothèses d'épaule État actuel. Paris: Elsevier Masson; 2008. p. 407–414.
48. Edwards TB, Williams MD, Labriola JE, Elkousy HA, Gartsman GM, O'Connor DP. Subscapularis insufficiency and the risk of shoulder dislocation after reverse shoulder arthroplasty. J Shoulder Elb Surg. 2009;18(6):892–6.
49. Baulot E, Valenti P, Garaud P, Boileau P, Neyton L, Sirveaux F, et al. Résultats des prothèses inversées. Rev Chir Orthop Réparatrice Appar Mot. 2007;93(6, Supplement 1):63–92.
50. Valenti P, Katz D, Kilinc A, Elkholti K, Gasiunas V. Mid-term outcome of reverse shoulder prostheses in complex proximal humeral fractures. Acta Orthop Belg. 2012;78:442–9.
51. Werner CML, Steinmann PA, Gilbart M, Gerber C. Treatment of painful pseudoparesis due to irreparable rotator cuff dysfunction with the Delta III reverse-ball-and-socket total shoulder prosthesis. J Bone Joint Surg. 2005;87(7):1476–86.
52. Lévigne C, Boileau P, Favard L, Garaud P, Molé D, Sirveaux F, et al. Scapular notching in reverse shoulder arthroplasty. J Shoulder Elb Surg. 2008;17(6):925–35.
53. Cazeneuve J-F, Cristofari DJ. Delta III reverse shoulder arthroplasty: Radiological outcome for acute complex fractures of the proximal humerus in elderly patients. Orthop Traumatol Surg Res. 2009;95(5):325–9.
54. Sirveaux F, Favard L, Oudet D, Huquet D, Walch G, Mole D. Grammont inverted total shoulder arthroplasty in the treatment of glenohumeral osteoarthritis with massive rupture of the cuff results of a multicentre study of 80 shoulders. J Bone Joint Surg Br. 2004;86(3):388–95.
55. Boileau P, Balg F. Prothèse totale d'épaule inversée: principes biomécaniques, concept et évolution: the reverse shoulder prosthesis: biomechanical principles, concept and evolution. In: Boileau P, Walch G, éditeurs. Prothèses d'épaule État actuel [Internet]. Paris: Elsevier Masson; 2008 p. 153–168.
56. Kempton LB, Balasubramaniam M, Ankerson E, Wiater JM. A radiographic analysis of the effects of prosthesis design on scapular notching following reverse total shoulder arthroplasty. J Shoulder Elb Surg. 2011;20(4):571–6.

Dislocations and Fracture Dislocations of the Shoulder Girdle

11

Danny Ryan and Mustafa Rashid

Introduction

The shoulder is the most commonly dislocated joint in the body [1], with an incidence between 1 and 2% in the population per year [2, 3]. Studies have highlighted the group at highest risk of sustaining a traumatic shoulder dislocation to be males between the ages of 21 and 30 years, with further risk conferred with overhead activities and participation in contact sports [3–6]. While the humerus may dislocate posteriorly, approximately 98% of dislocations occur anteriorly [2–8].

Shoulder Anatomy: Glenohumeral Joint

The glenohumeral joint is a ball and socket joint, comprising of the shallow 'cup' of the glenoid, and the relatively larger, spherical, humeral head. This configuration alone is inherently unstable, and a combination of both static and dynamic stabilisers are required to maintain the position of the humeral head in joint.

Static Stabilisers

There are three main static stabilisers contributing to shoulder stability:

1. Osseous anatomy
2. Labrum
3. Glenohumeral ligaments

Osseous Anatomy

The glenoid is roughly 20–30 mm wide (greatest width is found inferiorly) with a concave surface area that is approximately one-third of the surface of the humeral head. In 75% of people it demonstrates 3–7° of retroversion to the scapular plane, but in the remainder of the population this may be to a lesser degree, or even a slight amount of anteversion may be present. Superior tilt is in the region of 3–5°, and anteversion in the coronal plane 30–40°.

The head of the humerus is inclined superiorly, with a head neck angle of 130–140°, and is retroverted by 20–30° relative to the transepicondylar axis. Furthermore, the head is positioned in an eccentric, posterior position relative to the axis of the diaphysis of the humerus.

D. Ryan, MA, MB, BChir (Cantab), PGCME, FRSA, MRCSEng (✉)
Trauma and Orthopaedic Surgery, Gloucestershire Royal Hospital, Gloucester, UK
e-mail: danny.ryan@cantab.net

M. Rashid, MB, ChB, MRCS, MSc
Nuffield Department of Orthopaedics, Rheumatology, and Musculoskeletal Sciences (NDORMS), Oxford, UK

G. Huri, N.K. Paschos (eds.), *The Shoulder*, Orthopaedic Study Guide Series, DOI 10.1007/978-3-319-51979-1_11

Labrum

Both the articular cartilage of the glenoid and the surrounding labrum contribute to the congruency of the joint. The cartilage thickens as it approaches the edge of the glenoid, and, in combination with the labrum, increases the concavity of the surface by an additional 5–9 mm, thereby reducing translation and improving conformity.

The labrum itself is a fibrocartilaginous structure, which is triangular in cross-section, appearing similar to the meniscus in the knee. Superiorly, it is a relatively mobile structure, but inferiorly it has a firmer attachment and more rounded cross-section. It contributes roughly a third of the additional height of the concavity, which is deeper superiorly and inferiorly than at the anterior and posterior edges. The labrum also provides the attachment for the glenohumeral ligaments.

Glenohumeral Ligaments

The superior, middle and inferior glenohumeral ligaments blend with the joint capsule to provide tension at varying degrees of humeral motion, in order to maintain centering of the humeral head within the concave surface of the glenoid.

Inferior Glenohumeral Ligament (IGHL)

The IGHL is composed of an anterior and posterior band, taking the majority of its attachment from the labrum, with only around 15% from the glenoid rim, and inserting inferior to the greater and lesser tuberosities. The area between the distinct bands, extending from the inferior two-thirds of the glenoid rim to the inferior third of the humeral head, is known as the axillary pouch: this section of ligament creates a hammock under the humeral head. In 90° abduction and external rotation the anterior band tightens, thus preventing anterior and inferior translation of the humeral head, while in flexion and internal rotation the posterior band is tightest. The IGHL is the primary stabilizer of the glenohumeral joint in abduction.

Middle Glenohumeral Ligament (MGHL)

The MGHL arises from the supraglenoid tubercle, at the anterosuperior aspect of the glenoid rim, and between the 1 and 3 o'clock positions of the anterosuperior labrum. It attaches to the lesser tuberosity of the humerus, where it blends with the insertion of subscapularis. The MGHL is the primary stabilizer against anterior dislocation between 0 and 90° of abduction, after which the IGHL takes over this role as described above.

Superior Glenohumeral Ligament (SGHL)

The SGHL also has its origin at the supraglenoid tubercle, anterior to the long head of biceps, running in an anterosuperior direction to attach to the lesser tuberosity. It prevents inferior translation of the arm in adduction. The SGHL covers the long head of biceps, and is augmented by the coracohumeral ligament, which runs from the dorsolateral coracoid to the lesser (anterior band) and greater (posterior band) tuberosities. The anterior band tightens in external rotation, and the posterior band in internal rotation, providing resistance to anteroinferior translation during these movements. The SGHL and coracohumeral ligaments lie in the rotator interval, the capsular interval between the anterior edge of the supraspinatus tendon and the superior edge of subscapularis.

Further factors that add to static stability include a negative intra-articular pressure (providing a 'suction-cup' effect between the humeral head and glenoid) and the size differential between the surface areas of the glenoid and humeral head, creating high forces across the joint.

Dynamic Stabilisers

Dynamic stability of the glenohumeral joint aims to minimize translation during rotation of the humeral head through concavity compression force. In addition to the structural relationship between the humeral head and surface of the glenoid and the glenohumeral ligament contributions at the extremes of motion, the musculature providing the compressive force pushing the humeral head into the glenoid is also vitally important. Three groups of muscles contribute to the dynamic stability of the glenohumeral joint:

1. Rotator cuff
2. Long head of biceps
3. Scapular stabilisers

Rotator Cuff

Contraction of the rotator cuff results in compression of the humeral head into the glenoid fossa, providing resistance to translation. This force is particularly potent in mid-range motion.

Long Head of Biceps

The long head of biceps originates from the superior labrum, providing stability against translation of the humeral head in superoinferior and anteroposterior directions.

Scapular Stabilisers

The position of the scapula is important in determining glenoid version and tilt. The rotatory force couple, which maintains a normal scapulothoracic rhythm, is balanced by upper and lower components (Table 11.1). In combination with the pectoral muscles (responsible for scapulohumeral rhythm) stability of the shoulder is maintained.

The deltoid muscle also contributes to concavity compression force with the arm in 90° of abduction, and provides a superior shear force when the arm is adducted. Finally, proprioceptive feedback from capsular stretch aids in normal muscle function and dynamic stability.

Table 11.1 Scapular stabilisers

Upper component	Lower component
Levator scapulae	Trapezius (lower fibres)
Trapezius (upper fibres)	Serratus anterior (upper fibres)
Serratus anterior (upper fibres)	

Anterior Dislocation of the Glenohumeral Joint

Examination

The majority of shoulder dislocations occur anteriorly [2–8], usually as a result of a force in external rotation and abduction. Clinically, patients often present with a first-time traumatic anterior dislocation, acutely, in severe pain that is poorly localized around the proximal humerus and glenohumeral joint. One must be careful to take a thorough history to elucidate the mechanism of injury, past medical and surgical history, time of last meal, allergies and other relevant information that may contraindicate a general anaesthetic. It is also important to note that a subset of patients may present in a polytrauma setting, with a high-energy injury. In this case, simultaneous assessment and resuscitation in accordance with the Advanced Trauma Life Support principles should be commenced without delay. The shoulder dislocation will have to be addressed after the patient's life and limb threatening injuries are treated, and their vital signs stabilised.

In the normal anatomical position, the most lateral edge of the proximal humerus is the contour of the deltoid as it descends laterally to attach to the deltoid tuberosity of the humerus. In an anterior dislocation, the humerus lies anterior to the glenoid and medial to its normal position. Hence, the most lateral edge of the shoulder now becomes the lateral edge of the acromion, which appears flatter and more 'square' in contour when viewed anteriorly. This is often an indication that the glenohumeral joint is dislocated anteriorly.

Neurovascular examination should be performed and documented both prior to, and following, any attempted reduction. The most commonly injured nerve is the axillary nerve, owing to its course around the surgical neck of the humerus, closely followed by the suprascapular nerve [9]. These injuries tend to be neuropraxias, which will resolve spontaneously following reduction [10, 11], however, in one series, 48% of patients had documented nerve injuries following dislocation when using electromyography (EMG) to aid diagnosis [12]. Risk of nerve injury is increased with increasing age, associated fracture and presence of haematoma [10]. Vascular injury, whilst rare, can easily be missed owing to good collateral circulation around the shoulder. Vascular injuries are often associated with neurological injury, and extensive bruising and swelling in the axilla should raise suspicion, warranting further investigation. Injuries to the circumflex humeral arteries, as well as axillary artery transection and delayed presentations of pseudoaneurysms have all been reported in the literature [13–16].

Imaging

Anteroposterior radiographs may be difficult to interpret [17, 18], particularly in posterior dislocation, so a modified axillary view should be sought. 29% of shoulder dislocations have an associated fracture, with up to 59% being missed on initial assessment [19, 20]. Early computed tomography (CT) scan can be useful for determining injuries to the bony anatomy which may require early surgery, while magnetic resonance imaging (MRI) has a place in diagnosis of associated soft tissue injuries after the dislocation has been reduced.

Reduction Techniques

As with dislocation of any joint, early closed reduction should be performed in order to reduce tension on neurovascular structures [12]. This can be carried out under sedation in the Emergency Room, or under general anaesthetic, with or without muscle relaxant, in the Operating Room. Several methods have been described, and these are summarized in Table 11.2 below. Care should be taken to avoid fracture of the proximal humerus during reduction.

If closed reduction is successful, neurovascular examination should be repeated, and the patient placed in a broad arm sling. After 1–2 weeks, mobilization with physiotherapy can begin, focusing on correct scapular posture, appropriate coordinated scapulothoracic motion exercises and range of motion. The 'at risk' position of 90° abduction and 90° external rotation should be avoided to prevent early recurrence.

Table 11.2 Methods of closed reduction for anterior dislocation of the shoulder

Hippocratic	Longitudinal traction applied to the arm with the foot placed in the axilla
Kocher	With the elbow flexed to 90°, apply traction with external rotation, followed by adduction and internal rotation (NB. High risk of fracture and neurovascular complications [21])
Stimson	Patient prone, apply 4.5 kg weight to the affected arm [22]
Rockwood	Place a sheet around patient's chest and apply traction in direction of deformity, with rotation to disengage humeral head from glenoid rim
Milch	Patient supine, abduct and externally rotate patient's arm into overhead position and 'thumb' humeral head into glenoid fossa
Scapular manipulation	Patient prone, 5–10 lbs of traction applied to arm. Push tip of scapula medially, with lateral rotation of superior aspect of scapula [23]

The position of sling immobilization is controversial: Itoi et al. showed a reduced rate of recurrence for bracing in external rotation versus neutral rotation for 3 weeks (42 vs. 26%) [24], though these results were not replicated by a similar randomized controlled trial in Norway [25].

If closed reduction is not achievable, open reduction via a deltopectoral approach should be performed. This approach begins at the interval between the deltoid and pectoralis major muscles, which is the internervous plane between the axillary nerve and medial and lateral pectoral nerves.

Associated Injuries

Soft Tissue

The anteroinferior glenoid labrum and anterior band of the IGHL are most commonly injured in a young patient presenting with a first-time anterior shoulder dislocation. This defect was first described by Bankart, with an incidence of 86–100%, and is known as a Bankart lesion [3].

During anterior dislocation of the shoulder, the posterior and superior rotator cuff become stretched. As age increases, the cuff degenerates and becomes less pliable, and rates of cuff tear as high as 54–61% have been reported in those over 40 years of age (although it cannot be completely certain that the tears were not present prior to dislocation) [26–28]. Correlations between full thickness tears of supraspinatus, night pain and inability to abduct to 90° have been described [26], and, if a rotator cuff tear is suspected, this should be investigated at follow-up (with MRI or ultrasound scan), given improved outcomes with earlier intervention to repair the rotator cuff [29].

Humeral avulsion of the glenohumeral ligament (HAGL—usually affects older patients than those with a Bankart lesion), anterior labral periosteal sleeve avulsion (ALPSA) and glenoid labral articular defects (GLAD—articular cartilage shears off with the labrum) can also occur.

MRI or magnetic resonance arthrogram (MRA) are the preferred methods of imaging to detect soft tissue lesions. The latter requires injection of contrast into the glenhumeral joint, and has been shown to be 90% sensitive and 100% specific for Bankart lesions [30].

Fractures

The overall fracture rate associated with shoulder dislocation is 29%, with independent risk factors being:

- First-time dislocation
- Age over 40 years
- Mechanism of injury [26]

Fractures of the humerus, glenoid, or both, can occur.

The most common fracture affecting the humerus is the Hill-Sachs lesion: a chondral defect affecting the posterosuperior aspect of the head of the humerus, caused by impaction against the anterior rim of the glenoid. Greater tuberosity fractures were seen in over 15% of patients in a study involving nearly 4000 patients, mostly in patients over 50 years of age [31], while proximal humerus (as classified by Neer) and surgical neck fractures arising less commonly (both are also a risk during reduction).

Anteroinferior fractures of the glenoid rim, the result of either avulsion of the labrum or impaction of the humeral head as it dislocates, are known as bony Bankart lesions. CT is the optimal imaging modality for assessment of bony injuries, giving information in terms of location, size and depth.

Management

As discussed earlier, following an acute anterior dislocation of the shoulder, treatment with a sling (in external or neutral rotation) and physiotherapy are often the first-line treatment. However, rates of recurrent dislocation can be as high as 87% at 2 years following first dislocation [5, 32], with some surgeons proposing early stabilization for those at risk of developing instability [33].

Instability symptoms can be revealed either by a history of recurrent dislocation episodes, or during clinical examination. The 'apprehension test' is performed by placing the patient's arm into 90° of abduction and external rotation, and, when positive, is accompanied by a feeling that the shoulder may dislocate. The 'relocation sign' reduces apprehension through the application of an antero-posterior force, with both tests being indicative of unidirectional instability.

Risk Factors

A number of studies have demonstrated younger age at time of dislocation (<25 years) to correlate with risk of recurrence, with other intrinsic risk factors including sex (males are 3.2 times more likely to suffer recurrent instability than women), hypermobility and bony and soft tissue lesions at the time of injury [34]. For example, a large Hill-Sachs can 'engage' with the glenoid rim, leading to dislocation through leverage of the head out of the joint, or a large glenoid rim fracture can affect conformity of the joint and lead to recurrent dislocation (glenoid rim fractures are seen in 49% of recurrent dislocators).

Extrinsic, or modifiable, factors include: participation in contact sports and occupation involving activity above chest height [5, 35].

Recurrent Instability

The rationale for reducing the incidence of recurrence through surgical intervention originated following evidence that rates of re-dislocation reduced following early arthroscopic lavage, versus traditional non-operative management (20 vs. 60%) [36]. A number of randomized controlled trials have demonstrated superiority of early arthroscopic surgery techniques over non-operative management for young, active, first-time dislocators (22 vs. 92% and 14 vs. 80%, respectively) [37, 38]. This evidence was supported by a Cochrane review (239 patients, mean age of 22 years-old), showing that instability was statistically significantly lower in the operative group [39].

Operative Techniques

Decision-making in terms of operative approach is dependent on assessment of patient factors and injury pattern. Specific soft tissue or bony lesions that are the direct cause of instability should be identified and addressed to provide an optimal outcome.

In the young (<25 years), athletic patient with a Bankart lesion, arthroscopic stabilization has been shown to yield excellent outcomes and return to previous activity levels, with low rates of recurrent dislocation [5]. A 'double-breasting' of the anterior capsule is performed, and the Bankart lesion reattached to the glenoid using suture anchors, thus providing an anterior restraint to the humeral head. The additional benefit of arthroscopic surgery over more traditional open techniques is the ability to perform a full diagnostic visualization of the joint, thus allowing identification of lesions, such as a HAGL, that might otherwise be missed.

In the presence of bony deficiency of the glenoid (15–20%), the risk of failure following arthroscopic Bankart repair is high. For these patients, the Bristow and Latarjet procedures have been described. The coracoid process is osteotomised and transferred to the site of the anteroinferior area of glenoid bone loss: the original description of the Bristow repair involved passing the coracoid fragment and conjoint tendon underneath subscapularis, but the Latarjet approach of passing the coracoid through subscapularis has gained increasing popularity, conferring the triple benefit to stability of:

1. Repair of the capsule
2. Restoring the surface area of the glenoid
3. Providing constraint to the joint when the arm is abducted and externally rotated to reinforce the antero-inferior capsule

For large, 'engaging' lesions of the humeral head (Hill-Sachs defects of >25% surface area), the 'Remplissage technique' can be employed to reduce risk of dislocation, where infraspinatus and posterior capsule are sutured into the defect. Alternatively, rotational osteotomy of the head or allograft reconstruction of the defect (e.g. using iliac crest bone graft) may be performed, and arthroplasty forms a last resort in lesions that cannot be reconstructed by any other means.

No operative procedure is without risk, however, and, as with all surgical intervention, benefit to the patient must be weighed against potential complications. Recurrence, although much lower than with conservative treatment, remains the greatest risk following stabilization, followed by infection and neurovascular injury. Furthermore, future risk of degenerative arthritis has not yet been quantified with these techniques, as has been seen with now historical, techniques such as the Putti-Platt and Magnuson-Stack approaches, which resulted in over-tightening of the joint and increased loading of the glenoid.

Posterior Dislocation of the Glenohumeral Joint

Posterior dislocations of the glenohumeral joint account for around 2% of shoulder dislocations [40, 41]. Mechanism of injury is commonly a fall directly onto the shoulder, such as during a seizure, resulting in an anteroposterior force to the humeral head. Alternatively, adduction and axial loading of the arm may also result in posterior dislocation. It is estimated that almost 50% of posterior dislocations may be missed on initial examination [42].

Examination

A history of the causative event should be taken: clinical examination will reveal a decreased range of movement, particularly external rotation, as the head of the humerus is trapped posterior to the glenoid. The arm will be held in internal rotation.

Imaging

Posterior dislocations can be subtle on AP radiographs of the shoulder. A 'light bulb' sign may be seen, in which the humeral head appears symmetrical, with the greater tuberosity missing owing to the internal rotation of the head [43]. An axillary or scapular Y view is necessary for assessment of the position of the humeral head relative to the glenoid.

CT may be useful in cases where diagnosis is uncertain and for assessment of associated bony injuries.

Ultrasound or MRI scan can be used for evaluation of the rotator cuff in cases where there is suspicion of a tear.

Associated Injuries

65% of posterior dislocations have an associated fracture or rotator cuff tear, and in the absence of a fracture, the risk of a cuff tear increases by 4.6 times [44].

Soft Tissue

The posterior band of the inferior glenohumeral ligament (IGHL) is the primary restraint to internal rotation, and may be avulsed or torn during posterior dislocation.

Avulsion of the postero-inferior labrum, or a posterior Bankart lesion, can also occur as a result of acute dislocation. Occasionally, the labrum may appear intact superficially, but the deep portion is avulsed (known as a Kim lesion).

Labral cysts and capsular pouches are more commonly the result of chronic posterior instability.

Fractures

Following posterior dislocation, the anteromedial aspect of the humerus becomes impacted against the posterior glenoid rim. This can result in indentation, or fracture, of this surface of the humeral head, known as a Reverse Hill-Sachs, or McLaughlin, lesion. If the lesion is less than 25% of the articular surface of the humeral head, this is considered to be small, 25–50% medium and more than 50% large [45].

Posterior glenoid rim fractures may also be present, caused either by the humeral head abutting against it at the time of dislocation, or as an avulsion fracture associated with the postero-inferior labrum.

Lesser tuberosity fractures are rare in isolation, and should raise suspicion of a posterior dislocation when seen on X-ray. The subscapularis muscle forms the primary dynamic restraint in external rotation, and can cause avulsion of the lesser tuberosity at the time of injury.

Management: Closed Reduction

Closed reduction can be performed under sedation or general anaesthetic. The technique for closed reduction was first described by Hippocrates, who advocated internal rotation of the arm, flexion of the elbow and reduction of the shoulder from behind. Longitudinal traction may be preferred, with the addition of flexion and adduction of the shoulder. If the humeral head is impacted on the posterior aspect of the glenoid rim, internal rotation may be required to disimpact the head before traction is applied. Care should be taken to avoid fracture of the humeral head or neck during this manoeuvre. If stable following reduction, the arm should be immobilized in a broad arm sling for 3–4 weeks (in neutral rotation or 10–20° of external rotation) before commencement of physiotherapy.

Management: Open Reduction

If closed reduction is not possible, open reduction via the deltopectoral approach should be performed. Owing to the deformity of the glenohumeral anatomy, the biceps tendon can be used for reference, in order to safely identify the lesser tuberosity and rotator interval prior to making a capsulotomy and accessing the humeral head.

Management: Recurrent Instability and Internal Fixation

Following a traumatic posterior dislocation, patients may proceed to develop recurrent instability. It is important to distinguish those with true structural abnormalities, as described above, from patients with muscle patterning problems, multidirectional instability (with global capsular insufficiency) or dislocations secondary to a psychological issue.

A clear history of trauma, clinical examination and appropriate investigation can be used to determine patients appropriate to undergo surgical intervention for recurrent instability.

Clinical examination should include:

- 'Posterior stress test', where the arm is place in 90° flexion and internal rotation and a posterior force applied (a clunk is felt as the shoulder subluxes and reduces).
- 'Kim test', with the patient seated, the arm is placed in 90° of abduction, and gradually flexed to 45° while an axial load is applied to the elbow, forcing the humerus in a postero-inferior direction. Pain indicates a positive test.
- 'Drawer test', the shoulder is abducted to 30° and a posterior force applied to the head of the humerus. Posterior laxity is evident in instability.

As mentioned previously, CT is helpful in determining bony abnormalities, while MRI, with arthrogram, is useful in the diagnosis of soft tissue abnormalities.

Patients in whom recurrent instability develops with posterior Bankart or Kim lesions can be treated with posterior labral/Bankart repair and capsular shift. This can be performed either through an open approach or arthroscopically.

In the presence of no bony injury, or a small (<25% articular surface) reverse Hill-Sachs lesion, instability is unlikely. Medium and large lesions can lead to symptomatic instability, for which two open procedures have been described.

1. McLaughlin Procedure—Transfer of the subscapularis into the humeral head at the site of the bony defect [46].
2. Neer Procedure—Osteotomy of the lesser tuberosity and transfer into the bony defect [47].

Rotational osteotomy, intended to maintain the bony defect anterior to the glenoid, and allograft/autograft reconstruction have also been described with similar results [48–51].

Arthroplasty (hemiarthroplasty or total shoulder replacement) is a final option for large lesions (>50%) where there is poor bone stock or significant arthritis of the humeral head and glenoid [52, 53].

Chronic Posterior Dislocation

Chronic posterior dislocation, following an unrecognized acute posterior dislocation, poses a particular treatment dilemma. Closed reduction may not be possible 3 weeks after injury [45], and in the elderly, non-operative treatment is an option, giving reasonable outcomes [54, 55]. For patients with chronic dislocation <6 months old, open reduction with a McLaughlin or Neer procedure is the preferred option, but for those >6 months old, arthroplasty should be considered [55].

Acromioclavicular Joint Injuries

Anatomy

The clavicle provides the main osseous connection between the thorax and the shoulder girdle. It maintains the lateral position of the shoulder, resisting the combined actions of trapezius and pectoralis major. Medially, the clavicle circum-ducts around the sternoclavicular joint and, laterally articulates with the medial clavicular facet of the acromion.

The acromioclavicular joint (ACJ) contains a fibrocartilaginous disc, that can be either complete or partial (meniscoid) in nature. Stability of the ACJ is detmerined by the capsular (acromioclavicular) and extracapsular (coracoclavicular) ligaments. The strongest acromioclavicular ligament is the superior ligament, which is also augmented by the attachments of deltoid and trapezius. The majority of anteroposterior stability of the ACJ is provided by the acromioclavicular ligaments, with superoinferior stability conferred by the coracoclavicular ligaments. The conoid (medial) and trapezoid (lateral) ligaments originating at the base of the coracoid process, attaching to the inferior surface of the clavicle. They are the primary suspensory ligaments of the upper limb.

ACJ Dislocation

ACJ dislocation is most common among young men, and is often the result of direct injury to the shoulder tip or a fall onto the elbow: force spreads through the acromioclavicular ligaments initially, followed by the coracoclavicular ligaments, and, in a complete injury, through the coracohumeral ligaments. The result is inferior translation of the upper extremity, clinically presenting as prominence of the distal end of the clavicle.

Classification

Classification systems relating to the ACJ are based on the degree of damage to the acromioclavicular and coracoclavicular ligaments. Tossy, Mead and Sigmond [56] and Allman [57] described three categories of ACJ disruption based on an AP radiograph of the shoulder, with Rockwood [58] later adding a further three:

1. Acromioclavicular ligaments sprained, coracoclavicular ligaments intact.
2. Acromioclavicular ligaments ruptured, coracoclavicular ligaments sprained.
3. Both acromioclavicular and coracoclavicular ligaments ruptured. Clavicle displaced *superiorly*.
4. Both acromioclavicular and coracoclavicular ligaments ruptured. Clavicle displaced *posteriorly*, button-holing through trapezius muscle.
5. Both acromioclavicular and coracoclavicular ligaments ruptured. Marked superior dislocation of the clavicle. Deltoid and trapezius detached.
6. Both acromioclavicular and coracoclavicular ligaments ruptured. Clavicle displaced *inferior* to acromion and coracoid process.

Management

Types 1 and 2

The majority of type 1 and 2 ACJ injuries can be managed conservatively, with a broad arm sling, for 1–2 weeks. However, it has been argued that these injuries are not as benign as previously thought, with one series showing only 50% of patients to be asymptomatic after 6 years [59]. Nearly one third of patients developed chronic ACJ pathology requiring subsequent surgery, with a similar number reporting activity-related pain. Athletes and manual labourers, particularly those involved in overhead activities or with carrying objects on their shoulders, may require later surgery.

Type 3

The management of type 3 ACJ injuries is controversial: currently there is limited evidence for the superiority of either operative or non-operative treatment in the treatment of these injuries. Meta-analyses and systematic reviews on the current evidence have found that, while operative management is associated with improved cosmetic outcome, it also has a higher complication rate, longer recovery and greater time for return to work and sport [60–62].

Types 4, 5 and 6

Owing to the significant displacement of these injuries, operative management is generally recommended, as instability and impingement symptoms can persist with non-operative management.

Numerous techniques are available for restoration of ACJ alignment. In 1972 Weaver and Dunn [63] described their classic procedure, involving excision of the lateral clavicle and transfer of the coracoacromial ligament from the acromion to the lateral end of the clavicle. This has undergone several modifications [64], with newer developments such as the Tightrope (Arthrex) and Surgilig (Surgicraft) offering further options for securing the ACJ in an anatomical position using attachment through, or around, the coracoid. The lateral clavicle hook plate is also an option, but in the majority of cases the plate will require removal at a later stage to avoid impingement. In patients with chronic symptoms or post-traumatic osteolysis, excision of the acromioclavicular joint and distal 5–10 mm of the clavicle, the Mumford procedure, performed through a 'bra-strap' incision, provides satisfactory outcomes [65].

Summary

- Dislocations of the shoulder girdle are common injuries, particularly anterior glenohumeral dislocations.
- Appropriate imaging and clinical examination should be performed both before and following attempted reduction.
- Reduction should be performed expediently in the emergency room, or operating theatre.
- If closed reduction is not possible, open reduction should be performed through a deltopectoral approach.
- Initial management is in a sling in external or neutral rotation
- In young patients (<25 years) who take part in contact sports, risk of recurrence is high, and early stabilization should be considered.
- There is a strong association between dislocations of the glenohumeral joint and soft tissues injuries and fractures. If instability occurs, these must be investigated and dealt with appropriately to restore stability.
- Management of acromioclavicular joint injuries remains controversial, with the possibility for operative anatomical reduction and early or late ligament reconstruction, or late excision of the joint and distal clavicle being shown to yield satisfactory results. Patient factors must be taken into account when considering operative treatment.

Questions

1. What is the most common fracture type after shoulder dislocation?
   A. Bony Bankart
   B. Greater tuberosity
   C. Surgical neck of humerus
   D. Hill-Sachs
   E. Coracoid
   D

2. You decide to operate a 21 year old male patient with recurrent shoulder dislocation arthroscopically. Which of the following do you expect to see damaged most common intraoperatively?
   A. Posterior band of IGHL
   B. SGHL
   C. MGHL
   D. Rotator cuff
   E. Anterior band of IGHL
   E

3. 40 year old female patient with a traumatic anterior left shoulder dislocation admitted to hospital after a fall from the stairs one year ago. A closed reduction was performed and no other pathology was observed. She has been suffering from recurrent dislocations since then. A glenoid defect of %30 was detected on her CT. What would be your first choice of treatment?
   A. Conservative treatment with PT
   B. Diagnostic arthroscopy
   C. Laterjet procedure + arthroscopy
   D. Remplissage procedure
   E. Shoulder arthroplasty

What's new?

There is a conflict about the stabilization of AC joint dislocations with hook plate. The study of Canadian Orthopaedic Trauma Society which shows no difference between non-operative and operative treatment of acute AC joint dislocation, may change our treatment algorithm.

Multicenter Randomized Clinical Trial of Nonoperative Versus Operative Treatment of Acute Acromio-Clavicular Joint Dislocation. Journal of Orthopaedic Trauma, November 2015, Canadian Orthopaedic Trauma Society.

References

1. Itoi E, Hatakeyama Y, Kido T, Sato T, Minagawa H, Wakabayashi I, et al. A new method of immobilization after traumatic anterior dislocation of the shoulder: a preliminary study. J Shoulder Elb Surg. 2003;12:413–5. doi:10.1016/S1058-2746(03)00171-X.
2. Hovelius L. Incidence of shoulder dislocation in Sweden. Clin Orthop Relat Res. 1982;166:127–31.
3. Gooding B, Geoghegan J, Manning P. The management of acute traumatic primary anterior shoulder dislocation in young adults. Shoulder Elb. 2010;2:141–6.
4. Owens BD, Dawson L, Burks R, Cameron KL. Incidence of shoulder dislocation in the United States Military: demographic considerations from a high-risk population. J Bone Joint Surg Am. 2009;91:791–6. doi:10.2106/JBJS.H.00514.
5. Robinson CM, Howes J, Murdoch H, et al. Functional outcome and risk of recurrent instability after primary traumatic anterior shoulder dislocation in young patients. J Bone Joint Surg Am. 2006;88:2326–36.
6. Llaa RL, Brand R, Marti RK, et al. A prospective arthroscopic study of acute first-time anterior shoulder dislocation in the young: a five year follow-up study. J Shoulder Elb Surg. 2003;12:529–34.
7. Kroner K, Lind T, Jensen J. The epidemiology of shoulder dislocation. Arch Orthop Traum Surg. 1989;108:288–90.
8. Smith T. Immobilization following traumatic anterior glenohumeral joint dislocation. A literature review. Injury. 2006;37:228–37. doi:10.1016/j.injury.2005.06.005.
9. Arnander M, Tennent D. Shoulder dislocations—missed associated injuries. J Trauma Orthop. 2014; 2(3):44–6.
10. Travlos J, Goldberg I, Boome RS. Brachial plexus lesions associated with dislocated shoulders. J Bone Joint Surg Br. 1990;72(1):68–71.
11. Visser CP, et al. The incidence of nerve injury in anterior dislocation of the shoulder and its influence on functional recovery. A prospective clinical and EMG study. J Bone Joint Surg Br. 1999;81(4):679–85.
12. Christofi T, Kallis DA, Raptis M, Rowland M, Ryan J. Management of shoulder dislocations. Trauma. 2007;9:39–46.
13. Drury JK, Scullion JE. Vascular complications of anterior dislocation of the shoulder. Br J Surg. 1980;67(8):579–81.
14. Helm AT, Watson JS. Compression of the brachial plexus in a patient with false aneurysm of the axillary artery as a result of anterior shoulder dislocation. J Shoulder Elb Surg. 2002;11(3):278–9.
15. Kelley SP, Hinsche AF, Hossain JF. Axillary artery transection following anterior shoulder dislocation: classical presentation and current concepts. Injury. 2004;35(11):1128–32.
16. Plaga BR, et al. Axillary artery injury secondary to inferior shoulder dislocation. J Emerg Med. 2010; 39(5):599–601.
17. Bloom MH, Obata WG. Diagnosis of posterior dislocation of the shoulder with use of Velpeau axillary and angle-up roentgenographic views. J Bone Joint Surg Am. 1967;49(5):943–9.
18. Garth Jr WP, Slappey CE, Ochs CW. Roentgenographic demonstration of instability of the shoulder: the apical oblique projection. A technical note. J Bone Joint Surg Am. 1984;66(9):1450–3.
19. Kahn JH, Mehta SD. The role of post-reduction radiographs after shoulder dislocation. J Emerg Med. 2007;33(2):169–73.
20. Ogawa K, Yoshida A, Ikegami H. Isolated fractures of the greater tuberosity of the humerus: solutions to recognizing a frequently overlooked fracture. J Trauma. 2003;54(4):713–7.
21. Kirker JR. Dislocation of the shoulder complicated by rupture of the axillary vessels. Repeat of a case. J Bone Joint Surg. 1952;34B:72–3.
22. McRae R. Pocketbook of orthopaedics and fractures. 2nd ed. Philadelphia: Churchill Livingstone Elsevier; 2006. p. 276–80.
23. Kothari RU, Dronen SC. Prospective evaluation of the scapular manipulation technique in reducing anterior shoulder dislocation. Ann Emerg Med. 1992;21: 1349–52.
24. Itoi E, Hatakeyama Y, Sato T, et al. Immobilization in external rotation after shoulder dislocation reduces the risk of recurrence. J Bone Joint Surg Am. 2007;89:2124–31.
25. Liavaag S, Brox JI, Pripp AH, et al. Immobilization in external rotation after primary shoulder dislocation did not reduce the risk of recurrence. J Bone Joint Surg Am. 2011;93(10):897–904.
26. Berbig R, et al. Primary anterior shoulder dislocation and rotator cuff tears. J Shoulder Elb Surg. 1999; 8(3):220–5.
27. Neviaser RJ, Neviaser TJ, Neviaser JS. Concurrent rupture of the rotator cuff and anterior dislocation of the shoulder in the older patient. J Bone Joint Surg Am. 1988;70(9):1308–11.
28. Simank HG, et al. Incidence of rotator cuff tears in shoulder dislocations and results of therapy in older

patients. Arch Orthop Trauma Surg. 2006;126(4): 235–40.
29. Bassett RW, Cofield RH. Acute tears of the rotator cuff. The timing of surgical repair. Clin Orthop Relat Res. 1983;175:18–24.
30. Han Oh J, Yoon Kim J, Choi JA, et al. Effectiveness of multidetector computed tomography arthrography for the diagnosis of shoulder pathology: comparison with magnetic resonance imaging with arthroscopic correlation. J Shoulder Elb Surg. 2010;19(1):14–20.
31. Robinson C, Shur N, Sharpe T, et al. Injuries associated with traumatic anterior glenohumeral dislocations. J Bone Joint Surg Am. 2012;94:18–26.
32. Rowe CR. Prognosis in dislocations of the shoulder. J Bone Joint Surg Am. 1956;38:957–77.
33. Boone JL, Arciero RA. First-time anterior shoulder dislocations: has the standard changed? Br J Sports Med. 2010;44:355–60.
34. Olds M, Ellis R, Donaldson K, et al. Risk factors which predispose first-time traumatic anterior shoulder dislocations to recurrent instability in adults: a systematic review and meta-analysis. Br J Sports Med. 2015;49:913–23.
35. Sachs R, Lin D, Stone M-L, et al. Can the need for future surgery for acute traumatic anterior shoulder dislocation be predicted? J Bone Joint Surg Am. 2007;89:1665.
36. Wintzell G, Haglund-Akerlind Y, Nowak J, Larsson S. Arthroscopic lavage compared with nonoperative treatment for traumatic primary anterior shoulder dislocation: a 2-year follow-up of a prospective randomized study. J Shoulder Elb Surg. 1999;8:399–402.
37. Wheeler JH, Ryan JB, Arciero RA, et al. Arthroscopic versus non-operative treatment of acute shoulder dislocations in young athletes. Arthroscopy. 1989;5: 213–7.
38. Arciero RA, WheelerJH RJB, et al. Arthroscopic Bankart repair versus nonoperative treatment for acute, initial anterior shoulder dislocations. Am J Sports Med. 1994;22:589–94.
39. Handoll HHG, Almaiyah MA. Surgical versus nonsurgical treatment for acute anterior shoulder dislocation. Cochrane Database Syst Rev 2004; CD004325.
40. Cave EF, Burke JF, Boyd RJ. Trauma management. Chicago: Year Book Medical Publishers; 1974. p. 437.
41. Becker R, Weyand F. Rare, bilateral posterior shoulder dislocation: a case report. Unfallchirurg. 1990;93: 66–8.
42. Heller KD, Forst J, Forst R. Differential therapy of traumatically-induced persistent posterior shoulder dislocation: review of the literature. Unfallchirurg. 1995;98:6–12.
43. Arndt J, Sears A. Posterior dislocation of the shoulder. Am J Roentgenol. 1965;94:639–45.
44. Rouleau DM, Hebert-Davies J. Incidence of associated injury in posterior shoulder dislocation: systematic review of the literature. J Orthop Trauma. 2012;26(4):246–51.
45. Cicak N, Bilic R, Delimar D. Hill-Sachs lesion in recurrent shoulder dislocation: sonographic detection. J Ultrasound Med. 1998;17:557–60.
46. Cicak N. Posterior dislocation of the shoulder. J Bone Joint Surg Br. 2004;86-B:324–32.
47. McLaughlin HL. Posterior dislocation of the shoulder. J Bone Joint Surg Am. 1952;34-A:584–90.
48. Hughes M, Neer II CS. Glenohumeral joint replacement and postoperative rehabilitation. Phys Ther. 1975;55:850–8.
49. Keppler P, Holz U, Thielemann FW, Meinig R. Locked posterior dislocation of the shoulder: treatment using rotational osteotomy of the humerus. J Orthop Trauma. 1994;8:286–92.
50. Gerber C, Lambert SM. Allograft reconstruction of segmental defects of the humeral head for the treatment of chronic locked posterior dislocation of the shoulder. J Bone Joint Surg Am. 1996;78-A: 376–82.
51. Connor PM, Boatright RJ, D'Alessandro DF. Posterior fracture-dislocation of the shoulder: treatment with acute osteochondral grafting. J Shoulder Elb Surg. 1997;6:480–5.
52. Page AE, Meinhard BP, Schulz E, Toledano B. Bilateral posterior fracture-dislocation of the shoulders: management by bilateral shoulder hemiarthroplasties. J Orthop Trauma. 1995;9:526–9.
53. Cheng SL, Mackay MB, Richards RR. Treatment of locked posterior fracture-dislocations of the shoulder by total shoulder arthroplasty. J Shoulder Elb Surg. 1997;6:11–7.
54. Loebenberg MI, Cuomo F. The treatment of chronic anterior and posterior dislocations of the glenohumeral joint and associated articular surface defects. Orthop Clin North Am. 2000;31:23–34.
55. Gerber C. Chronic, locked anterior and posterior dislocation. In: Warner JJP, Ianotti JP, Gerber C, editors. Complex and revision problems in shoulder surgery. Philadelphia: Lippincott-Raven; 1997. p. 99–113.
56. Tossy JD, Mead NC, Sigmond HM. Acromioclavicular separation: useful and practical classification for treatment. Clin Orthop. 1963;28:111–9.
57. Allman Jr FL. Fractures and ligamentous injuries of the clavicle and its articulation. J Bone Joint Surg Am. 1967;49:774–84.
58. Rockwood CA, Williams GR, Youg DC. Disorders of the acromioclavicular joint. In: Rockwood CA, Masten II FA, editors. The shoulder. Philadelphia: Saunders; 1998. p. 483–553.
59. Mouhsine E, Garofalo R, Crevoisier X, Farron A. Grade I and II acromioclavicular dislocations: results of conservative treatment. J Shoulder Elb Surg. 2003;12(6):599–602.
60. Smith TO, et al. Operative versus non-operative management following Rockwood grade III acromioclavicular separation: a meta-analysis of the current evidence base. J Orthop Traumatol. 2011;12:19–27.

61. Spencer Jr EE. Treatment of Grade III acromioclavicular joint injuries: a systematic review. Clin Orthop Relat Res. 2007;455:38–44.
62. Ceccarelli E, Bondì R, Alviti F, Garofalo R, Miulli F, Padua R. Treatment of acute grade III acromioclavicular dislocation: a lack of evidence. J Orthop Traumatol. 2008;9(2):105–8. doi:10.1007/s10195-008-0013-7.
63. Weaver JK, Dunn HK. Treatment of acromioclavicular injuries, especially complete acromioclavicular separations. J Bone Joint Surg. 1972;54-A:1187.
64. Copeland S. Operative shoulder surgery. New York: Churchill Livingstone; 1995.
65. Fraser-Moodie JA, Shortt NL, Robinson CM. Injuries to the acromioclavicular joint. J Bone Joint Surg Br. 2008;90-B:697–707.

Scapula and Glenoid Fractures

12

Egemen Turhan, Mehmet Kaymakoglu, Gazi Huri, and Mahmut Nedim Doral

Introduction

Scapula fractures are not frequently seen even in trauma centers. They comprise only less than 1% of all fractures and 3–5% of fractures involving shoulder region [1, 2]. This low rate is explained with its close position to elastic chest wall, surrounding thick shoulder girdle muscles and soft tissues and high mobility of shoulder girdle. Therefore, scapula fractures are highly associated with high energy trauma such as vehicle accidents or falling from height. Although rare bilateral cases were seen in the literature, scapula fractures almost occur unilaterally as a matter of course [3]. Scapula fractures can be misdiagnosed in polytrauma patients because of less attention given when other concomitant severe injuries exist.

Treatment strategies varies from conservative to open reduction and fixation, as well as arthroscopy assisted techniques which became more popular in the last decade especially in glenoid fractures. Management of these fractures would be challenging for some surgeons due to its rarity and lack of experience. Lack of large patient groups makes the agreement on the treatment and indications difficult. Thus, numerous surgical or conservative management strategies can be found in the literature. Open reduction techniques is associated with good end results, on the other hand arthroscopy assisted techniques are applied only by experienced artroscopists. In this chapter we discuss the nature of scapula fractures, its classifications and current treatment strategies.

E. Turhan (✉) • M. Kaymakoglu • G. Huri
M.N. Doral
Orthopaedics and Traumatology Department, Hacettepe University, Ankara, Turkey
e-mail: dregementurhan@yahoo.com

Anatomy

Scapula is like a rudder of the shoulder girdle. It stabilizes the shoulder and on the other hand helps the glenohumeral joint's circumduction which has the highest range of motion of the entire body. It has a flat, triangular shape with a spine on posterosuperior side extending from medial side to glenoid fossa. Scapular spine touches slightly posterior side of the glenoid fossa, goes towards superiorly and forms the acromion. On the sagittal plane it is slightly concave to correspond the shape of thoracic wall. This concavity is named subscapular fossa. Coracoid process stems from the superior side and heads towards anteriorly and laterally. Suprascapular notch, in which suprascapular nerve and artery run through, lies just medial to the coracoid.

Medial, lateral and superior borders of the scapula are thicker, as many muscles has insertion on these areas. Medial border is the site of

G. Huri, N.K. Paschos (eds.), *The Shoulder*, Orthopaedic Study Guide Series,
DOI 10.1007/978-3-319-51979-1_12

muscles that connect the scapula to axial skeleton (e.g. levator scapula, rhomboid muscles, serratus anterior) Lateral border is the origo site of teres major, teres minor and some bundles of subscapularis on the anterior lip. Trapezius muscle is the main muscle group that attaches to the superior border. Posterior bundles of deltoid also attaches to the spine of scapula. Infraspinatus and supraspinatus cover the two self-titled fossas on the posterior and anterior concavity is filled with subscapularis muscle. These three muscle is responsible for rotating the humerus and named 'rotator cuff' together with teres minor muscle.

Shoulder Suspensory Complex

Scapula provides stability to the shoulder with a complex bony and soft tissue ring called 'Superior Shoulder Suspensory Complex'. This complex is made of various ligaments and bone structures. The bone structure composed of two struts: superior and inferior. Superior strut is made of the middle third of the clavicle and the inferior strut is formed by the upper border of the junction of scapular neck and body. Bony/soft tissue complex was divided into three units by Goss: acromioclavicular joint and ligaments, coracoclavicular ligaments and junction of glenoid, coracoid and acromion [4]. This structure shows us the importance of soft tissue linkage between the scapula and axial skeleton. We will discuss its injuries in Goss classification section.

Classification

Petit who is a french surgeon in eighteenth century, was the first phycisian described the scapula fractures [5]. We can simply divide the scapula fractures into four groups, as Ada and Miller et al. did in 1991 [6]. These groups consist fractures of processes, scapular neck fractures, glenoid fossa fractures and body fractures. Today, many classification systems exist but there is no consensus about which one should be used [7–9]. Most widely used classification systems are AO/OTA New International Classification System for Scapula Fractures, Ideberg classification for glenoid fossa fractures and the Goss Classification for shoulder suspensory complex injuries.

AO/OTA Classification

In 2013, AO represented its new modified classification system called 'New International Classification System for Scapula Fractures' (Fig. 12.1). One year later, Neuhaus et al. found the interobserver reliability of New Classification System higher than the previous AO/OTA Classification [10].

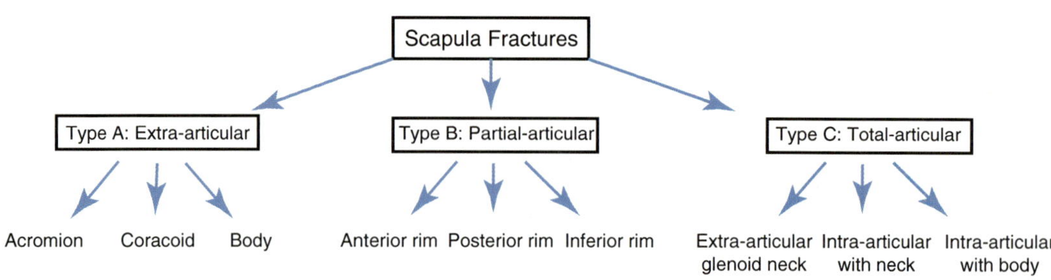

Fig. 12.1 AO/OTA classification

Table 12.1 Ideberg classification

Type 1: Anterior glenoid rim fracture. Type 1A with a fracture fragment of 5 mm or less, and type 1B with a fracture fragment larger than 5 mm.
Type 2a: Inferior glenoid fracture involving part of the neck
Type 3: Superior glenoid fracture extending through the base of the coracoid process.
Type 4: Horizontal fracture involving both scapula neck and body. Fracture line always runs inferior to the spine of the scapula.
Type 5: Horizontal fracture (as in type 4), with an additional complete or incomplete neck fracture.

Ideberg Classification

Ideberg et al. published a classification system for glenoid fractures in 1995, after reviewing more than 100 glenoid fractures [11]. He found that the most common fracture of glenoid fossa is associated with shoulder dislocation and avulsion fracture of anterior margin of glenoid is the most broken site of glenoid. You can find a summary of Ideberg Classification below (Table 12.1) [11].

Goss Classification

Goss summarized superior shoulder suspensory complex (SSSC) injuries and defined a classification system in 1995 [12]. He divided these injuries into two; single disruptions with only one ligament torn in SSSC ring and double unstable disruptions which requires surgical stabilization [4]. He stated that double disruptions make the shoulder girdle unstable and result in displacement of the fracture site. If any suspicious injury about SSSC occurs, careful clinical examination, weight-bearing AP X-rays and a CT-scan is needed to reveal the exact injury. You can find Goss' specification in Table 12.2. Physicians must be careful at assessing the type of SSRC disruption, as fracture of one bony strut with a double disruption of SSRC can create 'Floating Shoulder'. For example, glenoid neck and clavicle fracture with torn CC ligaments can demonstrate this circumstance.

Table 12.2 Goss classification

Single disruptions
• Type A: Single disruption by a break
• Type B: Single disruption by ligament injury
Double disruptions
• Type C: Double ligament injury
• Type D: Double break
• Type E: Combined bone and ligament disruption
• Type F: Both struts disrupted
• Type G: One strut and one ring disruption

Treatment of Scapula Fractures

An orthopaedic surgeon has various treatment strategies among patients with scapula fractures. The main principle of scapula fracture treatment is to preserve range of motion of shoulder joint. Because of the complex structure of shoulder joint with many ligaments and soft tissues e.g. rotator cuff, pain is the main complaint after the treatment, as many associated injuries can occur even after a simple glenohumeral dislocation [13]. Instability and preventing osteoarthritis is the main indications for surgical treatment. Generally, non displaced fractures of the scapula tend to be treated more conservatively. Intraarticular fractures namely glenoid fractures are treated surgically, especially if there is a step in articular surface or if the broken part is more than 25% of the whole glenoid.

Main principles in assessment of scapula fractures should not be forgotten; a concise neurological and vascular examination should be performed for each patient in ER. Because of high incidence of concomitant injuries in scapula fractures, care should be taken for the whole body. Physicians should never be forget that polytrauma patients and high energy injuries have the highest risk for scapula fractures, hence other fractures and organ injuries usually accompany a scapula fracture. Many missed scapula fracture cases were published in the literature [14].

Conservative treatment is applied with a 2–3 week long immobilization with a sling. After this period, the patient must be referred to a physiotherapist to start pendular exercises to avoid frozen shoulder. After 1 month the patient can start active range of motion exercises and finally, strengthening of shoulder muscles [15]. There are some good results in the literature with conservative treatment of scapula fractures. Bozkurt et al. reported acceptable results in patients with scapula neck fractures in which conservative treatment were applied [16].

There is a debate in ***operative treatment*** indications. The main treatment strategy is open reduction and internal fixation for displaced body and neck fractures, however many authors recommend arthroscopically assisted fixation for glenoid and even coracoid fractures. Imaging with a CT scan should be performed to assess the exact type of fracture before surgery. Below, we will discuss each individual scapula fracture type.

Scapula Neck Fractures

Neck fractures is the hardest type to decide whether conservative or surgical treatment is appropriate. The main consensus is that if the coracoacromial or coracoclavicular ligaments are intact, the fracture are accepted as more stable. Authors recommend open reduction for fractures with the suspensory ligaments (CA-CC) are torn [17]. Usually, the glenoid displaces anteriorly and medially because of the tonus of muscles attached to glenoid. This rotational displacement can be measured with 'glenopolar angle'

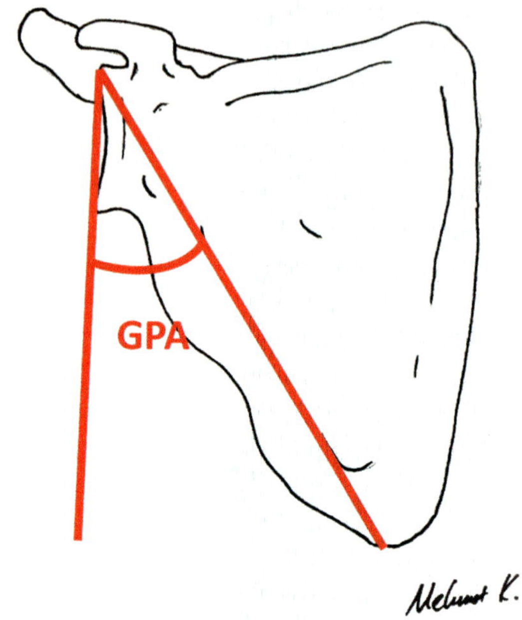

Fig. 12.2 Glenopolar angle

(Fig. 12.2). Normal values are 30–45° and less than 20° is indicative for operative treatment. Plate fixation is recommended for the open reduction and internal fixation. Well-known Judet approach can be used for this type of fracture.

Judet Approach

Judet described this approach in 1964 for operative treatment of scapula fractures [18]. It creates a bow-like incision line starting from glenoid to superomedial corner of scapula and extends down till the inferior border of scapula. It gives opportunity to reach almost all areas of scapula. It is indicated in scapular spine, neck, body and posterior glenoid rim fractures. During the incision process, the skin is raised like a flap and deltoid muscle is retracted laterally. After that dissection of infraspinatus and teres minor is made and an interval between this muscles is created (Fig. 12.3).

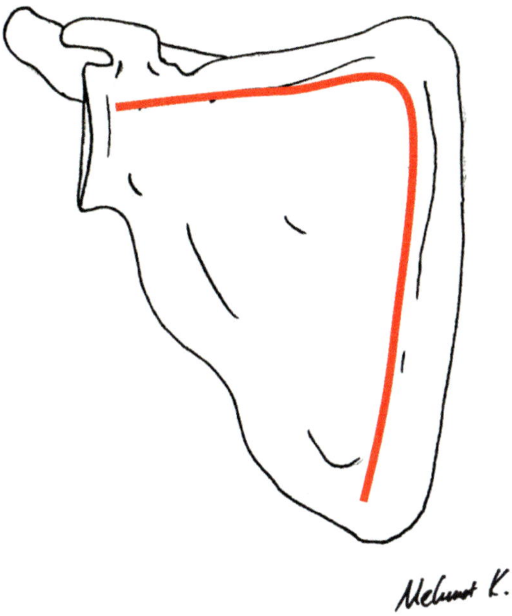

Fig. 12.3 Judet approach

Glenoid Fractures

Glenoid fossa fractures differs from other type of scapula fractures with joint involvement. This feature manifests itself with sensitive criteria of joint congruity for surgical fixation. Surgery is recommended for about 5 mm articular step or 20–30% involvement of articular surface. Deltopectoral approach can be used for fixation of glenoid. The most common type of glenoid fracture is the anteroinferior rim displacement after shoulder dislocation. This gived the idea to some authors that arthroscopy can be used in fixation of bony lesions. Recently, many papers were published good results with arthroscopically assisted fixation. Sugaya et al. stated that successful fixation with suture anchors in patients with an average of 27% bone loss of glenoid can be performed [19].

Body Fractures

Body fractures are generally managed conservatively, if there is no any malalignment between glenoid and lateral border of the scapula. Attention to the spine of scapula must be given as trapezius and deltoid muscles can displace the fracture line and cause malunion and pain. Open reduction and fixation are being used more these years, as recent papers give courage to trauma surgeons about how good end results ORIF has. A 3D-CT scan must be performed to evaluate the exact pattern of the fracture line [20].

Our Case

Thirty-four year old male patient was evaluated after a traffic accident in ER. His left shoulder was tender and had a very limited range of motion. After his full complete examination, his first AP shoulder X-ray is below:

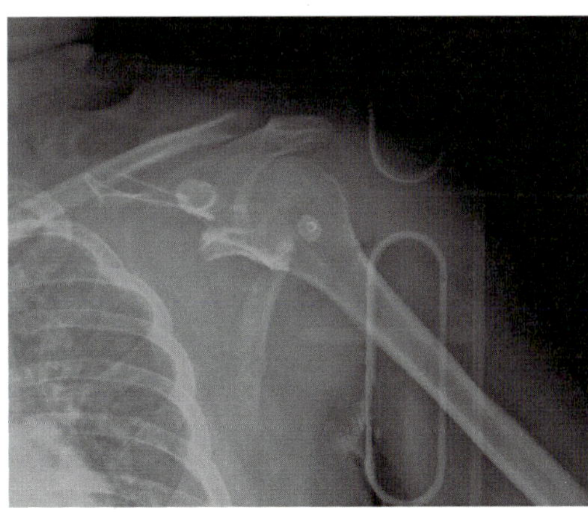

Picture 1.

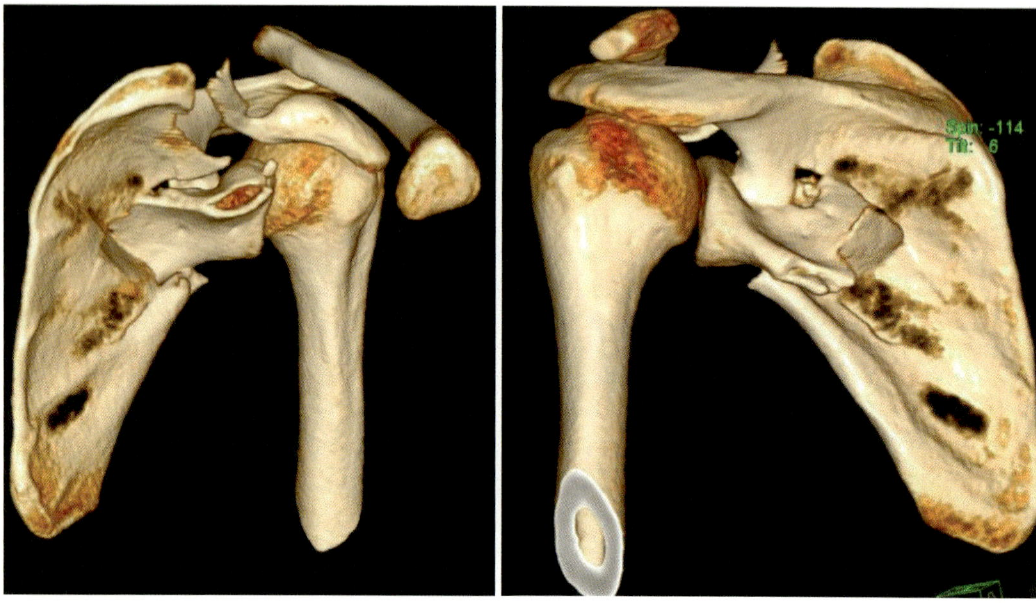

Picture 2–3. After the first examination and plain radiograph, a CT-scan was performed to understand the exact fracture pattern. Glenoid fracture with distal AC joint dislocation was seen on CT-scan.

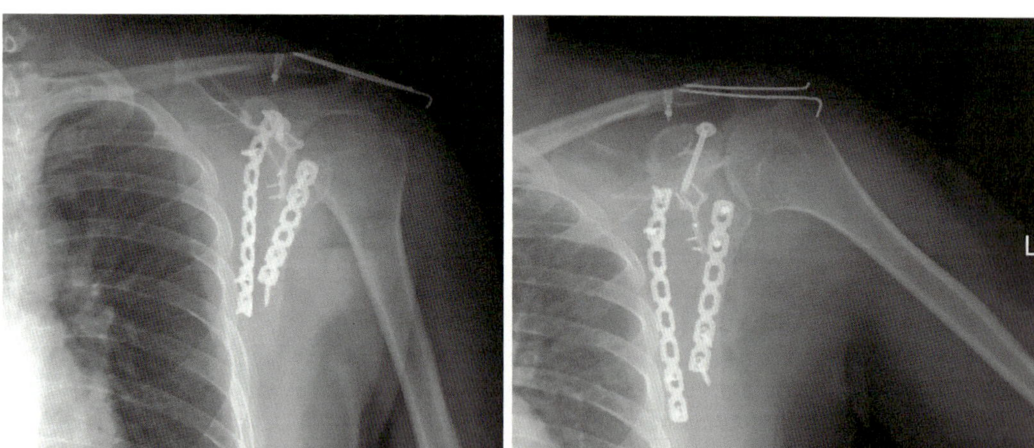

Picture 4–5. Open reduction and internal fixation was performed with two recon plates, one cannulated screw and two K-wires. CC ligament repair was made with one anchor.

Questions

1. In which situation would you prefer conservative treatment in a patient with shoulder girdle injury?
   A. Displaced clavicle fracture with CC ligaments torn
   B. Glenoid neck fracture with glenopolar angle less then 20 degrees
   C. AC seperation type 2
   D. Glenoid fossa fracture with 40% involvement of articular surface
   E. Displaced clavicle fracture + coracoid process fracture
   C

2. You examine a 60 year old male patient with left shoulder pain after a traffic accident. After the evaluation you diagnose a displaced glenoid fossa fracture and perform an OR-IF with deltopectoral approach. The patient was well after the operation but complains about his left shoulder pain aggrevated with motion after 6 months. You cannot see any non-union or implant failure on his x-rays. Which of the following is the most probable misdiagnosis at his referral to hospital after trauma?
   A. Vascular injury
   B. Servical neck injury
   C. Brachial plexus injury
   D. Rotator cuff injury
   D. Rotator cuff injury is the most common misdiagnosed injuries after shoulder trauma.

References

1. Reggio AW. Fractures of the shoulder girdle. In: Wilson PD, editor. Experience in the management of fractures and dislocations, based on an analysis of 4390 cases. Philadelphia: Lippincott Williams & Wilkins; 1938. p. 370–4.
2. Thompson DA, Flynn TC, Miller PW, et al. The significance of scapular fractures. J Trauma. 1985;25(10):974–7.
3. Tuček M, Bartoníček J, Novotný P, Voldřich M. Bilateral scapular fractures in adults. Int Orthop. 2013;37:659–65.
4. Goss TP. Double disruptions of the superior shoulder suspensory complex. J Orthop Trauma. 1993;7(2):99–106.
5. Bartoníček J, Kozánek M, Jupiter JB. Early history of scapular fractures. Int Orthop. 2016;40(1):213–22.
6. Ada JR, Miller ME. Scapular fractures. Analysis of 113 cases. Clin Orthop Relat Res. 1991;269:174–80.
7. Bartonicek J, Fric V. Scapular body fractures: results of the operative treatment. Int Orthop. 2011;35:747–53.
8. Tscherne H, Christ M. Konservative und operative Therapie der Schulterblattbrüche. Hefte Unfallheilkd. 1975;126:52–7.
9. Mayo KA, Benirschke SK, Mast JW. Displaced fractures of the glenoid fossa. Clin Orthop Relat Res. 1998;346:122–30.
10. Jaeger M, Lambert S, Südkamp NP, Kellam JF, Madsen JE, Babst R, Andermahr J, Li W, Audigé L. The AO Foundation and Orthopaedic Trauma Association (AO/OTA) scapula fracture classification system: focus on glenoid fossa involvement. J Shoulder Elb Surg. 2013;22(4):512–20.
11. Ideberg R, Grevsten S, Larsson S. Epidemiology of scapular fractures. Incidence and classification of 338 fractures. Acta Orthop Scand. 1995;66(5):395–7.
12. Goss TP. Scapular fractures and dislocations: diagnosis and treatment. J Am Acad Orthop Surg. 1995; 3(1):22–33.
13. Atef A, El-Tantawy A, Gad H, Hefeda M. Prevalence of associated injuries after anterior shoulder dislocation: a prospective study. Int Orthop. 2016;40(3):519–24.
14. Martin SD, Weiland AJ. Missed scapular fracture after trauma. A case report and a 23-year follow-up report. Clin Orthop Relat Res. 1994;299:259–62.
15. Cole PA, Gauger EM, Schroder LK. Management of scapular fractures. J Am Acad Orthop Surg. 2012;20:130–41.
16. Bozkurt M, Can F, Kirdemir V, Erden Z, Demirkale I, Başbozkurt M. Conservative treatment of scapular neck fracture: the effect of stability and glenopolar angle on clinical outcome. Injury. 2005;36(10):1176–81.
17. Romero J, Schai P, Imhoff AB. Scapular neck fracture the influence of permanent malalignment of the glenoid neck on clinical outcome. Arch Orthop Trauma Surg. 2001;121(6):313–6.
18. Judet R. Traitement chirurgical des fractures de l'omoplate. Acta Orthop Belg. 1964;30:673–8.
19. Sugaya H, Kon Y, Tsuchiya A. Arthroscopic repair of glenoid fractures using suture anchors. Arthroscopy. 2005;21(5):635.
20. Esenkaya I, Unay K. Anatomical frame plate osteosynthesis in Ada-Miller type 2 or 4 scapular fractures. Acta Chir Orthop Traumatol Turc. 2011;45:151–61.

Part V

Specific Shoulder Disorders

Inflammatory Arthropathy of the Shoulder

13

Kadir Büyükdoğan, Gazi Huri, Ashnaa Rao, and Mahmut Nedim Doral

Inflammatory Arthropathy is the term used to describe a group of diseases that results in chronic inflammation. The shoulder is commonly affected by the chronic systemic diseases such as rheumatoid arthritis (RA) and spondyloarthritis (SpA) and mainly manifest with inflammation of the joints as well as joint pain and stiffness [1]. In a patient with inflammatory arthropathy, the immune response is ongoing and lacks the ability to self-regulate or stop, and the body can attack the lining of the joints, and the joints become swollen, stiff and painful. Usually, the joints of the hands and feet or axial skeleton are affected first, but many people with inflammatory are severely affected in their shoulders.

Introduction

The shoulder is involved in up to 70% of the patients with rheumatoid arthritis (RA) and 25% of the spondyloarthritis (SpA) patients [1]. Patients generally report symptoms of pain and restriction of movements [2]. Synovitis, bursitis and tendinitis decreases muscle strength, cause persistent pain, reduced range of motion and joint destruction, which may lead to functional loss and difficulties with daily activities [3].

Among seronegative spondyloarthropathies, psoriatic arthritis and ankylosing spondylitis (AS) are the most common processes to affect the glenohumeral joint [4]. In some AS patients, the entire superolateral aspect of the humeral head is destroyed by the erosive process and results in a characteristic defect of the humeral head, the so-called hatchet sign. Ankylosing spondylitis has similar radiographic findings with rheumatoid arthritis, except for the findings of subchondral sclerosis, irregular bony proliferation about the erosions and at tendon attachment sites and rarely ankylosis of the joint [5].

Rheumatoid arthritis is the most common inflammatory arthropathy to involve the shoulder. The prevalence of rheumatoid arthritis is believed to be in the range from 0.4 to 1.3% worldwide. This prevalence of rheumatoid arthritis has increased over time likely as a result of changes in the environment and an increasing emphasis that is placed on the treatment and early diagnosis of rheumatoid arthritis. It is also estimated that two out of three patients that are diagnosed with rheumatoid arthritis have shoulder involvement. Shoulder symptoms are more common in patients with positive rheumatoid-factor serology and joint destruction, particularly at the hands and wrists [6]. It is also common for the joint involvement in

K. Büyükdoğan, M.D. (✉)
Steadman Philippon Research Institute,
Vail, Colorado, USA
e-mail: kadirbuyukdogan@gmail.com

G. Huri, M.D. • M.N. Doral, M.D.
Department of Orthopaedics and Traumatology,
Hacettepe University, Ankara, Turkey

A. Rao, M.D.
Johns Hopkins School of Medicine,
Baltimore, Maryland, USA

G. Huri, N.K. Paschos (eds.), *The Shoulder*, Orthopaedic Study Guide Series,
DOI 10.1007/978-3-319-51979-1_13

rheumatoid arthritis to be symmetrical. So if one shoulder is affected, it is likely that the other one will be as well [7]. Under the title of inflammatory arthropathies of shoulder rheumatoid arthritis will be discussed in this chapter.

Clinical Presentation

Symptoms associated with rheumatoid arthritis in the shoulder are tenderness and warmth in the joints, stiffness in the shoulders, rheumatoid nodules under the skin in the shoulder and arm area, weight loss, low-grade fever and fatigue. Patients often are unaware of the early loss of motion, perhaps because of their ability to compensate with motion at adjacent joints or with the contralateral extremity. Other symptoms include joint damage, redness, pain, swelling, loss of function, and inflammation. As disease progresses, patients may find it difficult to perform activities of daily living, even they have a well-functioning elbow and hand [8]. Besides glenohumeral joint, RA may affect acromioclavicular joint (AC) and sternoclavicular joint as well. There are studies reporting the AC joint involvement occur with 28–40% incidence. However in long term two-thirds of the patients with RA showed involvement of the AC joints. Erosions were located most often on the inferior margin of the joint [9].

If both the glenohumeral and AC joints are affected then there would be pain throughout the shoulder. It is also common to have night pain and limited range of shoulder motion [7]. Shoulders involved with RA have frequently damage to rotator cuff. One-quarter to one-half of patients with rheumatoid arthritis of the shoulder joint have at least one large rotator cuff tear [10, 11]. Furthermore, tendinitis, pannus formation, fatty degeneration of the rotator cuff muscles and muscle atrophy result in superior migration of humeral head and subacromial impingement (Fig. 13.1). This may cause further pain which in turn, initiates a vicious cycle of inactivity, progression of the disease and further joint destruction [12].

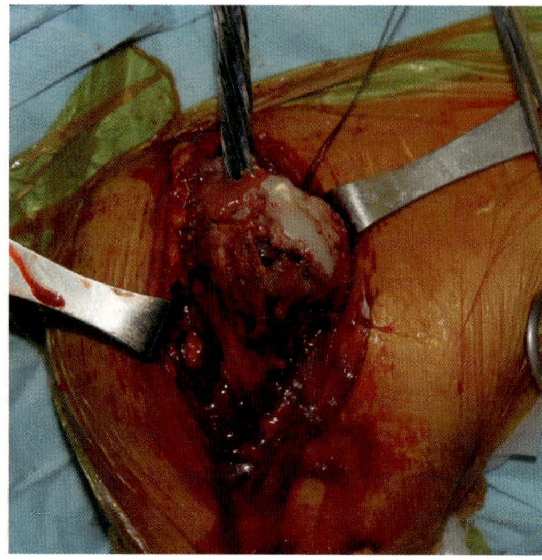

Fig. 13.1 Note the erosion of the superolateral aspect of the humeral head because of pannus formation

Radiology

Earliest radiographic characteristics of RA in a plain film is regional osteopenia of the humeral head or glenoid. With disease progression, marginal erosions and cysts become apparent at the inferior margin of the joint lines. Inflammation is greatest at sites of soft-tissue insertion usually adjacent to the greater tuberosity. At least 3 months of active disease usually are required before irreversible joint changes, such as cartilage thinning and bone erosion, can be seen. The AC joint space may be narrowed or widened. Erosions of the AC joint may occur on either side of the joint but are more common on the clavicle [7]. Glenoid erosions can be central or peripheral. Glenohumeral joint space narrowing is common with progressive RA. Superior subluxation of the humeral head on the glenoid fossa may indicate substantial cuff atrophy or damage.

An ultrasound can also be used to observe some of the manifestations of rheumatoid arthritis. Some of the features that sonography findings include are synovial proliferation and inflammation of the superficial joints, bursitis and tenosynovitis of biceps tendon. Computed tomography may be indicated to determine the extent of humeral head defects and glenoid articular erosions. This is particularly important in evaluating glenoid erosion to determine implant type.

Currently MRI is commonly used and is particularly sensitive to detect the features of rheumatoid arthritis. In comparison with US, contrast-enhanced MRI is significantly more sensitive in evaluating rheumatoid shoulders, and less operator dependent in detecting tenosynovitis, bursitis and cuff tears [13]. Some of the features that are demonstrated with an MRI in rheumatoid arthritis are synovial hyperaemia, synovial hyperplasia, pannus formation, decreased thickness of cartilage, subchondral cysts and erosions, juxta-articular bone marrow edema, and joint effusions [14]. In the late stages of RA, some parts of hypertrophic villi may detach and appear as rice body in joint cavity. Usually they are diagnosed on MR as multiple intra-articular or intrabursal bodies that demonstrate decreased T1 and T2 signal intensity. Although rice bodies are not pathognomonic to RA their removal can result in a marked improvement in symptoms [15].

Classification

RA of the shoulder was classified by Laine and later by Neer into three stages based on clinical and radiographic findings [16, 17]. In stage I, slight limitation of shoulder motion is present, with mild to moderate pain and tenderness. Radiographs show only generalized osteopenia. Stage II is characterized by moderate limitation of shoulder motion and moderate to severe pain. Radiographs show osteopenia, erosive bony changes, and joint space narrowing. In stage III, severe functional deficits are present; range of motion is painful and limits activities of daily living. Radiographic findings include advanced erosive changes of the glenohumeral joint. Neer classified RA shoulder as dry, wet, and resorptive stages and these stages are approximately equivalent to those of Laine.

Conservative Management

There is no known cure for rheumatoid arthritis, however the treatment of rheumatoid arthritis is focused on relieving pain, reducing inflammation, slowing or stopping joint damage and improving shoulder function. Non-surgical management of RA is indicated when synovial inflammation is the primary manifestation before significant bony changes occur. Management usually consist of the combination of corticosteroids, Non-steroidal Anti-inflammatory Agents (NSAIDs), DMARDs (Disease Modifying Anti-Rheumatic Drugs) and Tumor necrosis factor (TNF) inhibitors.

NSAIDs help to reduce acute inflammation and pain while improving overall shoulder function. These agents also have analgesic properties, however, these agents do not independently change the course of the disease of rheumatoid arthritis and do not prevent joint destruction. Corticosteroids can be given intravenously, orally and intramuscularly. If patient does not respond to these therapies, intraarticular injection should be considered [18]. They are an anti-inflammatory and have immunoregulatory activity. Corticosteroids often result in dramatic pain relief but multiple injections can have a deleterious effect on connective tissue structures, including the articular cartilage and the rotator cuff tendons, and therefore should be avoided [19].

Aside from medications, other treatment options include the reduction of joint stress, physical therapy as well as occupational. Probably, the only therapeutic intervention that is not questioned is patient education about the nature of RA, which provides him with the knowledge to cope effectively with the chronicity of his disease [7]. The optimal treatment for some patient with rheumatoid arthritis may involve a combination of medical, social, and emotional support.

Surgical Management

Surgical intervention for rheumatoid shoulder is considered when conservative management fails to relieve pain and maintain function. The timing of surgical management should be dictated by the degree of symptoms, clinical presentation and degree of joint destruction. Due to polyarticular involvement of RA, multiple surgical procedures should be needed. There must be adequate interval between surgical procedures to allow patient ambulate easily without assistive devices or avoid weight bearing.

Synovectomy is indicated for patients with primarily active synovitis without evidence of extensive articular destruction. Synovectomy provide symptomatic relief when main complaint is pain but it seldom results in a significant increase in range of motion [18]. Modern DMARDs and biological therapies have made the use of this procedure rare in contemporary practice.

RA is a progressive disease causing bony erosions and structurally deformed joints, arthroplasties may be considered the only beneficial treatment option for end-stage arthritis. Arthroplasty has been highly successful for relief of pain but much less consistent for improvement of motion. The diagnosis of RA is the most important predictive factor for the end-result, with a stronger influence than the condition of the rotator cuff or whether a hemiarthroplasty or a total arthroplasty is performed [20, 21]. The design and type of implant does not appear to influence outcome, but resurfacing is not appropriate when severe joint destruction renders the humeral head too small or soft [22]. There is also a high infection rate in patients with RA is likely related to the disturbances of the immune system responsible for this autoimmune disease [23, 24].

Indications for shoulder hemiarthroplasty (HA) include extensive humeral head involvement with minimal involvement of the glenoid surface. If there is an extensive humeral head and glenoid involvement with associated osteopenia there raise concerns regarding the secure fixation of a glenoid component. Additionally hemiarthroplasty can be used in the presence of extensive articular cartilage deterioration with a massive irreparable rotator cuff tear. In younger patients (<65 years) who wish to maintain an active lifestyle, concerns about glenoid component loosening have led some to avoid the use of glenoid components [18]. However, long-term pain relief is less reliable than with glenoid resurfacing because of owing to poor bone quality, glenoid erosion after hemiarthroplasty is more frequent than in patients with osteoarthritis. In contrast to glenoid loosening, glenoid erosion is almost always painful and leads to poor results requiring surgical revision [21].

Total shoulder arthroplasty (TSA) is considered a good option for treatment of the rheumatoid shoulder when the rotator cuff is intact or moderately worn, with no more than one defective tendon and the glenoid bone stock is preserved. Several investigators have reported that total shoulder arthroplasty results in pain relief and satisfactory increases in range of motion, and markedly improved functional status [25, 26]. The osteopenia, high incidence of rotator cuff tears and immunosuppressive medications commonly seen in these patients can lead to concerns about glenoid component loosing. Nevertheless, glenoid loosening is not progressive over long periods and is well tolerated by the majority of patients. Thus, the rate of glenoid revision operations in rheumatoid patients seldom exceeds 5% in mid- and long-term studies [21]. There are reports comparing results of hemiarthroplasty and total shoulder arthroplasties in rheumatoid shoulders. Both HA and TSA provide pain relief and improved motion in patients with rheumatoid arthritis. In patients with an intact rotator cuff, pain relief and range of motion are more improved with TSA compared with HA. There is a high rate of component lucency, but component revision is uncommon [26]. Other authors report similar results even in the presence of a selection bias favoring the use of total shoulder arthroplasty in the presence of a functional or reparable rotator cuff [27].

In order to compensate for the loss of rotator cuff force, reverse shoulder prosthesis might be a treatment option in RA patients [8]. However there are concerns on reverse shoulder prosthesis for RA patients. Early glenoid loosing is a problem due to the combination of poor bone and the increased stress on the glenoid component inherent with this type of prosthesis [28]. However there are reports reverse shoulder arthroplasty for the rheumatoid shoulder with a deficient rotator cuff can provide noteworthy improvement for most patients and the range of motion improvement was superior to the typical range reported after anatomical replacements [23, 29, 30]

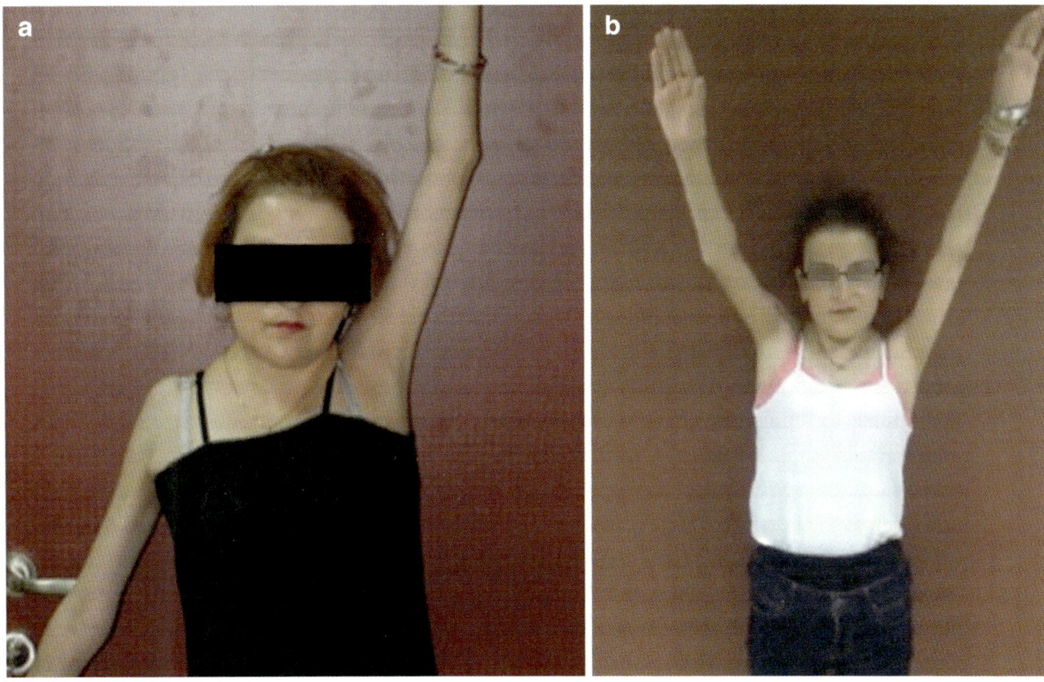

Fig. 13.2 This photograph (**a**) reveals the restricted range of motion of right shoulder in RA patient; (**b**) post-op 8 month after reverse shoulder arthroplasty. Notice the significant improvement in elevation of shoulder

(Fig. 13.2). Longer follow-ups will provide valuable information on durability and late complications of reverse shoulder prosthesis [29]. Reverse total prosthesis should be reserved for the treatment of very disabling shoulder arthropathy with a massive rotator cuff rupture, and it should be used exclusively in patients over 70 years old with low functional demands [31]. The indication for a revision is key to deciding on the correct implant. It is reported that revision from a hemiarthroplasty to a total shoulder replacement for glenoid wear with an intact rotator cuff can yield good results. Although short term results are promising there is paucity in literature about revision of reverse shoulder prosthesis in long term.

Summary

Management of inflammatory shoulder requires a multi-disciplinary approach. There is a wide clinical presentation of these inflammatory diseases and while planning the management, clinical and radiological stages of disease should be considered. In conclusion, systemic considerations of this progressive disease, rehabilitation, immunologic and mental status of patients, implant choice is extremely important in inflammatory shoulder management.

Questions

1. Which of the following is the earliest radiographic sign of rheumatoid involvement of the shoulder?
   (a) Subchondral cyst in humeral head
   (b) Subchondral cyst in glenoid
   (c) Regional osteopenia of humeral head or glenoid
   (d) Superior migration of humeral head
   (e) Marginal erosions of humeral head

   Answer C. The earliest radiographic sign of rheumatoid involvement of the shoulder region is regional osteopenia of the humeral head or glenoid. Marginal erosions and subchondral cysts may be evident with disease progression. Superior migration of the humeral head usually reflects a later involvement of the rotator cuff.

Ref:

7. Gibson KR. Rheumatoid arthritis of the shoulder. Physical therapy. 1986;66(12): 1920-9.

1. Which of the following findings is more evident in patients with rheumatoid arthritis when compared to patients with primary osteoarthritis of the shoulder?
   (a) Subchondral sclerosis in glenoid
   (b) Osteophytes in humeral head
   (c) Concentric glenoid erosion
   (d) Asymmetric glenohumeral joint space narrowing
   (e) Sclerosis in humeral head

Answer C. Concentric glenoid erosion is a characteristic radiographic presentation of inflammatory arthropathies of the shoulder and generally results in medialized glenohumeral joint line. Asymmetric glenohumeral joint narrowing, subchondral sclerosis and osteophytes in humeral head or glenoid typically seen in primary osteoarthritis patients.
Ref:

18. Chen AL, Joseph TN, Zuckerman JD. Rheumatoid arthritis of the shoulder. J Am Acad Orthop Surg. 2003;11(1):12-24.

1. Which of the following conditions is typically associated with limited erosion of the lateral aspect of humeral head, the so-called hatchet sign?
   (a) Rheumatoid Arthritis
   (b) Ankylosing spondylitis
   (c) Psoriatic arthritis
   (d) Systemic lupus erythematosus
   (e) Primary osteoarthritis of the shoulder

Answer B. In some AS patients, the superolateral aspect of the humeral head is destroyed by the erosive process and results in a characteristic defect of the humeral head. This sign helps to differentiate AS from rheumatoid arthritis.
Ref:

(5) Sankaye P, Ostlere S. Arthritis at the shoulder joint. Seminars in musculoskeletal radiology. 2015;19(3):307-18.

References

1. Lambert RG, Dhillon SS, Jhangri GS, Sacks J, Sacks H, Wong B, et al. High prevalence of symptomatic enthesopathy of the shoulder in ankylosing spondylitis: deltoid origin involvement constitutes a hallmark of disease. Arthritis Rheum. 2004;51(5):681–90.
2. Pahle JA, Kvarnes L. Shoulder synovectomy. Ann Chir Gynaecol Suppl. 1985;198:37–9.
3. Bilberg A, Bremell T, Balogh I, Mannerkorpi K. Significantly impaired shoulder function in the first years of rheumatoid arthritis: a controlled study. Arthritis Res Ther. 2015;17:261.
4. Farid N, Bruce D, Chung CB. Miscellaneous conditions of the shoulder: anatomical, clinical, and pictorial review emphasizing potential pitfalls in imaging diagnosis. Eur J Radiol. 2008;68(1):88–105.
5. Sankaye P, Ostlere S. Arthritis at the shoulder joint. Semin Musculoskelet Radiol. 2015;19(3):307–18.
6. Gabriel SE, Michaud K. Epidemiological studies in incidence, prevalence, mortality, and comorbidity of the rheumatic diseases. Arthritis Res Ther. 2009;11(3): 229.
7. Gibson KR. Rheumatoid arthritis of the shoulder. Phys Ther. 1986;66(12):1920–9.
8. Christie A, Dagfinrud H, Engen Matre K, Flaatten HI, Ringen Osnes H, Hagen KB. Surgical interventions for the rheumatoid shoulder. Cochrane Database Syst Rev. 2010;1:CD006188.
9. Lehtinen JT, Kaarela K, Belt EA, Kautiainen HJ, Kauppi MJ, Lehto MU. Incidence of acromioclavicular joint involvement in rheumatoid arthritis: a 15 year endpoint study. J Rheumatol. 1999;26(6):1239–41.
10. Rozing PM, Nagels J, Rozing MP. Prognostic factors in arthroplasty in the rheumatoid shoulder. HSS J. 2011;7(1):29–36.
11. Rozing PM, Brand R. Rotator cuff repair during shoulder arthroplasty in rheumatoid arthritis. J Arthroplasty. 1998;13(3):311–9.
12. van der Zwaal P, Pijls BG, Thomassen BJ, Lindenburg R, Nelissen RG, van de Sande MA. The natural history of the rheumatoid shoulder: a prospective long-term follow-up study. Bone Joint J. 2014;96-b(11): 1520–4.
13. Nelson MC, Leather GP, Nirschl RP, Pettrone FA, Freedman MT. Evaluation of the painful shoulder. A prospective comparison of magnetic resonance imaging, computerized tomographic arthrography, ultrasonography, and operative findings. J Bone Joint Surg Am. 1991;73(5):707–16.
14. Hermann KG, Backhaus M, Schneider U, Labs K, Loreck D, Zuhlsdorf S, et al. Rheumatoid arthritis of the shoulder joint: comparison of conventional radiography, ultrasound, and dynamic contrast-enhanced magnetic resonance imaging. Arthritis Rheum. 2003;48(12):3338–49.
15. Narvaez JA, Narvaez J, Roca Y, Aguilera C. MR imaging assessment of clinical problems in rheumatoid arthritis. Eur Radiol. 2002;12(7):1819–28.

16. Laine VA, Vainio KJ, Pekanmaki K. Shoulder affections in rheumatoid arthritis. Ann Rheum Dis. 1954;13(2):157–60.
17. Neer CS. The rheumatoid shoulder. In: Cruess RL, Mitchell N, editor. The surgical management of rheumatoid arthritis. Philadelphia: JB Lippincott; 1971. p. 117–27.
18. Chen AL, Joseph TN, Zuckerman JD. Rheumatoid arthritis of the shoulder. J Am Acad Orthop Surg. 2003;11(1):12–24.
19. Rozental TD, Sculco TP. Intra-articular corticosteroids: an updated overview. Am J Orthop (Belle Mead NJ). 2000;29(1):18–23.
20. Lehtinen JT, Belt EA, Kauppi MJ, Kaarela K, Kuusela PP, Kautiainen HJ, et al. Bone destruction, upward migration, and medialisation of rheumatoid shoulder: a 15 year follow up study. Ann Rheum Dis. 2001; 60(4):322–6.
21. Hedtmann A, Werner A. [Shoulder arthroplasty in rheumatoid arthritis]. Der Orthopade 2007;36(11): 1050–61.
22. Levy O, Funk L, Sforza G, Copeland SA. Copeland surface replacement arthroplasty of the shoulder in rheumatoid arthritis. J Bone Joint Surg Am. 2004; 86-a(3):512–8.
23. Ekelund A, Nyberg R. Can reverse shoulder arthroplasty be used with few complications in rheumatoid arthritis? Clin Orthop Relat Res. 2011;469(9): 2483–8.
24. Wall B, Nove-Josserand L, O'Connor DP, Edwards TB, Walch G. Reverse total shoulder arthroplasty: a review of results according to etiology. J Bone Joint Surg Am. 2007;89(7):1476–85.
25. Sojbjerg JO, Frich LH, Johannsen HV, Sneppen O. Late results of total shoulder replacement in patients with rheumatoid arthritis. Clin Orthop Relat Res. 1999;366:39–45.
26. Barlow JD, Yuan BJ, Schleck CD, Harmsen WS, Cofield RH, Sperling JW. Shoulder arthroplasty for rheumatoid arthritis: 303 consecutive cases with minimum 5-year follow-up. J Shoulder Elbow Surg. 2014;23(6):791–9.
27. Collins DN, Harryman II DT, Wirth MA. Shoulder arthroplasty for the treatment of inflammatory arthritis. J Bone Joint Surg Am. 2004;86-a(11):2489–96.
28. Gerber C, Pennington SD, Nyffeler RW. Reverse total shoulder arthroplasty. J Am Acad Orthop Surg. 2009;17(5):284–95.
29. Hattrup SJ, Sanchez-Sotelo J, Sperling JW, Cofield RH. Reverse shoulder replacement for patients with inflammatory arthritis. J Hand Surg [Am]. 2012; 37(9):1888–94.
30. Young AA, Smith MM, Bacle G, Moraga C, Walch G. Early results of reverse shoulder arthroplasty in patients with rheumatoid arthritis. J Bone Joint Surg Am. 2011;93(20):1915–23.
31. Guery J, Favard L, Sirveaux F, Oudet D, Mole D, Walch G. Reverse total shoulder arthroplasty. Survivorship analysis of eighty replacements followed for five to ten years. J Bone Joint Surg Am. 2006;88(8):1742–7.

Joint Sepsis

14

Mesut Atabek, Gazi Huri, and Ugur Gonc

Pathogenesis, epidemiological and microbiological features of shoulder sepsis are similar to other bone and joint infections, but shoulder joint has some different specific properties. Different surgical procedures for the shoulder may cause postoperative infections. This chapter includes both primary and secondary infections.

Following the development of arthroscopic techniques, the infection rates have decreased compared to open surgery. However high infection rates can still be seen after major shoulder surgeries such as reverse shoulder arthroplasty (RSA). On the other hand arthroscopic surgery also has its own specific infections. Propionibacterium acnes (P. acnes) is suspected to be a causative agent for primary shoulder osteoarthritis [1].

Generally late diagnosis and insufficient treatment cause poor results after joint infections. Shoulder infections in pediatric age group have different properties compared to other joints. Although shoulder joint usually tolerate complications more easily than hip and knee joints in pediatric patients, normal function and anatomy must be the aim of the treatment. Early diagnosis and the virulence of the pathogen usually determine the shoulder functions.

The pathogens enter the joints through various ways and a damage in the tissue makes it easier. The articular cartilage is acellular. Leucocyte migration is usually not enough to protect the cartilage. Both host dependent and pathogen dependent factors are important for the development of infection. Host dependent factors may be local or systemic.

The local factors include trauma, previous surgeries and procedures like intraarticular injections. The skin condition before surgery and proper skin preparation are important concepts of infection prophylaxis. The implants used in arthroplasty, arthroscopy or trauma management may cause susceptibility to infection. Bone cement used in arthroplasty or the polysaccharide biofilm layer formed over implants may avoid macrophages or antibiotics to reach the infected area and provide a suitable environment for bacterial colonization. With antibiotic prophylaxis, infection rates have decreased after total shoulder arthroplasty. However hematoma formation in the potential space occurring after RSA may provide a suitable environment for microorganisms.

Systemic factors increasing susceptibility to infection include any condition causing immune system depression like diabetes mellitus, rheumatoid arthritis, liver cirrhosis, chronic kidney failure, vascular diseases, neoplastic diseases, hematological disorders, drug abusers, systemic

M. Atabek, M.D. (✉) • U. Gonc, M.D.
Orthopaedics and Traumatology Division, Liv Hospital, Ankara, Turkey
e-mail: mesutatabek@yahoo.com

G. Huri, M.D.
Department of Orthopaedics and Traumatology, Hacettepe University, Ankara, Turkey

G. Huri, N.K. Paschos (eds.), *The Shoulder*, Orthopaedic Study Guide Series,
DOI 10.1007/978-3-319-51979-1_14

trauma, advanced age and HIV infection. Patients with HIV infection are more prone to some specific pathogens.

The pathogen microorganisms may enter the shoulder joint through three ways: spontaneous hematogenous spread, spread of metaphyseal osteomyelitis to intraarticular region and direct inoculation by joint penetration after trauma or surgical procedures.

Clinical Findings

Most common clinical findings are pain, limitation of motion, functional impairment and swelling around the shoulder joint. The patients usually tend to hold their shoulder in adduction and internal rotation due to limited joint motion. Increased fever and deterioration of the general status may also be observed.

Increased joint space or findings related to osteomyelitis may be seen in direct radiographic examination.

Laboratory Findings

Leukocytosis and increased erythrocyte sedimentation rate (ESR) or C-reactive protein (CRP) levels may be observed. These findings may be suppressed in immunocompromised and rheumatoid patients. Infection must be suspected in rheumatoid patients when there is an acute deterioration.

Synovial fluid analysis and culture are important in the diagnosis of infection (Tables 14.1 and 14.2)

Cell count more than 50,000/mm^3 and polymorphonuclear leucocyte (PMN) ratio more than 75% are important parameters in synovial fluid analysis indicating septic arthritis. Protein levels are usually elevated. Glucose levels may be decreased especially in adults. Increased monocyte count usually indicates micobacterial infection.

Unexpected findings may be observed after prosthetic infections. White blood cell count (WBC) is normal in 93% of patients. Preoperative CRP, ESR levels and intraoperative histological findings may be negative respectively in 75, 86 and 92% of infected patients [2].

A recent study suggests that WBC and PMN count and lactate level in synovial fluid are effective methods demonstrating joint infections after prosthetic surgery [3].

In another study, significant high serum Interleukin-6 (IL-6), ESR and CRP levels were observed after prosthetic infections, whereas there was no statistically significant difference in

Table 14.1 Synovial fluid findings in acute septic arthritis

Joint fluid examinations	Noninflammatory fluids	Noninfectious (inflamamatory)	İnfectious (inflammatory)
• Color	• Colorless, pale yellow	• Yellow to white	• Yellow
• Turbidity	• Clear, slightly turbid	• Turbid	• Turbid, purulent
• Viscosity	• Not reduced	• Reduced	• Reduced
• Mucin clot	• Tight clot	• Friable	• Friable
• Cell count (per mm^3)	• 200–1000	• 3000–10,000	• 10,000–100,000
• Predominant cell type	• Mononuclear predominant	• PMN[a]	• PMN
• Synovial fluid-blood glucose ratio	• 0.8–1.0	• 0.5–0.8	• <0.5
• Lactic acid	• Same as plasma	• Higher than plasma	• Often very high
• Gram stain for organism	• None	• None	• Positive[b]
• Culture	• Negative	• Negative	• Positive[b]

Adapted from Schmid FR: Principles of diagnosis and treatment of bone and joint infections. In McCarty DJ (ed): Arthritis and Allied Conditions: A textbook of Rheumatology. Philadelphia: Lea-Febiger, 1985, p: 1638 [112]

[a]*PMN* polymorphonuclear leucocyte

[b]İn some cases especially in gonococcal infection, no organism may be demonstrated

Table 14.2 Synovial fluid characteristics and arthritis-related laboratory findings

Characteristic	Normal	Nonainflamatory arthritis[a]	Inflamatory arthritis[b]	Septic arthritis (native joint)[c]	Prosthetic hip or knee infection[d]
• Appearance	• Clear	• Clear	• Opaque or translucent	• Opaque yellow or green	• Clear or opaque
• WBC/mm^3	• <1000	• <1000	• 5000–75,000	• >50,000	• >1100–3000
• Polymorphonuclear cells	• <25%	• <25%	• >50%	• >75%	• >64–80%
• Culture	• Negative	• Negative	• Positive	• Positive	• Positive

Adapted from Deirmengian CA, Patel R. Clinical and Laboratory Evaluation, Chapter 5. In Cierny III G, Mclaren AC, Wongworawat MD (eds): Orthopaedic Knowledge Update, Musculoskeletal Infection. Rosemont, AAOS, 2009. p: 57–65 [113]

WBC white blood cell count

[a]Associated conditions: degenerative joint disease, trauma, pigmented villonodular synovitis, neuropathy, systemic lupus erythematosus, acute rheumatic fever

[b]Associated conditions: Rheumatoid arthritis, crystal-induced arthritis, seronegative arthropathy, systemic lupus erythematosus, acute rheumatic fever

[c]An immunocompromised patient may not have elevated synovial WBC. A normal or noninflammatory WBC does not preclude active septic arthritis

[d]Data are unavailable for other types of prosthetic joints. Underlying inflammatory arthritis may cause false-positive results

WBC count. IL-6 level less than 10 pg/mL was considered as normal. However this study was performed for knee and hip arthroplasty and was not specific for shoulder [4]. Coffey et al. suggested to use IL-6 level also for the diagnosis of shoulder prosthetic infections [5]. Serum IL-6 level was found to have 100% sensitivity and 95% specificity [4]. It can be used for timing the surgery in two-stage revisions [5]. In contrast to these studies a recent study reported that IL-6 cannot be used for shoulder infections due to low sensitivity and specificity [6, 7].

Another parameter is serum procalcitonin. Its level is usually higher in bacterial infections than other types of infection [8].

Alpha-defensin is an antimicrobial peptide. A recent study showed that its high level in synovial fluid analysis correlates with infection and can be used as a diagnostic tool [9].

Both aerobic and anaerobic cultures and cultures for acid-fast bacilli should be taken. Gram and acid-fast staining should be performed during surgery. The probability of tuberculosis should be kept in mind in patients with monoarticular arthritis and tenosynovitis.

Polymerase chain reaction (PCR) can be performed for Kingella kingae in infants and for Staphylococcus aureus (S. aureus) in adults if the cultures are negative [10].

According to Mirra, detection of more than five PMN in each area in intraoperative frozen sections is in favor of acute inflammation and infection [11]

Pediatric Shoulder Sepsis

Bone and joint infections are important problems in pediatric age group. Both bacterial or fungal osteomyelitis can be observed. Generally acute hematogenous osteomyelitis is seen in pediatric patients. Secondary infections due to trauma, open wounds and surgical implants are mostly common in adults. Osteomyelitis related to vascular insufficiency may be seen in elderly patients with co-morbidities [12].

Acute Hematogenous Osteomyelitis

In children this type of osteomyelitis usually occurs after bacteremia. Rich metaphyseal circulation, inoculation of the bacteria in capillary loops and adhesion in cartilagenous matrix may cause osteomyelitis. Due to its bacterial adhesion capacity S. aureus is the most common agent [12]. In children under 18 month of age, the joint can also be infected through transepiphyseal vessels. One third of the neighbor joint can be affected in osteomyelitis whereas there is no significant difference after 18 months of age [13]. In experimental animal studies more bone infection was observed in traumatized regions of bacteremic animals. This finding may explain why trauma is the etiologic factor in 30% of the cases in children [14]. Although the real incidence is not known recent studies showed that the incidence of acute and subacute hematogenous osteomyelitis has decreased [15].

S. aureus is the most common agent of osteomyelitis in each age group. The infection was due to community-acquired methicillin resistant S. aureus (CA-MRSA) in more than half of 59 patients with musculoskeletal infection [16].

In young infants Streptococcus agalactiae and gram (−) enteric bacteria may be other causative agents. In preschool or early school periods Streptococcus pyogenes is responsible for 10% of acute hematogenous osteomyelitis. Streptococcus pyogenes, Streptococcus pneumonia and Kingella kingae are more frequently seen in older children [17].

Joint involvement is more common than bony infections after Streptococcus pneumoniae infections [18]. The incidence of bone and joint infections due to Streptococcus pneumoniae, as well as Haemophilus influenza type b has decreased significantly after vaccination programmes [19].

Osteomyelitis due to anaerobic microorganisms like Bacteroides, Fusobacterium, Clostridium or Peptostreptococcus is rare in healthy children. Anaerobic infections can be seen after to bites, chronic sinusitis, mastoiditis or dental infections. Mycobacterium, Bartonella, Coxiella Burnetti or fungal infections are other rare agents causing musculoskeletal infections.

Salmonella and S. aureus are usually responsible for osteomyelitis in sickle cell disease but rarely Escherichia coli, Shigella, Haemophilus influenza type b and Streptococcus pneumoniae can be observed as causative agent.

Chronic recurrent multifocal osteomyelitis is an inflammatory process and can be confused with osteomyelitis due to clavicular involvement [20].

Septic Arthritis of Glenohumeral Joint

Four percent of whole joint infections occurs in glenohumeral joint [21, 22]. General infection symptoms like irritability, apathy, diarrhea and fever are important findings in newborn period. In their series Ernat et al. reported restricted shoulder motion, pain, swelling and even sepsis in 9% of cases [23]. Direct radiographies were normal in half of the cases. Osteomyelitis was observed in magnetic resonance (MR) evaluation in 75% of patients. Cultures were negative in 36% and blood cultures were positive in 25% of patients. Average hospitalization time was 2 weeks and average number of procedures was 1.5. MRSA positive patients had more hospitalization time and more direct radiographic findings due to increased incidence of osteomyelitis [23]. In another study 57% of patients with shoulder septic arthritis had accompanying infections in other regions like ear, respiratory system, skin or nervous system [24]. Risk factors for poor prognosis were reported as late diagnosis, younger patients less than 3 months of age, metaphyseal osteomyelitis, non-operative treatment and high virulence of the agent (penicillinase producing microorganisms) [19, 25–27].

Insufficient treatment may cause recurrence, bacteremia, distant septic emboli, anemia, septic shock and even death. Articular cartilage degeneration, contractures, subluxation and growth retardation may develop after delayed treatment. Inflammation, bacterial products and lysosomal enzymes cause cartilage damage. Increased intraarticular pressure leads to ischemia. Additional thrombotic process facilitates the infection. Local spread may lead to osteomyelitis after joint destruction.

Delayed treatment may cause permanent changes and disability. Accompanying osteomyelitis may lead to growth retardation due to damage of proximal humeral physis. In one study,

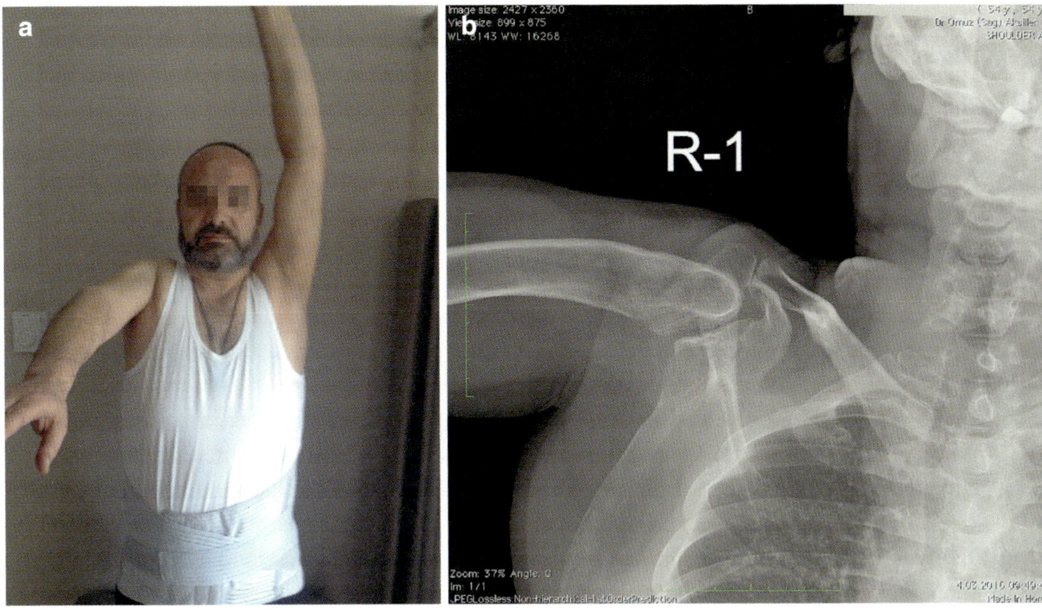

Fig. 14.1 The picture reveals (**a**) significant loss of shoulder range of motion and (**b**) avascular necrosis of humerus head in a shoulder with septic arthritis sequel

only 7% of patients less than 18 months of age had normal shoulder after 6 years of follow-up and between 0 and 9 cm of shortness was present in the patients [24]. Age is very important. Since proximal humerus physis is responsible 80% of the growth of upper extremity, impairment due to infection may lead to shortness, humeral head deformity and inferior subluxation [27] (Fig. 14.1). After 14 years of follow-up of ten patients with neonatal shoulder septic arthritis, patients with delayed treatment showed more humeral shortness and humeral head deformity. On the other hand the patients had good shoulder function except for some limitation of external rotation [28].

In Schmidt et al.'s series five out of nine patients had accompanying osteomyelitis [29]. Similarly Ernat et al. detected accompanying osteomyelitis with MR evaluation in 75% of patients [23]. This rate was 67% in Belthut et al.'s series [30].

The treatment options for pediatric septic arthritis are arthrotomic or arthroscopic debridement and aspiration [27, 31].

Smith et al. compared arthrotomy and aspiration in 61 patients and found no significant difference between groups, but Salmonella was the pathogen in most of the cases. In Smith's prospective randomized study there was no significant difference between arthrotomy and aspiration in terms of clinical and radiological finding [32]. Bos et al. treated ten patients with neonatal shoulder septic arthritis by aspiration. Two patients needed further arthrotomy. More deformity was observed in patients who had delayed treatment, but the functional impairment was insignificant [28].

Ernat et al. treated all of their patients by arthrotomic debridement. High percentage of osteomyelitis was observed in their patients in preoperative MR imagings so they preferred arthrotomy to reach the abscess and advised routine preoperative MR evaluation in every patient [23].

Forward and Hunter treated three pediatric shoulder septic arthritis arthroscopically by using small wrist arthroscope. They reported arthroscopic debridement as an effective minimally invasive technique with good cosmetic and functional results [33].

A recent study comparing hip and shoulder septic arthritis confirmed that the treatment was longer and more complicated in shoulder and the diagnosis was usually late. Two out of nine patients with shoulder septic arthritis were presented with septic shock unlike hip septic arthritis group. Due to more significant symptoms in lower extremity, like limping because of pain, the suspicion and early diagnosis of septic arthritis were easier. Pathological fracture due to shoulder septic arthritis was first reported in this study in two patients. Recurrent debridement was needed in three patients with MRSA infection. Chronic osteomyelitis was more common in shoulder group and required long term antibiotic treatment [30].

Shoulder Sepsis in Adults

Glenohumeral Septic Arthritis

Glenohumeral septic arthritis is a rare problem. In adults it is usually observed after fifth decade and men are more effected. Co-morbidities like diabetes mellitus, chronic kidney failure, chronic liver failure or malignancies increase the risk [34]. Fourteen percent of the patients with septic arthritis have a history of intraarticular injection or aspiration, and this problem may be life threatening [35].

One study showed that in about 62% of patients one stage surgery was enough for septic arthritis treatment. However, more than one debridement could be needed in patients with diabetes mellitus, inflammatory arthropathy, major joint involvement, and if the PMN count in synovial fluid was 85,000 and the pathogen was S. aureus [36].

Arthroscopic classification of septic arthritis was first described by Gachter et al. [37] and modified by Jeon et al. [38]:

- Stage I indicates opacity of fluid, redness of the synovial membrane, and possible petechial bleeding.
- Stage II includes purulent material, severe inflammation, and fibrinous deposition.
- Stage III has thickening of the synovial membrane with cartilage erosion.
- Stage IV is the most aggressive of the stages, with subchondral delamination.

Arthroscopic shoulder septic arthritis treatment is effective especially in Gachter stage I patients [38]. Abdel et al. treated 50 patients with shoulder septic arthritis by athroscopic debridement, 57% of which was immunocompromised and most of the patients were elderly. S. aureus was the most common agent. Fourty-four percent of patients had MSSA and 20% of the patients had MRSA infection. Secondary procedures with arthrotomy were needed in 32% of patients [31]. Open surgical treatment may be performed in patients with delayed diagnosis or when arthroscopic debridement is unsuccessful. It is difficult to preserve the joint after bony and cartilage degeneration or development of avascular necrosis. Resection arthroplasty or arthrodesis may be needed in these patients. In late periods the infection can be treated by resection or application of antibiotic-impregnated cement spacers, but the functional results are usually not good. Garofalo et al. reported only a slight improvement of functional results after RSA applications [39]. Reinfection rates were found to be low in patients who had primary arthroplasty for the treatment of sequels of infection. However the surgical technique was more difficult due to bony loss and soft tissue problems related to infection, and the results were worse compared patients who had primary arthroplasty for the treatment of osteoarthritis [40]. Recent studies reported satisfactory short term results in patients without co-morbidities after arthroplasty applications with low reinfection rates [41, 42].

Post-arthroscopy Septic Arthritis

Infection after shoulder arthroscopy is very rare, but it is a serious complication. The incidence of post-arthroscopy infections is less than 1%. However there has been an increase in incidence due to widespread application of arthroscopic procedures in recent years and implants used [43]. Infection is a less common complication after shoulder arthroscopy compared to other complications [44–46]. P. acnes is the most common pathogen. This infection presents slowly within weeks with minimal symptoms. P. acnes infection is more specific to shoulder joint and the diagnosis is usually difficult with standard culture mediums.

Patients who had rotator cuff repair are more prone to post-arthroscopy infection. Previous surgeries and patients more than 60 years of age are important risk factors [46]. Yeronasian et al. reported 0.27% of incidence for post-arthroscopy infections. Patients older than 60 years of age had twice infection rates compared to patients under 40 years of age. There was no gender difference. Infection was observed more in rotator cuff repairs with an incidence of 0.29% whereas it was only 0.16% after capsulorraphies [46]. Previous studies showed that men had more infection rates which may be due to skin flora [47, 48]. High rates of positive cultures for P. Acnes were detected in patients who had arthroscopic revision surgeries due to pain or restricted motion [49].

Deep infection is rare after post-arthroscopy infections. The infection rate increases when arthroscopic surgery is followed by open surgery. The risk factor are similar to other infections. The treatment includes debridement and antibiotics.

The rate of skin colonization with P. acnes is high at arthroscopic portals, especially in men. The rate of deep tissue inoculation with P. acnes after shoulder arthroscopy may be high despite standard skin preparation and antibiotic prophylaxis although the reported infection rates are low in the literature [50].

Acromioclavicular Septic Arthritis

Septic arthritis mostly effects major joints. Acromioclavicular (A-C) septic arthritis is very rare. The symptoms are swelling, redness and pain over A-C joint. The patients usually have shoulder pain and functional impairment. Local spread after septic arthritis of A-C joint is possible. The rate is higher in immunocompromised patients. Local risk factors include trauma, osteoarthritis, surgery, intraarticular injections and systemic risk factors include rheumatoid arthritis, diabetes mellitus, AIDS, corticosteroid or cytostatic users and drug abusers [51, 52]. Rarely this infection can be observed in patients with good immune condition [53]. The literature usually includes case reports. S. aureus and streptococcus species are the most common agents [54]. Haemophilus parainfluenza may be a rare responsible pathogen [55]. The incidence was reported as 2–10/100,000. Ultrasound is practical diagnostic tool. MR may also be used for diagnosis and detection of the spread of infection. Sometimes the source of bacteremia can be determined. In one case reported foot ulcers were present in the patient [51, 56]

Sternoclavicular Septic Arthritis

Sternoclavicular (S-C) septic arthritis is only 1% of whole joint infections [57]. It is very rare and only 23% of patients are healthy. Predispositional factors are present in most of the cases. According to a review bacteremia was present in 62% of patients. The risk factors included intravenous drug use (21%), distant site infection (15%), diabetes mellitus (13%), trauma (12%), and infected central venous line (9%) [57]. Computerized tomography (CT) or MR can be used to assess for the presence of chest wall phlegmon, retrosternal abscess or mediastinitis. Half of the cases had S. aureus, pseudomonas aueruginosa and Group C streptococcus as causative agent [57, 58]. In Nusselt et al.'s series of five patients, one patient had laryngeal cancer, one patient had port-explantation linked to a rectum carcinoma, one patient had spondylodiscitis and one patient had brain stem infarct with reduced general condition. Only one patient had no underlying medical problem [58].

Chest pain is the main complaint in patients, rather than shoulder pain. This infection is important due to the close relationship of S-C joint with other organs and related complications [59]. Fatal complications like mediastinitis is possible. CT and MR is usually necessary to determine the spread and seriousness of the infection. Early diagnosis is important. In early stages simple drainage, debridement and antibiotic treatment is usually enough [58]. However, more radical debridement is needed in complicated patients with clavicula or manibrum sterni osteomyelitis. S-C joint resection is an option for accompanying osteomyelitis with good functional results [60]. Song et al. proposed resection should be the main treatment, since in their five patients out of six cases simple debridement was insufficient [59]. Pectoralis major flap reconstruction may be needed in chronic cases with widespread osteomyelitis [61].

Prosthetic Infections

In the French literature, the first shoulder arthroplasty which was made of platinum and rubber, was performed by Jean Pean for shoulder tuberculosis, but the prosthesis was removed after 2 years due to infection [62, 63]. Infection after shoulder arthroplasty is a painful and potentially fatal complication [64].

The incidence of infection after shoulder arthroplasty is between 0 and 4% ([65][66, 67]). The incidence is a little bit higher after RSA which was reported in the literature as 0–18.8% [68–73]. In Sperling et al.'s series the incidence of infection after revision shoulder arthroplasty cases was 3%, whereas it was only 0.8% after primary cases [67].

Although the treatment of shoulder prosthetic infections is uncertain, the guidelines for hip and knee prosthetic infections are usually used to determine the treatment principles. The loosening of the humeral component must be regarded as infection unless proven otherwise. In case of an infection after prosthetic implantation, any recent procedures like dental procedures or urinary catheterization causing bacteremia should be questioned as well as the indication of the primary operation and any problems that had occurred during arthroplasty application.

The diagnosis of infection after shoulder arthroplasty is difficult. Clinical symptoms like erythema, fistula formation, fever, septicemia and reduced general condition are rarely observed. Pain and functional impairment are the most important clinical findings. Increased ESR and CRP levels and leucocyte count in synovial fluid are important laboratory findings but laboratory findings may be normal in most of the cases [2]. The microbiological investigation of the aspirated synovial fluid and identification of the pathogen by culture is critical for the diagnosis and effective treatment of the infection.

The causative agent must be identified by joint aspiration before planning a revision surgery. The growth in the culture may take some time [2]. If the growth is late it may be due to contamination unless there are infection symptoms [9]. However positive cultures alone are enough for the diagnosis of infection. Evaluation of positive cultures in P. acnes infections have some controversies. The diagnosis is usually made by evaluating the clinical symptoms, laboratory and microbiological tests, radiography and indium scanning together.

The risk of prosthetic infection is more in patients with co-morbidities like diabetes mellitus, rheumatoid arthritis or systemic lupus erythromatosus. In different studies immunosuppressive therapy, systemic cortisone use, repeated cortisone injections and previous surgeries were found to be responsible for the prosthetic infections in 66% of cases [67, 74, 75]. Ince et al. observed diabetes mellitus, steroid use or malignancy in 44% of patients who had revision surgery for prosthetic infections [76]. In another series of ten patients, two patients had malignancy, one patient had liver cirrhosis, three patients had cranial injury, one patient had chronic polyarthritis and one patient was having hemodialysis [63].

The average number of previous surgeries before revision surgery was found as four in Beekman et al.'s series of shoulder prosthetic infections. All patients had clinical findings of infection like swelling, redness or sinus formation. No radiographic findings of loosening were observed in patients and this was confirmed during the operation. After revision surgery antibiotics treatment was continued for 6 weeks until ESR and CRP levels have decreased [68].

Acute deep infection after fixation of proximal humerus fractures is an important complication with poor functional outcomes and increased rate of nonunion [47]. The risk of prosthetic infection is high when arthroplasty is performed for the treatment of failed fracture fixation or its complications [71, 77, 78]. Klatte et al. observed growth in the culture in five patients out of 32 who had arthroplasty after failed fracture fixation. The procedures were regarded as one stage revision with arthroplasty, and no reinfection was observed. They concluded that the risk of occult infection was high in patients with proximal humerus fractures compared to hip and knee [79].

The prosthetic infections in shoulder may differ in many ways from knee and hip joints. Although staphylococcus species were reported as primary pathogen in some studies like other prosthetic infections [5, 76], in many other studies P. acnes was responsible for most of the infections [67, 80, 81].

P. acnes is a gram (+) anaerobic bacillus and is a common pathogen in post-surgical shoulder infections. This microorganism is found in pilosebaceous glands of the skin in high concentrations [82]. It is usually located in fat rich body regions with hair follicles, especially in moist areas of shoulder and axilla [83]. Shoulder infections with P. acnes is well defined and understood, but the pathogenesis is not clear. The diagnosis in prosthetic infections is difficult and usually delayed due to low virulence and slow progression of the infection [84]. In one study about revision arthroplasty cases in shoulder, P. acnes was detected in intraoperative cultures despite good surgical field preparation and prophylaxis, especially more commonly in men. It was concluded that P. acnes could be related to primary arthroplasty failure [85]. This finding was also supported in other study about primary shoulder surgical procedures and the authors thought the surgical field was contaminated with P. acnes due to exposition of pilosebaceous glands after the incision [114].

The cultures can be positive for P. acnes without any sign of obvious infection. This contamination as thought to be a probable reason of primary osteoarthritis [1].

Further diagnostic techniques like implant sonication or PCR can be used for P. acnes infections but there is no such a study for shoulder infections [86]. Some tests with high specificity for the detection of Ig G related to P. acnes can also be used, but these tests are defined for general infections and are not specific to shoulder [87].

Anaerobic bone and joint infections are uncommon. These are usually polymicrobial. P. acnes is the reason in 22% of the cases, especially around shoulder joint. MALDI-TOF MS (Matrix-assisted laser desorption ionization time-of-flight mass spectrometry) can be used for the diagnosis and the choice of proper antibiotic treatment of anaerobic bone and joint infections [88].

In one study about the patients having the first shoulder surgical procedure, growth in the culture was observed two times more in anterolateral approach compared to deltopectoral approach, and three times more in men. This finding was not found to be related to subacromial injections [89].

In another study of 12 patients who had secondary procedures after shoulder arthroplasty due to post-operative hematoma formation, 6 patients had positive intraoperative cultures [70]. Post-operative hematoma causes poor results requiring additional procedures and it may be related to deep infection in most of the patients.

Detritic synovitis can be confused with P. acnes infections. The macroscopic appearance of the synovial fluid is similar. This condition is related to aseptic loosening and one stage revision surgery is usually sufficient [90].

Treatment

Sperling et al. classified shoulder infections as acute, subacute and chronic infections [67]. Then they improved this classification by including the treatment algorithm and described AAOS classification [66]:

Type I: Positive Cultures at Time of Revision Surgery

Organism-specific antibiotic treatment is instituted with close clinical observation. There are no good data to determine the optimal length of antibiotic treatment.

Type II: Acute Infection within 30 days After Surgery

Surgical debridement and prosthetic retention is utilized, although there are minimal data available on the outcomes of this approach.

Type III: Acute Hematogenous Infection More Than 30 days After Surgery

Surgical debridement with retention of the implants or two-stage treatment with use of an antibiotic spacer impregnated with gentamycin and vancomycin between explantation and reimplantation is recommended.

Type IV: Chronic Infection

Surgical debridement with implant removal, temporary placement of an antibiotic spacer impregnated with gentamycin and vancomycin, and reimplantation approximately 8 weeks later are recommended.

Different options are described for the treatment of prosthetic infections like debridement with antibiotic therapy, arthroscopic debridement, one stage or two stage revisions, resection arthroplasty, arthrodesis, keeping the antibiotic-impregnated cement spacers or even amputation [91]. Variable results of these treatment modalities are present in the literature for infection control. Weber et al. was able to treat infection with VAC-irrigation in one patient, although there is no enough study supporting this method [63].

Debridement with Antibiotic Therapy

Over 65% of reinfection risk is present with this method [41, 92]. Coste et al. performed debridement in eight patients, two of which had arthroscopic debridement. The patients with arthroscopic debridement and four out of six patients with open debridement had unsuccessful results [65].

Resection Arthroplasty

Although infection rates are low, the functional results are usually poor after resection arthroplasty. It can be a choice as a salvage procedure [41, 92, 93].

Two Stage Revision

The primary aim in prosthetic infections is the control of the infection which requires a sufficient bone and soft tissue debridement. This debridement sometimes may include the rotator cuff and a RSA may be a better choice in one stage or two stage revisions in order to obtain a good functional result. Sabesan et al. reported 6% of reinfection rate and satisfactory functional results after two stage revisions with RSA [94]. Low reinfection after revisions with RSA was also reported in other studies [93].

In a multicentre retrospective study no reinfection was observed after two stage revisions [95]. This was also a finding in Sperling et al.'s of three patients who had two stage revision and these patients had active abduction of 100 ° postoperatively. In contrary, Strickland et al. observed 38% of reinfection rate after two stage revisions and the patients had an average abduction of 89 ° and average external rotation of 48 ° [96].

Coffey et al. proposed to use commercially produced antibiotic-impregnated cement spacers in two stage revisions, since the amount and the release of antibiotics were more controlled in these implants. Theses spacers were produced by using custom reusable molds and had the advantages of less glenoid erosion due to smooth surface and less surgical time [5]. Stine et al. reported breakage of the spacer in 3 out of 18 patients and reimplantation was needed in these patients. During the debridement, it was observed that the bony defect was extending below the surgical neck [97].

Keeping the Antibiotic-Impregnated Cement Spacer

This method can be a treatment option in low demand elderly patients but the shoulder functions are usually poor. It can be used only if the infection control is sufficient [98, 99]. Four out of 15 patients refused revision surgery after spacer implantation in Coffey et al.'s series [5]. Although no clinical difference was found between this technique and resection arthroplasty [100], some studies reported pain free shoulder functions in daily activities [97]. Limited weight bearing in the upper extremity may be an advantage for this kind of spacer application.

One Stage Revision

In the literature, one stage revision surgery for the treatment of shoulder prosthetic infections has comparable results with two stage revisions or resection arthroplasty. Ince et al. used one staged revision in their patients and observed no reinfections. The diagnosis of the pathogen was possible preoperatively in 81% of patients and staphylococcus infections were present in most of the cases. ESR and CRP levels were elevated in most of the patients. Successful results were reported in 6 out of 16 patients. Although no reinfection was observed, secondary procedures were needed due to other reasons in three patients, and the functional results were poor with an average abduction of 52 ° [76].

Klatte et al. observed 6% of reinfection in their patients who had one stage revision after 4.75 years of follow-up. Highest Constan-Murley scores were detected after revisions with RSA. The authors emphasized the importance of detecting the pathogen and its antibiotic sensitivity preoperatively. They advocated that the hospitalization time was less (average of 10.6 days) and the duration of antibiotic therapy was short in one stage revisions and this method was an effective option [101].

Beekmann et al. used RSA for one stage revision surgery in 11 patients. Only one patient had reinfection. They advocated that one stage revision had the advantages of less glenoid erosion due to cement spacer, short duration of treatment, less morbidity and less cost. Revision with RSA was an effective method for infection control with good functional results [68]. Poor functional results was reported after one stage revisions with total shoulder prosthesis [76].

According to Cuff et al. radical debridement is mandatory for the treatment of prosthetic infections which usually includes the debridement of the rotator cuff and the revision should be performed by RSA. In their series, there was no difference between one stage or two stage revisions. The average active abduction was 110° after RSA. The complication rate was 32% which may be related to complexity of the cases [93]. The deltoid muscle and its innervation must be intact in order to be able to use RSA for revision.

Shoulder Arthrodesis

Arthrodesis may be used after failed arthroplasty. The incidence of infection after shoulder arthrodesis is between 3 and 5% [102]. It can be a treatment option for chronic shoulder infections [103].

Infection Prevention

Antibiotic prophylaxis is recommended for most of the orthopedic procedures where implants are used. Most commonly used antibiotic is cefazolin with a suggested dose of 1 g started just before the operation and continued for 24 h in clean cases [62, 104]. The type of the antibiotic may change due to allergic status of the patient or in specific conditions.

Besides standard prophylaxis for orthopedic procedures, some studies are also present specific to shoulder joint. Intraoperative intraarticular application of gentamicin was observed to reduce infection rate from 3 to 0.29% [105]. Lorenzetti et al. found that application of a cyanoacrylate microbial sealent may reduce intraoperative positive cultures, thereof subsequent infections in revision shoulder arthroplasties [106].

Using antibiotic-impregnated bone cement for primary RSA was found to be effective in the prevention of deep infection. The infection rate was 3% after revisions with RSA when antibiotic-impregnated bone cement was not used, whereas no infection occurred in patients when antibiotic-impregnated bone cement was used [107].

In one study, topical application of benzoyl peroxide preoperatively reduced positive intraoperative cultures for P. acnes. This may decrease the infection rate [108].

Skin preparation with 2% chlorhexidine gluconate-impregnated cloths was found to be more effective in prevention of coagulase (−) staphylococcus growth compared to standard soaps [109]. Similarly Saltzman et al. observed that skin preparation with 2% chlorhexidine gluconate and 70% isopropyl alcohol was more effective than iodine and iodophor-isopropyl alcohol for infection prevention [110]. However these studies are related to the results of the cultures and their real effects on preventing the infections are controversial. Lee et al. showed existence of P. acnes in 70% of patients despite skin preparation with 2% chlorhexidine gluconate and 70% isopropyl alcohol [111].

Questions

1. What is the most sensitive and specific diagnostic parameter for prosthetic infections?
   A. CRP
   B. IL-6
   C. a-defensin
   D. ESR
   E. Leukocytosis
   C

2. What is the most common pathogen for septic arthritis of shoulder after arthroscopic surgery?
   A. Staf. Aureus
   B. Strep. Pneumonia
   C. P. acnes
   D. E. coli
   E. MRSA
   C

3. Which treatment method for prosthetic infection is associated with the most common recurrence rates?
   A. Debridement with antibiotherapy
   B. One stage revision
   C. Two stage revision
   D. Resection arthroplasty
   E. Shoulder arthrodesis
   A

What's new?

Propionibacterium acnes is almost specific for shoulder. A diagnostic controlled study was performed by Hudek et al. in order to clarify whether P. acnes is a true infection or contamination?

Propionibacterium acnes in shoulder surgery: true infection, contamination, or commensal of the deep tissue? Journal of Shoulder and Elbow Surgery, 2014 December, Hudek et al.

References

1. Levy O, Iyer S, Atoun E, Peter N, Hous N, Cash D, Musa F, Narvani AA. Propionibacterium acnes: an underestimated etiology in the pathogenesis of osteoarthritis? J Shoulder Elbow Surg. 2013;22(4):505–11.
2. Topolski MS, Chin PY, Sperling JW, Cofield RH. Revision shoulder arthroplasty with positive intraoperative cultures: the value of preoperative studies and intraoperative histology. J Shoulder Elbow Surg. 2006;15(4):402–6.
3. Lenski M, Scherer MA. Diagnostic potential of inflammatory markers in septic arthritis and periprosthetic joint infections: a clinical study with 719 patients. Infect Dis (Lond). 2015;47(6):399–409.
4. Di Cesare PE, Chang E, Preston CF, Liu CJ. Serum interleukin-6 as a marker of periprosthetic infection following total hip and knee arthroplasty. J Bone Joint Surg Am. 2005;87(9):1921–7.
5. Coffey MJ, Ely EE, Crosby LA. Treatment of glenohumeral sepsis with a commercially produced antibiotic-impregnated cement spacer. J Shoulder Elbow Surg. 2010;19(6):868–73.
6. Frangiamore SJ, Saleh A, Grosso MJ, Kovac MF, Higuera CA, Iannotti JP, Ricchetti ET. α-Defensin as a predictor of periprosthetic shoulder infection. J Shoulder Elbow Surg. 2015;24(7):1021–7.
7. Grosso MJ, Frangiamore SJ, Saleh A, Kovac MF, Hayashi R, Ricchetti ET, Bauer TW, Iannotti JP. Poor utility of serum interleukin-6 levels to predict indolent periprosthetic shoulder infections. J Shoulder Elbow Surg. 2014;23(9):1277–81.
8. Paosong S, Narongroeknawin P, Pakchotanon R, Asavatanabodee P, Chaiamnuay S. Serum procalcitonin as a diagnostic aid in patients with acute bacterial septic arthritis. Int J Rheum Dis. 2015;18(3):352–9.
9. Frangiamore SJ, Saleh A, Grosso MJ, Alolabi B, Bauer TW, Iannotti JP, Ricchetti ET. Early versus late culture growth of propionibacterium acnes in revision shoulder arthroplasty. J Bone Joint Surg Am. 2015;97(14):1149–58.
10. Levy PY, Fournier PE, Fenollar F, Raoult D. Systematic PCR detection in culture-negative osteoarticular infections. Am J Med. 2013;126(12):1143.e25–33.
11. Mirra JM, Amstutz HC, Matos M, Gold R. The pathology of the joint tissues and its clinical relevance in prosthesis failure. Clin Orthop Relat Res. 1976;117:221–40.
12. Lew DP, Waldvogel FA. Osteomyelitis. Lancet. 2004;364(9431):369–79.
13. Perlman MH, Patzakis MJ, Kumar PJ, Holtom P. The incidence of joint involvement with adjacent osteomyelitis in pediatric patients. J Pediatr Orthop. 2000;20(1):40–3.
14. Morrissy RT, Haynes DW. Acute hematogenous osteomyelitis: a model with trauma as an etiology. J Pediatr Orthop. 1989;9(4):447–56.
15. Blyth MJ, Kincaid R, Craigen MA, Bennet GC. The changing epidemiology of acute and subacute haematogenous osteomyelitis in children. J Bone Joint Surg Br. 2001;83(1):99–102.
16. Martínez-Aguilar G, Avalos-Mishaan A, Hulten K, Hammerman W, Mason Jr EO, Kaplan SL. Community-acquired, methicillin-resistant and methicillin-susceptible Staphylococcus aureus musculoskeletal infections in children. Pediatr Infect Dis J. 2004;23(8):701–6.

17. Yagupsky P. Kingella kingae: from medical rarity to an emerging paediatric pathogen. Lancet Infect Dis. 2004;4(6):358–67.
18. Tan TQ, Mason Jr EO, Barson WJ, Wald ER, Schutze GE, Bradley JS, Arditi M, Givner LB, Yogev R, Kim KS, Kaplan SL. Clinical characteristics and outcome of children with pneumonia attributable to penicillin-susceptible and penicillin-nonsusceptible Streptococcus pneumoniae. Pediatrics. 1998;102(6):1369–75.
19. Gutierrez K. Bone and joint infections in children. Pediatr Clin North Am. 2005;52(3):779–94.
20. Bleckwenn M, Sommer B, Weckbecker K. Chronic recurrent multifocal osteomyelitis manifested as painful clavicular swelling: a case report. BMC Res Notes. 2014;7:786.
21. Gillespie R. Septic arthritis of childhood. Clin Orthop Relat Res. 1973;96:152–9.
22. Nade S. Acute septic arthritis in infancy and childhood. J Bone Joint Surg Br. 1983;65(3):234–41.
23. Ernat J, Riccio AI, Fitzpatrick K, Jo C, Wimberly RL. Osteomyelitis is commonly associated with septic arthritis of the shoulder in children. J Pediatr Orthop. 2015;19. [Epub ahead of print]
24. Lejman T, Strong M, Michno P, Hayman M. Septic arthritis of the shoulder during the first 18 months of life. J Pediatr Orthop. 1995;15(2):172–5.
25. Fabry G, Meire E. Septic arthritis of the hip in children: poor results after late and inadequate treatment. J Pediatr Orthop. 1983;3(4):461–6.
26. Frank G, Mahoney HM, Eppes SC. Musculoskeletal infections in children. Pediatr Clin North Am. 2005;52(4):1083–106.
27. Saisu T, Kawashima A, Kamegaya M, Mikasa M, Moriishi J, Moriya H. Humeral shortening and inferior subluxation as sequelae of septic arthritis of the shoulder in neonates and infants. J Bone Joint Surg Am. 2007;89(8):1784–93.
28. Bos CF, Mol LJ, Obermann WR, Tjin a Ton ER. Late sequelae of neonatal septic arthritis of the shoulder. J Bone Joint Surg Br. 1998;80(4):645–50.
29. Schmidt D, Mubarak S, Gelberman R. Septic shoulders in children. J Pediatr Orthop. 1981;1(1):67–72.
30. Belthur MV, Palazzi DL, Miller JA, Phillips WA, Weinberg J. A clinical analysis of shoulder and hip joint infections in children. J Pediatr Orthop. 2009;29(7):828–33.
31. Abdel MP, Perry KI, Morrey ME, Steinmann SP, Sperling JW, Cass JR. Arthroscopic management of native shoulder septic arthritis. J Shoulder Elbow Surg. 2013;22(3):418–21.
32. Smith SP, Thyoka M, Lavy CB, Pitani A. Septic arthritis of the shoulder in children in Malawi. A randomised, prospective study of aspiration versus arthrotomy and washout. J Bone Joint Surg Br. 2002;84(8):1167–72.
33. Forward DP, Hunter JB. Arthroscopic washout of the shoulder for septic arthritis in infants. A new technique. J Bone Joint Surg Br. 2002;84(8):1173–5.
34. Lossos IS, Yossepowitch O, Kandel L, Yardeni D, Arber N. Septic arthritis of the glenohumeral joint. A report of 11 cases and review of the literature. Medicine (Baltimore). 1998;77(3):177–87. Review
35. Kelly PJ, Coventry MB, Martin WJ. Bacterial arthritis of the shoulder. Mayo Clin Proc. 1965;40:695–9.
36. Hunter JG, Gross JM, Dahl JD, Amsdell SL, Gorczyca JT. Risk factors forfailure of a single surgical debridement in adults with acute septic arthritis. J Bone Joint Surg Am. 2015;97(7):558–64.
37. Stutz G, Kuster MS, Kleinstück F, Gächter A. Arthroscopic management of septic arthritis: stages of infection and results. Knee Surg Sports Traumatol Arthrosc. 2000;8(5):270–4.
38. Jeon IH, Choi CH, Seo JS, Seo KJ, Ko SH, Park JY. Arthroscopic management of septic arthritis of the shoulder joint. J Bone Joint Surg Am. 2006;88(8):1802–6.
39. Garofalo R, Flanagin B, Cesari E, Vinci E, Conti M, Castagna A. Destructive septic arthritis of shoulder in adults. Musculoskelet Surg. 2014;98(Suppl 1):S35–9.
40. Schoch B, Allen B, Mileti J, Sperling JW, Cofield RH. Shoulder arthroplasty for the treatment of postinfectious glenohumeral arthritis. J Shoulder Elbow Surg. 2014;23(9):1327–33.
41. Mileti J, Sperling JW, Cofield RH. Shoulder arthroplasty for the treatment of postinfectious glenohumeral arthritis. J Bone Joint Surg Am. 2003;85-A(4):609–14.
42. Morris BJ, Waggenspack Jr WN, Laughlin MS, Elkousy HA, Gartsman GM, Edwards TB. Reverse shoulder arthroplasty for management of postinfectious arthropathy with rotator cuff deficiency. Orthopedics. 2015;38(8):e701–7.
43. Yeranosian MG, Petrigliano FA, Terrell RD, Wang JC, McAllister DR. Incidenceof postoperative infections requiring reoperation after arthroscopic knee surgery. Arthroscopy. 2013;29(8):1355–61.
44. Moen TC, Rudolph GH, Caswell K, Espinoza C, Burkhead Jr WZ, Krishnan SG. Complications of shoulder arthroscopy. J Am Acad Orthop Surg. 2014;22(7):410–9.
45. Weber SC, Abrams JS, Nottage WM. Complications associated with arthroscopic shoulder surgery. Arthroscopy. 2002;18(2 Suppl 1):88–95.
46. Yeranosian MG, Arshi A, Terrell RD, Wang JC, McAllister DR, Petrigliano FA. Incidence of acute postoperative infections requiring reoperation after arthroscopic shoulder surgery. Am J Sports Med. 2014;42(2):437–41.
47. Athwal GS, Sperling JW, Rispoli DM, Cofield RH. Deep infection after rotator cuff repair. J Shoulder Elbow Surg. 2007;16(3):306–11.
48. Herrera MF, Bauer G, Reynolds F, Wilk RM, Bigliani LU, Levine WN. Infection after mini-open rotator cuff repair. J Shoulder Elbow Surg. 2002;11(6):605–8.
49. Horneff III JG, Hsu JE, Voleti PB, O'Donnell J, Huffman GR. Propionibacterium acnes infection in shoulder arthroscopy patients with postoperative pain. J Shoulder Elbow Surg. 2015;24(6):838–43.

50. Chuang MJ, Jancosko JJ, Mendoza V, Nottage WM. The incidence of propionibacterium acnes in shoulder arthroscopy. Arthroscopy. 2015;31(9):1702–7.
51. Hammel JM, Kwon N. Septic arthritis of the acromioclavicular joint. J Emerg Med. 2005;29(4):425–7.
52. Zimmermann III B, Erickson AD, Mikolich DJ. Septic acromioclavicular arthritis and osteomyelitis in a patient with acquired immunodeficiency syndrome. Arthritis Rheum. 1989;32(9):1175–8.
53. Iyengar KP, Gudena R, Chitgopkar SD, Ralte P, Hughes P, Nadkarni JB, Loh WY. Primary septic arthritis of the acromio-clavicular joint: case report and review of literature. Arch Orthop Trauma Surg. 2009;129(1):83–6.
54. Chirag AS, Ropiak CR, Bosco Iii JA, Egol KA. Septic arthritis of the acromioclavicular joint—a report of four cases. Bull NYU Hosp Jt Dis. 2007;65(4):308–11.
55. Hong MJ, Kim YD, Ham HD. Acute septic arthritis of the acromioclavicular joint caused by Haemophilus parainfluenzae: a rare causative origin. Clin Rheumatol. 2015;34(4):811–4.
56. Blankstein A, Amsallem JL, Rubinstein E, Horoszowski H, Farin I. Septic arthritis of the acromioclavicular joint. Arch Orthop Trauma Surg. 1985;103(6):417–8.
57. Ross JJ, Shamsuddin H. Sternoclavicular septic arthritis: review of 180 cases. Medicine (Baltimore). 2004;83(3):139–48.
58. Nusselt T, Klinger HM, Freche S, Schultz W, Baums MH. Surgical management of sternoclavicular septic arthritis. Arch Orthop Trauma Surg. 2011;131(3):319–23.
59. Song HK, Guy TS, Kaiser LR, Shrager JB. Current presentation and optimal surgical management of sternoclavicular joint infection. Ann Thorac Surg. 2002;73:427–31.
60. Chun JM, Kim JS, Jung HJ, Park JB, Song JS, Park SS, Lee HS, Ahn TS. Resection arthroplasty for septic arthritis of the sternoclavicular joint. J Shoulder Elbow Surg. 2012;21(3):361–6.
61. Al-Mufarrej F, Martinez-Jorge J, Carlsen BT, Saint-Cyr M, Moran SL, Mardini S. Use of the deltoid branch-based clavicular head of pectoralis major muscle flap in isolated sternoclavicular infections. J Plast Reconstr Aesthet Surg. 2013;66(12):1702–11.
62. Richards RR. Sepsis of the shoulder: molecular mechanism and pathogenesis. In: Rockwood Jr CA, Matsen III FA, Wirth MA, Lippitt SB, editors. The shoulder, vol. 2. 3rd ed. Philadelphia; 2004. p. 1233–55.
63. Weber P, Utzschneider S, Sadoghi P, Andress HJ, Jansson V, Müller PE. Management of the infected shoulder prosthesis: a retrospective analysis and review of the literature. Int Orthop. 2011;35(3):365–73.
64. Cofield RH, Edgerton BC. Total shoulder arthroplasty: complications and revision surgery. Instr Course Lect. 1990;39:449–62.
65. Coste JS, Reig S, Trojani C, Berg M, Walch G, Boileau P. The management of infection in arthroplasty of the shoulder. J Bone Joint Surg Br. 2004;86(1):65–9.
66. Sperling JW, Hawkins RJ, Walch G, Zuckerman JD. Complications in total shoulder arthroplasty. J Bone Joint Surg Am. 2013;95(6):563–9.
67. Sperling JW, Kozak TK, Hanssen AD, Cofield RH. Infection after shoulder arthroplasty. Clin Orthop Relat Res. 2001;382:206–16.
68. Beekman PD, Katusic D, Berghs BM, Karelse A, De Wilde L. One-stage revisionfor patients with a chronically infected reverse total shoulder replacement. J Bone Joint Surg Br. 2010;92(6):817–22.
69. Boileau P, Watkinson D, Hatzidakis AM, Hovorka I. Neer Award 2005: the Grammont reverse shoulder prosthesis: results in cuff tear arthritis, fracture sequelae, and revision arthroplasty. J Shoulder Elbow Surg. 2006;15(5):527–40.
70. Cheung EV, Sperling JW, Cofield RH. Infection associated with hematoma formation after shoulder arthroplasty. Clin Orthop Relat Res. 2008;466(6):1363–7.
71. Kılıç M, Berth A, Blatter G, Fuhrmann U, Gebhardt K, Rott O, Zenz P, Irlenbusch U. Anatomic and reverse shoulder prostheses in fracture sequelae of the humeral head. Acta Orthop Traumatol Turc. 2010;44(6):417–25.
72. Seebauer L. Total reverse shoulder arthroplasty: European lessons and future trends. Am J Orthop. 2007;36(12 Suppl 1):22–8.
73. Werner CM, Steinmann PA, Gilbart M, Gerber C. Treatment of painful pseudoparesis due to irreparable rotator cuff dysfunction with the delta III reverse-ball-and-socket total shoulder prosthesis. J Bone Joint Surg Am. 2005;87(7):1476–86.
74. Wirth MA, Rockwood Jr CA. Complications of total shoulder-replacement arthroplasty. J Bone Joint Surg Am. 1996;78(4):603–16.
75. Zeller V, Ghorbani A, Strady C, Leonard P, Mamoudy P, Desplaces N. Propionibacterium acnes: an agent of prosthetic joint infection and colonization. J Infect. 2007;55(2):119–24.
76. Ince A, Seemann K, Frommelt L, Katzer A, Loehr JF. One-stage exchange shoulder arthroplasty for periprosthetic infection. J Bone Joint Surg Br. 2005;87(6):814–8.
77. Wall B, Nové-Josserand L, O'Connor DP, Edwards TB, Walch G. Reverse total shoulder arthroplasty: a review of results according to etiology. J Bone Joint Surg Am. 2007;89(7):1476–85.
78. Martinez AA, Bejarano C, Carbonel I, Iglesias D, Gil-Albarova J, Herrera A. The treatment of proximal humerus nonunions in older patients with reverse shoulder arthroplasty. Injury. 2012;43-2:S3–6.
79. Klatte TO, Sabihi R, Guenther D, Kamath AF, Rueger JM, Gehrke T, Kendoff D. High Rates of Occult Infection After Shoulder Fracture Fixation: Considerations for Conversion Shoulder Arthroplasty. HSS J. 2015;11(3):198–203.

80. Levy PY, Fenollar F, Stein A, Borrione F, Cohen E, Lebail B, Raoult D. Propionibacterium acnes postoperative shoulder arthritis: an emerging clinical entity. Clin Infect Dis. 2008;46(12):1884–6.
81. Pottinger P, Butler-Wu S, Neradilek MB, Merritt A, Bertelsen A, Jette JL, Warme WJ, Matsen III. FA. Prognostic factors for bacterial cultures positive for Propionibacterium acnes and other organisms in a large series of revision shoulder arthroplasties performed for stiffness, pain, or loosening. J Bone Joint Surg Am. 2012;94(22):2075–83.
82. Leeming JP, Holland KT, Cunliffe WJ. The microbial ecology of pilosebaceous units isolated from human skin. J Gen Microbiol. 1984;130(4):803–7.
83. Patel A, Calfee RP, Plante M, Fischer SA, Green A. Propionibacterium acnes colonization of the human shoulder. J Shoulder Elbow Surg. 2009;18(6):897–902.
84. Dodson CC, Craig EV, Cordasco FA, Dines DM, Dines JS, Dicarlo E, Brause BD, Warren RF. Propionibacterium acnes infection after shoulder arthroplasty: a diagnostic challenge. J Shoulder Elbow Surg. 2010;19(2):303–7.
85. Matsen III FA, Russ SM, Bertelsen A, Butler-Wu S, Pottinger PS. Propionibacterium can be isolated from deep cultures obtained at primary arthroplasty despite intravenous antimicrobial prophylaxis. J Shoulder Elbow Surg. 2015;24(6):844–7.
86. Achermann Y, Vogt M, Leunig M, Wüst J, Trampuz A. Improved diagnosis ofperiprosthetic joint infection by multiplex PCR of sonication fluid from removed implants. J Clin Microbiol. 2010;48(4):1208–14.
87. Marmor S, Bauer T, Desplaces N, Heym B, Roux AL, Sol O, Rogé J, Mahé F, Désiré L, Aegerter P, Ghout I, Ropers J, Gaillard JL, Rottman M. Multiplex antibody detection for noninvasive genus-level diagnosis of prosthetic joint infection. J Clin Microbiol. 2016;54(4):1065–73.
88. Walter G, Vernier M, Pinelli PO, Million M, Coulange M, Seng P, Stein A. Bone and joint infections due to anaerobic bacteria: an analysis of 61 cases and review of the literature. Eur J Clin Microbiol Infect Dis. 2014;33(8):1355–64.
89. Hudek R, Sommer F, Kerwat M, Abdelkawi AF, Loos F, Gohlke F. Propionibacteriumacnes in shoulder surgery: true infection, contamination, or commensal of the deep tissue? J Shoulder Elbow Surg. 2014;23(12):1763–71.
90. Gorbaty JD, Lucas RM, Matsen III FA. Detritic synovitis can mimic a propionibacterium periprosthetic infection. Int Orthop. 2016;40(1):95–8.
91. Unglaub F, Guehring T, Fuchs PC, Perez-Bouza A, Groger A, Pallua N. Necrotizing fasciitis following therapeutic injection in a shoulder joint. Orthopade. 2005;34(3):250–2. German
92. Braman JP, Sprague M, Bishop J, Lo IK, Lee EW, Flatow EL. The outcome of resection shoulder arthroplasty for recalcitrant shoulder infections. J Shoulder Elbow Surg. 2006;15(5):549–53.
93. Cuff DJ, Virani NA, Levy J, Frankle MA, Derasari A, Hines B, Pupello DR, Cancio M, Mighell M. The treatment of deep shoulder infection and glenohumeral instability with debridement, reverse shoulder arthroplasty and postoperative antibiotics. J Bone Joint Surg Br. 2008;90(3):336–42.
94. Sabesan VJ, Ho JC, Kovacevic D, Iannotti JP. Two-stage reimplantation for treating prosthetic shoulder infections. Clin Orthop Relat Res. 2011;469(9):2538–43.
95. Romanò CL, Borens O, Monti L, Meani E, Stuyck J. What treatment for periprosthetic shoulder infection? Results from a multicentre retrospective series. Int Orthop. 2012;36(5):1011–7.
96. Strickland JP, Sperling JW, Cofield RH. The results of two-stage re-implantation for infected shoulder replacement. J Bone Joint Surg Br. 2008;90(4):460–5.
97. Stine IA, Lee B, Zalavras CG, Hatch III G, Itamura JM. Management of chronic shoulder infections utilizing a fixed articulating antibiotic-loaded spacer. J Shoulder Elbow Surg. 2010;19(5):739–48.
98. Jerosch J, Schneppenheim M. Management of infected shoulder replacement. Arch Orthop Trauma Surg. 2003;123(5):209–14.
99. Themistocleous G, Zalavras C, Stine I, Zachos V, Itamura J. Prolonged implantation of an antibiotic cement spacer for management of shoulder sepsis in compromised patients. J Shoulder Elbow Surg. 2007;16(6):701–5.
100. Verhelst L, Stuyck J, Bellemans J, Debeer P. Resection arthroplasty of the shoulder as a salvage procedure for deep shoulder infection: does the use of a cement spacer improve outcome? J Shoulder Elbow Surg. 2011;20(8):1224–33.
101. Klatte TO, Junghans K, Al-Khateeb H, Rueger JM, Gehrke T, Kendoff D, Neumann J. Single-stage revision for peri-prosthetic shoulder infection: outcomes and results. Bone Joint J. 2013;95-B(3):391–5.
102. González-Díaz R, Rodríguez-Merchán EC, Gilbert MS. The role of shoulder fusion in the era of arthroplasty. Int Orthop. 1997;21(3):204–9.
103. Clare DJ, Wirth MA, Groh GI, Rockwood Jr CA. Shoulder arthrodesis. J Bone Joint Surg Am. 2001;83-A(4):593–600.
104. Neu HC. Cephalosporin antibiotics as applied in surgery of bones and joints. Clin Orthop Relat Res. 1984;190:50–64.
105. Lovallo J, Helming J, Jafari SM, Owusu-Forfie A, Donovan S, Minnock C, Adib F. Intraoperative intra-articular injection of gentamicin: will it decrease the risk of infection in total shoulder arthroplasty? J Shoulder Elbow Surg. 2014;23(9):1272–6.
106. Lorenzetti AJ, Wongworawat MD, Jobe CM, Phipatanakul WP. Cyanoacrylate microbial sealant may reduce the prevalence of positive cultures in revision shoulder arthroplasty. Clin Orthop Relat Res. 2013;471(10):3225–9.
107. Nowinski RJ, Gillespie RJ, Shishani Y, Cohen B, Walch G, Gobezie R. Antibiotic-loaded bone cement reduces deep infection rates for primary reverse total shoulder arthroplasty: a retrospective, cohort study of 501 shoulders. J Shoulder Elbow Surg. 2012;21(3):324–8.

108. Sabetta JR, Rana VP, Vadasdi KB, Greene RT, Cunningham JG, Miller SR, Sethi PM. Efficacy of topical benzoyl peroxide on the reduction of Propionibacterium acnes during shoulder surgery. J Shoulder Elbow Surg. 2015;24(7):995–1004.
109. Murray MR, Saltzman MD, Gryzlo SM, Terry MA, Woodward CC, Nuber GW. Efficacy of preoperative home use of 2% chlorhexidine gluconate cloth before shoulder surgery. J Shoulder Elbow Surg. 2011;20(6):928–33.
110. Saltzman MD, Nuber GW, Gryzlo SM, Marecek GS, Koh JL. Efficacy of surgical preparation solutions in shoulder surgery. J Bone Joint Surg Am. 2009;91(8):1949–53.
111. Lee MJ, Pottinger PS, Butler-Wu S, Bumgarner RE, Russ SM, Matsen III. FA. Propionibacterium persists in the skin despite standard surgical preparation. J Bone Joint Surg Am. 2014;96(17):1447–50.
112. Schmid FR. Principles of diagnosis and treatment of bone and joint infections. In: McCarty DJ, editor. Arthritis and allied conditions: a textbook of rheumatology. Philadelphia: Lea-Febiger; 1985. p. 1638.
113. Deirmengian CA, Patel R. Clinical and laboratory evaluation: Chapter 5. In: Cierny G III, Mclaren AC, Wongworawat MD, editors. Orthopaedic knowledge update, musculoskeletal infection. Rosemont: AAOS; 2009. p. 57–65.
114. Phadnis J, Gordon D, Krishnan J, Bain GI. Frequent isolation of propionibacterium acnes from the shoulder dermis despite skin preparation and prophylactic antibiotics. J Shoulder Elbow Surg. 2016;25(2):304–10.

Avascular Necrosis

15

Gazi Huri, Mehmet Kaymakoğlu,
Yusuf Bora Bozduman, Ersin Mutlu,
and Mahmut N. Doral

We aimed to discuss an unusual but neglected disease of the shoulder in this chapter with an example of a real case. Avascular necrosis of the humeral head is mostly not noticed by the physicians even in high risk potential patients. Consideration of this disease in differential diagnosis of shoulder problems in high risk patients would avoid its potential catastrophic consequences.

Epidemiology

Osteonecrosis of the humeral head should be investigated in two main groups: traumatic and non-traumatic. The course of traumatic osteonecrosis depends on the type and extent of the fracture, whereas non-traumatic osteonecrosis have various etiologic causes.

Osteonecrosis of the humeral head was first described in 1960 by Heimann and Freiberger [1]. İnitially described cases were osteonecrosis of the humeral head after high-dosage corticosteroid therapy for pemphigus and thrombotic thrombocytopenic purpura.

Osteonecrosis of the humeral head is an uncommon disease. But it is the second most necrotic symptomatic joint affectation after that of the femoral head [2]. It is more prevalent in young patients between second and fifth decades. Osteonecrosis of the humeral head occurs twice as common in men than women but women with osteonecrosis diagnosed with an autoimmune disease develop this condition more often than men with the same disease due to more corticosteroid intake.

Predicting the exact incidence of the non-traumatic humeral head osteonecrosis is difficult because of common asymptomatic course of the disease. Matsen described the incidence of the disease 4.6% among glenoarthritic patients [3]. Some authors also describe it as a common cause of shoulder arthroplasty. Cruess et al. found involvement of 18 humeral head osteonecrosis among 95 patients with corticosteroid induced osteonecrosis of femoral head [4]. Another study revealed 7% incidence of humeral osteonecrosis from a group of 1056 patients managed for osteonecrosis of any joint [5]. High incidence (>80%) of corticosteroid use, bilateral disease and hip involvement was also found in the same cohort group.

Proximal humeral fractures consists of 4–5% of all fracture types and and 11% of all these fractures are three or four part fractures [6]. Prevalence of post-traumatic osteonecrosis group is more predictable but still difficult due to

G. Huri, M.D. (✉) • M. Kaymakoğlu, M.D.
Y.B. Bozduman, M.D. • E. Mutlu, M.D.
M.N. Doral, M.D.
Orthopaedics and Traumatology Department, Hacettepe University School of Medicine, 06100 Ankara, Turkey
e-mail: gazihuri@hacettepe.edu.tr

G. Huri, N.K. Paschos (eds.), *The Shoulder*, Orthopaedic Study Guide Series,
DOI 10.1007/978-3-319-51979-1_15

different treatment regimens among the cohort groups. Several researches gives us an opinion whether we come up against an avascular necrosis depending on the severity and location of the fracture. Neer et al. reported the avascular necrosis risk more than 50% in four-part fractures of humeral head [7]. Three part-fractures have a risk of osteonecrosis from 0 to 25% and four-part fractures from 0 to 77% [8, 9]. Recent studies gives a lower but still significantly high incidence of risk, which varies from 3 to 37% with operative treatment. There is also concerns about whether the operative treatment increases the risk of avascular necrosis. A meta-analysis of seven studies reported that plate fixation of humeral head associated with an increased risk of osteonecrosis [10]. New operative methods are published in order to decrease this high incidence of risk [11].

Etiology

Several etiological factors have found to be associated with the avascular necrosis of humeral head. They are investigated in two main groups: traumatic and non-traumatic. However, the pathophysiological background of these two groups are similar; both produce a disturbance of vascular circulation of humeral head, increase the intraosseous pressure and cause sudden cell death [12] (Table 15.1).

Table 15.1 Most common etiologic factors for avascular necrosis of humeral head

Traumatic
Humeral head fractures
Dislocations
Surgery of the shoulder
Non traumatic
İdiopathic
Corticosteroids
Hemoglobinopathies (e.g. sickle cell)
Hypercoagulabilities
Cushing's disease
Dysbarism (Caisson disease)
Gaucher's disease
Alcohol
Tobacco
Systemic lupus erythematosus
Scleroderma
Romatoid arthritis
Inflammatory bowel diseases
Lipid metabolism disorders
Radiation
Human immunodeficiency virus
Chemotherapeutic drugs
Transplantations

Corticosteroids are the most common cause of non-traumatic avascular necrosis. They are widely used in many systemic disórders, autoimmune diseases, transplantations which have a huge patient population potential. Despite the decrease of the incidence of osteonecrosis among patients with long term systemic corticosteroids due to lower steroid dosing, total number of patients is not decreased comparing with the last decades. The mechanism has not been identified yet, but possible fat embolism and intraosseous pressure mechanisms are accused by researchers [13].

Hemoglobinopathies like sickle cell disease and hypercoagulabilities produce microinfarcts and interrupt the blood circulation of the head. Jones et al. found high incidence of coagulation abnormalities in 45 patient with non-traumatic avascular necrosis [14].

Dysbarism affects the sea-divers who rapidly rise to the surface from deep [15]. Solubility of gases in blood decreases and gas embolisms occur in different tissues of the body. Life threatening situations can occur and avascular necrosis should be considered as an occupational disease in these patients [16].

Lipid loaded Gaucher cells in the bone marrow can increase intraosseous pressure, provoke coagulation and occlusion of intraosseous vessels leading to osteonecrosis [17].

Alcohol intake and smoking are known etiologic causes of avascular necrosis pathogenesis [18].

Pathophysiology

An orthopaedic surgeon must have a precise knowledge about the vascular anatomy of humeral head to understand the mechanism of avascular necrosis (Fig. 15.1). Displaced fractures

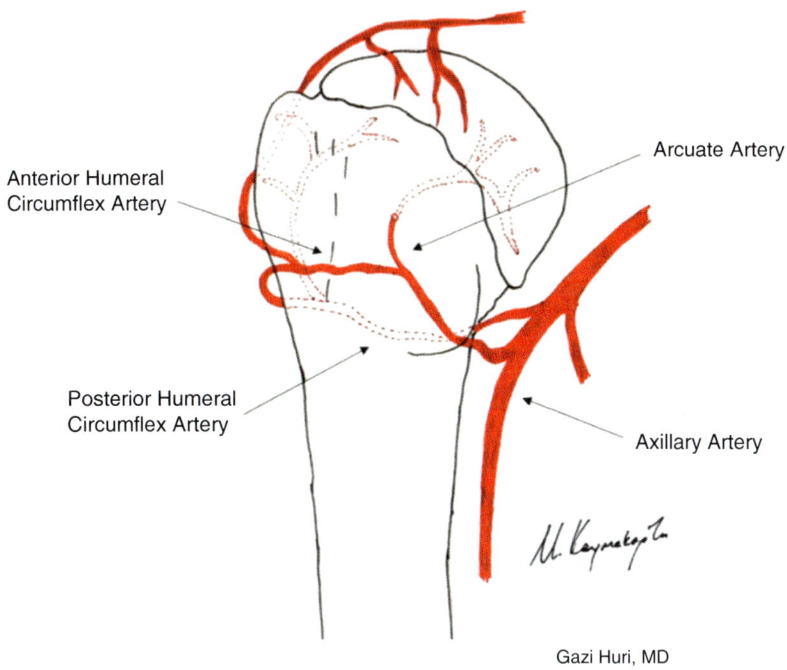

Fig. 15.1 Vascular anatomy of humeral head

of this region causes interruption of the blood supply and the incidence is not rare. Many researcher like Gerber et al. emphasized in the past that anterior humeral circumflex artery brings the main blood flow to the humeral head [19, 20]. Ascending branch of anterior humeral circumflex artery (arcuate artery) was believed to be the main nutrient of the head and researches focused on injury of this artery in posttraumatic osteonecrosis until the last decade. After the discovery of durability of posterior circumflex artery even in displaced fractures [21], Hettrich et al. published the quantitative assessment of vascular supply of the humeral head in a cadaveric study with MRI [22]. He found that PHCA perfuses more of the AHCA does, in three of four quadrants of the head. Realibility of this study comes from its three-dimensional visualization capability despite the previous two-dimensional studies. Hertel et al. investigated the predictors of ischemia after the fracture occurs. His colleagues found that the length of the dorsomedial metaphyseal extension and the integrity of the medial hinge are the determinants of vascular integrity during the fracture. Four years later, Bastian and Hertel reported that most of the posttraumatic ischemia does not lead up to osteonecrosis [23]. This study showed the importance of a successful reduction with osteosynthesis to achieve a possible revascularization in the humeral head.

Clinical Evaluation and Diagnosis

A patient complaining from shoulder pain should be carefully evaluated. A detailed history should be taken, including the habits like alcohol or smoking. Corticosteroid or other drug use should be noted. If an avascular necrosis of humerus detected, bilateralism and the other joints should be also investigated [24]. Most of the patients with non-traumatic avascular necrosis are young and have a dull ache in their shoulder which is hard to localize. The physician must be careful about that some of the patients with avascular necrosis are asymptomatic or have little complaints. Range of motion of the shoulder should be examined and differential diagnosis like rotator cuff rupture must be made with careful clinical tests. Standard shoulder radiography with at least from two direction is the first radiologic examination. One should note that radiography is not sensitive to evaluate the osteonecrosis. Stage 3 or worse lesions can be detected in radiography. The extent and stage of the avascular lesion can be best assessed with MRI. Other anatomic sites (e.g. hips, ankles) should be screened because of multifocal nature of the disease.

Case

26 year old female patient admitted to our orthopaedic clinic with left shoulder pain. Through her history, she described that she has the pain nearly about 6 months but in the last 2 months the pain got worse. She has diagnosis of scleroderma and she used to take steroids for 8 years. In physical examination, she had painful full range of motion of the left shoulder and her pain radiates to her arm. Her muscle strength were 5/5 and has a normal neurovascular examination. We first evaluated a standard radiography of her left shoulder. Radiography showed a mottled sclerosis area but the curvature of humeral head remains intact.

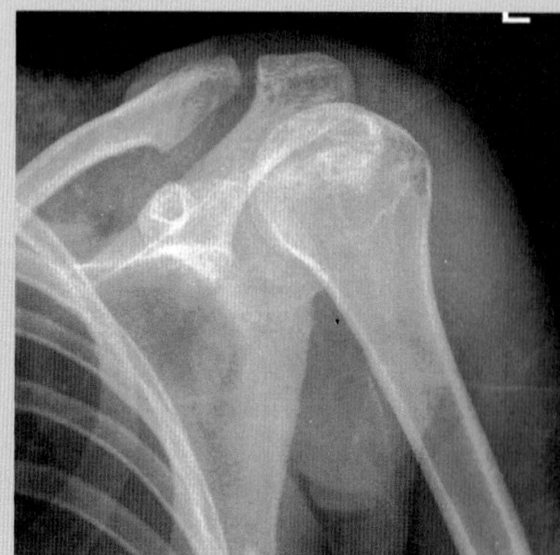

The progression of the disease depends mainly on presenting symptoms and stage of the osteonecrosis at initial diagnosis. A study group from Japan evaluated the necrotic angle and its correlation with the outcome of the disease [25]. They found that if the necrotic angle is greater than 90° at initial diagnosis, avascular lesion does not progress to osteoarthritis. In the same study, lower collapse rates was found compared with osteonecrosis of femoral head. This situation is attributed to that glenohumeral joint is not a weight bearing joint. However it is well known that late-stage disease (Ficat 3-4-5) progress to advanced osteoarthritis to a large extent at a point that arthroplasty is required [26]. Hatrup and Cofield reported 55% of patients with stage 4 disease and 79% of stage 5 disease required shoulder arthroplasty in 3 years of follow-up [27]. In the same cohort group, traumatic patients underwent surgery more likely than non-traumatic group.

Patients treated with corticosteroids are likely to experience avascular necrosis of humeral head. An average of 3 years for stage 2 patients and 10 years for stage 1 patients are needed for head collapse [28]. Surprisingly, they observed regression of some lesions just in stage 1 asymptomatic patients for whom observation or pharmalogical therapy is recommended.

Case

MRI is obtained for further investigation. On MRI, avascular lesion is located on superomedial portion of the humeral head which is close to glenohumeral joint surface and clarifies the cause of the pain. Radiological report does not showed any collapse or subchondral fracture, which makes it a stage 2 lesion depend on the Ficat classification system. We planned a core decompression with arthroscopy.

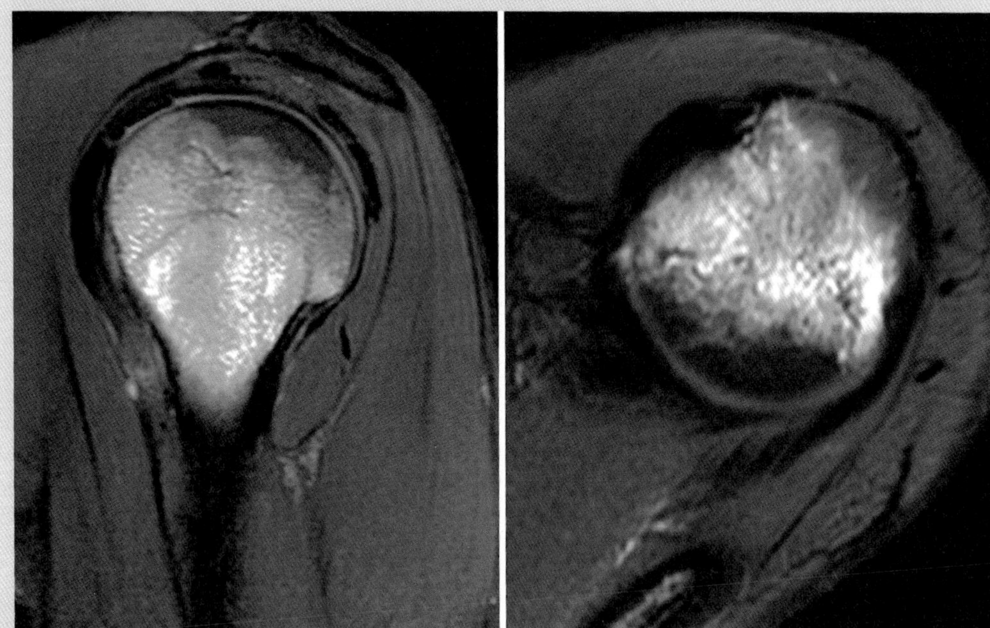

Classification

Ficat and Arlet were the first researchers that attempted to classify the femoral head osteonecrosis in 1964 [30], when MRI has not been invented yet. Cruess modified this classification system to humeral head avascular necrosis in 1978 [29]. After multiple modifications and adding, it became today's classification system that are widely used in orthopaedic surgery. Today it is also named as Cruess classification (Table 15.2), attributing to his modifications on the classification system.

Table 15.2 Cruess classification (with permission from [29])

Stage 1	Normal radiography. MRI changes
Stage 2	Mottled sclerosis on head
Stage 3	Crescent sign on X-ray—subchondral fracture on MRI
Stage 4	Collapse
Stage 5	Glenoid involvement

Ficat and Arlet classification system based on the collapse progression. Stage 1 shows no radiologic changes whereas Stage 5 possess both the glenoid and humeral head collapse. Stage 1 and 2 are named as 'early stages' and 3, 4 and 5 as 'late stages'. Radiological changes begins with 'Stage 2' and humeral head collapse begins at 'Stage 3'. Crescent sign is typical at this stage and indicative of subchondral fracture. Further subchondral collapse makes the lesion 'Stage 4'. Degenerative changes in the glenoid cavity occurs at 'Stage 5'. Ficat system is a very basic system depending on radiological changes. It lacks any of the measurements that can be made on femoral head.

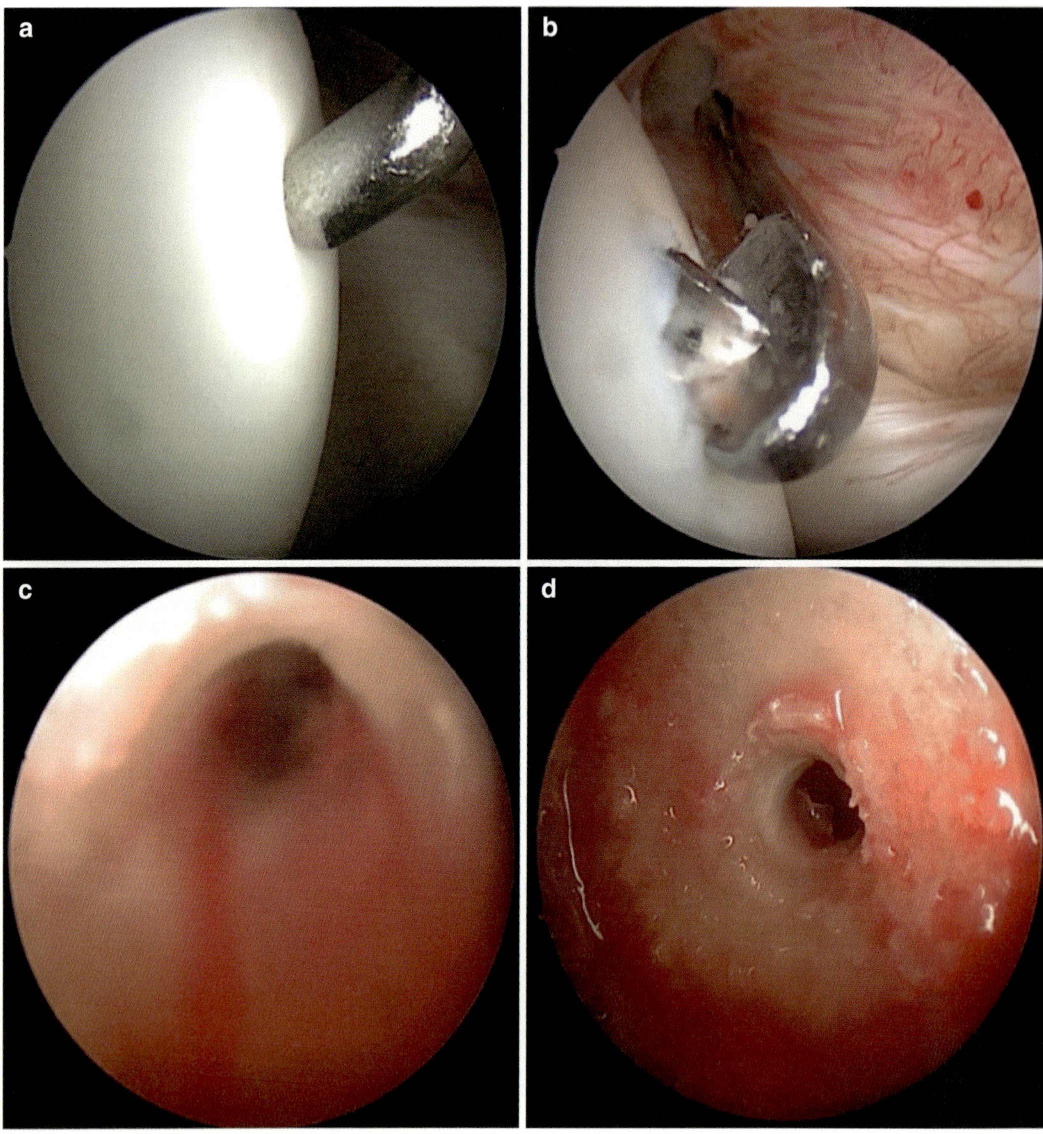

(a) Palpation of the humeral head avascular region with a probe reveals how the cartilage is softened.
(b) Using an ACL tibial guide, for retrograde drilling of avascular lesion with an 2.7 mm drill.
(c) 'Bonoscopy' (intraosseous endoscopy) was made following drilling. The non-bleeding zone is clearly seen in the picture.
(d) Bonoscopy provides active bleeding that was seen during the procedure. It would make the healing process faster with progenitor cells.

Treatment

Conservative

There are many treatment options in current literature. Surgical solutions are widely used by physicians, as there are conflicts about pharmacological treatment results.

Pathophysiological pathways are mainly targeted in pharmacological treatments like lipid lowering with statins, prostacyclin analogues, anticoagulants or bisphosphonates [31]. Most studies were performed for avascular necrosis of the femoral head but could be tried for humeral head due to same pathological causes.

Use of medical management is limited because of their ineffectiveness after the disease progresses in late stages and once an anatomical defect is formed, surgery becomes the only alternative treatment choice. Lai et al. described the effectiveness of bisphosphonates in order to prevent the collapse of effected avascular zone [32]. Statins are considered to be useful to prevent the osteonecrosis in patients who receive corticosteroid treatment [33].

Surgical

Many surgical methods are available and used in current surgical management of osteonecrosis of humeral head. We discuss the main surgical treatment modalities that are widely used in practice.

Although a good open reduction is related with lower avascular necrosis risk, there are doubts about operative treatment of proximal humerus fractures increases the rate [34]. This could be due to damage to periosteal vessels and main vasculature. Minimal invasive methods (e.g. arthroscopy assisted) are recommended for this type of fracture. Neviaser et al. reported the avascular necrosis rates after open reduction fixation with lateral locking plate [11]. Their results are breathtaking with nearly 0% avascular necrosis rate with a short term follow up. They also used anterolateral approach instead of deltopectoral approach. Hepp et al. compared the two approaches and found an increased trend of avascular necrosis in deltopectoral group.

Core decompression is the most known option for every early stage osteonecrosis of bone. Hungerford is the first who describe this method in femoral osteonecrosis [39]. Today core decompression is the first step method for early stage osteonecrosis (Stage 1-2). Harreld reported excellent results with percutaneous small diameter core decompression with improvements in UCLA scores and pain [35]. LaPorte received the same success in the early stage osteonecrosis with the open technique using a 6–10 mm trephine [36].

Arthroscopy have the advantage of being a minimal invasive method and it allows the surgeon to examine the cartilage tissue and debridement of joint degeneration. It gives the opportunity of exact staging and diagnose of the disease. Dines was the first who published the results of core decompression with arthroscopy using an ACL-guide [37]. Early results of this study have good results with immediate pain relief and improvements in clinical scores postoperatively.

However, it is a challenge to deal with the late stage osteonecrosis. Core decompression does not help lesion to regress and relieve the symptoms of the patients with stage 3 or more. Hemiarthroplasty can be considered for stage 3–4 patients. Raiss et al. published significant improvements in Constant-score and range of motions with a 3-year follow up [38]. Their study showed that non-traumatic group had better results than traumatic group. Total shoulder arthroplasty (TSA) is another option in patients who have a global glenohumeral involvement of osteoarthritis. A study comparing the TSA and hemiarthroplasty revealed that there is no difference between two groups in outcomes but TSA group have significantly higher complication rate. Thus, TSA is recommended for only Stage 5 patients in which hemiarthroplasty fails to prevent the glenohumeral pain.

Questions

1. Which joint(s) should be evaluated further for osteonecrosis after a patient diagnosed with humeral head osteonecrosis?
   A. Ankle
   B. Wrist
   C. Hip
   D. Elbow
   E. Knee
   Hip.

2. What would be your first diagnostic option when a patient referred to your clinic with a symptomatic avascular necrosis of the humeral head?
   A. MRI
   B. Arthroscopy
   C. X-ray
   D. CT
   E. USG
   MRI

X-ray should be the first imaging option of every patient with a shoulder complaint but it is not sensitive to diagnose early stages of the osteonecrosis. MRI is the preferred and sensitive imaging method for almost every patient to determine the stage of the disease. Physicians should not forget that arthroscopic diagnosis is more sensitive than MRI if the stage of the disease is not clearly understood. It also gives the opportunity to treat if the disease is not end-stage.

3. 45 year old woman diagnosed with scleroderma underwent a hip replacement surgery 1 year ago. She has been using corticosteroids for 5 years and will continue to take them as a treatment regime for scleroderma. She complaints about mild left shoulder pain at nights but she does not need any painkillers. You noticed a small sclerosis area at humeral head on her X-ray. In which stage do you think that osteonecrosis of this patient is (depending on clinical and radiological features)?
   A. 1
   B. 2
   C. 3
   D. 4
   E. 5
   2.

What is new about this topic?

Archer et al. found no correlation between the time of surgery and rate of avascular necrosis in traumatic patients. This knowledge leads us primarily that type of injury is more important in avascular necrosis pathogenesis.

Rate of Avascular Necrosis and Time to Surgery in Proximal Humerus Fractures, Musculoskeletal Surgery 2016 September, Archer LA, Furey A.

References

1. Heimann WG, Freiberger RH. Avascular necrosis of the femoral and humeral heads after high-dosage corticosteroid therapy. N Engl J Med. 1960;263:672–5.
2. Jacobs B. Epidemiology of traumatic and nontraumatic osteonecrosis. Clin Orthop. 1978;130:51–67.
3. Matsen III FA, Rockwood CA, Wirth MA, Lippett SB. Glenohumeral arthritis and its management. In: The shoulder. Philadelphia: Saunders; 1998. p. 840–964.
4. Cruess RL. Steroid-induced avascular necrosis of the head of the humerus. J Bone Joint Surg Br. 1976; 58:313–7.
5. Mont MA, Paymao RK, Laporte DM, et al. Atraumatic osteonecrosis of the humeral head. J Rheumatol. 2000;27(7):1766–73.
6. Court-Brown CM, Garg A, McQueen MM. The epidemiology of proximal humeral fractures. Acta Orthop Scand. 2001;72:365–71.
7. Neer II CS. Displaced proximal humeral fractures. Part II. Treatment of the tree-part and four-part displacement. J Bone Joint Surg Am. 1970;52: 1090–103.
8. Esser RD. Treatment of three- and four-part fractures of the proximal humerus with a modified cloverleaf plate. J Orthop Trauma. 1994;8(1):15–22.

9. Hagg O, Lundberg BJ. Aspects of prognostic factors in comminuted and dislocated proximal humeral fractures. In: Bateman JE, Welsh RP, editors. Surgery of the shoulder. Philadelphia: B.C. Decker; 1984.
10. Xu J, Zhang C, Wang T. Avascular necrosis in proximal humeral fractures in patients treated with operative fixation: a meta-analysis. J Orthop Surg Res. 2014;9:31.
11. Neviaser AS, et al. Rate of avascular necrosis following proximal humerus fractures treated with a lateral locking plate and endosteal implant. Arch Orthop Trauma Surg. 2011;131:1617–22.
12. Hungerford DS, Lennox DW. The importance of increased intraosseous pressure in the development of osteonecrosis of the femoral head: implications for treatment. Orthop Clin North Am. 1985; 16(4):635–54.
13. Fisher DE. The role of fat embolism in the etiology of corticosteroid induced avascular necrosis: clinical and experimental results. Clin Orthop. 1978;130:68–80.
14. Jones LC, Mont MA, Lc TB, et al. Procoagulants and osteonecrosis. J Rheumatol. 2003;30(4):783–91.
15. MacCallum RI, Walder DN, Barnes R, Catto ME, Davidson JK, Fryer DI, et al. Bone lesions in compressed air workers. With special reference to men on the Clyde Tunnels 1958 to 1963. J Bone Joint Surg Br. 1966;48:207–35.
16. Uguen M. Dysbaric osteonecrosis in professional divers: two case reports. Undersea Hyperb Med. 2015; 42(4):363–7.
17. Sarris I, Weiser R. Pathogenesis and treatment of osteonecrosis of the shoulder. Orthop Clin North Am. 2004;35(3):397–404.
18. Matsuo K, Hirohata T, Sugioka Y, Ikeda M, Fukuda A. Influence of alcohol intake, cigarette smoking, and occupational status on idiopathic osteonecrosis of the femoral head. Clin Orthop. 1988;234:115–23.
19. Laing PG. The arterial supply of the adult humerus. J Bone Joint Surg Am. 1956;38:1105–16.
20. Gerber C, Schneeberger AG, Vinh TS. The arterial vascularization of the humeral head. An anatomical study. J Bone Joint Surg Am. 1990;72:1486–94.
21. Coudane H, Fays J, De La Selle H, Nicoud C, Pilot L. Arteriography after complex fractures of the upper extremity of the humerus bone: a prospective study—preliminary results. J Shoulder Elb Surg. 2000;9:548.
22. Hettrich CM, et al. Quantitative assessment of the vascularity of the proximal part of the humerus. J Bone Joint Surg Am. 2010;92:943–8.
23. Bastian JD, Hertel R. Initial post-fracture humeral head ischemia docs not predict development of necrosis. J Shoulder Elb Surg. 2008;17(1):2–8.
24. LaPorte DM, Mont MA, Mohan V, Jones LC, Hungerford DS. Multifocal osteonecrosis. J Rheumatol. 1998;25:1968–74.
25. Sakai T, et al. Extent of osteonecrosis on MRI predicts humeral head collapse. Clin Orthop Relat Res. 2008;466:1074–80.
26. L'Insalata JC, Pagnani MJ, Warren RF, Dines DM. Humeral head osteonecrosis: clinical course and radiographic predictors of outcome. J Shoulder Elb Surg. 1996;5:355–61.
27. Hattrup SJ, Cofield RH. Osteonecrosis of the humeral head: relationship of disease stage, extent, and cause to natural history. J Shoulder Elb Surg. 1999;8:559–64.
28. Hemigou P, Flouzat-Lachaniette CH, Roussignol X, Poignard A. The natural progression of shoulder osteonecrosis related to corticosteroid treatment. Clin Orthop Relat Res. 2010;468(7):1809–16.
29. Cruess RL. Experience with steroid induced avascular necrosis of the shoulder and etiologic considerations regarding osteonecrosis of the hip. Clin Orthop Relat Res. 1978;130:86–93.
30. Ficat RP, Arlet J. Forage-biopsie de la tete femorale dans l'osteonecrose primative. Observations histo-pathologiques portant sur huit forages. Rev Rhum. 1964;31:257–64.
31. Harreld KL. Osteonecrosis of the humeral head. J Am Acad Orthop Surg. 2009;17:345–55.
32. Lai KA, Shen WJ, Yang CY, et al. The use of alendronate to prevent early collapse of the femoral head in patients with nontraumatic osteonecrosis. A randomized clinical study. J Bone Joint Surg Am. 2005; 87(10):2155–9.
33. Pritchett JW. Statin therapy decreases the risk of osteonecrosis in patients receiving steroids. Clin Orthop. 2001;386:173–8.
34. Iyengar JJ, et al. Nonoperative treatment of proximal humerus fractures: a systematic review. J Orthop Trauma. 2011;25:612–7.
35. Harreld KL, Marulanda GA, Ulrich SD, Marker DR, Seyler TM, Mont MA. Small-diameter percutaneous decompression for osteonecrosis of the shoulder. Am J Orthop. 2009;38(7):348–54.
36. LaPorte DM, Mont MA, Mohan V, Pierre-Jacques H, Jones LC, Hungerford DS. Osteonecrosis of the humeral head treated by core decompression. Clin Orthop Relat Res. 1998;355:254–60.
37. Dines JS, Strauss EJ, Fealy S, Craig EV. Arthroscopic-assisted core decompression of the humeral hcad. Arthroscopy. 2007;23:103.
38. Raiss P, Kasten P, Baumann F, Moser M, Rickert M, Loew M. Treatment of osteonecrosis of the humeral head with cementless surface replacement arthroplasty. J Bone Joint Surg Am. 2009;91(2):340–9.
39. Hungerford DS. Bone marrow pressure, venography, and core decompression in isquemic necrosis of the femoral head. In: The Hip: Proceedings of the Seventh Open Scientific Meeting of the Hip Society. St. Louis, MO: CV Mosby; 1979. p. 1.

Soft Tissue Disorders

16

Dogac Karaguven and Osman Orman

Despite the fact that our knowledge about shoulder anatomy, biomechanics, diagnosis and treatment, an area about shoulder pain and disabilities are still in mist. Early 1900s these shoulder problems are roughly named shoulder periarticular disorders, after then some disorders are named like calcific tendinitis, frozen shoulder, bicipital tendinitis. Now we have a rich knowledge about these conditions—thanks to MRI and arthroscopy—but they are still not clear. In this chapter we will discuss these problems; frozen shoulder, calcific tendinitis, long head of the biceps tendon problems and snapping shoulder.

Snapping Scapula Syndrome

Introduction

Snapping scapula syndrome causes pain and crepitation in the superomedial region of scapula due to abnormal scapulothoracal movements which disrupt the relationship between scapula and the thorax, a bony or soft tissue mass in this region or chronic scapulothoracic bursitis [1].

Anatomy

Two bursae can be found in the scapulothoracic region; the infraserratus and the supraserratus bursa. The infraserratus bursa lies between the serratus anterior muscle and the chest while the supraserratus bursa lies between the serratus anterior muscle and the subscapularis muscle. Other burase can be found in the superomedial, inferomedial region of scapula and the medial side of spina scapulae where they are considered pathologic.

Pathoanatomy

Inflammation secondary to overuse of the shoulder girdle can cause scapulothoracic bursitis. Other than bursites, other soft tissue problems such as elastofibromas, fibrotic or abnormal muscles around the scapula can cause snapping scapula. Osteochondromas, rarely chondrosarcomas, abnormal scapular anatomy (contact with chest wall secondary to superomedial angle being greater than 140°), malunion in the scapula or the ribs can also cause this syndrome [1, 2].

D. Karaguven, M.D. (✉)
Department of Orthopaedics and Traumatology, Ufuk University, Ankara, Turkey
e-mail: dogackaraguven@gmail.com

O. Orman, M.D.
Orthopaedic and Traumatology/Hand Surgery, Baltalimani Metin Sabancı Bone and Joint Diseases Education and Research Hospital, Istanbul, Turkey

G. Huri, N.K. Paschos (eds.), *The Shoulder*, Orthopaedic Study Guide Series,
DOI 10.1007/978-3-319-51979-1_16

Diagnosis

Patients often complain of moderate to severe pain and crepitation. Pain is usually located on the superomedial of the scapula and is completely unrelated to activity. A mass can be palpated on the scapular region which can point to a tumoral growth or winging can be observed which is a sign of scapulothoracal diskinesia [1, 3].

Direct graphy, anteroposterior shoulder, axillary and lateral scapular imaging are valuable in discerning tumors of the soft tissue and bones, old traumas of the scapula and ribs and malunions. If tumoral growth is suspected, CT—three dimensional CT—or MRI must be performed following direct graphy [4].

Treatment

Primary treatment is nonsurgical such as activity modification, non-steroid antiinflammatory drugs and physical therapy. In physical therapy posture must be corrected, the muscles around the scapula must be stretched and strengthened. If inflammation is present, corticosteroid injection into the bursa is both diagnostic and therapeutic [5, 6].

Patients who do not benefit from these interventions may require surgery due to tumoral reasons for snapping scapula. Surgery usually involves excision of the inflamed bursa and 2–3 cm resection of the superomedial corner of the scapula until the bony protrusion is eliminated. Mass excision is applied in situations arising from a mass [7, 8].

Diseases of the Long Head of the Biceps

Introduction

Although diseases concerning the long head of the biceps (LHBT) were described approximately 300 years ago, the role of this tendon and its clinical relevance is subject to debate. Lippman defines the long head of the biceps as "an unimportant tendon unless something goes wrong with it" [9, 10]. LHBT is believed to slightly depress caput humeri in the normal shoulder and to be a weak stabilizer of the shoulder. LHBT disorders can be as isolated conditions, but they are mostly with other shoulder issues such as rotator cuff tears (90%) [11, 12]. Tendonitis, instability, subluxation, dislocation, partial or complete tears are the common disorders of the long head of biceps tendon.

History

- First proper biceps and bicipital groove anatomy descriptions appeared in the 1400s [10].
- First reported LHBT dislocation 1694 [10, 13].
- Biceps tendinitis recognized and described by F. Pasteur (1932) and Schrager (1938) [10, 14, 15].
- Neer described anterior impingement that causes wear on the rotator cuff and LHBT in 1972 [16].
- Walch described biceps pulley and pulley lesions in 1993 [17].

Anatomy

LHBT consists of three parts:

1. Origo which consists of the superior labrum and the biceps anchor. Although there are variations of the superior of the glenoid labrum and the supraglenoidal tubercle, it usually originates from the posterior. Attachment types: Tip1 attaches entirely to the posterior labrum; Tip 2 predominantly to posterior plus some anterior labrum; Tip 3 attaches equally to anterior and posterior; Tip 4 mostly anterior [18].
2. Intraarticular part, which is found in the rotator interval and the part. The average length of the LHBT from supraglenoid tubercule to the musculotendinous junction is 99 to 138 mm [19]. The origo part is usually flat fibrocartilage and gets round as it approaches bicipital groove. Blood supply is provided by the

osteotendinous branches of the thoracoacromial artery and musculotendinous branches from the brachial artery; there is a hypovascular area 1.2–3 cm from the tendon origo [20]. The intraarticular part of the LHBT is partially stabilized by the biceps pulley. This pulley mechanism is formed by the superior glenohumeral ligament (SGHL), corachoacromial ligament, deep fibers of the subscapularis and the supraspinatus tendon. [21]

3. Extra-articular part which is found in the bicipital groove. It is divided into three zones: [22]
   (a) Zone 1; bony groove starting from biceps pulley to the distal margin of the subscapularis. The bicipital groove is found between the tuberculum major and minor; the depth of this groove, although its depth and angle varies between individuals, is around 4.3 mm (range 4–7 mm) and the medial wall angle is 56° (range 40–70°) [23]. The biceps tendon is loosely stabilized by the transverse humeral ligament which is formed by fibers from the subscapularis muscle and the supraspinatus tendon in the Zone 1 of the bicipital groove.
   (b) Zone 2; is the region between the distal margin of the subscapularis and the proximal margin of the pectoralis major tendon. This part of the tendon cannot be visualized by arthroscopy or from open subpectoral exposure below.
   (c) Zone 3; subpectoral region. From zone 1 to zone 3; osseos bicipital groove becomes flattened and synovium disappears [23].

The function of LHBT is still an issue of debate. LHBT seems to slightly depress caput humeri in the normal shoulder and to be a weak stabilizer of the shoulder [23–26].

Pathology

The lesion can be on the origo of the tendon, on the part found in the rotator interval, in the bicipital groove or on the musculotendinous junction.

- At the origo; SLAP lesions appear at this part.
- Intraarticular—rotator interval—part; LHBT ruptures are usually found in the hypovascular area which is 2.5 cm from the origo and may be partial or complete [20]. LHBT tendinopathy is chronic inflammation, fibrotic degeneration, decrease in the number of axons in the distal portion of the tendon [27]. Another intraarticular lesion is the hourglass biceps that is caused by a hypertrophic intraarticular portion of the tendon that is unable to slide into the bicipital groove during elevation of the arm, which can be compared with the condition of trigger finger in the hand [28]. Instability, subluxation and dislocation of the LHB tendon is seen where the biceps pulley is disrupted. Supraspinatus tears that affects this pulley causes posterolateral instability and so subscapularis tears causes medial instability. Dislocation of the LHBT only happens medially through the disrupted subscapularis tendons deep fibers [29].
- Extraarticular—bicipital groove–part; although LHBT tears usually extend to the bicipital groove [30]. Loose bodies, scar tissue, partial LHBT tears, osseous stenosis, osteophytes, instability, synovitis, and inflamed vincula can be seen [30]. From zone 2 to zone 3 bicipital tunnel there is a narrowing that forms a bottleneck for many lesions such as loose bodies which leads to an aggregation of space occupying lesions in zone 2 and produces bicipital tunnel syndrome. [22, 30].

Classification

Diseases of the LHBT are classified differently by various authors. These classifications are made by the location of the lesion, the situation of the tendon and the rotator cuff. Partial or full rotator cuff tear may accompany 90% of the biceps tendon pathologies [11, 12]. The Habermeyer and Walch Classification which includes biceps tendon problems and accompanied rotator cuff tears can be found below (Table 16.1) [31].

Table 16.1 Habermeyer and Walch classification (with permission from 31)

1. Origo
2. Interval lesions
(a) Biceps tendinitis
(b) Isolated ruptures
(c) Subluxation
• Type I: superior
• Type II: Inside the groove
• Type III: tuberculum minor fracture/nonunion
3. Accompanied by rotator cuff tears
(a) Tendinitis
(b) Dislocation
• Type IA: Extra-articular partial subscapularis tear
• Type IB: Extra-articular subscapularis intact
• Type II: Intra-articular
(c) Subluxation
(d) Rupture

Table 16.2 Biceps Sling pathologies classified by Habermeyer

Group 1	Isolated lesion at SGHL
Group 2	Lesion at SGHL and particular articular side tears of the supraspinatus tendon (PASTA); results in lateral LHB tendon subluxation
Group 3	Deep surface tears of the subscapularis and SGHL; results in medial LHB tendon subluxation
Group 4	Deep surface tears of the subscapularis, SGHL and PASTA; results in medial and lateral instability of the LHBT

Habermeyer et al. also classified biceps sling pathologies and the LHB tendon's condition (Table 16.2 with permission from 21)

Etiology

To the contrary, the LHB tendon disorders are mostly multifactorial. Leading causes are the location and the blood supply of the tendon [10]. Abduction occasions an avascular zone in the intracapsular portion of LHBT. Repetitive overhead activities because of the occupational causes makes the tendon prone to rupture, dislocation and elongation [10, 32]. Intra articular biceps tendon lesions can happen with a fall on the overstretched hand that drives humeral head up into the labrum and the tendon [33]. As in the majority of the tendon problems in the younger patients, repeated trauma are the major inciting factors. In older patients, degenerative changes in the tendon are the predominant etiologic factor [10].

Diagnosis

Patients with LHBT lesions often complain of anterior shoulder pain, the pain can radiate along the biceps muscle or the origo of the deltoid. The pain is more pronounced during the night. Popping-snapping may be observed during throwing in patients with biceps tendon instability. Popeye sign can be observed in patients whose biceps is completely torn as the bulge of the muscle is displaced distally.

Physical examination is not completely reliable. Minor loss of motion in abduction and internal rotation in addition to tenderness on the bicipital groove (over the bicipital groove when the shoulder is at 10° internal rotation). There are some special examination methods such as Speed's test, Yergason's test, biceps instability test, Ludington's test, Hueter sign and the uppercut test:

- Speed test is the existence of pain during the flexion of shoulder against resistance while the elbow is on extension and supination.
- Yergason test is the existence of pain during supination of the forearm against resistance while the shoulder is neutral and elbow is flexed.
- Uppercut test is the existence of pain during shoulder flexion when the shoulder is neutral, elbow is flexed, and forearm is supinated while force is applied to the patient's fist.
- For Hueter sign, pronation and supination forces of the forearm is compared while the shoulder is neutral and the elbow is flexed; supination is weakened in patients with LHBT problems.
- In biceps instability test, a popping sensation is found during shoulder switching from external rotation to internal rotation while the shoulder is in 90° abduction and the elbow is in 90° flexion.

- In Ludington test the patient is asked to contract both biceps brachii in an isometric fashion while both hands are behind the head and biceps mass is evaluated; this test is used to detect partial or complete tearing of the LHBT.

In biceps tendon diseases Speed test and uppercut test being positive at the same time is highly specific [34].

Direct radiography can be used to evaluate the bicipital groove, tuberculum major and minor with special defined positions such as the Fisk method (both arms are placed on the casette while both forearms are supinated and the patient leans forward, x-rays are directed perpendicularly to the bicipital groove) [35] and the bicipital groove position (the shoulder is brought to full external rotation while the patient lies supine and x-rays are directed to the humerus coronal plane at 15°) [36].

LHBT tendinitis, tears, dislocations and bicipital groove can be diagnosed via ultrasonography. Acute tendinitis is characterized by the anechoic enlargement of the sheath, as the inflammation persists tendon becomes thick and diffuse hypoechoic. Complete ruptures are identified with the non-visualization of the within the bicipital groove (empty groove sign) however, partial LHB tears may be missed. Osseous abnormalities as osteophytes and spurs of the bicipital groove can also be recognized. Dynamic USG can be utilized for the diagnosis of biceps instabilities [37, 38]. USG findings correlated to arthroscopic findings are found to be %100 specific and %96 sensitive for subluxation and dislocation whereas it is %50 sensitive for other LHBT pathologies [37].

MRI and MRI arthrography can be helpful in diagnosis of biceps tendon lesions. The intraarticular part of the tendon can be visualised in the coronal and sagittal planes while the intra-bicipital groove part can be visualized in the axial planes [39]. Intraarticular fluid is increased and the periphery of the bicipital groove is edematous in biceps tendinitis [39]. Tendon hypertrophy and an increase in intensity can be seen in T1 and T2 if degenerative tendinitis is present. Tendon cannot be visualized in some bicipital groove (empty groove sign) slices if the tendon is ruptured (dislocation must be ruled out) [40]. LHBT is seen over the tuberculum minor in dislocation.

Arthroscopy is the gold standard for the diagnosis of LHBT pathologies. Lafosse has classified tendon pathologies according to arthroscopic findings. Grade 0 for normal tendons, Grade I for minor lesions affecting lesions less than 50% of the tendon, fraying and erosion and Grade II for major lesions affecting more than 50% of the tendon, fraying and erosion. The part inside the bicipital groove must be evaluated by applying traction with the probe during arthroscopic investigation. Moreover, cartilaginous irregularities of the humeral head around the bicipital groove may point to biceps tendon pathologies [29].

Treatment

The problem in the biceps tendon and any other shoulder pathologies which accompany it must be identified prior to the initiation of the treatment. Rotator cuff pathologies, glenohumeral arthritis or adhesive capsulitis accompany most of the biceps pathologies.

Non-operative

First line treatment of the LHBT pathologies are usually nonsurgical. Methods such as non-steroid anti-inflammatory (NSAID) treatment, activity modification, steroid injection and physical treatment can be utilized.

- Despite the common practice prescribing NSAIDs, there is little evidence that they are efficacious in treating chronic tendon injuries [41] and should include a discussion of the gastrointestinal, renal, and cardiovascular risks of NSAIDs. Steroids must be injected into the joint and bicipital groove, not into the tendon itself; multiple case reports discuss the risk of tendon rupture [41, 42].
- Corticosteroid injections alone provide short-term anti-inflammatory effects therefore a multiphase physical rehabilitation program should be initiated. Since these injections have

the potential to reach the glenohumeral joint used in combination ropivacaine with corticosteroid should be used as ropivacaine is found to be less chondrotoxic than bupivacaine [43].

- A recent protocol called regenerative injection therapy (RIT) which uses different injectates to induce an inflammatory response in an attempt to heal and regenerate damaged tissue is gaining favor. RIT treatments include prolotherapy (dextrose solution, sodium morrhuate), platelet-rich plasma (differing concentrations of platelets, white blood cells, red blood cells, and activated and inactivated platelets), and stem cells (circulating stem cells, adipose derived, bone marrow aspirate, bone marrow aspirate concentrate, amniotic membrane derived) [44].
- Multiphase physical rehabilitation program for LHBT disorders can be summarized as: Rehabilitation phase 1 focuses on pain management and pain-free passive range of motion with the inclusion of additional modalities as needed. Rehabilitation phase 2 focuses on pain-free active range of motion with basic strengthening against gravity. Rehabilitation phase 3 focuses on advanced rotator cuff and periscapular strengthening. Rehabilitation phase 4 focuses on return to activity and return to sport [44].

If the age of the patient with ruptured tendon is advanced, surgery is usually not advised. Patients who do not undergo operations may suffer from cosmetic problems (Popeye sign) pain-cramps (which resolve in 6–8 weeks) and weakness in forearm supination. Weakness in elbow flexion can also be observed, which is subject to debate in literature [45–47].

Operative

Surgery is advised in patients whose partial-thickness tear of the LHB tendon of >25% to 50%, medial LHB subluxation, and LHB subluxation in the setting of a tear of the subscapularis tendon or biceps pulley/sling [48, 49]. LHB tendinitis that is refractory to nonsurgical management is a relative indication for surgery [48]. Additionally a hourglass LHB or severely inflamed "lipstick" LHB findings that are recognized during arthroscopy are other indications for surgical management [28].

Surgery usually involves two methods; tenotomy and tenodesis. Many studies have compared these two methods and state that there are no significant differences other than the cosmetic deformity. Tenotomy can be performed with a relatively simple and reproducible technique that provides predictable pain relief and requires little postoperative rehabilitation with cosmesis problems known as "Popeye deformity" and fatigue discomfort are potential problems [50]. Yet both technique offers a high satisfactory pain relief. Tenotomy is advised for patients who are old, obese and with low expectancies while tenodesis is advised for patients who are younger than 40 and have higher expectancies [51].

- Arthroscopic debridement and biceps tenotomy: LHBT should evaluated dry without pump pressure because the infusion fluid may compress peritendinous vessels and cause inflamed synovium to appear normal. Intertubercular regions of the LHBT should brought by the probe into the joint because pathologic areas are mostly in the groove. Also the stability of the tendon must be examined with probe by attempting subluxate the tendon. Some surgeons may elect to debride the LHB tendon with a shaver in the patient with arthroscopic evidence of <30–50% of intraarticular LHB fraying without instability. Where the tenotomy is indicated it should be excised with extra tissue at the point of adhesion to the glenoid is advised for tenotomy. This method will prevent the retraction by pinching of the proximal tendon in the bicipital groove entrance and thus avoid the Popeye sign [52–54].
- Tenodesis is favored for younger, high demanding patients. The area and fixation technique for tenodesis varies. Tenodesis can be made inside the bicipital groove or outside the groove with excising the inflamated tendon proximal portions. Tuberculum minor, coracoid, bicipital

groove, humerus under the pectoralis major, biceps muscle and the pectoralis major itself are candidates for tenodesis areas. Fixation may be done via bone tunnels, keyholes, suture to bicipital groove, interference screws and suture anchors. Tenodesis can be performed with arthroscopical techniques, open techniques such as subpectoral open biceps tenodesis can be used [55–58]. Velcro bandage is applied for 3 weeks postoperatively, passive elbow and shoulder movements are initiated as soon as possible. Gentle active exercises are initiated at the first month while strengthening exercises are initiated at the second month.

Calcific Tendinitis of the Shoulder

Introduction

Calcific tendinitis of the shoulder is a common disorder and is characterized by the presence of degeneration and calcification inside or around the insertion points of rotator cuff tendons, which causes acute and chronic pain. It is caused by multifocal accumulation of calcium hydroxy apatite crystals and inflammation near these deposits. Radiologically evident calcification has been reported in 7.5–20% of adults with no symptoms and in 6.8% of those with shoulder pain [59]. The most frequently involved tendon is the supraspinatus tendon, and in 10% of patients the condition is bilateral. Calcification can also occur in the infraspinatus and more rarely in the subscapularis tendon. The disorder is commonly seen in women slightly more than men and between 30 and 60 years of age. Workers who work at sedentary jobs are affected more than those working at a higher tempo [60, 61]. Although the pathogenesis of calcific tendinitis is still a matter of controversy it may be seen in young individuals with endocrine disorders such as diabetes and thyroid disorders [62].

History

In 1872, Dupley was the first to recognize the subacromial bursa and assumed that it was the source of pain in shoulders and he named the condition as painful periarthritis of the shoulder [63]. Painter used roentgenography to demonstrate the radiologic appearance of the disease, but he supposed that calcific deposits were in the bursal area [64]. Codman realized that the calcific deposits actually developed either inside or near the tendons and Bosworth reviewed the radiographs in a large series of patients and reported an incidence of 27% of calcific tendinitis of the shoulder. The condition was asymptomatic in 35% of the cases and supraspinatus tendon involvement was detected in 51% [65].

Pathogenesis

The reason for the deposition of calcium hydroxyapatite crystals in the tendon is still a matter of controversy. Two primary mechanisms have been suggested. Codman proposed that degenerative changes were necessary before the tendon would calcify which has similarities with degenerative lesions of the rotator cuff and further Moseley supported this by defining an avascular zone in the tendons insertion site [66, 67]. Uhthoff and Loetr proposed a multiphasic disease theory which suggested that the deposition of calcium in the tissues was followed by spontaneous resorption resulting in the calcific tendinitis. This process relies on cellular mediation, which promotes both the infiltration and removal of calcium from the area. Uhthoff and colleagues described three stages in the disease process which are precalcific, calcific and postcalcific stages. Gousen and Hoet reported four phases (precalcific, formative, resorptive and recovery) [61, 68].

The disorder has four stages. The first, precalcific stage, involves metaplasia of fibrocartilaginous tissue within the tendon. Patients usually do not have any symptoms in this stage. In the second stage, the formative stage, calcification develops within the cuff. This process may be asymptomatic or may be associated with different degrees of pain at rest or when in movement, especially abduction. The third stage is the resorptive stage, which is characterized by vascular invasion, oedema, migration of phagocytic cells, and increased intratendinous pressure. It is the most incapacitating for patients because of the extravasation of the calcium crystals into the subacromial bursa which can cause persistent severe pain and restriction of movement that typically lasts for 1–2 weeks. During this stage, the patients may exhibit systemic symptoms such as fever and malaise [69]. Some patients may even have elevated erythrocyte sedimentation rates and neutrophilia. Joint sepsis and gout must be ruled out in such patients.

The postcalcific stage is characterized by granulation tissue which replaces the space left behind by the removal of calcium deposit. This phase may last several months and is associated with mild-moderate pain and restricted function.

Other theories introduced in recent years include involvement of other factors, abnormal thyroid gland, metabolic disease (e.g. diabetes) and genetic predisposition to the formation of calcium deposits [62].

Classification

The evaluation of calcific tendinitis is based mainly on imaging studies, such as: x-rays, ultrasound (US) and magnetic resonance (MR) of the shoulder. The radiographic findings of calcifying tendinitis were first described by Painter in 1907. Since then several classifications of calcifying tendinitis have been proposed. DePalma classified calcifying tendinitis into two types: type I, fluffy and amorphous; type II, defined and homogenous. Type I calcifications are most commonly seen in patients with acute symptoms, and type II calcifications are most commonly observed in patients with chronic symptoms [70]. Gärtner [71] proposed a radiographic classification based on the morphological appearance of the calcification and correlated this with the frequency of resorption after needling. Loew et al. [72] proposed the first MR classification based on the morphological appearance of the calcific tendinitis. However, Maier [73] assessed the intraobserver reproducibility and interobserver reliability of the various classification systems using plain radiographs and CT scans and determined that the scores showed insufficient reliability and reproducibility that still remained statistically insignificant to be recommend as a routine investigation.

Gartner and Heyer Classification of Calcific Tendinitis

Type I	• Well circumscribed, dense calcification, formative
Type II	• Soft contour/dense or sharp/transparent
Type III	• Translucent and cloudy appearance without clear circumscription, resorptive

Mole et al. [74] Classification of Calcific Tendinitis

Type A	• Dense, homogeneous, sharp contours
Type B	• Dense, segmented, sharp contours
Type C	• Heterogeneous, soft contours
Type D	• Dystrophic calcifications at the insertion of the rotator cuff tendon

Diagnosis

For clinical evaluation and management of calcifying tendinitis, it is essential to understand the pathogenic mechanism of this disease. The clinical presentation can range from an incidental finding on the x-ray without symptoms to functional disability with acute, severe pain. The presentation of the disorder can be divided into three clinical stages (acute, subacute, chronic). The acute phase is characterized by spontaneous resorption of calcium, in which the calcium deposits are thick and creamy if removed. In this stage the pain is usually predominant and the reason of the pain is the influx of the resorption products to the bursal area. In the chronic phase, calcium crystals are deposited in the matrix vesicles and the calcium appears chalklike in the excision material. Although in most patients pain is related with the acute phase of the disease, also the episodes of acute pain can be associated with the flare-ups of the chronic tendinopathy. Generally, the acute phase lasts about 2 weeks; however, pain and movement restriction may extend up to 3–8 weeks during the subacute phase [75].

The symptoms of calcific tendinitis can mimic the clinical presentation of subacromial impingement syndrome such as atraumatic pain (most severe in the resorptive phase), catching, crepitus, mechanical block, and pain when the affected arm is especially in abduction. Patients can have sleep difficulties because of the night pains. The pain tends to be at night and patients are concerned about interrupted sleep. Ruling out other causes of shoulder pain like cervical radiculopathy, bursitis and bicipital tendinitis are important because calcium deposits seen on radiographs may be asymptomatic in 20% of cases [70]. In physical examinations the shoulder is often swollen and warm. The pressure applied over the supraspinatus insertion may exacerbate the pain. In the acute phase, the pain tends to be severe and allows only limited shoulder motion, but in the subacute and chronic phases, pain can be mild and generally shoulder motion is allowed [60]. Rarely the pain is about the onset of rare complications not related to the evolution of the disease such as adhesive capsulitis, rotator cuff tears pathology of the long head of biceps or osteolysis of the greater tuberosity [76–78].

Neer classically described four types of pain. First is caused by chemical irritation of the tissue by calcium deposits, second is the increased tissue pressure because of the swelling, third is the impingement like pain due to bursal thickening or deposits irritation and the last is caused by chronic stiffening of the glenohumeral joint due to voluntary prolonged immobilization [79].

Standard radiographs in AP views in internal rotation and external rotation, outlet and axillary views are used for diagnosis and follow-up of calcific tendinosis. Calcium deposits located in the supraspinatus tendon can be seen on a true AP view and are usually found 1–1,5 cm from supraspinatus tendon insertion. Following the changes in the calcific deposits by radiographs is useful to assess the process of the disease. IR view used to localize infraspinatus and teres minor and ER view shows subscapularis calcification. The axillary view is used for identifying deposits located in the subscapularis tendon.

The calcification seen in arthropathies have a distinct appearance and must be distinguished from calcific tendinopathy. Arthrophathies can be recognized by acromioclavicular space narrowing, degenerative bony and articular changes and calcification that extends into the bone [68, 80].

CT may characterize the three dimensional shoulder anatomy. USG examination is a fundamental tool in diagnosis and also utilized for guidance during needle decompression and injection. Use of high resolution USG reveals the presence of deposits and also their locations in the tendon, sizes and texture. In the resting phase, the deposits appear hyperechoic and arc shaped, while they appear non-arc shaped in the resolving plane, which can also be correlated with the symptomatic and asymptomatic phases of the disease [81].

MRI has limited utility in the diagnosis of calcific tendinitis. The accuracy of MRI in identifying calcific deposits is around 95% and the deposits have low signal intensity on all sequences. MRI is more useful in cases of chronic calcific tendinosis since these may be associated with rotator cuff tears, adhesive capsulitis and osteolysis of greater tuberosity [82].

Treatment

There are several options in the management of calcific shoulder tendinitis including conservative approaches and surgical modalities. However, the condition is also self limiting without any treatment and spontaneous resolution is likely ranging from 9.3% after 3 years and in 27% after 10 years [65]. Among all options, conservative management should be the first line approach in all phases with the reported success of 90% [83]. Non- steroidal anti-inflammatory drugs, physical therapy, stretching and strengthening, steroid injections, ultrasound guided therapy and ESWL are currently considered options of conservative management. However, approximately 10% of patients are resistant to the above mentioned modalities and patients appear to remain in a prolonged formative phase with chronic symptoms [84]. Surgical options such as open or arthroscopic surgery are associated with complete clinical improvement in the majority of cases (80–100%), particularly in those refractory to conservative treatment [85].

The main rationale of conservative treatment is to maintain the motion integrity of the shoulder and to provide complete pain relief. Restricting complete motion of the affected arm using a sling along with NSAII treatment is the mainstay of treatment. Following complete control of the pain, range of motion, pendulum and muscle strengthening exercises are recommended options. Numerous studies have demonstrated the effectiveness of physical modalities on calcific tendinitis [86–89]. Steroid injection is one of the conservative options in these cases. Despite the beneficial effect of steroid injections in patients with impingement signs, the treatment has been criticized to inhibit the resorption of calcific depositions [90–92]. There are several factors that might influence the conservative treatment's success in literature. Bilateral calcific tendinitis, medial extension and high volume of calcific deposits and occurrence of deposits near the anterior portion of the acromion have been proposed as drawbacks, whereas type 3 calcific deposits and lack of sonographic sound may be attributed as favorable factors that significantly reduce the probability of treatment failure [93].

Extracorporeal shock wave therapy seems to be an effective treatment option for calcific tendinitis, which is based on the use of shock waves and pressure impulses capable of producing fragmentation of calcific deposits and reduction of pain. High energy shock wave therapy should be considered before surgery in patients with chronic calcific tendinitis after a minimum of 6 months of unsuccessful conservative treatment or clinical signs of subacromial impingement [94]. The efficacy of ESWL has been confirmed in several prospective studies and favorable results have been reported in terms of patient satisfaction [95–97].

Another treatment option is the ultrasound guided needle lavage technique, in which two needles are used to create an inflow–outflow irrigation system for lavage. It is believed to work by decompressing the intratendinous pressure of calcium deposit and addition lavage may help remove part of the deposit. A small amount of saline and anesthetic can be injected around the calcification and aspiration of calcific material can be done with the other needle. Finally, steroids will be injected to provide sudden relief. Needle aspiration of calcific deposits is known to be effective, especially during the resorptive phase, and reported clinical variable success rates in calcific tendinitis [98–101].

Surgical treatment is a remaining option for patients in which prolonged conservative therapy has failed and the deposits do not show signs of spontaneous resolution on radiographs. Mostly surgery is indicated when the severe disabling symptoms persist for more than 6 months, which usually corresponds to the chronic formative phase [102].

After favorable results have been described in the literature with open removal of calcific deposits, arthroscopy has become the preferred technique to treat the chronic formative phase of calcific tendinosis, offering results similar to open surgery but with less morbidity of deltoid, a shorter rehabilitation time, better functional results and cosmetic appearance [103–105].

However, there are some controversial issues concerning arthroscopic treatment such as repairing versus leaving the defect created by removing all calcium deposits, substraction of all deposits versus partial eradication and finally the need for a subacromial decompression in addition to removal of the calcific tendinitis. There are many studies showing favorable results in the literature on all debating issues [106].

Adhesive Capsulitis

The aim of this chapter is to describe history, etiology, pathogenesis, and treatment of adhesive capsulitis. Adhesive capsulitis is associated with painful global limitation of both active and passive shoulder motion resulting from progressive fibrosis and contracture of the joint capsule that mostly involves the rotator interval.

History of the Disease

- In 1934, Duplay [107] described this condition as "peri-arthritis scapulohumerale".
- Codman [108] first used the term "frozen shoulder" to indicate a condition of tendinitis with secondary involvement of the subacromial bursa.
- Neviase [109] described the pathological lesion of fibrosis, inflammation and capsular contracture for frozen shoulder and used the term "adhesive capsulitis".
- The current consensus definition is "a condition of uncertain etiology characterized by significant limitation of both active and passive shoulder motion that occurs in the absence of a known intrinsic shoulder disorder and radiographic findings other than osteopenia" [110]. Many other conditions such as rotator cuff tears, calcific tendonitis, and glenohumeral arthritis may cause stiff and painful shoulder. However, these conditions lack true capsular contracture and restriction in passive range of motion; and should not be considered as adhesive capsulitis [111].

Etiology

Key Points

- Adhesive capsulitis is commonly seen in middle aged female patients with diabetes mellitus.
- A thorough history and physical examination is needed to distinguish primary adhesive capsulitis from other conditions.

Adhesive capsulitis is a common condition that is seen in approximately 2–5% of the general population, and the patients are commonly female between 40 and 60 years of age [112]. The nondominant hand is more frequently involved, but the condition often presents itself bilaterally and affects the contralateral side years after the onset of symptoms in the first shoulder [113]. The same shoulder is not usually affected twice.

Adhesive capsulitis is usually seen in patients with diabetes mellitus, thyroid dysfunction, Dupuytrens contractures, autoimmune disease, and the treatment of breast cancer [114]. Cerebrovascular accident and myocardial infarction have been associated with adhesive capsulitis. It is more common in sedentary patients. It has been reported that 20–30% of patients have had a minor shoulder trauma, but it still remains unclear whether this is a posttraumatic condition [113]. The disease may also occur after open and arthroscopic rotator cuff repair, acromioplasty and fracture fixation.

The primary adhesive capsulitis is described as idiopathic capsular inflammation and fibrosis of shoulder [114]. Previous shoulder trauma, surgery or other diseases may cause the secondary adhesive capsulitis. In these cases, development of adhesive capsulitis is related to prolonged immobilization and pain. Diagnosing primary or secondary disease can be challenging and they commonly overlap. Patients with stage 2 primary adhesive capsulitis were found to have supraspinatus partial-thickness tears [115]. A thorough history and physical examination would help the surgeon to distinguish primary adhesive capsulitis from other conditions.

Pathogenesis

Adhesive capsulitis is thought to be a combination of synovial inflammation and capsular fibrosis [111]. Cytokines such as VEGF, TGF-b, PDGF, IL-1b and TNF-a have been implicated in playing a role in the pathogenesis [116, 117]. Abnormal expression of matrix metalloproteinase inhibitors is involved in the pathogenesis of the disease [118]. The histological examination reveals a vascular, collagenous tissue with dense fibroblasts and myofibroblasts. The active fibroblast process in adhesive capsulitis is similar to Dupuytren disease [119]. There are few theories about the high incidence of adhesive capsulitis in diabetic patients. Excessive glucose concentration in diabetic patients may lead to a faster rate of collagen glycosylation and cross-linking in the shoulder capsule that is limiting shoulder motion [120].

Table 16.3 Histologic Classification described by Hannafin

	Symptoms	Arthroscopic appearance	Biopsy
Stage 1	Gradual onset of night pain	Fibrinous synovitis, no adhesions	Hypervascular, hypertrophic synovitis
			Normal capsular tissue
Stage 2	Severe night pain, stiffness	Fibrous adhesions	Hypertrophic, hypervascular synovitis, perivascular, subsynovial capsular scar
		Some loss of axillary fold	
Stage 3	Increasing stiffness, pain at the end of motion	Complete loss of axillary fold	Hypercellular, collagenous tissue with a thin synovial layer
		Synovitis resolving	
Stage 4	Severe stiffness, minimal pain	Severe contraction and adhesions	

Classification

Based on the physical and arthroscopic examination, the disease progresses through four stages which, are described by Neviaser [121]. Hannafin described histologic progression throughout the various stages [122] (Table 16.3). Understanding these stages is important so as to apply appropriate treatment. Early loss of external rotation with intact rotator cuff strength is characteristic for stage 1 adhesive capsulitis. Stage 2 is referred to as "freezing stage" in which both internal and external rotation, flexion and abduction motion is limited. This stage lasts between 10 and 36 weeks. In stage 3 "frozen stage", the main complaint of patients is severe stiffness. This phase can last from 4 to 12 months. Stage 4 is referred as the chronic stage or the thawing stage, where pain is minimal and gradual motion is regained over the course of 5–26 months. It is important to note that no pathological signs are seen on x-rays at any stages.

Natural History

The natural history of the adhesive capsulitis remains controversial. Some authors have reported that the majority of patients will have complete recovery [123], and others have reported that patients will have prolonged pain and stiffness [113, 124]. These variable results may be due to different methods of outcome measure. External rotation is limited at the latest follow up that may not limit daily life activities [111].

Clinical Evaluation

Key Points

- Insidious onset of night pain is characteristic.
- External rotation is limited initially.

The history and physical examination are very important for differential diagnosis. Patients with adhesive capsulitis frequently do not seek medical advise for weeks to months due to insidious onset of symptoms. Patients may describe a vague pain at the deltoid insertion. Night pain and painful restricted elevation and external rotation are common. As the disease progresses, pain and restriction become more apparent.

Evaluation of passive range of motion is essential. Forward flexion, abduction, and internal and external rotation should be evaluated in a supine position. True mechanical restriction with passive motion that occurs with capsular contraction is characterized by a firm, reproducible endpoint and must be differentiated from resistance due to pain [111].

Imaging

Radiographs are usually used to exclude other shoulder pathologies like calcific tendonitis, osteoarthritis of the glenohumeral and acromioclavicular joint. Osteopenia of the proximal humerus can be seen on radiographs [125]. While the axillary fold is contracted in frozen shoulder, arthrography of the shoulder can reveal reduced joint volume.

Magnetic resonance imaging (MRI) and MR arthrography are reliable imaging indicators for adhesive capsulitis. Thickening of the coracohumeral ligament, axillary recess and joint capsule in the rotator interval are common findings on MRI [126, 127].

Treatment

Key Points

- Majority of patients can benefit from conservative treatments.
- Studies have shown successful result of manipulation under anesthesia and arthroscopic release in refractory cases.

Initial treatment options for adhesive capsulitis include NSAIDs, intra-articular steroid injections and physical therapy. The majority of patients will benefit from conservative treatment, but some patients may have prolonged pain and restriction. Patients should have a minimum of 6 months of supervised conservative treatment before any other invasive treatments are considered [111]. Surgical treatment should be reserved for recalcitrant cases.

Literature on NSAIDs for the treatment of adhesive capsulitis is limited. They are often prescribed in early stages to provide short-term pain relief. There is no data showing superiority of NSAIDs over placebos for adhesive capsulitis. Oral corticosteroids can improve night pain and range of motion in the short-term [128]. It has been shown that corticosteroid injections into the glenohumeral and subacromial space have had similar outcomes to physiotherapy and manipulation [129, 130].

Physical therapy is the most commonly used treatment option to improve range of motion in advanced stages of the disease. Although there is limited data supporting the use of physical therapy, many studies reports its benefits, and its use in the treatment of adhesive capsulitis is almost universal [111, 131]. Gentle stretching and active motion appear to be the most appropriate treatment in many cases.

Hydrodilation combined with a therapy program was shown to be a successful treatment for idiopathic frozen shoulder [132]. It involves increasing intracapsular pressure and expanding capsular volume through injection of fluid until capsular rupture [114]. Suprascapular nerve blockade has also been proposed to be an effective treatment [133]. However, more studies are required to assess the effectiveness of these techniques in the treatment of adhesive capsulitis.

Manipulation under general anesthesia should be considered if pain and stiffness persists for more than 6 months. The shoulder should be gently stretched in all planes. Due to high risk of fracture, manipulation should not be attempted in posttraumatic and postsurgical cases. Iatrogenic humerus fractures, glenohumeral dislocation, rotator cuff tears and hemorrhagic effusions are possible complications of forceful manipulation.

Many studies have shown that arthroscopic release is a safe and effective treatment for recalcitrant adhesive capsulitis [134, 135]. The advantages of performing arthroscopy before capsular release are diagnosing and staging the disease and recognizing secondary causes of symptoms [114]. The joint is visualized with a standard posterior portal. Capsular adhesions on the rotator interval should be released initially. It is suggested to release anterior, posterior, and inferior portions of the capsule [136]. Care must be taken not to damage the axillary nerve during inferior capsular release.

The indications for an open surgery are very limited and it is rarely performed. Open surgery may have morbidities like postsurgical stiffness and prolonged recovery.

Future Outlook

The treatment of adhesive capsulitis still remains controversial despite many studies. Further prospective, comparative studies are needed to determine best treatment strategies for patients.

Questions

1. What is the gold standart diagnostic method for the pathologies of long head of biceps tendon?
   A. Speed + uppercut test.
   B. CT.
   C. MRI.
   D. Arthroscopy.
   E. Ultrasound.

   D

2. Which one of the following is false about calcific tendinitis of shoulder?
   A. The most frequently involved tendon is the infraspinatus tendon.
   B. Sedantary lifestyle is associated with higher rates of calcific tendinitis.
   C. Calcium deposits seen on radiograph can be asymptomatic in 20% of patients.
   D. Physical therapy with NSAİD is the mainstay of treatment.
   E. Arthroscopy is the preferred treatment if conservative treatment is unsuccessful.

   A

3. A 50 year old female patient with an insidious onset of right shoulder pain for 5 week admitted to your clinic. You examine that she has a restricted passive external rotation of 20° and abduction of 90°. She describes that the pain usually reaches to top at nights. She has not got ext/int rotation lag sign and lift off test is normal. She complaints about not able to reach shelfs higher than head level. Glenohumeral joint space seems normal on her x-ray. What would be your pre-diagnosis?

A. Rotator cuff rupture.
B. Adhesive capsulitis.
C. Impingement syndrome.
D. Glenohumeral arthritis.
E. Calcific tendinosis.

B

What is new?

Adhesive capsulitis is associated with inflammatory processes such as metabolic syndrome and even cardiovascular events. New researches investigated how cytokines are changed in affected shoulder. May it open a new era for targeted therapy?

Intercellular adhesion molecule-1 (ICAM-1, CD54) is increased in adhesive capsulitis. J Bone Joint Surg Am. 2013 Feb, Kim YS et al.

Adhesive capsulitis: An age related symptom of metabolic syndrome and chronic low-grade inflammation, Medical Hypotheses, March 2016, Pietrzak M et al.

References

1. Gaskill T, Millett PJ. Snapping scapula syndrome: diagnosis and management. J Am Acad Orthop Surg. 2013;21:214–24.
2. Patzkowski JC, Owens BD, Burns TC. Snapping scapula syndrome in the military. Clin Sports Med. 2014;33:757–66.
3. Kuhne M, Boniquit N, Ghodadra N, et al. The snapping scapula: diagnosis and treatment. Arthroscopy. 2009;25:1298–311.
4. Mozes G, Bickels J, Ovadia D, et al. The use of three-dimensional computed tomography in evaluating snapping scapula syndrome. Orthopedics. 1999;22:1029–33.
5. Kuhn JE, Plancher KD, Hawkins RJ. Symptomatic scapulothoracic crepitus and bursitis. J Am Acad Orthop Surg. 1998;6:267–73.
6. Manske RC, Reiman MP, Stovak ML. Nonoperative and operative management of snapping scapula. Am J Sports Med. 2004;32:1554–65.
7. Millett PJ, Gaskill TR, Horan MP, et al. Technique and outcomes of arthroscopic scapulothoracic bursectomy and partial scapulectomy. Arthroscopy. 2012;28:1776–83.
8. Blond L, Rechter S. Arthroscopic treatment for snapping scapula: a prospective case series. Eur J Orthop Surg Traumatol. 2013;24(2):159–64.
9. Lippmann RK. Bicipital tenosynovitis. N Y State J Med. 1944;90:2235–41.
10. Rockwood CA, Matsen FA, Wirth MA, Lippitt SB, Fehringer EV, Sperling JW. The shoulder. 4th ed: Elsevier.
11. Alan Barber F, Field LD, Ryu RKN. Biceps tendon and superior labrum injuries: decision-making. J Bone Joint Surg Am. 2007;89(8):1844–55.
12. Beall DP, Williamson EE, Ly JQ, Adkins MC, Emery RL, Jones TP, Rowland CM. Association of biceps tendon tears with rotator cuff abnormalities: degree of correlation with tears of the anterior and superior portions of the rotator cuff. AJR Am J Roentgenol. 2003;180(3):633–9.
13. Cowper W. Myotomia reformatia. London: Sam Smith and Ben Walford; 1694. p. 75.
14. Pasteur F. Les algies de l'épaule et la physiotherapie. La teno-bursite bicipatle. J Radiol Electrol. 16:419–29.

15. Schrager VL. Tenosynovitis of the long head of the biceps humeri. Surg Gynecol Obstet. 66:785–90.
16. Neer II CS. Anterior acromioplasty fort he chronic impingement syndrome in the shoulder. J Bone Joint Surg Am. 1972;54:41–50.
17. Walch G. LA pathologie de la longue portion du biceps. Presented at Conference d'enseignement de la SOFCOT, Paris, December 1993.
18. Vangsness Jr CT, Jorgenson SS, Watson T, Johnson DL. The origin of the long head of the biceps from the scapula and glenoid labrum. An anatomical study of 100 shoulders. J Bone Joint Surg Br. 1994; 76(6):951–4.
19. Lafrance R, Madsen W, Yaseen Z, et al. Relevant anatomic landmarks and measurements for biceps tenodesis. Am J Sports Med. 2013;41(6):1395–9.
20. Cheng N, Pan W, Vally F, Le Roux C, Richardson M. The arterial supply of the long head of biceps tendon: anatomical study with implications for tendon rupture. Clin Anat. 2010;23:683–92. doi:10.1002/ca.20992.
21. Habermeyer P, Magosch P, Pritsch M, et al. Anterosuperior impingement of theshoulder as a result of pulley lesions: a prospective arthroscopic study. J Shoulder Elb Surg. 2004;13(1):5–12.
22. Taylor SA, Fabricant PD, Bansal M, et al. The anatomy and histology of the bicipital tunnel of the shoulder. J Shoulder Elb Surg. 2015;24(4):511–9.
23. Cone RO, Danzig L, Resnick D, et al. The bicipital groove: radiographic, anatomic, and pathologic study. AJR Am J Roentgenol. 1983;141(4):781–8.
24. Malicky DM, Soslowsky LJ, Blasier RB, Shyr Y. Anterior glenohumeral stabilization factors: progressive effects in a biomechanical model. J Orthop Res. 1996;14:282–8.
25. Itoi E, Kuechle DK, Newman SR, et al. Stabilising function of the biceps in stable and unstable shoulders. J Bone Joint Surg Br. 1993;75(4):546–50.
26. Hwang E, Carpenter JE, Hughes RE, et al. Effects of biceps tension and superior humeral head translation on the glenoid labrum. J Orthop Res. 2014;32(11): 1424–9.
27. Singaraju V, Kang R, Yanke A, McNickle A, Lewis P, Wang V, et al. Biceps tendinitis in chronic rotator cuff tears: a histologic perspective. J Shoulder Elb Surg. 2008;17:898–904. doi:10.1016/j.jse.2008.05.044.
28. Boileau P, Ahrens PM, Trojani C, et al. Entrapment of the long head of the biceps: the "hourglass biceps". Another cause of pain and locking of the shoulder. Rev Chir Orthop Reparatrice Appar Mot. 2003;89(8):672–82.
29. Lafosse L, Reiland Y, Baier G, Toussaint B, Jost B. Anterior and posterior instability of the long head of the biceps tendon in rotator cuff tears: a new classification based on arthroscopic observations. Arthroscopy. 2007;23:73–80. doi:10.1016/j.arthro.2006.08.025.
30. Taylor SA, Khair MM, Gulotta LV, et al. Diagnostic glenohumeral arthroscopy failsto fully evaluate the biceps-labral complex. Arthroscopy. 2015;31(2):215–24.
31. Habermeyer P, Walch G. The biceps tendon and rotator cuff disease. In: Burkhead Jr WZ, editor. Rotator cuff disorders. Baltimore: Williams & Wilkins; 1996. p. 142–59.
32. Meyer AW. Unrecognized occupational destruction of the tendon of the long head of the biceps brachii. Arch Surg. 1921;2:130–44.
33. Snyder SJ, Karzel RP, Del Pizzo W, et al. SLAP lesions of the shoulder. Arthroscopy. 1990;6:274–9.
34. Kibler W, Sciascia A, Hester P, Dome D, Jacobs C. Clinical utility of traditional and new tests in the diagnosis of biceps tendon injuries and superior labrum anterior and posterior lesions in the shoulder. Am J Sports Med. 2009;37:1840–7. doi:10.1177/0363546509332505.
35. Fisk C. Adaptation of the technique for radiography of the bicipital groove. Radiol Technol. 1965;37:47–50.
36. Cone RO, Danzig L, Resnick D, Goldman AB. The bicipital groove: radiographic, anatomic, and pathologic study. AJR Am J Roentgenol. 1983;141: 781–8.
37. Armstrong A, Teffey S, Wu T, Clark A, Middleton W, Yamaguchi K, et al. The efficacy of ultrasound in the diagnosis of long head of thebiceps tendon pathology. J Shoulder Elb Surg. 2006;15:7–11. doi:10.1016/j.jse.2005.04.008.
38. Ptasznik R, Hennessy O. Abnormalities of the biceps tendon of the shoulder: sonographic findings. AJR Am J Roentgenol. 1995;164:409–14.
39. Tuckman GA. Abnormalities of the long head of the biceps tendon of the shoulder: MR imaging findings. AJR Am J Roentgenol. 1994;163:1183–8.
40. Klug JD, Moore SL. MR imaging of the biceps muscle–tendon complex. Magn Reson Imaging Clin N Am. 1997;5:755–65.
41. Childress MA, Beutler A. Management of chronic tendon injuries. Am Fam Physician. 2013;87(7):486.
42. Andres BM, Murrell GA. Treatment of tendinopathy: what works, what does not, and what is on the horizon. Clin Orthop Relat Res. 2008;466(7): 1539–54.
43. Piper SL, Kim HT. Comparison of ropivacaine and bupivacaine toxicity in human articular chondrocytes. J Bone Joint Surg Am. 2008;90(5):986–91.
44. Schickendantz M, King D. Nonoperative management (including ultrasound-guided injections) of proximal biceps disorders. Clin Sports Med. 2016;35:57–73.
45. Carroll R, Hamilton L. Rupture of biceps brachii. A conservative method of treatment. J Bone Joint Surg Am. 1967;49:101.
46. Mariani E, Cofield R, Askew L, Li G, Chao E. Rupture of the tendon of the long head of the biceps brachii: surgical versus nonsurgical treatment. Clin Orthop Relat Res. 1988;228:233–9.
47. Deutch S, Gelineck J, Johannsen H, Sneppen O. Permanent disabilities in the displaced muscle from rupture of the long head tendon of the biceps. Scand J Med Sci Sports. 2005;15:159–62. doi:10.1111/j.1600-0838.2004.00421.x.

48. Sethi N, Wright R, Yamaguchi K. Disorders of the long head of the biceps tendon. J Shoulder Elb Surg. 1999;8(6):644–54.
49. Barber FA, Byrd JW, Wolf EM, Burkhart SS. How would you treat the partiallytorn biceps tendon? Arthroscopy. 2001;17(6):636–9.
50. Frost A, Zafar MS, Maffulli N. Tenotomy versus tenodesis in the management of pathologic lesions of the tendon of the long head of the bicepsbrachii. Am J Sports Med. 2009;37(4):828–33.
51. Khazzam M, George M, Churchill S, Kuhn J. Disorders of the long head of biceps tendon. J Shoulder Elb Surg. 2012;21:136–45.
52. Bennett WF. Arthroscopic repair of anterosuperior (supraspinatus/subscapularis) rotator cuff tears: a prospective cohort with 2- to 4-yearfollow-up. Classification of biceps subluxation/instability. Arthroscopy. 2003;19(1):21–33.
53. Bradbury T, Dunn WR, Kuhn JE. Preventing the popeye deformity after release of the long head of the biceps tendon: an alternative technique and biomechanical evaluation. Arthroscopy. 2008;24(10): 1099–102.
54. Nho SJ, Strauss EJ, Lenart BA, Provencher MT, Mazzocca AD, Verma NN, Romeo AA. Long head of the biceps tendinopathy: diagnosis and management. J Am Acad Orthop Surg. 2010 Nov;18(11): 645–56.
55. Richards DP, Burkhart SS. Arthroscopic assisted biceps tenodesis for ruptures of the long head of biceps brachii: the cobra procedure. Arthroscopy. 2004;20(suppl 2):201–7.
56. Kim SH, Yoo JC. Arthroscopic biceps tenodesis using interference screw: end tunnel technique. Arthroscopy. 2005;21(11):1405.
57. Boileau P, Neyton L. Arthroscopic tenodesis for lesions of the long head ofthe biceps. Oper Orthop Traumatol. 2005;17(6):601–23.
58. Gartsman GM, Hammerman SM. Arthroscopic biceps tenodesis: operative technique. Arthroscopy. 2000;16(5):550–2.
59. Welfling J, Kahn M, Desroy M, Paolaggi J, De Seze S. Les calcifications de l'épaule. II. La maladie des calcifications tendineuses multiples. Rev Rhum Mal Osteoartic. 1965;32:325–34.
60. McKendry R, Uhthoff H, Sarkar K, Hyslop P. Calcifying tendinitis of the shoulder: prognostic value of clinical, histologic, and radiologic features in 57 surgically treated cases. J Rheumatol. 1981;9:75–80.
61. Uhthoff HK, Loehr JW. Calcific tendinopathy of the rotator cuff: pathogenesis, diagnosis, and management. J Am Acad Orthop Surg. 1997;5:183–91.
62. Harvie P, Pollard TC, Carr AJ. Calcific tendinitis: natural history and association with endocrine disorders. J Shoulder Elb Surg. 2007;16:169–73.
63. Duplay S. De la peri-arthrite scapulo-humerale et des raideurs de l'epaule qui en sont la consequence. Arch Gen Med. 1872;20:513–42.
64. Painter CF. Subdeltoid bursitis. Boston Med Surg J. 1907;156:345–9.
65. Bosworth BM. Calcium deposits in the shoulder and subacromial bursitis: a survey of 12,122 shoulders. J Am Med Assoc. 1941;116:2477–82.
66. Codman EA. On stiff and painful shoulders: the anatomy of the subdeltoid or subacromial bursa and its clinical importance. Subdeltoid bursitis. Boston Med Surg J. 1906;154:613–20.
67. Moseley HF, Goldie I. The arterial pattern of the rotator cuff of the shoulder. J Bone Joint Surg Br Vol. 1963;45:780–9.
68. Gosens T, Hofstee D-J. Calcifying tendinitis of the shoulder: advances in imaging and management. Curr Rheumatol Rep. 2009;11:129–34.
69. Ross G, Cooper J, Minos L, Steinmann SP. Acute calcific tendinitis of the shoulder mimicking infection: arthroscopic evaluation and treatment—a case report. Am J Orthop (Belle Mead NJ). 2006;35:572.
70. DePalma A. Long-term study of shoulder joints afflicted with and treatment for calcific tendonitis. Clin Orthop. 1961;20:61–72.
71. Gärtner J. Tendinosis calcarea—results of treatment with needling. Z Orthop ihre Grenzgeb. 1992;131: 461–9.
72. Loew M, Sabo D, Wehrle M, Mau H. Relationship between calcifying tendinitis and subacromial impingement: a prospective radiography and magnetic resonance imaging study. J Shoulder Elb Surg. 1996;5:314–9.
73. Maier M, Schmidt-Ramsin J, Glaser C, Kunz A, Küchenhoff H, Tischer T. Intra-and interobserver reliability of classification scores in calcific tendinitis using plain radiographs and CT scans. Acta Orthop Belg. 2008;74:590.
74. Mole D, Kempf J, Gleyze P, Rio B, Bonnomet F, Walch G. [Results of endoscopic treatment of nonbroken tendinopathies of the rotator cuff. 2. Calcifications of the rotator cuff]. Rev Chir Orthop Reparatrice Appar Mot. 1992;79:532–41.
75. Angelo RL, Esch J, Ryu RK. The shoulder: Elsevier Health Sciences; 2010.
76. Porcellini G, Paladini P, Campi F, Pegreffi F. Osteolytic lesion of greater tuberosity in calcific tendinitis of the shoulder. J Shoulder Elb Surg. 2009;18:210–5.
77. Merolla G, Bhat MG, Paladini P, Porcellini G. Complications of calcific tendinitis of the shoulder: a concise review. J Orthop Traumatol. 2015:1–9.
78. Speed CA, Hazleman BL. Calcific tendinitis of the shoulder. N Engl J Med. 1999;340:1582–4.
79. Neer C. Less frequent procedures. In: Shoulder reconstruction. Philadelphia: WB Saunders; 1990. p. 421–85.
80. Le Goff B, Berthelot J-M, Guillot P, Glémarec J, Maugars Y. Assessment of calcific tendonitis of rotator cuff by ultrasonography: comparison between symptomatic and asymptomatic shoulders. Joint Bone Spine. 2010;77:258–63.
81. Martinoli C, Bianchi S, Prato N, Pugliese F, Zamorani MP, Valle M, Derchi LE. US of the shoulder: non-rotator cuff disorders. Radiographics. 2003;26(1):e23.

82. Zubler C, Mengiardi B, Schmid MR, Hodler J, Jost B, Pfirrmann CW. MR arthrography in calcific tendinitis of the shoulder: diagnostic performance and pitfalls. Eur Radiol. 2007;17:1603–10.
83. Gschwend N, Scherer M, Löhr J. [Tendinitis calcarea of shoulder joint (Tc) (author's transl)]. Orthopade. 1981;10:196–205.
84. Uhthoff HK, Sarkar K, Maynard JA. Calcifying tendinitis: a new concept of its pathogenesis. Clin Orthop Relat Res. 1976;118:164–8.
85. Rubenthaler F, Ludwig J, Wiese M, Wittenberg RH. Prospective randomized surgical treatments for calcifying tendinopathy. Clin Orthop Relat Res. 2003;410:278–84.
86. Rocks J. Intrinsic shoulder pain syndrome: rationale for heating and cooling in treatment. Phys Ther. 1979;59:153–9.
87. Klein I, Klemes I. Treatment of peritendinitis calcarea in the shoulder joint. Radiology. 1941;37: 325–30.
88. Feibel A, Fast A. Deep heating of joints: a reconsideration. Arch Phys Med Rehabil. 1976;57:513–4.
89. Sundstrom W. Painful shoulders: diagnosis and management. Geriatrics. 1983;38:77–80, 5, 6, 91, 6.
90. Noel E, Carrillon Y, Gaillard T, Bouvier M. Needle aspiration irrigation in calcifying tendinitis of rotator cuff. In: The cuff. Paris: Elsevier; 1997. p. 152–7.
91. Tillander B, Franzén LE, Karlsson MH, Norlin R. Effect of steroid injections on the rotator cuff: an experimental study in rats. J Shoulder Elb Surg. 1999;8:271–4.
92. Wolf 3rd W. Shoulder tendinoses. Clin Sports Med. 1992;11:871–90.
93. Ogon P, Suedkamp N, Jaeger M, Izadpanah K, Koestler W, Maier D. Prognostic factors in nonoperative therapy for chronic symptomatic calcific tendinitis of the shoulder. Arthritis Rheum. 2009;60:2978–84.
94. Mouzopoulos G, Stamatakos M, Mouzopoulos D, Tzurbakis M. Extracorporeal shock wave treatment for shoulder calcific tendonitis: a systematic review. Skelet Radiol. 2007;36:803–11.
95. Moretti B, Garofalo R, Genco S, Patella V, Mouhsine E. Medium-energy shock wave therapy in the treatment of rotator cuff calcifying tendinitis. Knee Surg Sports Traumatol Arthrosc. 2005;13:405–10.
96. Cacchio A, Paoloni M, Barile A, Don R, de Paulis F, Calvisi V, Ranavolo A, Frascarelli M, Santilli V, Spacca G. Effectiveness of radial shock-wave therapy for calcific tendinitis of the shoulder: single-blind, randomized clinical study. Phys Ther. 2006;86:672–82.
97. Daecke W, Loew M. Long-term effects of extracorporeal shockwave therapy in chronic calcific tendinitis of the shoulder. J Shoulder Elb Surg. 2002;11:476–80.
98. De Conti G, Marchioro U, Dorigo A, Boscolo N, Vio S, Trevisan M, Meneghini A, Baldo V, Angelini F. Percutaneous ultrasound-guided treatment of shoulder tendon calcifications: clinical and radiological follow-up at 6 months. J Ultrasound. 2010;13:188–98.
99. Aina R, Cardinal E, Bureau NJ, Aubin B, Brassard P. Calcific shoulder tendinitis: treatment with modified US-guided fine-needle technique. Radiology. 2001;221:455–61.
100. del Cura JL, Torre I, Zabala R, Legórburu A. Sonographically guided percutaneous needle lavage in calcific tendinitis of the shoulder: short- and long-term results. AJR Am J Roentgenol. 2007;189:W128–W34.
101. Farin P, Räsänen H, Jaroma H, Harju A. Rotator cuff calcifications: treatment with ultrasound-guided percutaneous needle aspiration and lavage. Skelet Radiol. 1996;25:551–4.
102. Rotini R, Bungaro P, Antonioli D, Katusic D, Marinelli A. Algorithm for the treatment of calcific tendinitis in the rotator cuff: indications for arthroscopy and results in our experience. Chir Organi Mov. 2004;90:105–12.
103. Gazielly D, Bruyere G, Gleyze P, Thomas T. Open acromioplasty with excision of calcium deposits and tendon suture. In: The cuff. Paris: Elsevier; 1997. p. 172–5.
104. Rochwerger A, Franceschi J, Viton J, Roux H, Mattei J. Surgical management of calcific tendinitis of the shoulder: an analysis of 26 cases. Clin Rheumatol. 1999;18:313–6.
105. Jerosch J, Strauss J, Schmiel S. Arthroscopic treatment of calcific tendinitis of the shoulder. J Shoulder Elb Surg. 1998;7:30–7.
106. El Shewy MT. Arthroscopic removal of calcium deposits of the rotator cuff: a 7-year follow-up. Am J Sports Med. 2011;39:1302–5.
107. Duplay S. De la periarthrite scapulahumerale. Rev Frat d Trav De Med. 1896;53:226.
108. Codman EA. The shoulder: rupture of the supraspinatus tendon and other lesions in or about the subacromial bursa. Boston: T Todd Company; 1934.
109. Neviaser JS. Adhesive capsulitis of the shoulder. J Bone Joint Surg Am. 1945;27(2):211–22.
110. Zuckerman J, Cuomo F, Rokito S. Definition and classification of frozen shoulder: a consensus approach. J Shoulder Elb Surg. 1994;3:S72.
111. Hsu JE, Anakwenze OA, Warrender WJ, Abboud JA. Current review of adhesive capsulitis. J Shoulder Elb Surg. 2011;20(3):502–14.
112. Binder AI, Bulgen DY, Hazleman BL, Roberts S. Frozen shoulder: a long-term prospective study. Ann Rheum Dis. 1984;43(3):361–4.
113. Hand C, Clipsham K, Rees JL, Carr AJ. Long-term outcome of frozen shoulder. J Shoulder Elb Surg. 2008;17(2):231–6.
114. Neviaser AS, Hannafin JA. Adhesive capsulitis: a review of current treatment. Am J Sports Med. 2010 Nov;38(11):2346–56.
115. Yoo JC, Ahn JH, Lee YS, Koh KH. Magnetic resonance arthrographic findings of presumed stage-2 adhesive capsulitis: focus on combined rotator cuff pathology. Orthopedics. 2009;32(1):22.
116. Rodeo SA, Hannafin JA, Tom J, Warren RF, Wickiewicz TL. Immunolocalization of cytokines and their receptors in adhesive capsulitis of the shoulder. J Orthop Res. 1997;15:427–36.

117. Ryu JD, Kirpalani PA, Kim JM, Nam KH, Han CW, Han SH. Expression of vascular endothelial growth factor and angiogenesis in th diabetic frozen shoulder. J Shoulder Elb Surg. 2006;15:679–85.
118. Bunker TD, Reilly J, Baird KS, Hamblen DL. Expression of growth factors, cytokines and matrix metalloproteinases in frozen shoulder. J Bone Joint Surg Br. 2000;82:768–73.
119. Bunker TD, Anthony PP. The pathology of frozen shoulder. A Dupuytren-like disease. J Bone Joint Surg Br. 1995;77:677–83.
120. Brownlee M, Cerami A, Vlassara H. Advanced glycosylation end products in tissue and the biomechanical basis of diabetic complications. N Engl J Med. 1988;318:1315–21.
121. Neviaser RJ, Neviaser TJ. The frozen shoulder: diagnosis and management. Clin Orthop Relat Res. 1987;223:59–64.
122. Hannafin JA, Chiaia TA. Adhesive capsulitis. A treatment approach. Clin Orthop Relat Res. 2000:95–109.
123. Miller MD, Wirth MA, Rockwood Jr CA. Thawing the frozen shoulder: the “patient” patient. Orthopedics. 1996;19:849–53.
124. Shaffer B, Tibone JE, Kerlan RK. Frozen shoulder. A long-term follow-up. J Bone Joint Surg Am. 1992;74:738–46.
125. Lundberg BJ, Nilsson BE. Osteopenia in the frozen shoulder. Clin Orthop Relat Res. 1968;60:187–91.
126. Sofka CM, Ciavarra GA, Hannafin JA, Cordasco FA, Potter HG. Magnetic resonance imaging of adhesive capsulitis: correlation with clinical staging. HSS J. 2008;4:164–9.
127. Tamai K, Yamato M. Abnormal synovium in the frozen shoulder: a preliminary report with dynamic magnetic resonance imaging. J Shoulder Elb Surg. 1997;6:534–43.
128. Binder A, Hazleman BL, Parr G, Roberts S. A controlled study of oral prednisolone in frozen shoulder. Br J Rheumatol. 1986;25:288–92.
129. Ryans I, Montgomery A, Galway R, Kernohan WG, McKane R. A randomized controlled trial of intra-articular triamcinolone and/or physiotherapy in shoulder capsulitis. Rheumatology (Oxford). 2005;44:529–35.
130. Jacobs LG, Smith MG, Khan SA, Smith K, Joshi M. Manipulation or intra-articular steroids in the management of adhesive capsulitis of the shoulder? A prospective randomized trial. J Shoulder Elb Surg. 2009;18:348–53.
131. Green S, Buchbinder R, Hetrick S. Physiotherapy interventions for shoulder pain. Cochrane Database Syst Rev. 2003;2:CD004258.
132. Callinan N, McPherson S, Cleaveland S, Voss DG, Rainville D, Tokar N. Effectiveness of hydroplasty and therapeutic exercise for treatment of frozen shoulder. J Hand Ther. 2003;16(3):219–24.
133. Dahan TH, Fortin L, Pelletier M, Petit M, Vadeboncoeur R, Suissa S. Double blind randomized clinical trial examining the efficacy of bupivacaine suprascapular nerve blocks in frozen shoulder. J Rheumatol. 2000;27:1464–9.
134. Baums MH, Spahn G, Nozaki M, Steckel H, Schults W, Klinger HM. Functional outcome and general health status in patients after arthroscopic release in adhesive capsulitis. Knee Surg Sports Traumatol Arthrosc. 2007;15:638–44.
135. Berghs BM, Sole-Molins X, Bunker TD. Arthroscopic release of adhesive capsulitis. J Shoulder Elb Surg. 2004;13:180–5.
136. Jerosch J. 360 Degrees arthroscopic capsular release in patients with adhesive capsulitis of the glenohumeral joint: indication, surgical technique, results. Knee Surg Sports Traumatol Arthrosc. 2001;9(3):178–86.

Part VI

Non-operative Management of Shoulder Disorders

Splints and Orthoses

17

Nilgün Bek

Introduction

Shoulder injuries are commonly seen in athletes, particularly in overhead athletes (baseball, handball, volleyball, swimming, track and field throwing events, and tennis), and considered important because it leads to disability. A considerable amount of these injuries are considered as the overuse injuries of muscles, tendons, and joints. These overuse injuries may stem from incorrect postures, inappropriate overloading, and overhead throws and striking activities [1].

In addition, traumatic injuries caused by car or motorcycle accidents, falling, over stretching, and crushing are common in shoulder joint and in periarticular tissues. Shoulder braces are mainly used for athletes with shoulder injuries as an adjunct to rehabilitation programs. Clinically, athletic trainers might use bracing or taping in corrective exercise programs as a complementary therapy or to restore normal length-tension relation in muscle during the exercise program as a main therapy itself. Therefore, a better understanding of the effects of these braces requires further clinical experiment on different types of subjects (healthy subjects, athletes) and with different designs (pre-operative, post-operative, acute and chronic conditions).

N. Bek, P.T., Ph.D.
Department of Physiotherapy and Rehabilitation, Faculty of Health Sciences, Hacettepe University, Ankara, Turkey
e-mail: nilgunbek@gmail.com

The Purposes of the Shoulder Braces

- Pain relief
- Prevention of the deformity and the risk of secondary injuries
- Improvement of the normal alignment
- Maintenance of the normal range of motion of the shoulder
- Facilitation of the normal movement and function
- Immobilization and resting
- Supporting
- Correction of the deformities
- Acceleration of the fracture healing
- Stretching for the contractures
- Providing the glenohumeral joint stability
- Preparation for the surgery
- Providing development in the functional activities
- Maintenance of the normal scapulohumeral kinematics
- Weight-lifting of the arm weight when needed

G. Huri, N.K. Paschos (eds.), *The Shoulder*, Orthopaedic Study Guide Series,
DOI 10.1007/978-3-319-51979-1_17

Features of the Braces

Materials of the shoulder braces should be rather esthetic in terms of color, look, fitting, and other specific features. The thermoplastic materials are often preferred for the fabrication of these braces. Thermoplastics should be perforated to prevent sweating. Contact surfaces of the braces should be well adjusted. Functional and necessary movements should not be prevented, and the body structure, which needs support, should be covered. For example, brace should cover the acromion to prevent the shoulder abduction movement, and should not cover olecranon in order to maintain the elbow extension movement. Furthermore, no parts of the brace should press on the axillary region to avoid neuraproxia of the axillary nerve. Also, trunk parts of the brace should not restrict thoracic expansion movement. If brace is enclosing some joints, generally it should have a mechanical articulation- at this stage, this mechanical joint movement should simulate the real joint movement. These mechanical joint axes should also adopt the identical plan of the real anatomic joint axes. All shoulder braces should have some suspension tools, such as elastic straps or harnesses, as it is very difficult to hold these braces on the shoulder and the arm because of the gravitational force. Finally, appropriate brace fitting should be chosen for an effective treatment, particularly with off-the-shelf braces.

Brace Approaches in Common Shoulder Problems

Fractures of the Clavicle

The clavicle has an important function, which is negatively affected by complications and fractures. It serves as a strut between the shoulder (and arms) and the thoracic cage. It allows the full range of arm motion and stabilizes the pectoral girdle. In addition, it serves as a firm structure for muscle origins and insertions [2, 3]. It also supports respiratory function, protects neurovascular structures, and is essential in the appearance of the individual. Clavicle fractures are especially seen amongst adolescents and, in this age group, it makes up of 4% of all bone fractures. The most common causes of clavicle fractures are falling over abducted arm or blunt shoulder trauma. Bruising and deformity are clear visual clues of a clavicle fracture, which makes diagnosis clear [3, 4]. The structure of the clavicle consists of medial and lateral flat expansions, linked by a thin, tubular middle part. While muscular attachments and ligaments support the medial and lateral segments, the middle segment is unfixed, so it is susceptible to fractures. More than 80% of the clavicle fractures occur in this section. Clavicle fractures are classified into three groups: middle third fractures, lateral third fractures, and medial third fractures [5]. In a comprehensive epidemiological study, 76% of all fractures were reported to be middle third fractures, and they were found to occur in participants with a median age of 13 years. Just over half (53%) of middle third fractures were reported non-displaced [6]. They are frequently subjected to conservative treatment methods that do not involve any kind of surgery [7]. The most common therapy methods are use of arm slings, strapping, figure-of-eight taping, and splints (Fig. 17.1). Lenza et al. published a review in which they investigated different conservative interventions for treating middle third clavicle fractures in adolescents and adults and compared randomized controlled trial results including conservative treatment methods [8]. For clavicle fractures, they recommended further research

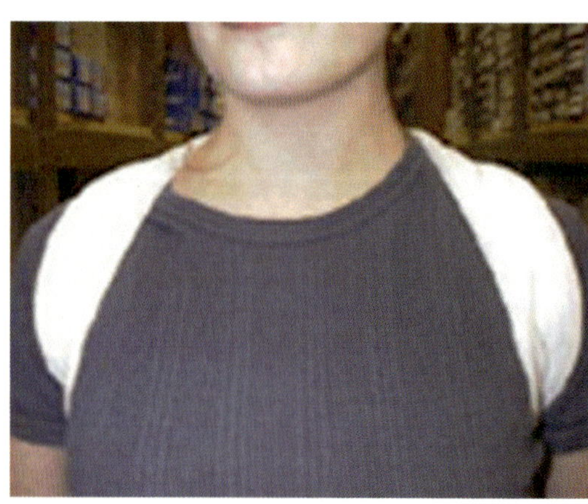

Fig. 17.1 Figure-of-eight brace

comparing contemporary and conservative therapy methods, such as arm sling and figure-of-eight brace.

Humeral Shaft Fractures

Fractures of the humeral shaft account for roughly 3% of all fractures. Most of humeral fractures can be treated non-operatively [7, 9] with a higher union rate of 90% [10–12]. Surgery is elected generally for fractures with a vascular component and nerve injury, in patients with multiple fractures, bilateral humeral shaft fractures, pathological fractures, comminuted segmental fractures, and open fractures. Functional bracing has essentially been replaced by all other conservative treatment methods and has become the "gold standard" for non-operative treatment with its easy applicability and adjustability characteristics, its ability to allow shoulder and elbow motion, and because it is relatively low cost and has reproducible results [9] (Fig. 17.2). The humeral functional brace works on the principles of the hydraulic effect of the brace (by compressing the soft tissues circumferentially to produce fracture alignment), active contraction effect of the muscles, and beneficial effect of the gravity. Furthermore it has been shown to be very effective for treating closed humeral shaft fractures [10–13]. The brace should be worn at all times and patients should be instructed to perform pendulum exercises immediately after the application of the initial cast or splint. Exercises should be maintained after the application of the brace [14]. After seeing clinical and radiographic signs of good callus formation and healing, the brace is removed. The criterion for clinical healing is having no pain and not having abnormal movement at the fracture site. The criterion for radiographic healing is the present formation of sufficient external bridging callus on both anteroposterior and lateral radiograms (bridging callus in at least three quadrants). Indications and contraindications were described by Sarmiento in 1999 as shown in Table 17.1 [15].

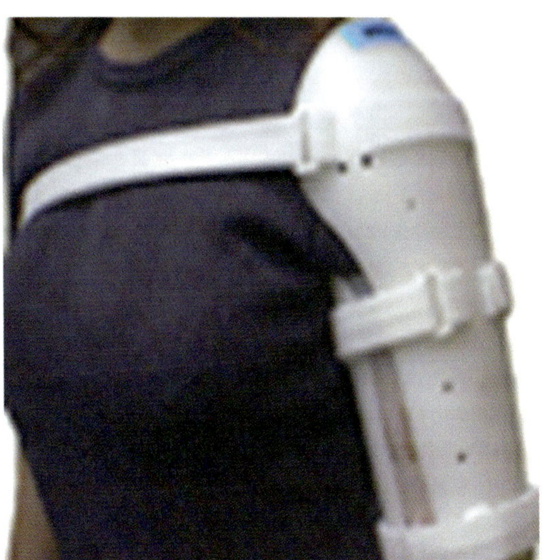

Fig. 17.2 Functional humeral brace

Table 17.1 Functional bracing of humeral shaft fractures (with permission from Ref. 15)

Indications
Closed diaphyseal fractures without marked distraction between the fragments
Closed fractures associated with initial radial nerve palsy similar to those described in the previous category
Open fractures without significant soft-tissue damage
Relative contraindications
Bilateral humeral fractures
Fractures in polytraumatized patients unless they are able to stand erect early and ambulate with external support on the opposite side

Functional humeral bracing is one of the rare methods accepted for treatment. However, treatment with braces causes some residual deformity and complications, such as varus angulation in humerus (which is marked more frequently in patients with short and obese arms), impairment in shoulder movement to a certain degree, decrease in the quality of life, and uncommon skin ulceration [16].

In the literature, there is a case study, which used an upper arm brace for **periprosthetic humeral fractures**. Due to the increasing number of implanted shoulder prostheses following trauma or arthritis in the recent past, an increase in the occurrence of periprosthetic humeral fractures is expected in the future. The current literature clearly recommends operative treatment with fixed angle plate osteosynthesis or a long-stemmed cement-free revision endoprosthesis. For example, a 70-year-old woman was diagnosed with a periprosthetic humeral fracture with an enclosed fracture endoprosthesis (Wright type B) in a study. The idea of the operative treatment with fixed angle plate osteosynthesis and the conservative therapy with a brace as an alternative to the operation were discussed with the patient. The patient decided on the conservative therapy with regular radiological course control. According to the results of this case report, we can say that conservative therapy of periprosthetic type B2 humeral fractures (according to Worland) using retention in an upper arm brace might lead to excellent radiological and functional results [17].

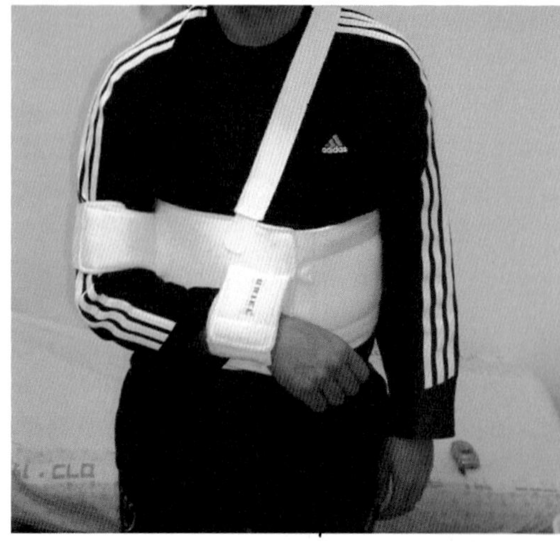

Fig. 17.3 The brace position on a primary traumatic anterior dislocation of the shoulder (in internal rotation) [19]

Shoulder Dislocations

Shoulder dislocations are common painful traumas. "Ball-and-socket" relationship is very loose in the glenohumeral joint; therefore, among all the joints in the body, it is the most commonly dislocated big joint [18]. The aim of the treatment of primary anterior traumatic dislocation of the shoulder is to prevent subsequent recurrent dislocation [19]. Following the initial joint reduction, the arm is immobilized in abduction and internal rotation position, which is the primary therapy in shoulder injuries [18]. However, it has been considered that this treatment method has no positive effect on its recurrence. But it is widely used. In recent years, researchers have started to investigate the effects of different shoulder positions. In particular, bracing in external rotation is often investigated. However, there is no consensus yet. Finestone et al. used the external rotation brace (ER) in 27 patients and an internal rotation brace (IR) in 24 patients in their study. They reported that new dislocations occurred at a mean interval of 12.4 months in the IR group, but found no significant difference in the rate of recurrence between those immobilized in external rotation or internal rotation [19]. In Figs. 17.3 and 17.4, both braces that were used in this study are shown [19].

Whelan et al. also investigated the effects of external rotation immobilization for primary shoulder dislocation. Their results showed no difference in the rate of recurrent instability between groups: 10 of 27 patients (37%) with the external rotation brace vs. 10 of 25 patients (40%) with

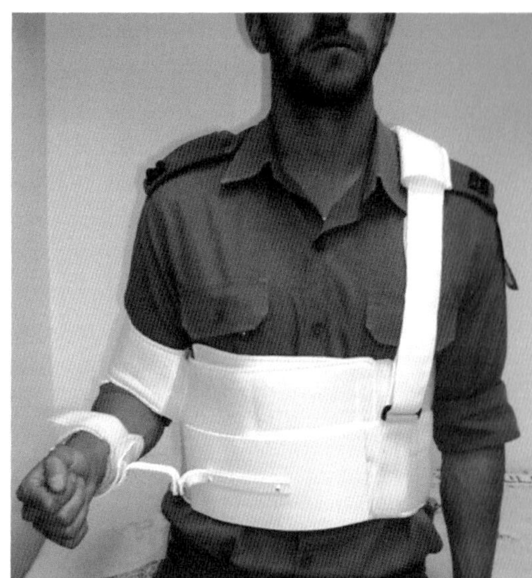

Fig. 17.4 The brace position in external rotation [19]

the sling redislocated or developed symptomatic recurrent instability ($p = 0.41$) [18].

According to the results of both studies, compliance of the external rotation brace was lower than traditional method because all patients were young and active men [18, 19].

Shoulder external rotation braces used for patients with a first-time shoulder dislocation are designed with a variety of arm positions in abduction as well as external rotation. However, few studies have focused on their immobilizing performance, comfort, or user-friendliness. Especially, there have been no robust data of shoulder abduction-external rotation (A-ER) braces in comparison to those of external rotation (ER) braces. The effects of different angular positions were investigated in shoulder external rotation braces in a study. Hata et al. tested four types of commercially available shoulder braces (two ER and two A-ER braces) in 30 healthy participants. The subjects were evaluated to assess the discomfort of bracing and difficulty of reapplication. In their study, results were compared between the two ER braces and the two A-ER braces as well as among the four braces. They reported that for both external rotation angle and subjective assessment, there were no significant differences between the ER and A-ER braces. Among the four braces, the measurement of arm position demonstrated no significant differences, except for the external rotation angles between the two ER braces. The A-ER braces were assessed to be significantly less comfortable than the ER braces in the subjective assessment. As a conclusion, immobilization using the A-ER braces could maintain the arm position in abduction-external rotation with comparable user-friendliness, although they tended to be less comfortable during daily activities compared to the ER braces [20]. In Fig. 17.5, four different braces used in this study are shown [20].

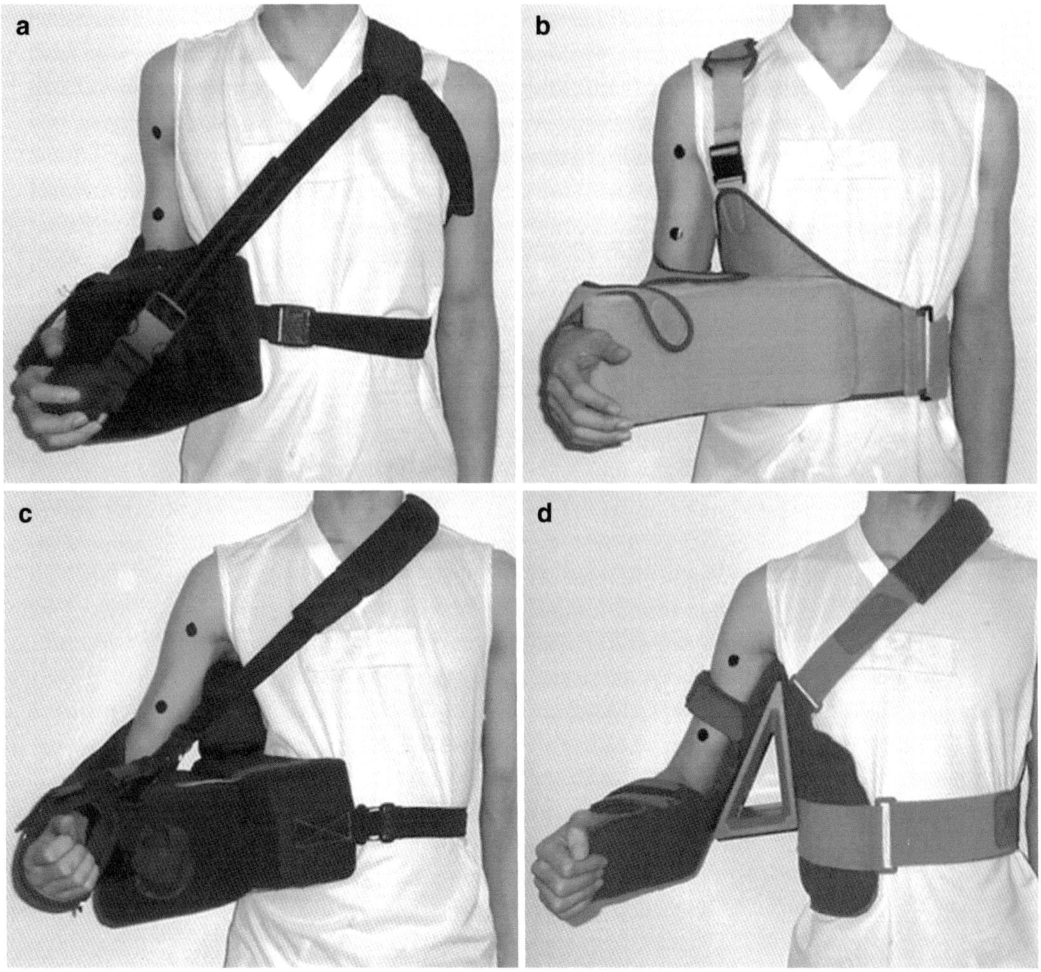

Fig. 17.5 (**a**) and (**b**) are the ER braces, and (**c**) and (**d**) are the A-ER braces [20].

The most up-to-date study in this area is a systematic review, which reports the following outcomes [21]:

- External rotation results in the anatomic reduction of the labrum in only 35% of cases.
- The failure to reduce the labrum may be a contraindication to ER bracing and further studies are proposed to determine whether acute MRI could be used to help identify patients in whom ER achieves labral reduction in a comfortable position.
- This approach also has the advantage of avoiding the significant inconvenience of ER bracing in those the labrum does not reduce and therefore theoretically less likely to benefit.
- It is a novel strategy with significant resource implications and therefore warrants further study.

Motion loss or the delay in motion recovery following arthroscopic shoulder stabilization is clinical problems leading to patient dissatisfaction to a certain degree; however, there exist no agreement upon which position is optimal for immobilization after surgery. **It is** unknown whether the position for shoulder immobilization has an effect on motion and functional recovery. In a study investigating the effect of external rotation bracing on motion and function, it was shown that ER bracing performed following arthroscopic shoulder stabilization has a relationship with a predictable ROM recovery and improvement in functional score [22].

External rotation shoulder braces have often been used in many shoulder problems, such as shoulder dislocations and Bancart lesions. Unfortunately, these are off-the-shelf braces with high costs. For example, the study mentioned above was published by Hatta et al., and used the following four braces: (1): the UltraSling ER with a 15° wedge (DonJoy, Vista, CA, USA); (2): the Shoulder Brace ER (Alcare, Tokyo, Japan); (3): the Össur SmartSling with axilla pillow (Össur, Reykjavik, Iceland); and (4): the Omo Immobil with shoulder positioning at 30° abduction and 30° external rotation (Otto Bock, Duderstadt, Germany) [20]. These are all well known expensive brands.

In recent years, a group of researchers in the Detroit Medical Center has been working on a low-cost alternative of external rotation shoulder brace for the treatment of acute shoulder dislocations. The low cost external rotation shoulder brace is therefore a more affordable option for the uninsured patient presenting with acute shoulder dislocation [23]. In Turkey, these braces should be fabricated in the same methods in order to augment the accessibility of the product for an appropriate treatment.

In the classical **Bankart Lesion**, there is avulsion of the antero-inferior labrum from the underlying glenoid fossa, and displacement and disruption of the periosteum of the scapula. In 1906, Perthes first described a lesion of the labrum in which there was an incomplete avulsion of its antero-inferior aspect with medial stripping of the periosteum, which remained intact. This lesion is now considered to be a variant of the Bankart lesion [19]. Seybold et al. used MRI to determine the effectiveness differences between classical Bankart lesions and Perthes lesions in terms of positioning (external rotation) with regard to the reduction in the labrum [24]. They found that external rotation was more effective in Perthes lesions, and it has the greatest effect when there was little or no deformation of the anterior labroligamentous structures. They also found that the incidence of Perthes and classical Bancart lesions was equal in their patients with primary traumatic dislocations [19].

Especially for the people who are involved in sports containing overhead movements, dislocations in the anterior glenohumeral joints may be troublesome. Braces that are used in glenohumeral joint stability are meant to protect the shoulder against repeating dislocation via setting a limitation for glenohumeral abduction and external rotation. Weise et al. investigated the effects of shoulder stability braces for limiting active and passive shoulder abduction and external rotation in football players. They compared the Denison and Duke Wyre harness with the Sawa shoulder brace. The Sawa shoulder brace was found to be most effective for the purpose of limiting abduction and external rotation during active and passive physiologic loading of the glenohumeral joint [25].

Rotator Cuff Problems

Shoulder abduction slings are frequently used for immobilization following rotator cuff surgeries. Shoulder abduction slings lower the pain by immobilization and boost the recovery. Abduction slings are made of cotton and/or other soft fabrics and they consist of an arm sling as well as shoulder and body straps. The weight of the arm is entirely on the shoulder strap, which also causes a substantial amount of pressure to the cervical region. The carotid sinus is a dilated area the base of the internal carotid just superior to the bifurcation of the common carotid which is located on either side of the neck at about the level of the superior border of thyroid cartilage. The aforementioned zone on which the shoulder strap applies pressure is where the carotid sinus is located (Fig. 17.6, [26]). The braces which are used in this study are shown in Fig. 17.6 [26].

Canbora et al. investigated the cardiovascular effects of the abduction shoulder sling in elderly patients who underwent rotator cuff surgery. They reported that abduction shoulder sling may trigger carotid hypersensitivity syndrome in short-necked and obese patients by exerting mechanical stimulation to the carotid sinus. Carotid hypersensitivity syndrome should be kept in mind in patients who present dizziness, presyncope, and palpitation during the postoperative period [26].

After many shoulder surgeries, such as rotator cuff repair, the shoulder is generally immobilized with braces as mentioned previously. Using the brace has always the potential of disuse muscle atrophy. Alenabi et al. reported that horizontal support of elbow and wrist flexion and extension activates the rotator cuff muscles minimally and thereby prevent other disorders that may occur in other muscular structures [27]. In addition, Alenabi et al. added in another study that possibly the rotator cuff muscles are minimally activated by elbow, wrist, and finger movements with the immobilization of the shoulder by a brace.

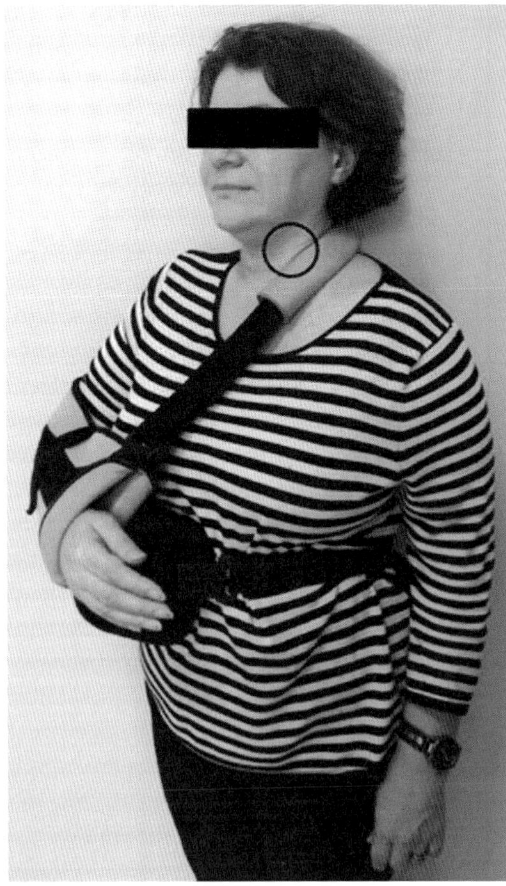

Fig. 17.6 The strap of the brace was applied pressure on carotid sinus. Reprinted with permission from Canbora, K., Kose, O., Gurkan, U. et al. Arch Orthop Trauma Surg (2013) 133: 1557. doi:10.1007/s00402-013-1840-4

Therefore we could recommend elbow, wrist, and finger movements in order to minimize disuse atrophy in shoulder girdle muscles after shoulder immobilization with brace [28].

Lee et al. defines round-shoulder posture as protraction, downward rotation, and anterior inclination of scapula position along with increased cervical lordosis and upper thoracic kyphosis. They recommended stretching exercises for the pectoralis major as well as a shoulder brace to cope with problems coming up with round-shoulder posture, such as altered scapular kinematics and muscle imbalance. Also, they emphasized posterior tilting exercise after pectoral is major stretching for eliciting greater lower trapezius muscle activation [29].

Questions

Indications for functional bracing of humeral shaft fractures

A. Closed diaphyseal fractures without marked distraction between the fragments
B. Closed fractures associated with initial radial nerve palsy similar to those described in the previous category
C. Closed bilateral fractures
D. Open fractures without significant soft-tissue damage

The effectiveness of external rotation in classical Bankart lesions and Perthes lesions with regard to the reduction in the labrum is believed to be:

A. External rotation is more effective in Bankart lesions
B. External rotation was more effective in Perthes lesions
C. External rotation is similarly effective
D. External rotation should be used in Perthes lesions while internal rotation should be used in Bankart lesions

For shoulder dislocations external rotation bracing results in anatomic reduction of the labrum

A. In 5% of cases
B. In 35% of cases
C. In 55% of cases
D. In 95% of cases

References

1. Cole AK, McGrath ML, Harrington SE, Padua DA, Rucinski TJ, Prentice WE. Scapular bracing and älteration of posture and muscle activity in overhead athletes with poor posture. J Athl Train. 2013;48(1):12–24.
2. Kotelnicki JJ, Bote HO, Mitts KG. The management of clavicle fractures. JAAPA 2006;19(9):50, 53–4, 6.
3. Lazarus MD. Fractures of the clavicle. In: Bucholz RW, Heckman JD, editors. Rockwood and Green's fractures in adults. 5th ed. Philadelphia: Lippincott-Wilkins; 2001. p. 1041–78.
4. Stanley D, Trowbridge EA, Norris SH. The mechanism of clavicular fracture. A clinical and biomechanical analysis. J Bone Joint Surg. 1988;70(3):461–4.
5. Allman Jr FL. Fractures and ligamentous injuries of the clavicle and its articulation. J Bone and Joint Surg. 1967;49(4):774–84.
6. Nordqvist A, Petersson CJ, Redlund-Johnell I. Mid-clavicle fractures in adults: end result study after conservative treatment. J Orthop Trauma. 1998;12(8):572–6.
7. Crenshaw Jr AH, Perez EA. Fractures of the shoulder, arm and forearm. In: Canale ST, Beaty JH, editors. Campbell's operative orthopaedics. 11th ed. Philadelphia: Mosby; 2007. p. 3389–98.
8. Lenza M, Belloti JC, Andriolo RB, Faloppa F. Conservative interventions for treating middle third clavicle fractures in adolescents and adults (review). Cochrane Libr 2014;5:1–37
9. Rutgers M, Ring D. Treatment of diaphyseal fracture of humerus using functional brace. J Orthop Trauma. 2006;20:597–601.
10. Sarmiento A, Kinman PB, Galvin EG, et al. Functional bracing of fractures of the shaft of the humerus. J Bone Joint Surg. 1977;59A:596–601.
11. Blafour GW, Mooney V, Ashby ME. Diaphyseal fractures of the humerus treated with a ready-made fracture brace. J Bone Joint Surg. 1982;64A:11–3.
12. Zagorski JB, Latta LL, Zych GA, et al. Diaphyseal fractures of the humerus treated with prefabricated braces. J Bone Joint Surg Am. 1988;70:607–10.
13. Bell MJ, Beauchamp CG, Kellam JK, et al. The results of plating humeral shaft fractures in patients with multiple injuries. J Bone Joint Surg. 1985;67B:293–6.
14. Kapil Mani KC, Gopal Sagar DC, Rijal L, Govinda KC, Shrestha BL. Study on outcome of fracture shaft of the humerus treated non-operatively with a functional brace. Eur J Orthop Surg Traumatol. 2013;23(3):323–8.
15. Sarmiento A, Latta LL. Functional fracture bracing. J Am Acad Orthop Surg. 1999;7(1):66–75.
16. Ali E, Griffiths D, Obi N, Tytherleigh-Strong G, Van Rensburg L. Nonoperative treatment of humeral shaft fractures revisited. J Shoulder Elbow Surg. 2015;24(2):210–4.
17. Adler D, Siekmann H. [Conservative therapy with a brace for periprosthetic humeral fractures. Clinical and radiological results after 19 months]. [Article in German]. Orthopade 2014;43(6):575–81.
18. Whelan DB, Litchfield R, Wambolt E, Dainty KN. External rotation immobilization for primary shoulder dislocation: a randomized controlled trial. Clin Orthop Relat Res. 2014;472(8):2380–6.
19. Finestone A, Milgrom C, Radeva-Petrova DR, Rath E, Barchilon V, Beyth S, Jaber S, Safran O. Bracing in external rotation for traumatic anterior dislocation of the shoulder. J Bone Joint Surg Br. 2009;91(7):918–21.
20. Hatta T, Sano H, Yamamoto N, Itoi E. Immobilizing performances, comfort, and user-friendliness of the shoulder abduction-external rotation braces. Ups J Med Sci. 2013;118(2):105–10.
21. Jordan RW, Saithna A, Old J, MacDonald P. Does external rotation bracing for anterior shoulder dislocation actually result in reduction of the labrum? A systematic review. Am J Sports Med. 2015;43(9):2328–33.

22. Yin B, Levy D, Meadows M, Moen T, Gorroochurn P, Cadet ER, Levine WN, Ahmad CS. How does external rotation bracing influence motion and functional scores after arthroscopic shoulder stabilization? Clin Orthop Relat Res. 2014;472(8):2389–96.
23. Lacy K, Cooke C, Cooke P, Schupbach J, Vaidya R. Low-cost alternative external rotation shoulder brace and review of treatment in acute shoulder dislocations. West J Emerg Med. 2015; 16(1):114–20.
24. Seybold D, Schliemann B, Heyer CM, Muhr G, Gekle C. Which labral lesion can be best reduced with external rotation of the shoulder after a first-time traumatic anterior shoulder dislocation? Arch Orthop Trauma Surg. 2008;29:318–24.
25. Weise K, Sitler MR, Tierney R, Swanik KA. Effectiveness of Glenohumeral-Joint Stability Braces in Limiting Active and Passive Shoulder Range of Motion in Collegiate Football Players. J Athl Train. 2004;39(2):151–55.
26. Canbora K, Kose O, Gurkan U, Polat A, Erdem S, Haklar U. Cardiovascular effects of abduction shoulder sling in elderly patients; is it really safe? Arch Orthop Trauma Surg. 2013;133(11):1557–60.
27. Alenabi T, Jackson M, Tetreault P, Begon M. Electromyographic activity in the shoulder musculature during resistance training exercises of the ipsilateral upper limb while wearing a shoulder orthosis. J Shoulder Elbow Surg. 2014;23:140–48.
28. Alenabi T, Jackson M, Tetreault P, Begon M. Electromyographic activity in the immobilized shoulder musculature during ipsilateral elbow, wrist, and finger movements while wearing a shoulder orthosis. J Shoulder Elbow Surg. 2013;22:1400–07.
29. Lee J, Cynna H, Yoona T, Koa C, Choia W, Choia S, Choi B. The effect of scapular posterior tilt exercise, pectoralis minor stretching, and shoulder brace on scapular alignment and muscles activity in subjects with round-shoulder posture. J Electromyogr and Kinesiol. 2015;25(1):107–14.

Shoulder Rehabilitation

18

Irem Duzgun, Leyla Sumeyye Eraslan, Taha Ibrahim Yildiz, and Serdar Demirci

Due to the fact that the shoulder joint has roles of both stability and mobility, while planning rehabilitation programme these two characteristics must be considered. In different shoulder pathologies primary effected parts could be stabilization or mobilization, however, it should be borne in mind that these are interlinked. Planned and followed physiotherapy approaches should include these two components.

Conservative or surgical treatment approaches can be preferred depending on the shoulder pathology. Although the preferred treatment is conservative in frozen shoulder, impingement syndrome, and Grade I rotator cuff tears; in instabilities surgical treatments are more preferred. However, physiotherapy applied both in conservative and surgical treatments bears utmost importance. Through correct physiotherapy approaches, recurrence of the issue can be prevented by alleviation of the symptoms of patients, increasing functionality and placement of correct biomechanics. For this reason, nature of the pathology and underlying causes should be analyzed well and physiotherapy and rehabilitation programme to be followed should be determined accordingly. In order to be able to do this, it is necessary for the physiotherapist to evaluate the patient very well. The assessments to be conducted in clinic in short;

Pain: This is generally the most frequently observed symptom in shoulder pathologies. It is recommended to assess the pain especially during resting, in activity and at night. The circumstances which patient is suffering from pain, provides us with the information about the pathology and thus physiotherapy approach we need to follow. If the patient suffers from pain at night time, this is an indicator of inflammation and the application to be conducted should avoid effects that would increase inflammation. Pain in resting can also be considered in the same manner. However, if the patient suffers from pain only during an activity, this is considered as more of a mechanical cause and normal movement biomechanics are affected. For successful rehabilitation, source of the abnormal movement should be revealed.

Range of motion: This is an important symptom in the differential diagnosis of the pathology. In assessing joint movement, pain-free active joint movement, active joint movement, and passive joint movement should definitely be evaluated. In impingement syndrome, while there is a decrease observed in joint movement due to pain, there is no limitation in passive joint movement. However, in frozen shoulder, limitation in passive joint motion is among the most significant determinants. In cases when frozen shoulder is developed secondary to impingement syndrome, rotator cuff tear or humerus fracture,

I. Duzgun, P.T., Ph.D. (✉) • L.S. Eraslan, P.T., M.Sc.
T.I. Yildiz, P.T., M.Sc. • S. Demirci, P.T., M.Sc.
Department of Physiotherapy and Rehabilitation, Hacettepe University, Ankara 06100, Turkey
e-mail: iremduzgun@yahoo.com

G. Huri, N.K. Paschos (eds.), *The Shoulder*, Orthopaedic Study Guide Series,
DOI 10.1007/978-3-319-51979-1_18

rehabilitation should primarily be planned bearing in mind frozen shoulder. However, in terms of the evaluation of functionality, active total elevation and active internal rotation assessment should not be overlooked.

Muscle strength: In painful conditions, assessment of the shoulder muscle strength would not produce reliable information. In muscle strength test, the presence of pain in patient would cause determination of muscle strength lower than its normal value. Evaluation of muscle strength following a decrease in pain is of importance in terms of revealing strength imbalance and planning exercise programmes suitable for the conditions.

Assessment of scapular movement: Assessment of scapular movement is important for establishing exercises to be prescribed. In clinic, scapular movement can be assessed by visually and by Lateral Scapular Slide (Kibler) test [1]. In laboratory environment, 3D analysis systems allow for an objective measurement in the assessment of scapular movement. However, due to the fact that such systems are costly and the assessment takes quite a long time, they are utilized more in scientific studies. Despite that the lateral scapular slide test can easily be conducted in clinic, varying results have been reported so far on it's reliability [1, 2]. It may especially be preferred in unilateral scapular dyskinesia to have an idea. Test is conducted in three different positions. In the first position, distance between the inferior angle of scapula and columna vertebralis is measured by a measuring tape when the patient is in standing position and arms are on the side of body. The distance between the inferior angle of scapula and columna vertebralis is also assessed and compared with the healthy side for second position the arms are on hips and for the third position the arm is at 90° abduction and internal rotation.

Palpation: This is important for evaluating the sensitivity of soft tissues. Especially assessing the tenderness of rotator cuff muscles, long head of biceps brachii, pectoralis minor and posterior capsule with palpation is important for manual therapy methods to be used.

Functional activity level: How much of activities of daily living (ADLs) can patients perform is actually among the most important indicators as to the success of the therapy. For this, various surveys are being used. Among the most commonly used of these are DASH-T [3], ASES patient survey [4], Constant-Murley score [5], SPADI [6] Penn Shoulder Score [7] etc.

In the light of these assessments, appropriate physiotherapy programme is planned.

One of the primary targets of the treatment is to reduce pain. To this end, various physiotherapy applications may be adopted. Hot/cold pack applications, electrotherapy modalities, and manual therapy are frequently preferred. If the patient suffers from pain especially at night, application of cold should be preferred in order to reduce the inflammation. Other than this, cold should be preferred on patients in third stage of frozen shoulder because of the applications would cause loading on the joint, even if they don't suffer pain at night. In previous studies, effects of hot applications in the treatment of frozen shoulder were manifested [8]. However, in cases which inflammation indication is present, cold applications are recommended [9]. If the shoulder pain of your patient develops secondary to strain in interscapular muscles, hot applications on this region would be beneficial.

In pain control, TENS application is among the effective electrotherapy methods. While the previous studies showed that the application of ultrasound in patients with impingement syndrome is not effective, laser applications were manifested to have an effect in the short term [10].

Of the manual therapy approaches, deep friction massage is believed to be effective in relieving the pain secondarily by decreasing the perception of pain and secondary to relieving the soft tissue tension [11].

Increasing the joint movement is the second target of physiotherapy programmes. However, source of movement limitation must be analyzed very well. Since, in impingement syndrome, there would be a limitation in movement due to pain, relieving pain would provide an increase in joint movement automatically. In such patients, instead of burdening with exercises to increase joint movement, relieving the pain and assisting with regulating biomechanics would be much more reasonable. However, stretching exercises and mobilization techniques would be beneficial in cases of which limitation exists in passive joint movement caused by not only pain but also on thickening and shortening of joint capsule, such as frozen shoulder.

Among the most effective physiotherapy applications in increasing joint movement are exercise and mobilization techniques [12–14]. It would be beneficial to start physiotherapy and rehabilitation applications with scapular mobilization techniques, manual posterior capsule and pectoralis minor stretching. It is also believed that relieving tension of the surrounding soft tissue with soft tissues mobilization techniques would be effective in increasing range of motion.

Our next target after suppressing the pain and increasing range of motion, should be correcting the muscular imbalance. It would be beneficial to begin strengthening exercises on surrounding muscles of scapula. It should be borne in mind that scapula is the foundation of upper extremity movements. Planning the rehabilitation on a non-robust foundation would lower the chance of success.

Among the important points of the exercise programme to be recommended is to correct the muscle imbalance between upper trapezius and its middle and lower parts [15, 16]. Generally, patients with affected shoulders try to compensate the movement with the over-activation of the upper trapezius especially in elevation during arm movements. This movement must absolutely be blocked in rehabilitation. Exercises should be oriented towards increasing middle and lower trapezius trapezius without activating the upper part. Especially the middle trapezius, serratus anterior and rhomboid muscles bear importance in enabling external and upward rotation of scapula along with it's medial stabilization. The lower trapezius has a duty in enabling the posterior tilt of scapula along with inferior stabilization. Strengthening of these muscles is important in providing correct biomechanics. Scapular retraction exercises conducted without activating the upper trapezius could be used to this end (Fig. 18.1a, b).

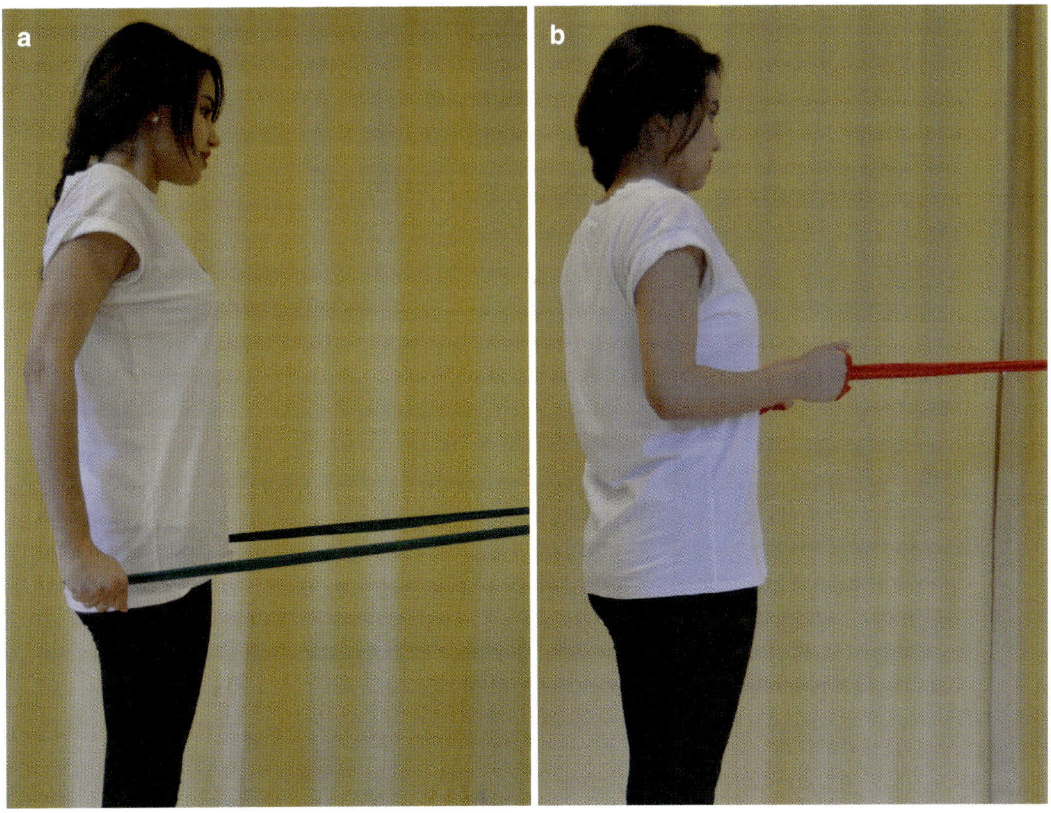

Fig. 18.1 (**a**) Scapular retraction with elbows in extension; (**b**) scapular retraction with elbows in flexion

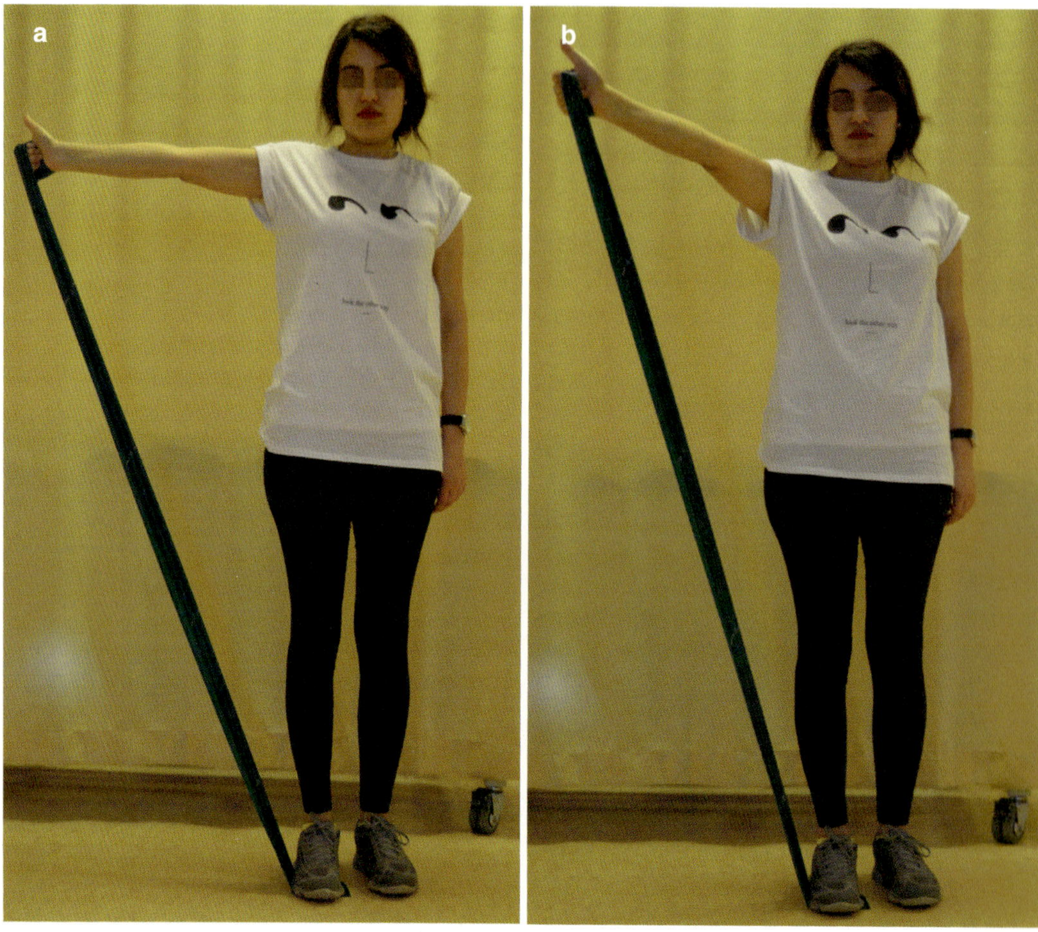

Fig. 18.2 (**a**) Shoulder abduction with theraband; (**b**) elevation in scapular plane with theraband

It is important to provide pain-free active joint motion for strengthening of the muscles surrounding glenohumeral joint. It should be ensured not to cause an increase in pain especially during resistance exercises prescribed for the strengthening of deltoid and rotator cuff muscles. For strengthening, exercises with weights or theraband exercises can be preferred (Fig. 18.2a, b).

Studies showed that proprioception is affected following injury [17–19]. Retraining of proprioception is quite important in rehabilitation. Especially it is a must in rehabilitation of patients with instability. Actually, it is known that all the movements causes a proprioceptive input. However, if we are aiming to retraining of proprioception, it is accepted the need of a sensory bombardment of contractile and non-contractile tissues (Fig. 18.3a–c).

Physiotherapy and Rehabilitation in Various Shoulder Pathologies

Conservative Physiotherapy and Rehabilitation

Scapular Dyskinesia

In order to be successful in the treatment of scapular dyskinesia, anatomic characteristics must be optimal. Before planning the rehabilitation, a good assessment is an absolute necessity and the treatment must be planned according to the underlying cause.

While, in the development of scapular dyskinesia, a loss of flexibility occurs in certain tissues, some experience a decrease in strength. Fundamentally, eliminating these two issues would increase the success of rehabilitation.

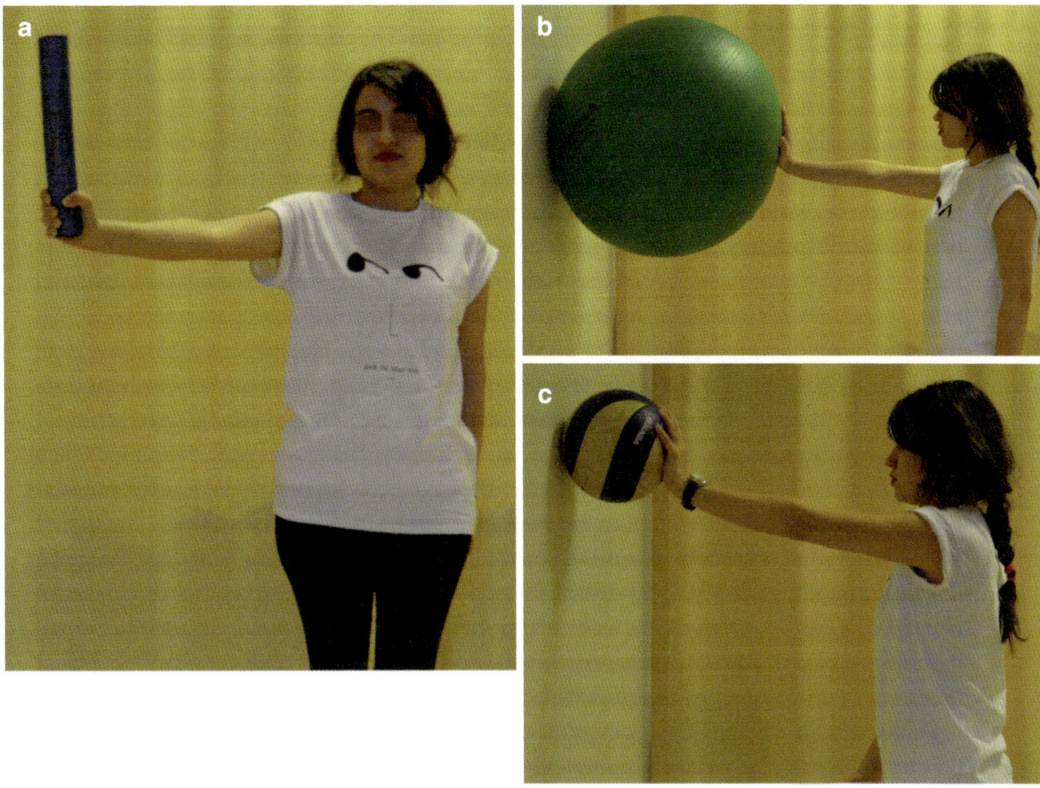

Fig. 18.3 (**a–c**) Proprioceptive exercises

Advancing from proximal to distal is recommended in scapular dyskinesia rehabilitation [20]. Primary aim of rehabilitation is to ensure an optimal scapular position, and that is posterior tilt, external rotation, and upward rotation during elevation. Ensuring body stabilization would assist in enabling proximal control in the three dimensional control of scapular movements. Especially the major muscles of body and lower extremity should be integrated into the rehabilitation [21]. While hip and body flexion help in facilitating scapular protraction, body rotation and hip and body extension help in facilitating scapular retraction [20]. Deficits in strength or flexibility of such proximal segments as body, pelvis, and hip must absolutely be considered [20].

Serratus anterior is the most important muscle in external rotation of scapula. Lower trapezius muscle plays a role in enabling the stabilization of scapula. Scapular stabilization protocols should focus on re-training of these muscles. Progress should be made from short *"arc"* kinetic chain exercises towards long *"arc"* exercises.

In order to strengthen rotator cuff muscles, scapula should be stabilized, which is in retraction position. After accomplishing scapular control in shoulder rehabilitation, the next aim should be rotator cuff. For this closed kinetic chain and co-contractions of shoulder muscles may be used [21].

Reducing the Loss of Flexibility

It would be beneficial to begin physiotherapy and rehabilitation applications with scapular mobilization techniques, manual posterior capsule and pectoralis minor stretchings. Also, it is believed that relieving the tension of the surrounding soft tissues with soft tissue mobilization techniques is effective in increasing the range of joint motion.

Loss of flexibility in soft tissues around scapula is correlated with abnormal scapular position. Especially increasing the flexibility of pectoralis minor, posterior capsule, and levator scapula is an important parameter of scapular rehabilitation.

Manual posterior capsule stretching is among important applications in shoulder rehabilitation. In cases which posterior capsule is stretched, scapula and humerus move as an unit. Trying to increase glenohumeral joint movement without restoring posterior capsule flexibility would cause repositioning of the scapula to abnormal lateral position, thus surrounding tissues would be loaded with an unnecessary stress. Posterior capsule stretching can be prescribed as home exercises of *"sleeper stretch"* (Fig. 18.4) and as cross body exercises (Fig. 18.5) or it can be applied as manual stretching (Fig. 18.6).

Soft tissue mobilization techniques and stretching exercises can be used in releasing pectoralis minor muscle. Various exercises have been defined that are effective in increasing the length of pectoralis minor [22, 23].

Unilateral corner stretch (shoulder in 90° abduction and external rotation in passive horizontal abduction) was shown to be more effective than manual stretch while sitting, and manual stretch while lying on back [24]. However, these positions are painful especially at the early stages of shoulder problems. Before prescribing stretching exercises, manual stretching of pectoralis minor is effective (Figs. 18.7 and 18.8).

It is believed that stretching levator scapula manually and with exercise is effective in both regulating scapular mechanics and in relieving neck pain (Fig. 18.9).

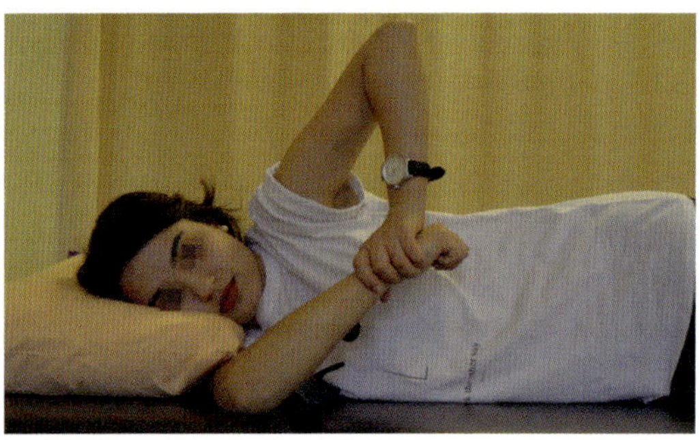

Fig. 18.4 "Sleeper stretch"

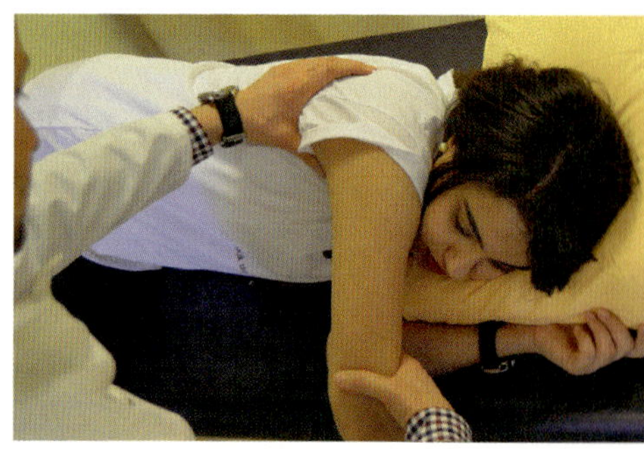

Fig. 18.6 Manual posterior capsule stretching

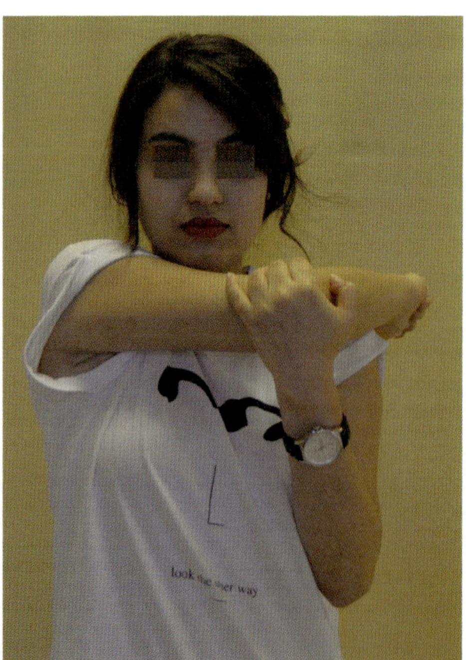

Fig. 18.5 Cross body stretching

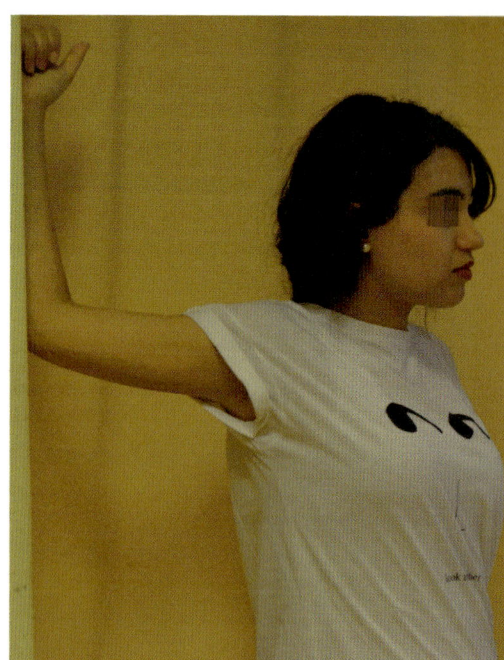

Fig. 18.7 Unilateral corner stretch

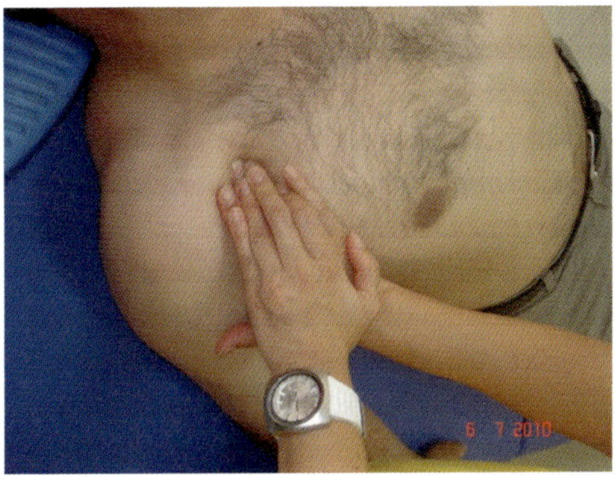

Fig. 18.8 Manual pectoralis minor releasing

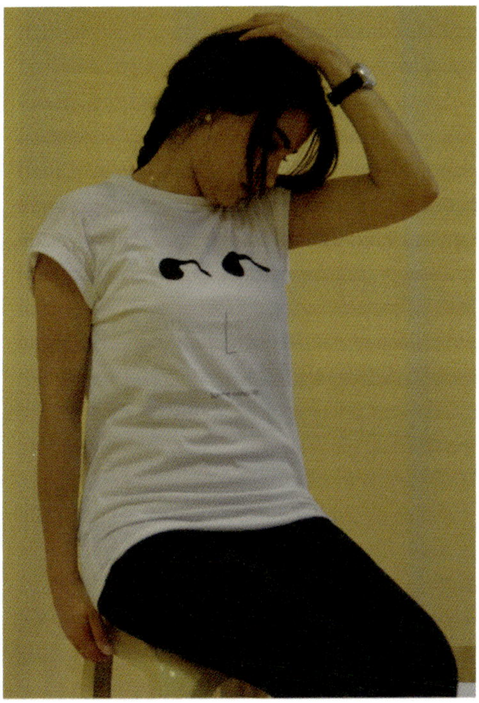

Fig. 18.9 Levator scapula stretching

Reducing Loss of Strength

Our next target following stretching shortened tissues should be correcting muscle strength imbalance. In strengthening exercises, it would be beneficial to primarily begin from muscles surrounding scapula. It must be borne in mind that scapula is the foundation of upper extremity movements. Planning rehabilitation on a foundation that is not robust would lower the chance of success.

Phase 1: Conscious Muscle Control

Muscle performance problems arise from neuromuscular deficit (loss of co-contraction or couples) or strength deficit. While serratus anterior, middle and lower trapezius muscles weaken the activity of upper trapezius muscle increases. Therefore, one of the important points of exercise programme to be prescribed is to correct the muscle imbalance between the upper trapezius and its middle and lower parts [16].

In general, patients with affected shoulders try to compensate with excessive activation of upper trapezius during arm movements especially in elevation. Such movement must absolutely be blocked during rehabilitation. While doing the exercises, they should be towards increasing the activity of middle and lower parts of trapezius without activating the upper part. Especially the middle trapezius muscle, serratus anterior and rhomboid muscles bear importance in ensuring external rotation of scapula and its upward rotation along with medial stabilization of scapula. Lower trapezius has a role in ensuring the posterior tilt of scapula along with inferior stabilization. Strengthening of these muscles is crucial in establishing the correct biomechanics. Scapular retraction exercises conducted without activating the upper trapezius can be used for this purpose (Fig. 18.1a, b).

Taping is among the methods used to ensure correct scapular movements. In individuals with "*Impingement*" syndrome, while there are studies showing that upper trapezius activation is reduced and lower trapezius activation is increased by scapular taping [8–10] (Fig. 18.10), there are also studies that report just the opposite, that it does not constitute a change [25] and that it even inhibits lower trapezius [26]. What is generally accepted is

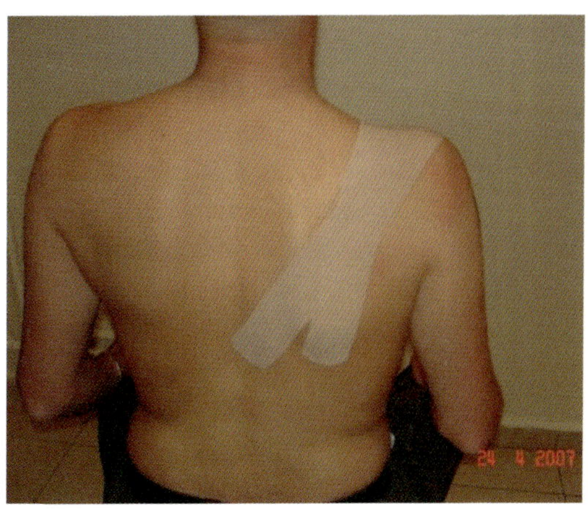

Fig. 18.10 Scapular taping

that it reduces the upper trapezius activity. Through this effect, it is believed to assist in correcting the muscle strength imbalance that is aimed in the rehabilitation of shoulder problems. In addition, taping is also believed to be effective in increasing the proprioceptive input [27]. This change may be correlated with ensuring neuromuscular control.

An important approach to adopt in this stage is ensuring correct posture. Scapular movements of posture is effective in creating both shoulder and neck problems. Therefore, ensuring a correct posture would be instrumental in both reduction of symptoms and prevention of the recurrence. Prescribing posture exercises would be influential in reducing such problems and also carrying out all other exercises in correct posture would provide the involvement of body stabilization.

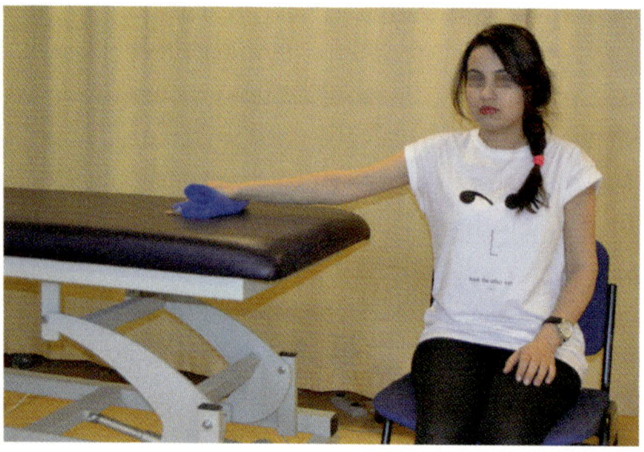

Fig. 18.11 Inferior glide exercise

Phase 2: Ensuring Muscle Control and Strength Necessary for the Activities of Daily Living

In this phase, in scapular muscle training, muscle control and co-contractions or muscle strength should be focused [28].

It would be beneficial to begin scapular co-contraction training with simple movements and to move gradually to harder exercises. In open and closed kinetic chain exercises, exercises done with or without weight bearing may be used for this purpose.

In their electromyographic study, Kibler et al. [29] defined exercises that can be used at the earlier stages of shoulder rehabilitation. *"Low row"*, *"inferior glide"* (Fig. 18.11), *"lawnmover"* (Fig. 18.12a, b), and *"robbery"* (Fig. 18.13a, b)

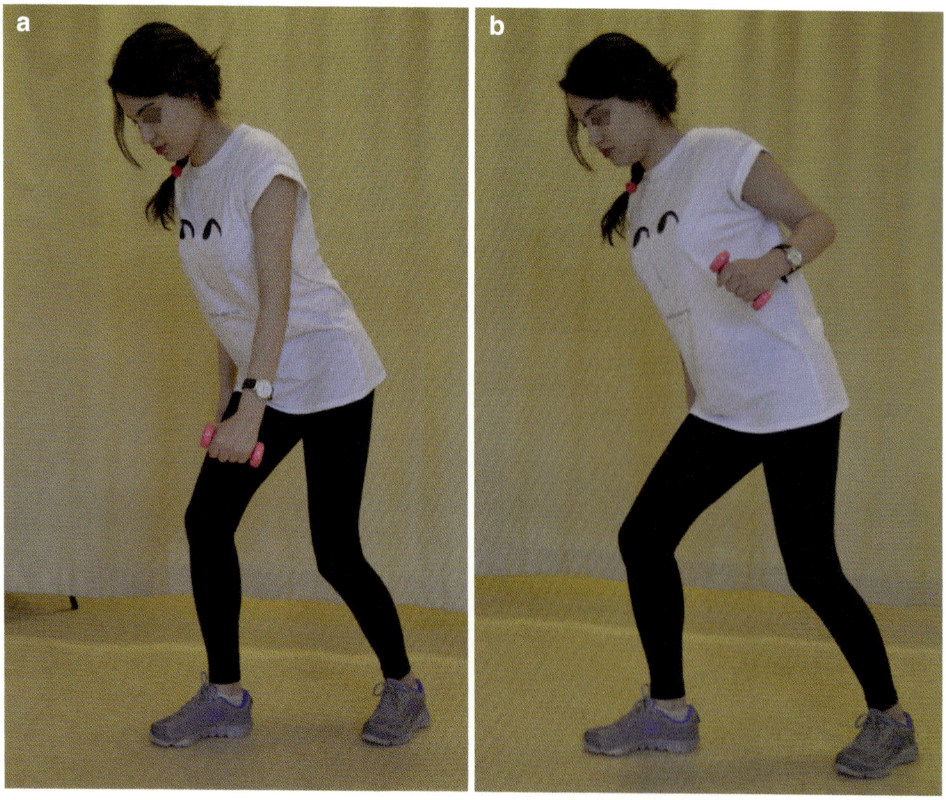

Fig. 18.12 (**a**) Beginning position of Lawnmover exercise; (**b**) ending position of Lawnmover exercise

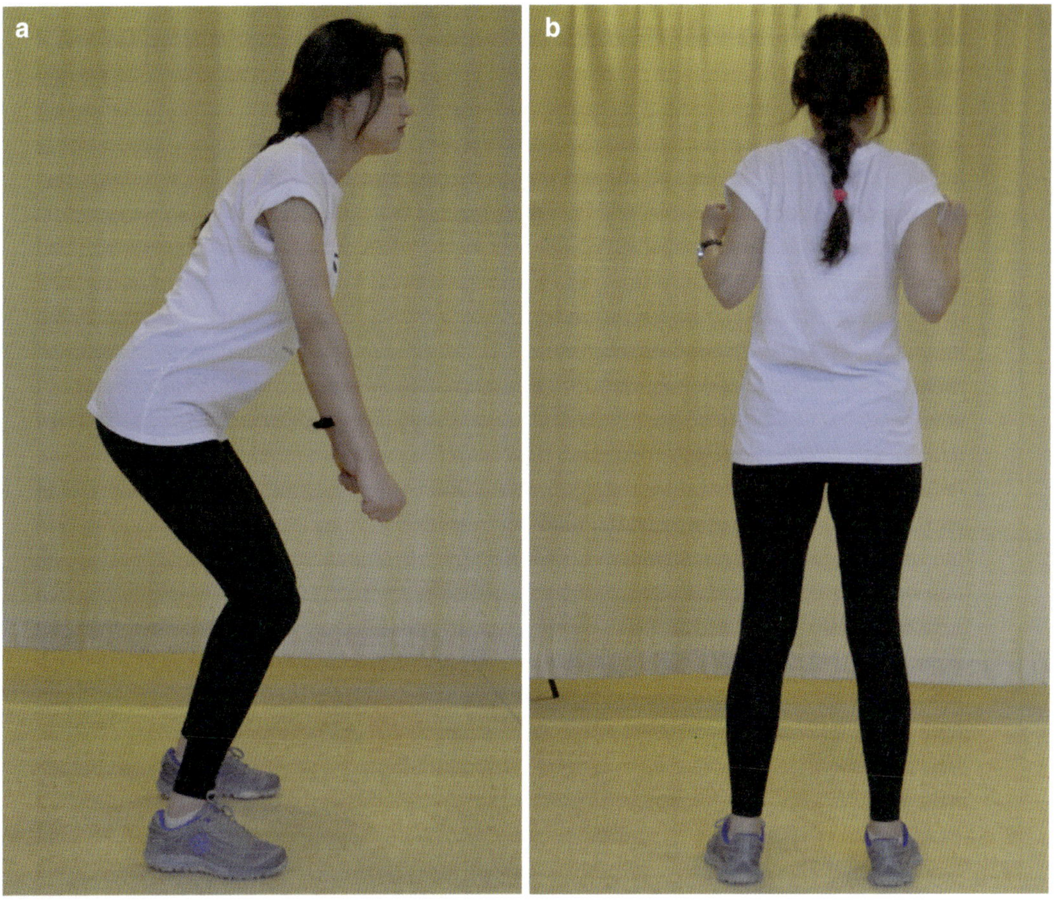

Fig. 18.13 (**a**) Beginning position of Robbery exercise; (**b**) ending position of Robbery exercise

exercises can be utilized to increase the activation of scapula stabilizer muscles during early rehabilitation phase.

Closed kinetic chain exercises are believed to help in increasing dynamic stability of glenohumeral joint, and also the input of intra-articular and periarticular proprioceptors and co-contraction rotator cuff muscles. However, it is important to conduct this training in correct scapular position [30]. In increasing scapular muscle activity it is recommended to begin with scapular retraction exercises with hands on the wall and retraction of scapula Fig. 18.14) and progress through push-ups on wall (Fig. 18.15), on the side of a table (Fig. 18.16), and then to continue with horizontal (Fig. 18.17a, b) scapular retraction and push-up exercises. It is possible to increase the activation of scapular muscles by having a mobile floor (Fig. 18.18) [31–33].

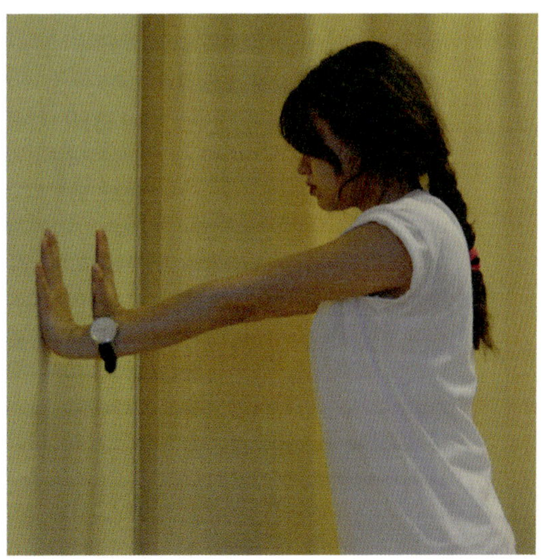

Fig. 18.14 Scapular retraction exercise on wall

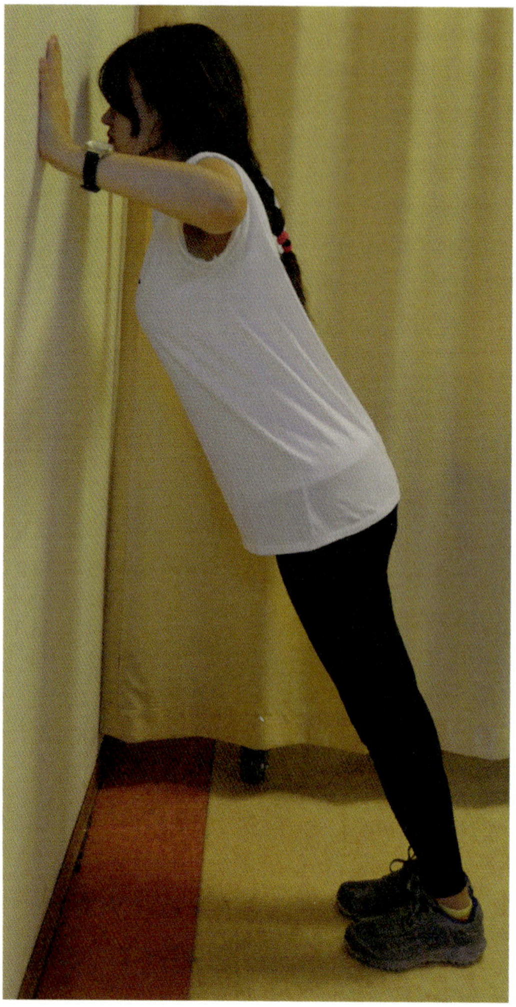

Fig. 18.15 Push-ups o wall

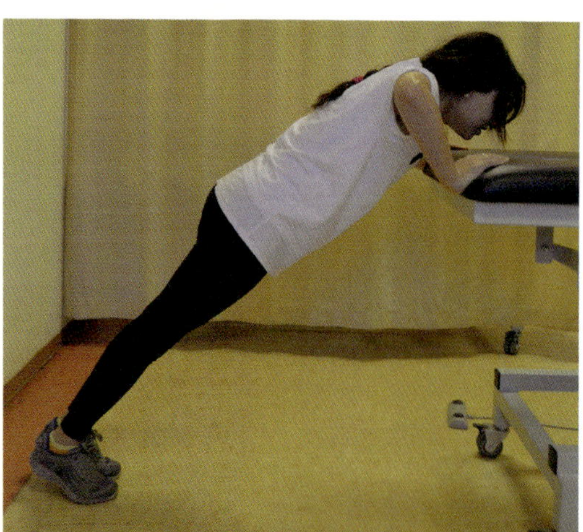

Fig. 18.16 Push-ups on the side of a table

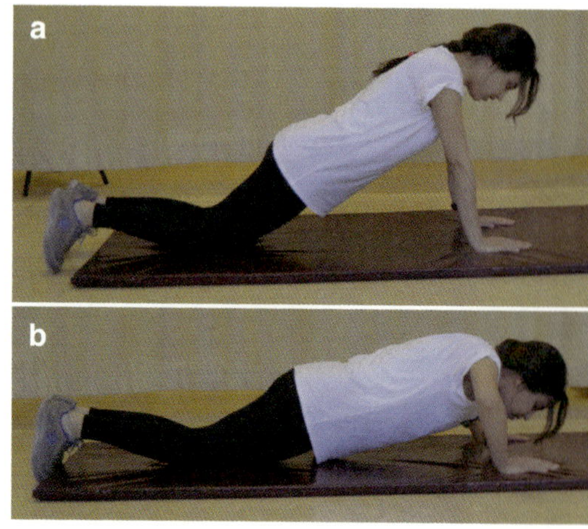

Fig. 18.17 (a) Beginning position of push-ups on knees; (b) ending position of push-ups on knees

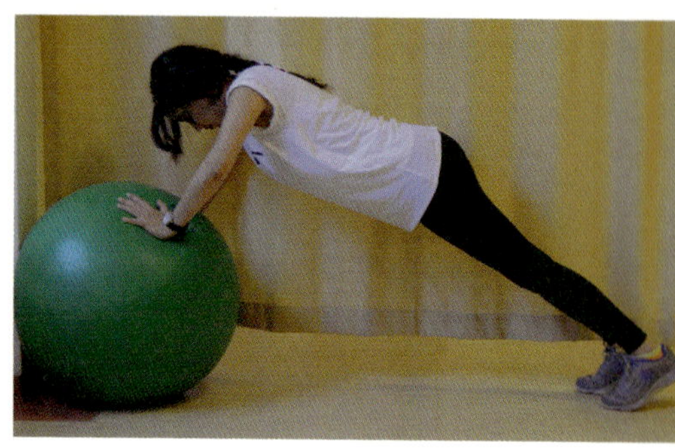

Fig. 18.18 Scapular retraction on ball

At this stage, while trying to increase serratus anterior, mid and lower trapezius muscle activity, avoiding upper trapezius activity continues. Cool et al. [16] notes that the exercises in Fig. 18.19a–d can be used for this purpose.

Phase 3: Scapular Control During Sports Activities

After restoring the strength balance, now the focus should be on the strengthening exercise. In this phase, sports-specific exercises can be used. Among the exercises preferred in this phase there are plyometric exercises such as throwing (Fig. 18.20) eccentric exercises done with the help of elastic resistance bands (Fig. 18.21a, b).

It is important not to overlook the scapulothoracic joint in the rehabilitation of upper extremity problems. It should be borne in mind that correct movement should be done on a sound foundation.

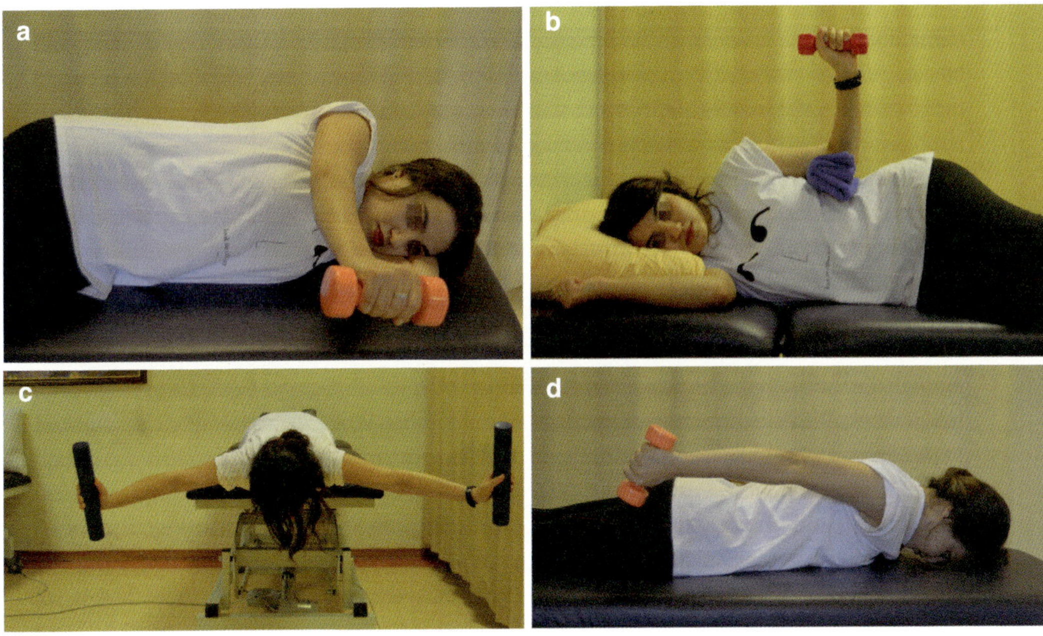

Fig. 18.19 (**a**) Scapular retraction at side lying position; (**b**) external rotation at side lying position; (**c**) scapular retraction exercises on prone; (**d**) shoulder extension on prone

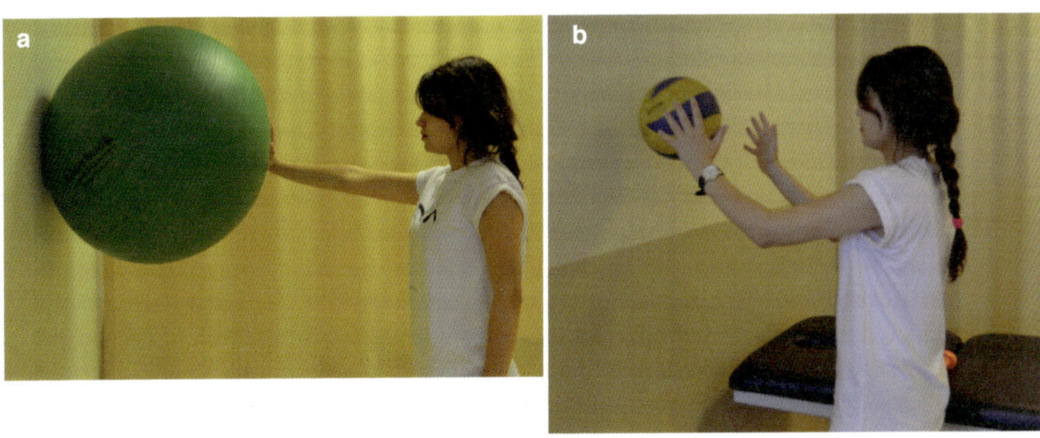

Fig. 18.20 (**a**, **b**) Plyometric exercises

Correct biomechanics are among important factors in preventing injuries.

Subacromial Impingement Syndrome

In impingement syndrome, understanding the underlying mechanisms and included structures enables us to administer more specific treatment approaches in treatment. Rehabilitation is a complex process and in this process we require a comprehensive assessment and multi-faceted treatment programme of pain, scapular dysfunction, and rotator muscle weakness [34]. A well-planned and early-onset treatment programme accelerates individuals' returning to activities and increases functionality. To this end, humeral head depressor mechanism weakness, posterior capsule tightness, and structures tightened in subacromial space contributing to impingement syndrome should be treated [35, 36]. Treatment should include reduction of pain and inflammation, cor-

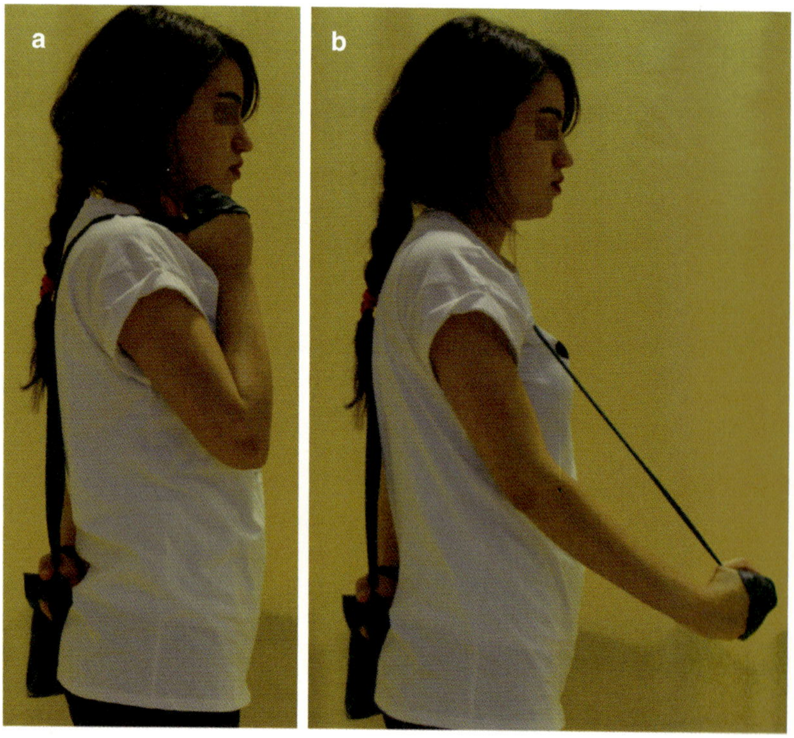

Fig. 18.21 (**a**) Beginning position of Biceps Brachi eccentric training; (**b**) ending position of Biceps Brachi eccentric training

rection of scapular humeral rhythm, increasing strength and endurance, re-education of movement, functional training, ergonomic modifications, and patient training [10].

In subacromial impingement syndrome, patients especially feel pain in overhead activities. Recurring overhead activities increase the damage in tendon and create a basis for inflammation. For this reason, it is necessary to commence the treatment with patient training and activity modification. Instead of expecting a complete limitation of movements from patients, it is important to educate and do modifications in activities that causes symptoms to increase such as limiting overhead activities, preventing elevation of shoulder over 90° and placing the hand under pillow [35]. In order to keep inflammation under control and relieving pain, various physical agents and electrotherapy modalities are utilized. If the patients suffers from pain especially at night, to control the inflammation and to decrease pain and edema (3–4 times a day/15 min) cold applications should be preferred [9]. Cold application is believed to create vasoconstriction effect, decrease metabolic activity and thus reduces inflammation. The most commonly used electrotherapy modalities in clinics are TENS, ultrasound, and laser. While TENS is among the effective electrotherapy applications in controlling the pain, studies showed that laser application is effective in the short term, and ultrasound application is not effective. Another method used in the treatment of subacromial impingement syndrome is acupuncture. However, since literature studies are limited and levels of evidence are low, it is not recommended as a standalone treatment method [10].

The most important aim in the period following keeping pain and inflammation under control is to restore shoulder joint movement within normal biomechanical limits and to ensure strength balance of shoulder girdle muscles. For the treatment, various types of exercises such as stretching exercises, isometric, isotonic, and isokinetic exercises should be selected considering the symptoms of the patient. The prescribed exercises should place the movement pattern of normal joint movement, reduce mechanical subacromial tensions, and include special endurance trainings that would ensure the maintaining of collagen tissue [37, 38].

In this process, decreases in the range of motion can be observed depending on capsular tensions. Measurement of glenohumeral joint internal-external rotation range of motion is an important part of assessment process, and can guide through the management of the treatment period. Posterior capsular tension and posterior rotator cuff muscle tendon unit tightness are defined as factors limiting glenohumeral joint internal rotation [34]. Posterior capsular tension increases translation of humeral head towards the front and upwards during shoulder elevation and causes impingement, and modifies humeral head kinematics. In addition, there are studies that show humeral head shifting to posteriosuperior in excessive posterior capsular tension [34, 39–41]. For this reason, capsular stretching exercises are quite important in regaining posterior capsular flexibility, and should be among the first exercises to think of (Fig. 18.5). Internal rotation stretching can be conducted both by using scapular plane and in various directions in glenohumeral abduction position. In internal rotation stretching, in order to reduce scapular compensation and control the shifting of humeral head towards anterior a hand is placed on humeral head and a posterior force is applied at varying degrees [34]. As home exercises, patients can be prescribed "sleeper stretch" and "cross body stretch". What is needed to be paid attention is the stabilization of scapula in order to increase the effect of stretching (Figs. 18.4 and 18.5).

Among the structures that need to be paid attention to in rehabilitation is the pectoralis minor muscle. Tension of this muscle impairs the shoulder mechanics and causes rounded shoulders and internal rotation of humerus, and narrows down the space where impingement occurs even more [42, 43]. In releasing pectoralis minor muscle, stretching exercises and soft tissue mobilization techniques can be used (Fig. 18.8). If there is a limitation in the joint movements of the patient, mobilization techniques can be utilized. The target joint for mobilization applications is initially the joint where the limitation is present, however, other joints in shoulder girdle (acromioclavicular, sternoclavicular, and scapula thoracic joint), and soft tissues of cervical and thoracic spine should be included in rehabilitation (Fig. 18.22). Studies showed that mobilization combining with exercise is more effective compared to exercise only [10]. In mobilization, patients that indicate having positive shoulder instability should be paid attention. These patients must be assessed well, and this must be taken into consideration for mobilization approaches. Unsuitable stretching and mobilization techniques risk shoulder stabilization and reduces the success of rehabilitation programme [34, 44, 45].

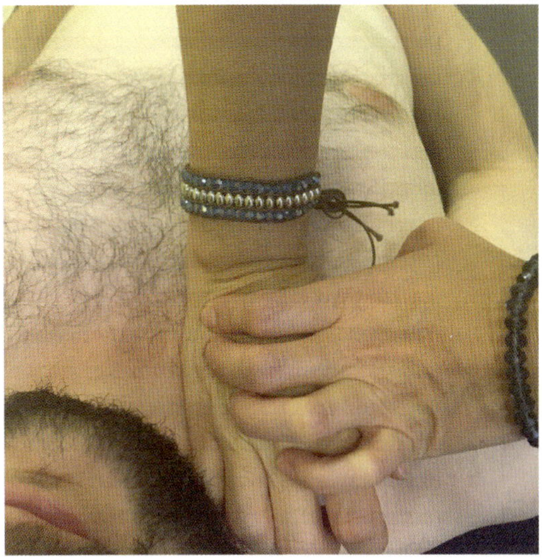

Fig. 18.22 Sternoclavicular joint mobilization

Following decreasing the pain in shoulder joint and gaining a near normal passive flexibility, strengthening exercises should be commenced [36]. Strengthening exercises should initially start with muscles around scapula. In patients with impingement symptoms and rotator cuff pathology, there exist sufficient evidence showing that scapular kinematics are affected [46].

In this problem, called "scapular dyskinesia", generally the upward rotation and posterior tilt of scapula is reduced while internal rotation is increased. Such change in scapular kinematics is observed in dynamic arm movement in addition to resting position. Conducting scapular dyskinesia rehabilitation in the manner described above is instrumental in reducing the symptoms [47–50].

When prescribing strengthening exercises for muscles around glenohumeral joint, not to increase the pain but to reduce subacromial tightness should be targeted. For this reason, strengthening training should be commenced initially with humeral head depressor muscles; and deltoid and supraspinatus muscle should be ignored [51].

In order to strengthen the shoulder internal and external rotator muscles that are humeral head depressors, resistive elastic bands or free weights can be used. During exercise, it must be ensured that deltoid muscle is in a relaxed position. For this reason, patient is asked to place a towel between arm and body and to complete the exercise without dropping the towel (Fig. 18.23a, b).

EMG studies showed that, in patients with shoulder impingement syndrome, a significant decrease occurs in supraspinatus and infraspinatus muscle activity [52]. In order to strengthen supraspinatus, "full can" exercises can be commenced in scapular position at this stage. In this exercise, less deltoid activity occurs compared to "empty can" exercise and it protects subacromial space and decreases upward translation of humerus. External rotation while side lying position is the exercise that creates the highest amount of activity in infraspinatus muscle (Fig. 18.19b) [53]. It can then be proceeded to scapular retraction and horizontal abduction exercises along with external rotation in facedown position. The next step is eccentric strengthening. In this step, movement is conducted against low resistance utilizing weights or exercise elastic bands. In the next stage of rehabilitation, primary elevator muscles of shoulder should be strengthened. For the strengthening, simple weights and elastic bands can be preferred (Fig. 18.24a, b).

In order to increase muscle activity of weak muscles and stimulate proprioception, kinetic chain exercise, proprioceptive neuromuscular facilitation techniques, and diagonal exercises should be included to the rehabilitation program. Scapular protraction, retraction on wall, push-up and press-up exercises can be carried out in various positions also by using other segments of the body. Studies showed that activity in various push-up positions; same side leg extension causes increase of serratus anterior muscle and opposite leg extension causes increase of lower trapezius muscle activity [54]. Plyometric exercises should be gradually proceeded to at the last stage. For the transition, the criteria are pain-free full range of joint motion, absence of sensitivity with palpation, and %80 muscle strength compared to the unaffected side.

Unwanted movements should be controlled during all these exercises, and conducting the exercise in isolation should be assisted. For this reason, exercises should first be done under the control of a physiotherapist, and then should be included in the home exercise programme of the patient.

Rehabilitation programme can be planned as in the example below.

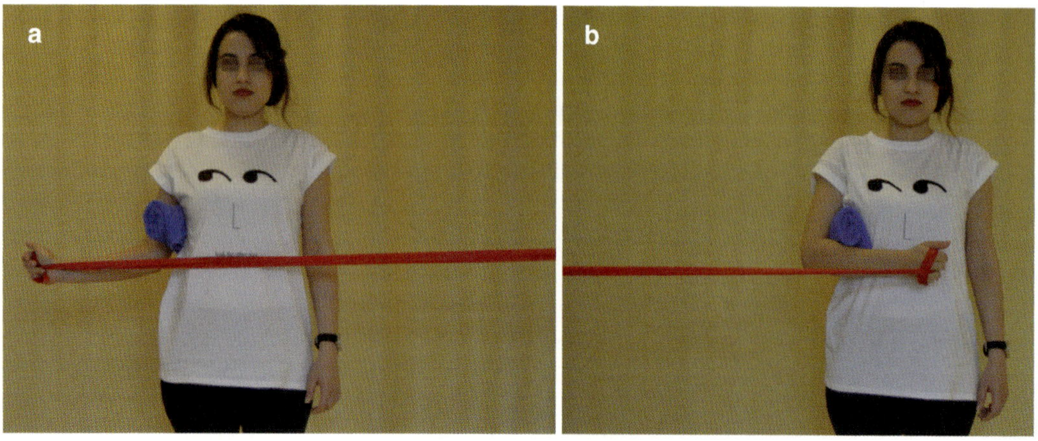

Fig. 18.23 (**a**) Resistive external rotation; (**b**) resistive internal rotation

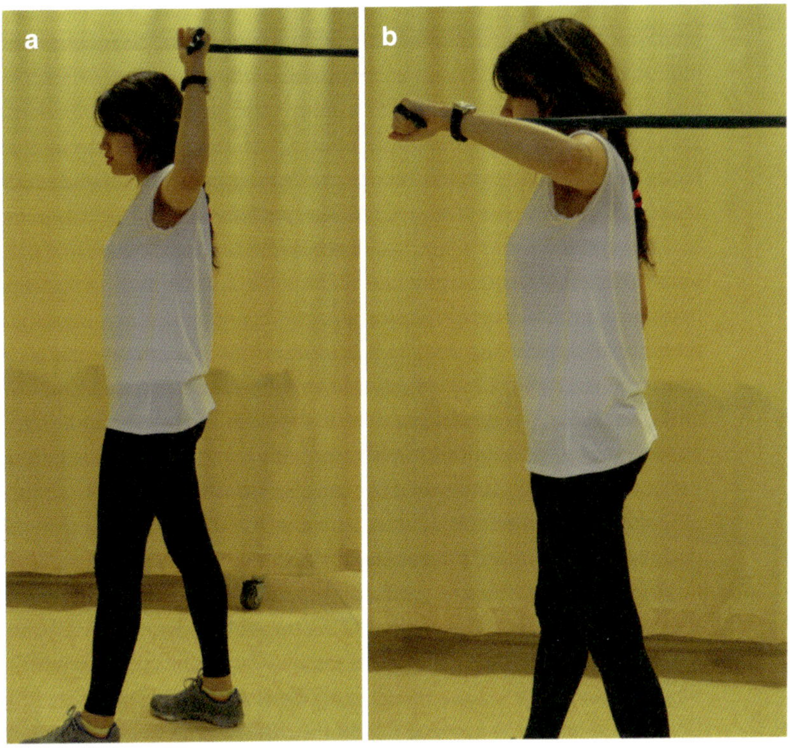

Fig. 18.24 (a, b) Rotator cuff strengthening during elevation

Phase I: Acute Inflammatory Phase

Our goals

- To reduce pain.
- To keep inflammation under control.
- To preserve glenohumeral joint mobility.
- To prevent muscular atrophy.
- To correct posture.
- Patient education.

Rehabilitation

- To limit activities overhead/causing shoulder pain.
- Cold pack application, 3–4 times/day, 15 min.
- Posture exercises.
- Posterior capsule stretching, every hour, 20 s.
- Soft tissue mobilization and manual posterior capsule stretching, one time/week, at the clinic.
- Scapular retraction with elbow in flexion, 4 times/day, 10 repeats.
- Scapular retraction with elbow in extension, 4 times/day, 10 repeats.

Phase II: Subacute Phase

To proceed to this phase, pain and inflammatory symptoms should be reduced, and Phase I rehabilitation should be well tolerated by the patient.

Our goals

- Widening the subacromial space.
- Increasing flexibility.
- Improving neuromuscular control.
- Correction of scapula humeral rhythm.

Rehabilitation

- Phase I exercises continue.
- Scapula protraction retraction exercise with hands on the wall, 4 times/day, 10 repeats.

- Internal/external rotation with shoulder in adduction (with towel between arm and body) and elbow in 90° flexion with elastic exercise band, 4 times/day, 10 repeats.
- Full can exercise with a weight of 0.5 kg (arm elevation in scapular plane), 4 times/day, 10 repeats.
- Scapular retraction in facedown position with 90° horizontal abduction.
- Dynamic hugging exercise with resistive band, 4 times/day, 10 repeats.

Phase III: Functional Phase

To proceed to this phase, pain and impingement symptoms should not be formed in all shoulder movements, there should be an increase in muscle performance, and a good scapular stabilization is necessary.

Our goals

- Increasing strength and endurance of upper extremity.
- Ensuring neuromuscular control all direction.
- Normalizing arthrokinematics of shoulder complex.

Rehabilitation

- Internal, external rotation with resistive band with shoulder at 90° abduction, elbow at 90° flexion, 4 times/day, 10 repeats.
- Shoulder in flexion, abduction with a weight of 0.5 kg, 4 times/day, 10 repeats.
- Diagonal shoulder exercises in PNF patterns with exercise band.
- Perturbation exercises in various positions.
- Plyometric exercises containing throwing programmes can be commenced at the end of this phase.

Frozen Shoulder

The aim of physiotherapy approaches for frozen shoulder is to reduce pain and increase range of joint motion and functionality. Placing correct biomechanics during rehabilitation can prevent recurrence of the problem. For this reason nature of the pathology and underlying causes should be well analyzed and exercises programme must be planned accordingly. In order to be able to do this, it is necessary for the physiotherapist to evaluate the patient very well.

In the light of such assessments, first of all, information about the phase of disease and what shall be carried out should be given to the patient. Informing the patient especially on the fact that patient doing prescribed home exercise programme does affect the success of the treatment. Studies showed that home exercise programs are effective in reducing symptoms [55, 56].

At the early phase of frozen shoulder (Phase 1–2), pain is the most significant problem for patients. At these phase limitation in joint movements is not observed due to capsule but because of pain. For this reason, various physiotherapy applications can be utilized. Especially cold applications, electrotherapy modalities and manual therapy are preferred. If the patient specifically suffers from pain at night, which is frequently observed at this stage, cold application should be preferred in order to reduce inflammation. Other than this, in patients at the third stage of frozen shoulder, treatment modalities would cause loading on the joint cold applications may also be preferred even though the patients do not suffer from pain at night. Studies showed the effects of heat applications in frozen shoulder treatment. Stretching exercises done with deep heat modality especially in the frozen phase were shown to be more effective compared to stretching exercises done with superficial heat modality or standalone stretching exercises [8]. However, in cases that inflammation findings are present, we believe that cold application would be more beneficial. If the shoulder pain of the patient occurs secondary to tension in interscapular muscles, heat to be applied on this region would also be quite beneficial.

Apart from this, TENS can be noted as effective electrotherapy methods for pain control. Along with the TENS application, long term low level stretching exercise were shown to be effective in reducing pain and increasing movement [57]. In a case study, it was reported that analgesic electric stimulation applied on subscapularis muscle breaks pain-muscle protection cycle and that it can increase the range of motion and functional level. During the application, one of the electrodes is placed on segmental innervation of subscapularis muscle (C5-T1), and the other on the belly of muscle [58]. In addition, it was also shown that laser application is effective in reducing pain and thus increasing function [59].

In clinics, various electrotherapy modalities are preferred for reducing symptoms. However, evidence is low in general on the effectiveness of such applications. While a low dose laser therapy for 6 days was found as more effective compared to the placebo group, it was also shown that its application with exercise was more effective than self exercise programme after 4 months [60]. The same review also reported that the level of evidence is low in other electrotherapy modalities. In another study, electroacupuncture and interferential current were compared, however, both groups were also prescribed exercises. They reported that an improvement was present but a difference was absent between the groups. Although, in the study, both types of current were effective in the treatment of frozen shoulder, it is not clear whether the effect shown was produced due to the current type or to exercise [61].

In manual treatment approaches, it is believed that deep friction massage is effective in reducing pain secondarily with relaxing the soft tissue along with the decreasing perception of pain. However, levels of evidence are also low in studies conducted on the subject. In a review study, Glucocorticoid injection is found more effective in terms of pain relief at early phase, and manual therapy could be more effective in the long term but further studies would be necessary [60].

While trying to relieve the pain on one hand, dealing with the reduced range of joint motion is needed on the other. Especially at the first and second phases of frozen shoulder, it is quite troublesome to both reduce the pain and prevent the range of joint motion from decreasing. While resting is recommended to reduce inflammation, joint becoming inactive would cause the limitation to increase. Physiotherapist should be quite careful at this stage. While conducting necessary applications to relieve pain, range of motion exercises should be commenced without causing too much pain. It should be borne in mind that stretching exercises and mobilization techniques would be beneficial in cases with limitation in passive joint movement such as frozen shoulder that is not only due to pain but also to thickening and shortening in joint capsule.

Among the most effective physiotherapy approaches for increasing joint movements are exercise and mobilization techniques. Although many authors and clinicians think that mobilization techniques are effective in reducing pain and increasing range of motion [62–64], sufficient evidence on this issue unfortunately does not exist. In a case series published on seven frozen shoulder patients, Vermullen [63] showed that the end range mobilization technique applied for 3 months was effective. In another study, Vermullen [64] compared mobilization techniques applied in higher and lower intensities, and noted that both groups had improvements but that better results were obtained in the mobilization technique adopted at a higher intensity with a smaller difference. Yang et al. [65] showed that the end range mobilization technique is more effective compared to mobilization applied at mid range In physiotherapy and rehabilitation approaches it would be beneficial to start with scapular mobilization techniques, manual posterior capsule and pectoralis minor stretching. However, it is believed that relieving the tension of the surrounding soft tissue through soft tissue mobilization techniques is effective in increasing the range of motion. In frozen shoulder reduced scapular upward rotation, posterior tilt and external rotation was reported in previous studies [66, 67]. As previously noted, increasing scapular movement through manual therapy methods would be effective in gaining the range of motion.

Thickening in the capsule is the most important problem in frozen shoulder. It was shown in the frozen shoulder that anterior or posterior capsule may be tightened but that more frequently posterior capsule is involved [68]. In cases in which posterior capsule is tense, scapula and humerus act as a whole. Trying to increase glenohumeral joint movement without ensuring posterior capsule flexibility would result in scapula shifting to lateral and this would cause the surrounding tissues to be loaded with excessive stress. Posterior capsule stretching can be prescribed as home exercise, and it should also be added to manual therapy programmes.

As it is the case in other shoulder pathologies, pectoralis minor is among the muscles that need attention in frozen shoulder rehabilitation. Short pectoralis minor is a frequently observed in frozen shoulder. As noted previously, releasing and stretching exercises through manual therapy can be prescribed.

After the surrounding soft tissue is relaxed, and the scapular movements are increased, now glenohumeral joint mobilization techniques can be adopted if there still exists a continuing movement limitation. Today numerous mobilization techniques are being used such as Cyriax, mulligan, Maitland, etc. According to our clinical experiences, if your patient has a pain-related movement limitation as is the case in impingement syndrome, Mulligan's mobilization techniques are quite effective; however, if there is a limitation of movement due to thickening in joint capsule as it is the case in frozen shoulder, Cyriax mobilization techniques are believed to be more effective (Fig. 18.25a, b). It was shown that especially "*end range*" mobilization techniques are effective in gaining joint movements [63].

In a rehabilitation programme, exercise is the most important keypoint of a physiotherapist to increase the range of joint motion in addition to manual therapy methods. Patients doing the exercises both in the clinic and as a home programme will increase the success of the treatment. In literature, there are studies showing the effectiveness of exercise.

Stretching exercises occupies an important place in rehabilitation. Muscles are attempted to relax through manual therapy must absolutely be supported by stretching exercises. However, stretching at a correct intensity would affect the success of the treatment [69]. Intensity of the stretching can be determined according to the irritability classification. In patients that are highly irritated, stretching exercises at lower intensity and for shorter periods would be sufficient to reduce pain, decrease muscle spasm, and increase range of motion by stimulating joint

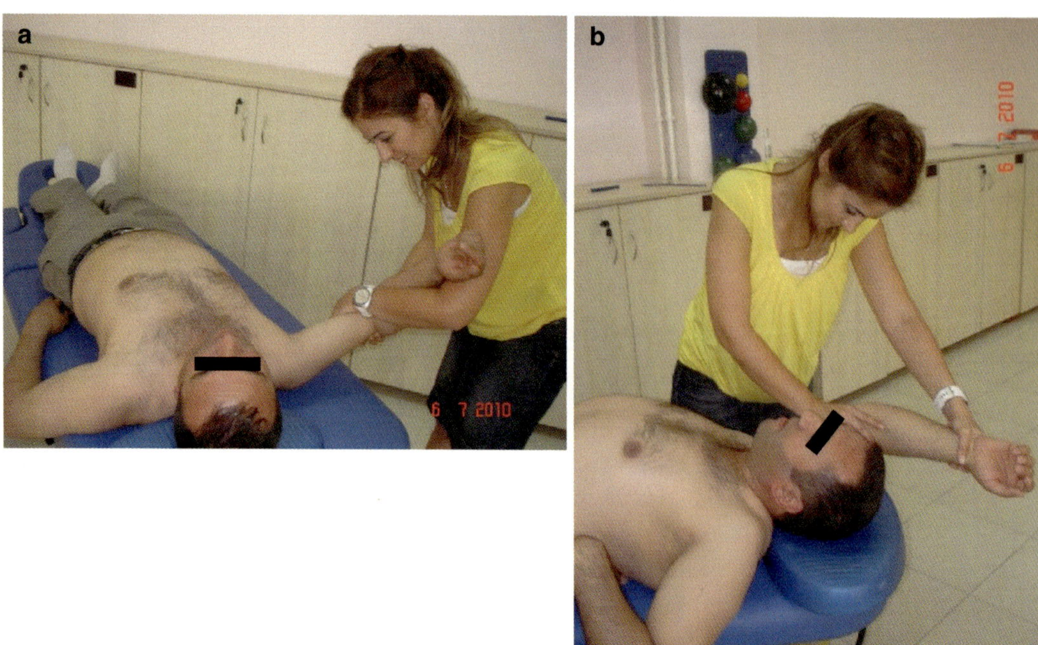

Fig. 18.25 Cyriax mobilization techniques (**a**) abduction during traction; (**b**) passive shoulder flexion

receptors [70]. At this point, stretches should be between 1 and 5 s and within the range of pain-free joint movement. Aggressive stretches done during this period may cause the extension of such period. When level of irritability of patients is decreased, it is possible to increase the intensity of stretches. It should be borne in mind that in this period, the tissue is in *"remodelling"* phase and it becomes stronger with collagen synthesis and increase of other extracellular components by the applied eccentric loading [71, 72].

Especially posterior capsule (Figs. 18.4 and 18.5), anterior capsule (Fig. 18.26), upper trapezius (Fig. 18.27), and pectoralis minor stretching exercises are recommended. In addition, latissimus dorsi muscle must not be forgotten. This muscle is responsible for shoulder internal rotation. Tightness of this muscle would affect the range of joint motion. Latissimus dorsi stretching exercise is effective in increasing the range of motion [73].

Exercises done by using the body weight at the edge of a table are quite effective in increasing the range of motion (Fig. 18.28a, b). Finger ladder exercise are frequently preferred in clinics. However, when this exercise is prescribed, attention must be paid. Many patients resort to hyperextension in lumbar region in order to reach further. When this exercise is done frequently in this position, it may cause back pain.

In some cases, in patient that continue to have a long-term range of motion limitation, they may not be able to use their arms comfortably in their activities of daily living even though the passive range of joint motion increases. The reason for this is lack of sufficient muscle strength against gravity. At this stage, exercises with active assistance should be preferred. *"Wand"* exercises are among the exercises to be prescribed for this purpose. It would be possible to increase active range of motion through active repetitive contractions by keeping the arm in the position following raising the arm with the help of a walking stick and stopping the assistance of the walking stick at varying angles (Fig. 18.29).

Our next goal following the decreasing the pain and increasing the range of joint motion

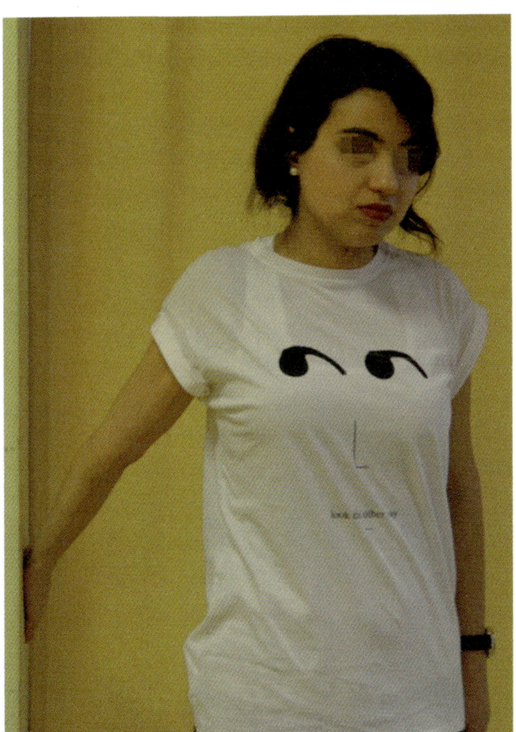

Fig. 18.26 Anterior capsule stretching

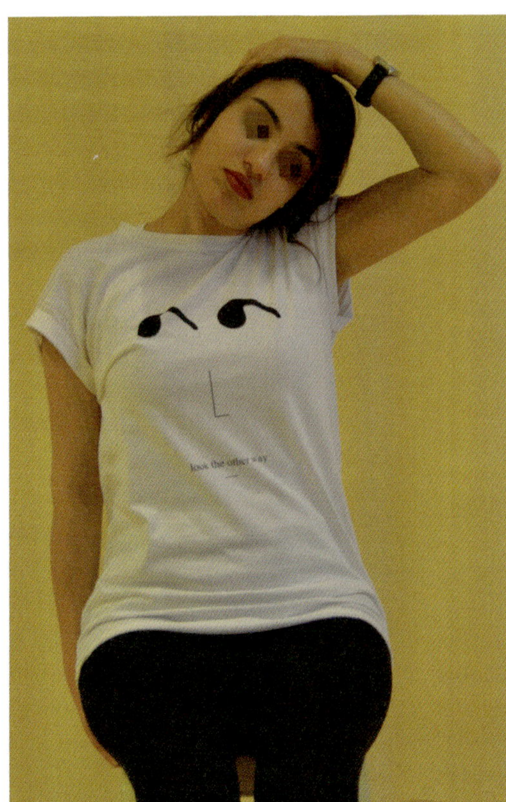

Fig. 18.27 Upper trapezius stretching

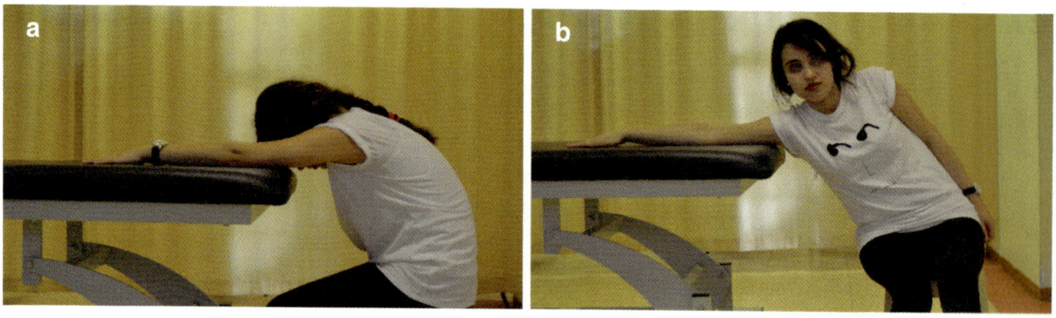

Fig. 18.28 (**a**) Flexion stretching at the edge of a table; (**b**) abduction stretching at the edge of a table

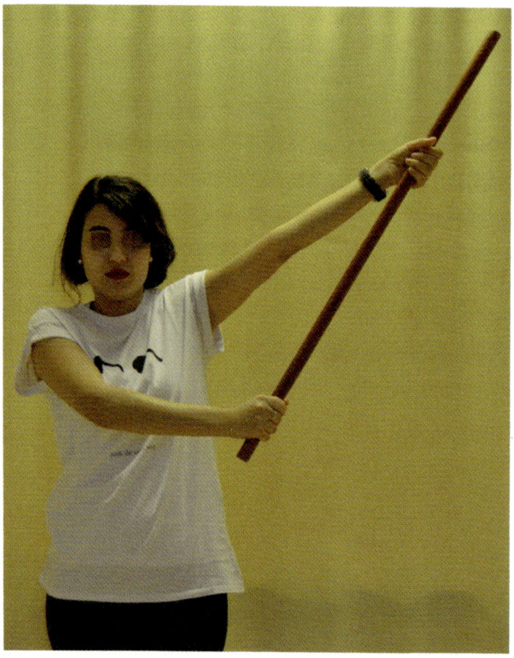

Fig. 18.29 "*Wand*" exercises

should be to correct the strength imbalance. As with the other shoulder pathologies, it would be accurate to start strengthening exercises from the muscles surrounding scapula and then move on to muscles surrounding the shoulder.

Proprioceptive exercises should also be prescribed in the rehabilitation programme. Closed kinetic chain exercises are believed to be effective in increasing the proprioceptive input both through stress loading on joint capsule and through forming co-contractions. Various sensory inputs can be ensured through different platforms used in these exercises (Fig. 18.30).

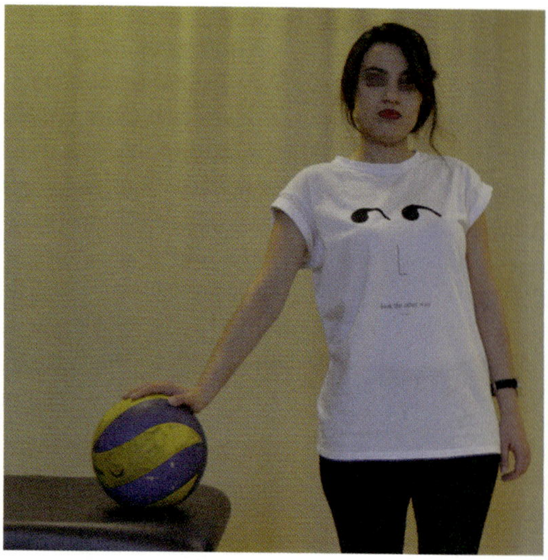

Fig. 18.30 Scapular clock exercise

Instabilities

In shoulder instability, it is important to fully understand the pathophysiology occurring in glenohumeral joint in order to plan a rehabilitation programme. Laxity increase in glenohumeral joint capsule, impairment of the integrity of joint capsule and glenohumeral ligaments, glenoid bone loss, deformities occurring on the longer head of the biceps muscle in SLAP lesions should be assessed well and appropriate approach must be selected.

In previous studies, it was reported that while planning a rehabilitation programme in shoulder instabilities, attention should be paid to such factors as the onset of pathology, the level of instability (subluxation, dislocation), prevalence (acute, chronic), direction of instability (anterior, posterior, multi-directional), accompanying pathologies, neuromuscular control, and pre-injury activity levels [74].

The first thing that should come to mind is the injury mechanism. In shoulder instabilities occurring due to a trauma, joint movements should be permitted within the pain threshold, due to the fact that pain is caused by tissue damage and muscle spasm, and pain and muscle spasm should be reduced. In atraumatic and recurrent dislocations, an insufficiency is observed in keeping humeral head inside the glenoid cavity, and for this reason, dynamic stability needs to be increased along with proprioceptive training.

On the other hand, severity of trauma, presence of injury in contractile tissue along with degeneration in glenohumeral joint capsule and in ligaments, the direction of dislocation is the key point in determining the rehabilitation programme.

Previous studies reported that the application of physiotherapy or immobilization in individuals at the ages between 21 and 30 that went through primary shoulder dislocation did not reduce the recurrence risk of shoulder dislocation. Primary surgical stabilization is recommended especially for individuals doing sports at higher intensities [75, 76]. Studies noted that post-surgery rehabilitation success after the first shoulder dislocation is higher compared to rehabilitation on individuals that do not go through surgery [77].

In posterior shoulder instability rehabilitation, increased internal rotation of scapula and horizontal adduction of the arm should be paid attention. In posterior shoulder dislocations that occur due to trauma, shortening that may develop in the posterior capsule after surgery should be prevented. For this purpose, arm slings that fix the arm lightly in external rotation should be used [78, 79].

In SLAP lesion, pathological changes occur in superior glenoid labrum and the long head of biceps muscle. At the early stages, degenerative changes are observed in labrum and the long head of biceps muscle. At later stages, impairment of the stability of shoulder joint and superior labral tear occur due to bicipital instability. For this reason, reducing the pain developing in shoulder during rehabilitation and increasing muscle activity in biceps muscle gradually bears importance [80, 81].

In multi-directional shoulder instabilities, such symptoms as pain, lack of confidence, and kinesiophobia occur due not being able to preserve centralization of humeral head into joint movement centre of glenoid cavity, during arm elevation. Pain developing in such individuals is not localized on a certain region but shows a widespread course. In general, conservative treatment is preferred in shoulder instability that occurs voluntarily and/or involuntarily.

Understanding recovery response of the tissue along with knowing the surgical technique adopted in shoulder instability, occupy an important place in rehabilitation.

Conservative Rehabilitation in Shoulder Instabilities

Phase 1 (0–2 Weeks):

Our objectives

- Reducing pain and inflammation.
- Ensuring pain-free range of joint motion.
- Preventing glenohumeral and scapulothoracic muscle atrophy.

Rehabilitation

- Applying ice to reduce pain.
- Passive range of shoulder joint motion with exercise ball.
- Active assistive shoulder flexion and abduction exercises.
- Scapular retraction exercises.
- Isometric strengthening exercises with pain control for shoulder girdle muscle.
- Progressive shoulder IR/ER exercises with pain control beginning from 0° abduction position.

Phase 2 (3–4 Weeks):

Objectives

- Gaining and increasing shoulder and scapular muscle control.

- Ensuring normal scapulothoracic arthrokinematics.
- Ensuring neuromuscular control.
- Improving proprioception.

Rehabilitation

- Isotonic strengthening exercises for shoulder girdle.
- Ensuring scapular control.
- Scapular retraction and closed kinetic chain exercises.
- Shoulder IR/ER strengthening exercises at progressive abduction angles (from 45° to 90°).
- Core stabilization exercises.
- Neuromuscular control exercises.
- Proprioceptive exercises.

Phase 3 (4–6 Weeks):
Objectives

- Increasing shoulder girdle and scapulothoracic muscular strength, and endurance.
- Ensuring dynamic stability.
- Ensuring pain-free total range of joint motion.

Rehabilitation

- Exercises applied in Phase 2 progressively continue.
- Isokinetic strengthening exercises.
- Thrower's ten exercises.
- Sports-specific exercises.

Attention to in conservative rehabilitation of shoulder instabilities

- Stretching exercises for SLAP 1 and 3 posterior and inferior capsules should be included in rehabilitation programme at earlier stages.
- At the early stages of multi-directional shoulder instabilities and posterior shoulder instabilities, closed kinetic chain exercises that cause increase in the retroversion of glenoid should be avoided [82].
- Strengthening of primary periscapular stabilizers muscles is important in the conservative rehabilitation approach of shoulder instability. In addition to the strengthening programme primarily for mid-lower trapezius, rhomboids and serratus anterior muscles, secondary muscles responsible for scapular stabilization such as pectoralis minor, latissimus dorsi, and pectoralis major should be included in the rehabilitation programme at later stages.
- Exercise programme should be progressive. The programme should start from the prone position first, and then should progress to ensure scapular stabilization in supine position, standing up, and increased arm elevation. To this end, the isometric strength of the person, manual resistance, theraband, theratubes, and free weights can be used.
- Strengthening exercises for rotator cuff muscles should be prescribed. Rhythmic stabilization exercises to be done by using co-contraction of agonist and antagonist muscles in the neutral position of glenohumeral joint and scapular in retraction should continue at later stages by increasing the arm abduction.
- Proprioceptive training of unstable glenohumeral joint is important. Proprioceptive training should start with closed kinetic chain exercises and scapular clock exercises at early stages, and at later stages, scapular and glenohumeral stability should be ensured at varying glenohumeral joint angles, and perturbation training and plyometric training should be given.

Postoperative Rehabilitation

If symptoms affect normal function of the patient, surgical treatment can be preferred in impingement syndrome that does not respond to conservative treatment, and in partial or full thickness rotator cuff tears and instabilities. However, an early repair can be implemented in young patients with acute rotator cuff tear.

In order to increase the surgical success and carry out and more effective rehabilitation, the characteristics of the patient should be brought to an optimal level. Absence of limitation in passive joint movement, especially before the surgery, would ensure a much more successful rehabilitation after the surgery. Otherwise, both preserving surgical structure and trying to increase the passive joint movement would cause a prolongation of the rehabilitation process. For this reason, physiotherapists should always be in communication with orthopaedists and implement preoperative rehabilitation on patients with passive joint movement limitation before the surgery. This way it will be possible to implement a faster rehabilitation programme through increasing activation of the muscle around scapula and of the shoulder and through learning exercises to be done after the surgery. Table 18.1 shows pre-surgery rehabilitation protocol implemented by Duzgun et al. [83].

Rehabilitation Following Subacromial Decompression

Impingement syndrome and partial tears can be treated by the debridement of both the lower and upper surface of tendon. Debridement allows for the repair of the injured segment of rotator cuff and stimulates recuperation response. Patients with partial tear are luckier in going back to activities in the post-surgery period.

Since, in these surgeries, no repair is applied on soft tissue, the objective in rehabilitation is to relieve the pain, relieve the tension of the soft tissue, and increase the range of motion. Cold application is quite effective for the decreasing pain and inflammation after the surgery [84]. Especially

Table 18.1 Rehabilitation protocol implemented before the surgery (with permission from ref. 83)

Week	Application	Frequency
1. Week	Cold application	4 times/day, 20 min
	Posterior capsule stretching	1 time/h
	Rest of the shoulder joint	
2. Week	Continue first week	
	Scapular mobilization and manual posterior capsule stretching	1 time/week, at clinic
	Scapular retraction with elbow flexion	4 times/day, 10 rep.
	Scapular retraction with elbow extension	4 times/day, 10 rep.
	Scapular retraction on the wall	4 times/day, 10 rep.
3. Week	Continue second week	
	Shoulder muscle strengthening with 0.5 kg weight	
	Flexion	4 times/day, 10 rep.
	Abduction	4 times/day, 10 rep.
	Full can (arm elevation at scapular plane)	4 times/day, 10 rep.
4–6 Weeks	Continue third week	
	Arm flexion, abduction and full can increased weight	4 times/day, 10 rep.
	External and internal rotation at 0° arm abduction with thera-band	4 times/day, 10 rep.

Table 18.2 Rehabilitation programme following rotator cuff repair (with permission from ref. 86)

Fast	Exercise	Protocol		Slow
Week		In clinic	At home	Week
0–1 weeks	Cold pack (before treatment)		Every 2 h, for 20 min	0–1 week
1–2 weeks	Cold pack	Once 20 min	Every 2 h, for 20 min	1–4 weeks
	Deltoid and biceps soft tissue mobilization	Kneading 5 min		
	Standing passive flexion near the table	10 rep × 1 set	10 rep × 2 set/day	
	Standing passive abduction near the table	10 rep × 1 set	10 rep × 2 set/day	
	Standing passive ER with stick	10 rep × 1 set	10 rep × 2 set/day	
	Active elbow flexion	10 rep × 1 set	10 rep × 2 set/day	
	Active elbow extension	10 rep × 1 set	10 rep × 2 set/day	
	Gripping exercises for hand	10 rep × 2 set	10 rep × 2 set/day	
	Active cervical flexion-extension	10 rep × 1 set	10 rep × 2 set/day	
	Active cervical lateral flexion	10 rep × 1 set	10 rep × 2 set/day	
	Active cervical rotation	10 rep × 1 set	10 rep × 2 set/day	

(continued)

Table 18.2 (continued)

Fast	Exercise	Protocol		Slow
Week		In clinic	At home	Week
2–3 weeks	Cold pack	Once 20 min	20 min × 4 times/day	4–6 weeks
	Supine passive flexion with stick	10 rep × 1 set	10 rep × 2 set/day	
	Supine passive scaption with stick	10 rep × 1 set	10 rep × 2 set/day	
	Passive ER with stick	10 rep × 1 set	10 rep × 2 set/day	
	Active elbow flexion	10 rep × 1 set	10 rep × 2 set/day	
	Active elbow extension	10 rep × 1 set	10 rep × 2 set/day	
	Scapular mobilization	Superior-inferior, medio-lateral directions 5 min		
	GH mobilization	Grade 1–2 ant-post gliding 5 min		
	Scapular clock	10 rep × 1 set		
3–4 weeks	Cold pack	Once 20 min	20 min × 3 times/day	6–8 weeks
	Scapular mobilization	Add rotation component 5–10 min		
	GH mobilization	Progress grade 3 to 4 10 min		
	Manual scapular resistive exercise	Retraction-protraction up-downward rot 10 rep × 1 set		
	If no resting pain			
	Active shoulder flexion until 90	6 rep × 1 set	6 rep × 2 set/day	
	Active shoulder IR at 0 abd	6 rep × 1 set	6 rep × 2 set/day	
	Active shoulder abduction until 90	6 rep × 1 set	6 rep × 2 set/day	
	Active shoulder 45 ER at 0 abd	6 rep × 1 set	6 rep × 2 set/day	
	Scapular retraction during elbow flexion with light tb	10 rep × 2 set	10 rep × 2 set/day	
	Scapular retraction during elbow extension with light tb	10 rep × 2 set	10 rep × 2 set/day	
	Resistive biceps with light tb	10 rep × 1 set	10 rep × 2 set/day	
	Resistive triceps with light tb	10 rep × 1 set	10 rep × 2 set/day	
	Supine serratus anterior strengthening	10 rep × 1 set with 1 kg	10 rep × 2 set/day	
4–5 weeks				8–10 weeks
	Cold pack	Once 20 min	20 min × twice/day	
	If it is necessary continue scapular and GH joint mobilization			
	Shoulder flexion with light tb until 90	10 rep × 1 set	10 rep × 2 set/day	
	Shoulder abduction with light tb until 90	10 rep × 1 set	10 rep × 2 set/day	
	Shoulder IR with light tb at 0 abd	10 rep × 1 set	10 rep × 2 set/day	
	Shoulder ER with light tb at 0 abd	10 rep × 1 set	10 rep × 2 set/day	
	Active shoulder flexion up to 90	10 rep × 1 set		
	Active shoulder abduction up to 90	10 rep × 1 set		
	Active shoulder IR at 45 abd	10 rep × 1 set		
	Active shoulder ER at 45 abd	10 rep × 1 set		
	Scapular retraction during flexion with moderate tb	10 rep × 1 set	10 rep × 2 set/day	
	Scapular retraction during extension with moderate tb	10 rep × 1 set	10 rep × 2 set/day	
	Posterior capsule stretching	3 rep × 1 set 30 s	3 rep × 2 set/day	
	Scaption thumb up with light tb	10 rep × 1 set	10 rep × 2 set/day	

Table 18.2 (continued)

Fast	Exercise	Protocol		Slow
Week		In clinic	At home	Week
5–6 weeks				10–14 weeks
	Cold pack	Once 20 min	20 min × twice/day	
	If it is necessary continue scapular and GH joint mobilization			
	Shoulder flexion with mod tb	10 rep × 1 set	10 rep × 2 set/day	
	Shoulder abduction with mod tb	10 rep × 1 set	10 rep × 2 set/day	
	Shoulder IR with mod tb	10 rep × 1 set	10 rep × 2 set/day	
	Shoulder ER with mod tb	10 rep × 1 set	10 rep × 2 set/day	
	Scapular retraction during elbow flexion with mod. Tb	10 rep × 1 set	10 rep × 2 set/day	
	Scapular retraction during elbow extension with mod. Tb	10 rep × 1 set	10 rep × 2 set/day	
	Posterior capsule stretching	3 rep × 1 set 30 s	3 rep × 2 set/day	
	Scaption thumb up with mod tb	10 rep × 1 set	10 rep × 2 set/day	
	Prone horizontal abd thumb up	10 rep × 1 set	10 rep × 2 set/day	
	Side lying IR stretching	3 rep × 1 set 30 s	3 rep × 2 set/day	
	Side lying ER with 1 kg		10 rep × 1 set	
	Stabilization training on the ball	5 min		
	Wall shoulder press up	10 rep × 1 set	10 rep × 2 set/day	
6–8 weeks				14–22 weeks
6 weeks	Cold pack	Once 20 min	20 min × once/day	14–18 weeks
	Shoulder flexion with moderate tb	10 rep × 1 set	10 rep × 2 set/day	
	Shoulder abduction with moderate tb	10 rep × 1 set	10 rep × 2 set/day	
	Shoulder IR with moderate tb	10 rep × 1 set	10 rep × 2 set/day	
	Shoulder ER with moderate tb	10 rep × 1 set	10 rep × 2 set/day	
	Posterior capsule stretching	3 rep × 1 set 30 s	3 rep × 2 set/day	
	Scaption thumb up with moderate tb	10 rep × 1 set	10 rep × 2 set/day	
	Prone horizontal abduction thumb up	10 rep × 1 set with 1 kg	10 rep × 2 set/day	
	Side lying IR stretching	3 rep × 1 set 30 s	3 rep × 2 set/day	
	Side lying ER with 2 kg	10 rep × 1 set	10 rep × 2 set/day	
	Wall-ball stabilization	5 min		
	Resistive PNF patterns	10 rep × 1 set with 2 kg		
7 weeks				18–22 weeks
	Wall shoulder push up	10 rep × 1 set	10 rep × 2 set/day	
	On the table press up	10 rep × 1 set	10 rep × 2 set/day	
	On the table push up	10 rep × 1 set	10 rep × 2 set/day	

at early stages, a 15-min ice application every 2 h is recommended. Passive joint motion can be commenced from the second day following the surgery. Since fundamentally no repair occurs in the soft tissue, although there exists no disadvantage to commence active movement, passive joint motion exercises to be done at the pain threshold would produce the desired effect without the patient suffering from too much pain due to post-surgery inflammation presence and the tightness surrounding soft tissue. Exercises done at the end of the table and on ball for the purpose of passive range of motion exercises are suitable in the post-surgical period (Fig. 18.31a, b).

In addition, releasing of the surrounding soft tissue by manual therapy applications conducted in this period would help in relieving the pain (Fig. 18.32a, b).

Under normal conditions, pain is expected to reduce from the fifth day after the surgery. Following the pain beginning to reduce, increase in active range of joint motion is aimed with active assisted exercises. Wand exercises are quite effective in this period (Fig. 18.33a, b).

In addition, this would be a step taken for producing a correct biomechanics through strengthening exercises for scapular retractors.

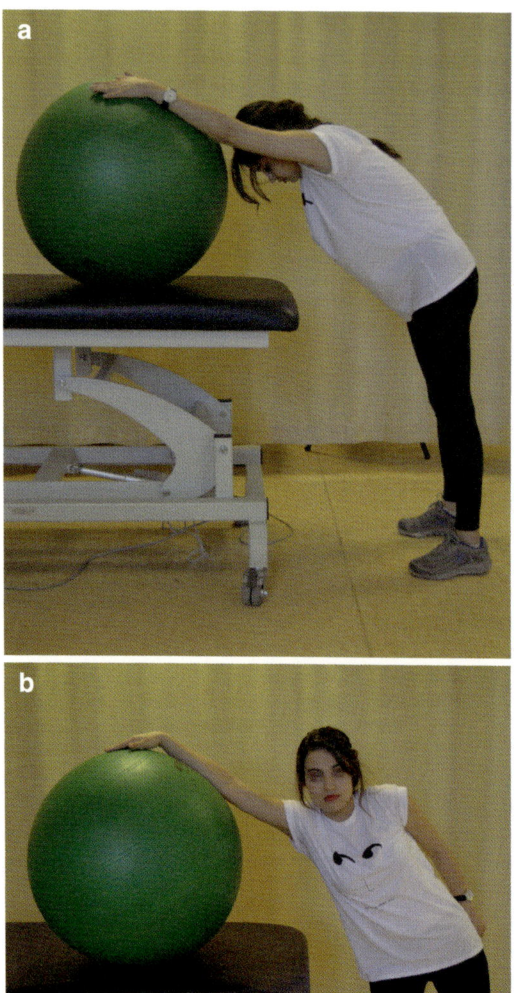

Fig. 18.31 (**a**) Flexion stretching on the ball; (**b**) abduction stretching on the ball

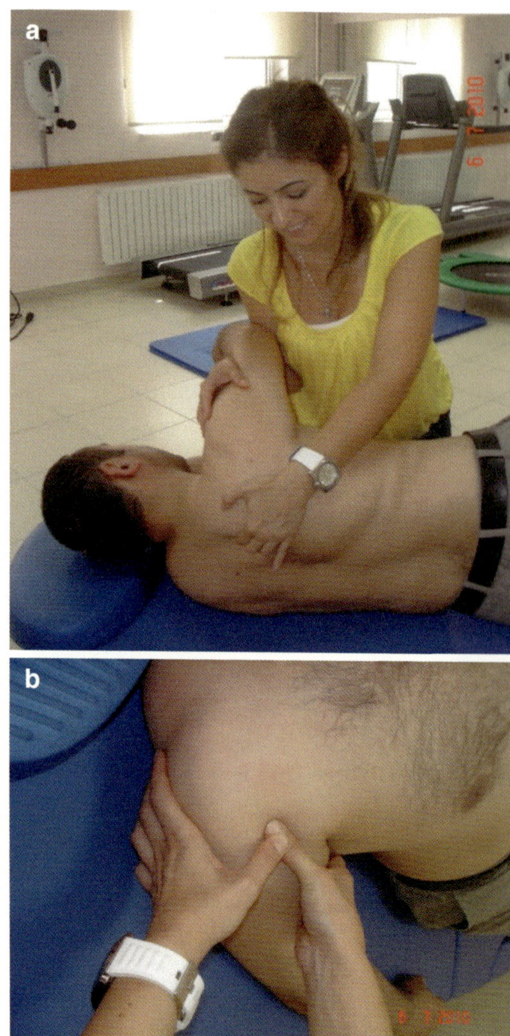

Fig. 18.32 (**a**) Scapular mobilization; (**b**) surrounding soft tissue mobilization

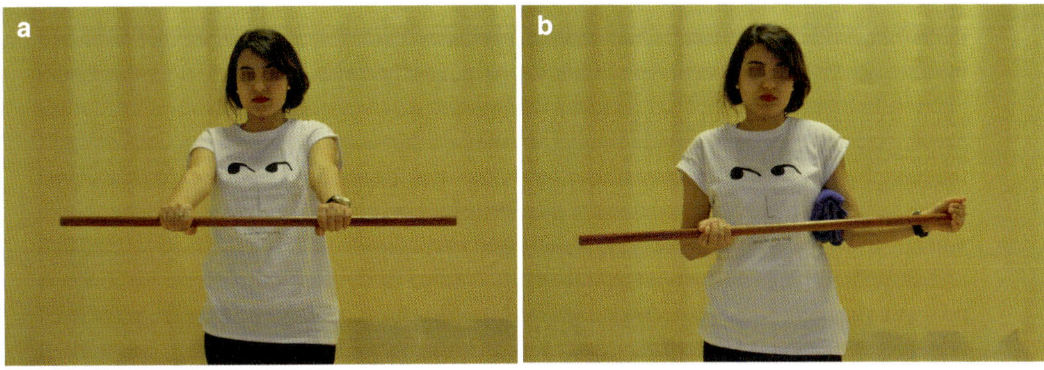

Fig. 18.33 (**a**) Wand exercise- flexion; (**b**) wand exercise- external rotation

In active assisted exercises, Active movement can be used to along with the reduction in pain, and the said period of time is between 2 and 3 weeks. Shoulder joint active movements can be commenced with elevation exercises in flexion, abduction, and scapular plane. For these movements, mild resistance exercises can be added following the reduction in pain. In clinic, the starting point is generally 0.5 kg and resistance is then planned to increase according to the adaptation of the patient.

In the next phase, can be proceeded first to the resistance internal rotation and then to resistance external rotation exercises.

The special attention that needs to be paid in resistance exercises is not to cause an increase in the pain of the patient. Increase in the paint points to the fact that the muscle is loaded with a higher load than it can actually bear, and thus resistance must absolutely be decreased. Proprioceptive exercises should definitely have a place in rehabilitation following the surgery. To sum up, rehabilitation following decompression surgeries is not at all different than conservative physiotherapy programmes. Taking into consideration the pain bears quite an importance in the progression of exercises [84].

Rehabilitation Following Rotator Cuff Repair

Following the repair, the protection of the repaired tissue is one of the prior objectives of rehabilitation. Since active movement would impose stress on the restored region especially at early stages, special attention should be paid. There is yet to be a consensus on this subject in literature. While some authors suggest that active movement should not be commenced before 6 weeks [85], certain studies show that active movement started at the third week does not have a damaging effect. In their study, Düzgün et al. [86] manifested that fast rehabilitation protocol applied with pre-surgery rehabilitation programme does not have a damaging effect in the sixth month. However, further studies are needed for long-term results. In a meta-analysis, it was reported that early range of joint motion exercises might be effective in preventing post-surgery rigidity in small and medium tears but special attention should be paid in massive tears [87]. In another meta-analysis, while re-tear rate in patients that were prescribed early passive joint motion exercise in small tears below 3 cm were lower compared to patients that were commenced late, commencing early passive joint exercises increase re-tear risk in tears greater than 5 cm [88]. The size of tear should be taken into consideration for exercises to be selected.

In classic rehabilitation protocols to starting passive movements during weeks 1–4, then active assisted exercises between weeks 4–6, and active movement between weeks 6–8 is accepted. Timing of commencing resistance exercises after active movement are within basic guidelines of rehabilitation. This means that it is of utmost importance to not to increase the pain by the prescribed resistance exercise.

In their study, Hayes et al. [89] showed that a difference does not exist between the treatment of patients in clinic and follow-ups through home programme following rotator cuff repair in terms of range of joint motion and muscle strength. Patience adhering to home programme is among the definite factors that affect the success of the treatment. However, it is believed that a follow-up at a physiotherapy clinic by physiotherapists for 2 days a week would increase the success of post-surgery rehabilitation.

When checked in general, although there exists no significant differences between manual therapy phases applied after soft tissue repair (rotator cuff repair, Bankart repair, SLAP repair), timing of the exercise and movements that needs to be paid attention to manifests differences. Manual therapy application phases following soft tissue repair are given below.

Phase 1: Maximum Protection Phase (1–10 Days)

This is the absolute immobilization period.

Treatment:

- Immobilization with a sling.
- Ice application.

Causes:

Immobilization is of utmost importance in the first 3–5 days since this allows for inflammation and proliferation phases. Throughout the inflammation phase (1–72 h), vasodilatation, edema, and debris phagocytosis are formed around the wound [69]. Movement is not permitted in order to protect the newly formed capillaries. Early and excessive movement causes inflammation phase to prolong and excessive scar tissue to occur.

Heat is the second factor to be avoided. It causes vascular stress on the newly formed capillaries. Ice application can be used to keep edema and pain under control.

On the 7th–10th days following the surgery, initial application of stress on the tissue can be started. Fibroblastic phase of recovery with fibroblasts in tissue has just begun [90]. This slow early movement, just as Grade 1–2 joint mobilization and passive joint movement in the preserved position, helps the formation of new regular collagen fibres, ensuring muscle relaxation, and prevention of adhesion formation [69].

Phase 2: Protective Mobilization (10 Days–4 Weeks)

Immobilization with sling continues.

Treatment:

- Continued Grade 1–2 mobilization.
- Active and passive scapular gliding.

Causes:

The aim of this phase is to form a functional scar and to decrease other compensatories and dysfunction. Early mobilization has a significant effect on the length, sliding, and tension force of the scar tissue. Recovery begins with fibroplasia following the end of inflammatory phase. As noted by Donatelli, Peacock et al. [14] showed that the wound recovery starts on the fourth day with the formation of scar tissue and is accelerated in the first 3 weeks [69].

Mobilization techniques may become effective throughout early fibroplasia depending on the re-development of collagen tissue.

Phase 3: Medium Protection Phase (4–6 Weeks)

Glenohumeral joint's pain and sensitivity at rest are decreased. Sutures were removed and superficial healing was ensured. Decrease in scapular movement in patients continues.

Treatment:

- Grade 3 and 4 Glenohumeral joint mobilization in posterioanterior direction.
- Soft tissue mobilization.
- Active assisted and active joint movements are commenced.

Causes:

Medium protection phase mostly allows for the transition from active assistive joint movement to active joint movement in the fourth week. Collagen formation continues at a high level up until the sixth week. In this phase, the purpose of rehabilitation is to ensure the prolongation of collagen that is newly synthesized, and increasing a regular collagen formation and also sliding between collagen fibres. When the tensile strength reaches its maximum, in the third week at the earliest, active joint movement is permitted.

Soft tissue mobilization carried out on the scar and its surroundings enables the incision scar to prolong and allows for proper muscle function and reduction in pain. In addition, Prevention of muscle atrophy and inhibition, and protecting from the negative effects of immobilization are among the purposes of this phase.

PNF resistance is commenced in scapular pattern. This way scapular muscle activity restoration and dynamic proximal stability is ensured. Isometric contractions in protected position begin in the fifth week. With isometric contractions, it is aimed to prevent muscle inhibition and ensure the recovery of soft tissue through dynamic tension [69].

Phase 4: Late Medium Protection Phase (6–12 Weeks)

In this phase, increase in the mobility of incision scar and scapular movements being within normal range are expected.

Collagen formation gradually decreases in the sixth week. Maturation or reformation (remodelling phase) begins in the third week and continues up until 12–18 months. It is important to bring scar extensibility to maximum since scar deformity may largely decrease in the 14th week [91]. Importance should be attached to strengthening in this phase.

Phase 5: Minimal Protection Phase (12–16 Weeks)

In this phase, joint movement conducted without multi - repetitive limitation ensures the scar to mature. Elimination of limitation is aimed through manual techniques adopted throughout this phase [69].

Phase 7: Back to Function (16 Weeks and Beyond)

In general, if abnormal pattern or pain is nonexistent in movements in the 16th week, functional phase is commenced. This phase is progressed based on the response. A higher functionality and maximal effort is required during exercises [69].

Generally, the key point in rehabilitation following rotator cuff repair is the improvement of the movement. If pain is present during movement, a severe muscle inhibition is responsible for this. Pain may occur as a result of an injury or due to surgery. In order to relieve pain, numerous modalities such as ultrasound, TENS, galvanic stimulation can be used. And also resting, ice application and avoidance painful movements should be advised [92]. After the pain is kept under control, exercises to increase the range of joint motion should be started. In order to increase shoulder joint movement active assisted exercises may be initiated following passive joint mobilisation. Cohen et al. [85] recommends beginning joint movement exercises in supine position while the arm is on the side of the patient, supported by pillows and elbow in flexion. With this position, forces through the shoulder joint are reduced through decreasing the gravity effect and shortening the upper extremity limb.

In this phase, Codman's exercises are preferred in numerous protocols. Patient must be ensured to relax their arm during Codman's exercises especially following rotator cuff repairs. It was shown in a study that EMG activation increases in muscle especially during Codman's exercises done extensively [93]. For this reason, attention should be paid during this exercise and Codman's exercises should be preferred on a smaller scale.

As the pain-free joint movement of the patient improves, exercises should be progressed to sitting and standing positions.

The time to start muscle strengthening exercises during rehabilitation is correlated with the correct diagnosis and establishment of treatment programme. In literature, it is recommended to start active movement and muscle strengthening exercises at the sixth week following the surgery in order to allow for the recovery of the repaired tendon and greater tubercle of the humerus in a patient that went through rotator cuff repair. Various exercises can be used to strength the muscles surrounding the shoulder. Closed kinetic chain exercises used in the beginning are the safest strengthening exercises. The advantage of closed kinetic chain exercises is that it ensures the co-contraction of both agonist and antagonist muscle groups. These exercises enhance shoulder stabilization function and limit the amount of shear strength going through the joint via normal physiologic motor patterns. Strengthening exercises are commenced below 90° flexion and extension. Following the recovery of the tissue and the joint movement is ensured, abduction and flexion movements with resistance are initiated. Strengthening of scapular stabilizers bears quite an importance and should be commenced in the early phases of the rehabilitation programme [79].

More aggressive strengthening are proceeded towards as the recovery continues. Internal/external rotation exercises are a form of open kinetic chain activity and doing these exercises by positioning the shoulder in scapular plane increases the performance since minimum load is imposed on the shoulder joint capsule in scapular plane and functional movements are conducted in this position [94]. The most widely used open kinetic chain exercises are plyometric exercises. Plyometric activities, which are a part of all sports activities, are defined as the tension and shortening cycle of the muscle. First the muscle is stretched eccentrically and then load is gradually born [95].

For this reason these exercises create more stress on the tissue and completion of tissue recovery and ensuring a complete motion is necessary to start plyometrics within the rehabilitation programme. TheraBand, exercise ball or free weights are accepted as plyometric exercise materials. In order to prevent an unwanted injury during such exercises, physiotherapist should always observe the patient.

Patient education is an important step in starting the rehabilitation programme. This is more important component that affects the motivation of the patient during rehabilitation. Patient education includes general information, contents of the exercise programme and steps that are necessary to do exercises correctly. In this way it is aimed to increase the motivation of the patient within the home programme. In order to ensure complete recovery, home exercise programmes are recommended. In this way recovery of the patient is accelerated and the cost is reduced. Many health insurance policies impose restrictions on physical therapy expenditures. The rehabilitation period is shortened through home exercise programme carried out regularly.

Table 18.2 shows fast and slow rehabilitation protocol following rotator cuff repair generated by Duzgun et al. [86]. In the study, patients with grade 2–3 rotator cuff tear were implemented into two different exercise protocols. In the fast protocol, patients that underwent rotator cuff repair were given pre-surgery exercise programme. When slow and fast protocols were compared in the sixth month following surgery, no difference in pain and functional activity was found [80]. However, in fast protocol, range of joint motion [83] and functional activity levels were shown to re-gain at the earlier stages.

It must be borne in mind that such factors as age, size of tear, fatty infiltration amount should be taken into consideration for the rehabilitation of patients following rotator cuff repair. While following the programme, responses of the patient to exercises must be observed well and accurate exercise timing should be ensured.

Rehabilitation After Anterior Capsulolabral Repair of the Shoulder

There are four main rules to ensure success in rehabilitation [96]:

1. Understanding the surgical technique: In anterior instabilities without labral injuries, surgeons stretch capsule and glenohumeral ligaments with capsular plication or capsular shift techniques. Suture anchors are used in cases with anteroinferior labral injuries. Three suture anchors are used in typical capsular shift application without Bankart repair. In the presence of Bankart lesions, shift or stretch of capsule is not necessary in general in bony Bankart or other labral injuries. Anatomic repair of capsulolabral complex is then applied.
2. Understanding how anatomic structures are under stress and how recovery is stimulated:

In standard anterior capsulolabral repairs weakening is present in anterior inferior capsule. The highest stress is imposed in external rotation in 90° abduction [97, 98]. Since the inferior glenohumeral joint capsule is under stress during forward flexion, flexion above 90° is prohibited up to post-surgery third week and 135° degree flexion is permitted in the sixth week. Since, in classic open Bankart repairs, insertion area of subcapularis muscle is shifted, attention should be paid to active internal rotation movement at early periods following surgery. However, such a protection is not necessary as no changes are made in subcapularis in standard arthroscopic capsulolabral repairs.

3. Selection of suitable exercises for the recovered tissue: Exercise should be chosen taking into consideration the recovery mechanism of the tissue. It must be borne in mind that overload may harm muscles that ensures dynamic or active stabilisation, protects the repaired region [99, 100], supports joint capsule, increases compression stress [101, 102] and shows resistance to shifting in joint [103].

Understanding the necessary immobilization period and progression rate of joint movement: Absolute immobilization must be ensured by a shoulder sling for the first 4 weeks following arthroscopic capsulolabral repair. Sling should only be removed during exercise or while sitting or standing up for a short time between the weeks 4 and 6. However, surgeon's preference should also be taken into consideration for immobilization period. Just like immobilization period, timing of the joint movement is also of importance. A total joint movement should be reached in weeks 8–12 following surgery. When we look at post-surgery rehabilitation phases:

Phase 1: Post-Surgery Weeks 0–6

The first 6 weeks are maximum protection phases. Range of joint movement shown in the table should not be exceeded. Attention should especially be paid to external rotation limits. Since rotator cuff muscles are not affected in arthroscopic stabilization, passive and active assistive range of joint motion exercises may conveniently be used at the early stages following surgery. Passive and active assistive exercises used at the early stages following rotator cuff repair are also suitable after these surgeries. What should specifically be borne in mind is to ensure controlled external rotation. Exercises should be commenced with a bar within limits while arms are on the side of body in order to prevent limitation in external rotation. Scapular retraction exercises can be commenced for controlling scapular movements but over-extension of the arm should be prevented during this exercise and this should be done at earlier stages without resistance or with lower intensities. There is no harm in strengthening rotator cuff muscles following arthroscopic stabilization, however, pain should be taken into consideration while prescribing such exercises. Submaximal isometric exercises are suitable in this phase with arm in neutral position.

Phase 2: Post-Surgery Weeks 6–12

In this phase, neuromuscular control of rotator cuff and scapular muscles is aimed to ensure within the permitted range of joint motion. Range of joint motion, submaximal tissue load and dynamic stabilization are increased in a gradual manner. Completion of the range of joint motion is aimed in all planes by 12 weeks except external rotation movement in 90° abduction. We already noted the importance of posterior capsule for normal arthrokinematics. In this phase, posterior capsule stretching exercises can be commenced.

Phase 3: Post-Surgery Weeks 12–24

In this phase, it is aimed to normalize neuromuscular functions through endurance, strength, and dynamic stability exercises. Proprioceptive exercises and sport specific exercises that the patient is involved must absolutely be included in the rehabilitation programme.

Rehabilitation Following Shoulder Posterior Capsulolabral Repair

A rehabilitation programme similar to anterior capsule repairs is implemented. However, shoulder sling should be in neutral or mild ER position in order to reduce the stress borne on posterior capsule at early stages.

Rehabilitation after posterior stabilization surgery

- More slower.
- More restrictive.
- More careful than rehabilitation after the anterior stabilization surgery.

At the same time, first 6–8 weeks excessive internal rotation, which could lead to increase in posterior capsuler laxity, must be prevented [104].

In the rehabilitation of posterior shoulder stabilities, Strengthening of posterior deltoid and external rotators of the shoulder, that play a significant role in posterior stability, is important.

Rehabilitation Following SLAP Repair

Lesion formation mechanism and SLAP type are important when determining the rehabilitation programme for SLAP lesions. In general, in traction injuries that occur as a result of a trauma, severe and eccentric contraction that may be possible in biceps muscle should be avoided. In degloving occurring in glenoid labrum due to repetitive shoulder activities, abduction-external rotation of the shoulder should be limited. The increase of the stretching stress forming in the insertion area of biceps brachii's long head on glenoid labrum at abduction - ER position of the shoulder should be borne in mind.

In postoperative SLAP rehabilitation, it is important to protect the recovered tissue in labrum, ensure increase of strength in the pain-free range of biceps muscle and restore of glenohumeral stability [105].

Treatment is conservative in general due to the biceps labral intersection being intact in Type 1 and Type 3 SLAP lesions. However, in some cases, debridement can be conducted without anatomic repair on labrum. Rehabilitation differs in Type 2 SLAP lesions. In Type 2 tears, biceps muscle is separated from glenoid insertion. In this case, arthroscopic surgical repair is applied. In SLAP lesions, especially the rehabilitation of Type 2 tears differ since biceps-labral tissue is effected only in Type 2. For these reasons, biceps should not be loaded at earlier stages.

Following surgical repair, it is necessary to protect the repaired tissue during rehabilitation, prevent excessive stresses to be borne on these tissues, and especially the overload on biceps muscle should be prevented. Rehabilitation programme to be implemented after surgery show similarities with post-Bankart repair rehabilitation. Ice application is essential to suppress inflammation and reduces pain at postoperative early stages. The patient should not lift or carry an object with the affected side for the first 2 weeks following surgery and isolated biceps movements should be prevented. In the postoperative fourth week, shoulder sling can be taken off and active movements can be commenced within pain-free range of joint motion. In the sixth week, strengthening exercises are commenced on rotator cuff and periscapular muscles. Biceps brachii strengthening may be started with light weights between weeks 8 and 12. Other strengthening and proprioceptive exercises are continued [106].

Rehabilitation Following Shoulder Arthroplasty

Total Shoulder Arthroplasty

In total shoulder arthroplasties, postoperative rehabilitation programme bears importance in terms of regaining the functionality of an atomic structure repaired with surgery. While previously rehabilitation programmes are initiated at later stages in order to preserve surgery and allow for the soft tissue to recover following total shoulder arthroplasties, recently it is aimed to begin rehabilitation programme at an early stage in a safely manner [107–109].

Postoperative rehabilitation programmes reported in literature generally beginning with passive and mild joint movements and progress through active and total joint movement to later on strengthening and endurance trainings. Overall rehabilitation program generally include three or four phases [107, 109–111]. An important issue here is to be aware of the rehabilitation principles and goals and planning the program accordingly. For a good rehabilitation

- Surgical procedure should be completely understood.
- Surgical region should be known well anatomically and biomechanically.
- Presence of a different surgery should be known in addition to arthroplasty.
- Recovery patterns of tissues should be understood and stresses imposed on the tissue should be appropriate.
- Needs and requirements of the patient should be known and rehabilitation programme should be prepared accordingly.

In general, postoperative rehabilitation programme can be compiled in four phases. However, there exists no sharp distinctions between these phases and although phases differ from each other through the time elapsed following the surgery, functional conditions of the individuals are also accepted as important in transition between phases.

Phase 1: Postoperative Early Stage

This stage of rehabilitation generally covers the first postoperative 4–6 weeks.

Objectives

- To preserve the surgery.
- To allow the soft tissue to recover.
- To control edema and inflammation.
- To preserve normal range of joint movement in the surrounding joints.
- To gradually increase passive joint movement.

Points to take into account

- Passive and then active moments should be started at the earliest possible stage in order to prevent adhesion formation and stimulate tissue recovery [112].
- However, since new capillaries that are formed as a result of angiogenesis occurs at the end of the inflammatory period and in the beginning of proliferation stage are indurable, a total immobilization can be recommended for the first 7–10 days [113].
- Shoulder sling should be used for the first 3–4 weeks, and should only be taken off during exercises and for personal hygiene.
- In order not to expose to loads on shoulder anterior capsule and subscapularis muscle, an external rotation higher than 30° with arm next to the body should not be allowed.
- Abnormal shoulder extension should be avoided in order to protect anterior capsule and subscapularis muscle.
- Active shoulder movements should be avoided for the first 4 weeks and active internal rotation should be avoided for the first 6 weeks.

Rehabilitation Programme

- Ice application in order to keep edema, inflammation, and pain under control [114].
- Passive shoulder flexion, abduction, and passive internal rotation exercises.
- Active movements of joints in distal.
- Active assisted wand exercises commencing from week 4.
- Scapular mobilization while being gentle at early stages.
- Isometric shoulder flexion-abduction-extension exercises can be commenced from the fourth week.
- Scapular retraction exercises can be commenced from the fourth week in order to obtain scapular stabilization again.

Phase 2: Early Strengthening Period

This generally covers the postoperative period of up to 6–8 weeks.

Objectives

- To gain total range of joint motion.
- Transition from passive and active assisted movements to active movement.
- If any, to control pain, edema, and inflammation.
- To correct postural defects.

Points to take into account

- Tissues cannot be loaded abnormal stress even though active movement started.
- External rotation range of joint motion should be increased at a slower pace.
- Shoulder sling should be continued to wear at night even though taken off during the day.
- Active exercises should be done without causing exhaustion in shoulder.

Rehabilitation Programme

- Active shoulder exercises should be commenced towards all directions.
- Neuromuscular electrical stimulation should be applied on patients that cannot do active exercises.
- Isometric internal rotation exercises can be initiated.
- Closed kinetic chain exercises can be commenced by conducting load transfer on wall.
- Ice application should be continued with frequency decreasing gradually.
- Postural exercises can be prescribed depending on the patient's needs.
- Gentle stretches can be started in order to increase range of joint motion excluding external rotation.
- Core stabilization exercises started.

Phase 3: Intermediate Strengthening Period

This generally covers the postoperative period of 8–12 weeks.

Objectives

- Regaining shoulder girdle dynamic stability.
- Attempting to regain neuromuscular control.
- Gradual shoulder girdle strengthening.
- Gradual return to activities of daily living.

Points to take into account

- Lifting heavy weights should be prevented.
- Sudden movements should be avoided.
- Excessive stretching of anterior capsule and subscapularis should be avoided.

Rehabilitation Programme

- Joint capsule stretch exercises can be started in order to correct joint biomechanics, and if necessary, to gain total range of joint motion.
- If necessary, range of joint motion exercises may be continued.
- Weight bearing exercise can be carried out on swiss ball.
- Progression through isotonic resistance exercises may be carried out excluding internal rotation.
- By the end of this period, it is possible to progress through internal rotation strengthening exercises.
- Scapular stabilization exercises are continued.
- Neuromuscular coordination exercises are continued.
- Core stabilization exercises are continued.

Phase 4: Advanced Strengthening and Home Programme Period

This covers the postoperative 12th week and beyond.

Objectives

- Gaining of complete upper extremity functionality.
- Gaining of complete shoulder and scapular control.
- Gradual return to recreational activities.
- Gaining maximum external rotation.
- Gaining normal rotator cuff and shoulder girdle muscle strength.

Points to take into account

- Strengthening and endurance exercises should be increased gradually.
- Sudden movements and activities causing excessive loads on anterior capsule should be avoided.

Rehabilitation Programme

- If necessary, capsular stretching exercises can be continued
- Proprioceptive neuromuscular exercises for shoulder and scapula are continued with progression.

- Rotator cuff strengthening can be commenced at varying degrees of shoulder joint.
- Patient may start working after post-operative 16th week.
- Depending on the condition of the patient, swimming can be commenced gradually at week 18–20.

Reverse Shoulder Arthroplasty

In reverse shoulder arthroplasty, rotator cuff muscles function is either at a minimum level or completely lost. In addition, biomechanical characteristics are also different than normal shoulder structure. Because of these, post operative rehabilitation is different from total shoulder arthroplasty. Rehabilitation can be planned in four stages following reverse shoulder arthroplasty [115].

Phase 1: Maximum Protection

This period covers the first 6 weeks.

Objectives

- To preserve surgery.
- To protect joint stability.
- To ensure gaining passive movement [115].
- To keep pain, edema, and inflammation under control.

Points to take into account

- At the onset of the treatment, individuals should be informed about the condition of the extremity, rehabilitation period, and objectives.
- Patients should use a shoulder sling that positions the arm on a scapular plane for 4 weeks on average and should take off the sling on leave for their personal hygiene and during exercises [116].
- In order to prevent dislocation, movements that load stress especially on the anterior of the joint and that increase the dislocation risk such as internal rotation, hyperextension, and hyperabduction should be at all times avoided during this period.
- At early stages, drains can be placed in patients in order to decrease the dislocation risk due to potential hematoma that may occur between acromion and prosthetics.
- At this stage, it is necessary to maintain pain and edema control.
- Active movements of surrounding joints are permitted.
- During this period, recovery of the soft tissue should be ensured. Considering the soft tissue healing, passive joint exercises should be commenced on the 7th–10th day following the surgery in order to prevent the inflammatory process to prolong, to stimulate tissue recovery, and to prevent adhesion formation [117, 118].
- Active assisted exercises can be commenced in week 5 depending on the condition of the patient in order to ensure deltoid functionality at early stages.
- Patients with insufficient deltoid function can be applied neuromuscular electrical stimulation.
- When considered the range of joint motion, a range of motion or at least 138° should be targeted although the previous studies produced varying data [115, 119].

Rehabilitation Programme

- An absolute immobilization is recommended in order to allow for soft tissue recovery for the first 10 days.
- A 15-min ice application is recommended every 2 h.
- Grade 1 mobilization techniques are implemented in order to relax the surrounding soft tissue.
- In supine position shoulder flexion and abduction movement in scapular plane are carried out by a physiotherapist in order to ensure passive range of joint motion.
- Flexion on table and passive abduction exercise on scapular plane are recommended as home programme 4 times a day with 10 repeat, between the weeks 1–4.
- Passive elevation exercise is recommended 4 times a day with 10 repeat, on sagittal plane and scapular plane with a swiss ball as home programme from the fourth week.

- Depending on the condition of the patient, wand exercises can be commenced with the patient lying on supine position from the fifth week onwards.

Phase 2: Early Stages Strengthening (6–12 Weeks)

Objectives

- At this stage, transition to active assisted and active movements from passive moments should be carried out.
- Joint stability mechanics should be improved and strengthening exercises should be commenced [115].

Points to take into account

- Individuals should avoid shoulder hyper-adduction and internal rotation while shoulder adduction. Range of joint motion exercises should continue at this phase as well.
- Active assisted rotational movements may be commenced on scapular plane.
- Active assisted shoulder elevation movements should be started and progress should be made towards active movement depending on the condition of the patient.
- Acromion stress fracture risk is present since active movement is initiated in deltoid muscle and attention should be paid in case of this [120].
- At this stage, Isometric exercises can be commenced and progress should be made in exercises and then moved on to isotonic exercises.
- In addition, scapular exercises may be started depending on the tolerance of the patient in order to regain the shoulder kinematics.
- At this stage, joint is vulnerable to injuries even though active movements are commenced. This should be explained to the patient, and the patient should be informed that they should not carry loads despite using the arm in daily life is permitted, they should avoid sudden movements and crossing the arm against the body and attempting to touch their back is forbidden.

Rehabilitation Programme

- Ice application and exercises done with swiss ball continue.
- Wand exercises are commenced on foot in sagittal and frontal plane.
- Active assistive internal-external rotation exercises on scapular plane are commenced and then switched to active rotations.
- Depending on the tolerance of the patient, active arm elevations are commenced in sagittal, scapular, and frontal planes.
- In order to increase active range of motion, elevation exercises are done in the form of repetitive contractions throughout the range of motion with the help of a stick.
- Scapular retraction exercises are commenced with elbow in flexion with the help of an exercise band.
- Isometric exercises are conducted for the purposes of strengthening in deltoid posterior segment.

Phase 3: Mid Strengthening Period (After the 12th Week)

When the patient possesses sufficient joint movement, they are able to conduct the movement pain-free, and when the patient is now able to do mildly resistant exercises, transition to the third phase is possible.

Objectives

- To increase the muscle strength of the extremity.
- To ensure shoulder girdle biomechanics regularity and patient gaining their independence [115].

Points to take into account

- At this stage, progressive strengthening exercises are commenced. However, exercises should be done with lower weights and in the manner of multiple repetitive movements in principle.
- Even though they gain their independence in daily life to a larger extent, patients should still avoid carrying heavy loads and sudden and straining movements.

Rehabilitation Programme

- Scapular retraction with resistive band, active arm elevation, and repeated contraction exercises with a stick continue.
- If the range of joint motion is not on the desired level, Pilates ball exercises are continued.
- Depending on the condition of the patient, resisted arm elevation exercises are commenced on sagittal, scapular and frontal plane.
- Active internal rotation of the arm is permitted with the body in sagittal plane, internal-external rotation exercises can be commenced on sagittal plane when standing up, in supine position with 90° abduction.

Phase 4: Long Term Home Follow-Up (4 Months and Above)

When patients gained pain-free range of motion and total independence in daily life, after physiotherapist and surgeon make a decision on the suitability of the individual in terms of functionality, they are prescribed home exercise programme and follow-up starts.

Points to take into account

At this stage, the vital point the patient needs to know is that, although pain is not present and functionality is ensured, the arm that received prosthetics was repaired in an non-anatomical manner, should never be compared with the other healthy arm, and that they should take this into account in daily life.

Rehabilitation Programme

- Exercises with weights or theraband on three planes in order to improve strength and endurance of deltoid muscle are gradually continued.
- In addition to scapular retraction exercises, push up exercises on wall can be done for scapular stabilization.
- Depending on the condition of the patient, internal-external rotation exercises with theraband can be prescribed.

Exam

1. Which of the following should be avoided during early stages of (0–6 weeks) post-operative bankart repair?
   (a) Passive shoulder elevation.
   (b) Shoulder internal-eksternal rotation with resistive band at 0° abduction.
   (c) Scapular retraction exercise with resistive band.
   (d) Passive shoulder external rotation at 90° shoulder abduction.

2. Which of the following is incorrect for posterior shoulder instability rehabilitation protocol?
   (a) Rotator cuff muscles strengthening exercises at the early stages.
   (b) Closed kinetic chain (push-up) exercises at the early stages.
   (c) Scapular retraction exercise exercises at the early stages.
   (d) Neuromuscular training at the early stages.

3. Which of these should not recommended during early stages of impingement rehabilitation?
   (a) Posterior capsule stretching exercise.
   (b) Cold-pack application.
   (c) Deltoid muscle strengthening.
   (d) Scapular retraction exercise.

References

1. Kibler WB, Uhl TL, Maddux JW, Brooks PV, Zeller B, McMullen J. Qualitative clinical evaluation of scapular dysfunction: a reliability study. J Shoulder Elb Surg. 2002;11(6):550–6.
2. Shadmehr A, Azarsa MH, Jalaie S. Inter- and intrarater reliability of modified lateral scapular slide test in healthy athletic men. Biomed Res Int. 2014;2014:384149.
3. Hudak PL, Amadio PC, Bombardier C. Development of an upper extremity outcome measure: the DASH (disabilities of the arm, shoulder and hand) [corrected]. The upper extremity collaborative group (UECG). Am J Ind Med. 1996;29(6):602–8.
4. Michener LA, McClure PW, Sennett BJ. American shoulder and elbow surgeons standardized shoulder

assessment form, patient self-report section: reliability, validity, and responsiveness. J Shoulder Elb Surg. 2002;11(6):587–94.
5. Constant CR, Murley AH. A clinical method of functional assessment of the shoulder. Clin Orthop Relat Res. 1987;214:160–4.
6. Roach KE, Budiman-Mak E, Songsiridej N, Lertratanakul Y. Development of a shoulder pain and disability index. Arthritis Care Res. 1991;4(4):143–9.
7. Leggin BG, Michener LA, Shaffer MA, Brenneman SK, Iannotti JP, Williams Jr GR. The Penn shoulder score: reliability and validity. J Orthop Sports Phys Ther. 2006;36(3):138–51.
8. Leung MS, Cheing GL. Effects of deep and superficial heating in the management of frozen shoulder. J Rehabil Med. 2008;40(2):145–50.
9. Schaser KD, Disch AC, Stover JF, Lauffer A, Bail HJ, Mittlmeier T. Prolonged superficial local cryotherapy attenuates microcirculatory impairment, regional inflammation, and muscle necrosis after closed soft tissue injury in rats. Am J Sports Med. 2007;35(1):93–102.
10. Michener LA, Walsworth MK, Burnet EN. Effectiveness of rehabilitation for patients with subacromial impingement syndrome: a systematic review. J Hand Ther. 2004;17(2):152–64.
11. Romanowski M, Romanowska J, Grzeskowiak M. A comparison of the effects of deep tissue massage and therapeutic massage on chronic low back pain. Stud Health Technol Inform. 2012;176:411–4.
12. Hannafin JA, Chiaia TA. Adhesive capsulitis: a treatment approach. Clin Orthop Relat Res. 2000;372:95–109.
13. Duzgun I, Baltaci G, Atay OA. Manual therapy is an effective treatment for frozen shoulder in diabetics: an observational study. Eklem Hastalik Cerrahisi. 2012;23(2):94–9.
14. Celik D. Comparison of the outcomes of two different exercise programs on frozen shoulder. Acta Orthop Traumatol Turc. 2010;44(4):285–92.
15. Lin JJ, Wu YT, Wang SF, Chen SY. Trapezius muscle imbalance in individuals suffering from frozen shoulder syndrome. Clin Rheumatol. 2005;24(6):569–75.
16. Cools AM, Dewitte V, Lanszweert F, Notebaert D, Roets A, Soetens B, et al. Rehabilitation of scapular muscle balance: which exercises to prescribe? Am J Sports Med. 2007;35(10):1744–51.
17. Hung YJ, Darling WG. Shoulder position sense during passive matching and active positioning tasks in individuals with anterior shoulder instability. Phys Ther. 2012;92(4):563–73.
18. Sole G, Osborne H, Wassinger C. The effect of experimentally-induced subacromial pain on proprioception. Man Ther. 2015;20(1):166–70.
19. Hung YJ. Effects of surgical repair on active shoulder position sense and 3-dimensional reaching accuracy in a patient with anterior shoulder instability. Physiother Theory Pract. 2014;30(3):165–70.
20. Kibler WB, Sciascia A. Current concepts: scapular dyskinesis. Br J Sports Med. 2010;44(5):300–5.
21. Kibler WB, McMullen J, Uhl T. Shoulder rehabilitation strategies, guidelines, and practice. Orthop Clin North Am. 2001;32(3):527–38.
22. Muraki T, Aoki M, Izumi T, Fujii M, Hidaka E, Miyamoto S. Lengthening of the pectoralis minor muscle during passive shoulder motions and stretching techniques: a cadaveric biomechanical study. Phys Ther. 2009;89(4):333–41.
23. Borstad JD, Ludewig PM. Comparison of three stretches for the pectoralis minor muscle. J Shoulder Elb Surg. 2006;15(3):324–30.
24. Borstad JD. Resting position variables at the shoulder: evidence to support a posture-impairment association. Phys Ther. 2006;86(4):549–57.
25. Cools AM, Witvrouw EE, Danneels LA, Cambier DC. Does taping influence electromyographic muscle activity in the scapular rotators in healthy shoulders? Man Ther. 2002;7(3):154–62.
26. Alexander CM, Stynes S, Thomas A, Lewis J, Harrison PJ. Does tape facilitate or inhibit the lower fibres of trapezius? Man Ther. 2003;8(1):37–41.
27. Lin JJ, Hung CJ, Yang PL. The effects of scapular taping on electromyographic muscle activity and proprioception feedback in healthy shoulders. J Orthop Res. 2011;29(1):53–7.
28. Cools AMJ, Struyf F, De Mey K, Maenhout A, Castelein B, Cagnie B. Rehabilitation of scapular dyskinesis: from the office worker to the elite overhead athlete. Br J Sports Med. 2014;48(8):692–U34.
29. Kibler WB, Sciascia AD, Uhl TL, Tambay N, Cunningham T. Electromyographic analysis of specific exercises for scapular control in early phases of shoulder rehabilitation. Am J Sports Med. 2008;36(9):1789–98.
30. Uhl TL, Carver TJ, Mattacola CG, Mair SD, Nitz AJ. Shoulder musculature activation during upper extremity weight-bearing exercise. J Orthop Sports Phys Ther. 2003;33(3):109–17.
31. Ludewig PM, Hoff MS, Osowski EE, Meschke SA, Rundquist PJ. Relative balance of serratus anterior and upper trapezius muscle activity during push-up exercises. Am J Sports Med. 2004;32(2):484–93.
32. Maenhout A, Van Praet K, Pizzi L, Van Herzeele M, Cools A. Electromyographic analysis of knee push up plus variations: what is the influence of the kinetic chain on scapular muscle activity? Br J Sports Med. 2010;44(14):1010–5.
33. Hardwick DH, Beebe JA, McDonnell MK, Lang CE. A comparison of serratus anterior muscle activation during a wall slide exercise and other traditional exercises. J Orthop Sports Phys Ther. 2006;36(12):903–10.
34. Ellenbecker TS, Cools A. Rehabilitation of shoulder impingement syndrome and rotator cuff injuries: an evidence-based review. Br J Sports Med. 2010;44(5):319–27.

35. Morrison DS, Greenbaum BS, Einhorn A. Shoulder impingement. Orthop Clin N Am. 2000;31(2):285–93.
36. Cakmak A. Subakromiyal sikişma sendromunda konservatif tedavi. Acta Orthop Traumatol Turc. 2003;37:1.
37. Tsui KH-S. Shoulder impingement syndrome. Hong Kong Bull Rheum Dis. 2005;5:14–8.
38. Krishnan SG, Hawkins RJ, Warren RF. The shoulder and the overhead athlete. Philadelphia: Lippincott Williams & Wilkins; 2004.
39. Tyler TF, Nicholas SJ, Roy T, Gleim GW. Quantification of posterior capsule tightness and motion loss in patients with shoulder impingement. Am J Sports Med. 2000;28(5):668–73.
40. Gerber C, Werner C, Macy J, Jacob H, Nyffeler R. Effect of selective capsulorrhaphy on the passive range of motion of the glenohumeral joint. J Bone Joint Surg Am. 2003;85-A(1):48–55.
41. Koffler KM, Bader D, Eager M, Moyer R, Kelly JD. The effect of posterior capsule tightness on glenohumeral translation in the late-cocking phase of pitching: a cadaveric study (SS-15). Arthroscopy. 2002;18(5):11–3.
42. Ludewig PM, Reynolds JF. The association of scapular kinematics and glenohumeral joint pathologies. J Orthop Sports Phys Ther. 2009;39(2):90–104.
43. Borstad JD, Ludewig PM. The effect of long versus short pectoralis minor resting length on scapular kinematics in healthy individuals. J Orthop Sports Phys Ther. 2005;35(4):227–38.
44. Ellenbecker TS. Shoulder rehabilitation: non-operative treatment. Stuttgart: Thieme; 2011.
45. Wilk KE, Obma P, Simpson CD, Cain EL, Dugas J, Andrews JR. Shoulder injuries in the overhead athlete. J Orthop Sports Phys Ther. 2009;39(2):38–54.
46. Timmons MK, Thigpen CA, Seitz AL, Karduna AR, Arnold BL, Michener LA. Scapular kinematics and subacromial-impingement syndrome: a meta-analysis. J Sport Rehabil. 2012;21(4):354.
47. Ludewig PM, Cook TM. Alterations in shoulder kinematics and associated muscle activity in people with symptoms of shoulder impingement. Phys Ther. 2000;80(3):276–91.
48. Endo K, Ikata T, Katoh S, Takeda Y. Radiographic assessment of scapular rotational tilt in chronic shoulder impingement syndrome. J Orthop Sci. 2001;6(1):3–10.
49. Hébert LJ, Moffet H, McFadyen BJ, Dionne CE. Scapular behavior in shoulder impingement syndrome. Arch Phys Med Rehabil. 2002;83(1):60–9.
50. McClure PW, Michener LA, Karduna AR. Shoulder function and 3-dimensional scapular kinematics in people with and without shoulder impingement syndrome. Phys Ther. 2006;86(8):1075–90.
51. Hinterwimmer S, Von Eisenhart-Rothe R, Siebert M, Putz R, Eckstein F, Vogl T, et al. Influence of adducting and abducting muscle forces on the subacromial space width. Med Sci Sports Exerc. 2003;35(12):2055–9.
52. Reddy AS, Mohr KJ, Pink MM, Jobe FW. Electromyographic analysis of the deltoid and rotator cuff muscles in persons with subacromial impingement. J Shoulder Elb Surg. 2000;9(6):519–23.
53. Reinold MM, Escamilla R, Wilk KE. Current concepts in the scientific and clinical rationale behind exercises for glenohumeral and scapulothoracic musculature. J Orthop Sports Phys Ther. 2009;39(2):105–17.
54. Maenhout A, Van Praet K, Pizzi L, Van Herzeele M, Cools A. Electromyographic analysis of knee push up plus variations: what is the influence of the kinetic chain on scapular muscle activity? Br J Sports Med. 2009;44(14):1010–5.
55. Bulgen DY, Binder AI, Hazleman BL, Dutton J, Roberts S. Frozen shoulder: prospective clinical study with an evaluation of three treatment regimens. Ann Rheum Dis. 1984;43(3):353–60.
56. Carette S, Moffet H, Tardif J, Bessette L, Morin F, Fremont P, et al. Intraarticular corticosteroids, supervised physiotherapy, or a combination of the two in the treatment of adhesive capsulitis of the shoulder: a placebo-controlled trial. Arthritis Rheum. 2003;48(3):829–38.
57. Rizk TE, Christopher RP, Pinals RS, Higgins AC, Frix R. Adhesive capsulitis (frozen shoulder): a new approach to its management. Arch Phys Med Rehabil. 1983;64(1):29–33.
58. Gulick DT, Borger A, McNamee L. Effect of analgesic nerve block electrical stimulation in a patient with adhesive capsulitis. Physiother Theory Pract. 2007;23(1):57–63.
59. Favejee MM, Huisstede BMA, Koes BW. Frozen shoulder: the effectiveness of conservative and surgical interventions-systematic review. Br J Sports Med. 2011;45(1):49–56.
60. Page MJ, Green S, Kramer S, Johnston RV, McBain B, Buchbinder R. Electrotherapy modalities for adhesive capsulitis (frozen shoulder). Cochrane Database Syst Rev. 2014;10:CD011324.
61. Cheing GLY, So EML, Chao CYL. Effectiveness of electroacupuncture and interferential electrotherapy in the management of frozen shoulder. J Rehabil Med. 2008;40(3):166–70.
62. Nicholson GG. The effects of passive joint mobilization on pain and hypomobility associated with adhesive capsulitis of the shoulder. J Orthop Sports Phys Ther. 1985;6(4):238–46.
63. Vermeulen HM, Obermann WR, Burger BJ, Kok GJ, Rozing PM, van Den Ende CH. End-range mobilization techniques in adhesive capsulitis of the shoulder joint: a multiple-subject case report. Phys Ther. 2000;80(12):1204–13.
64. Vermeulen HM, Rozing PM, Obermann WR, le Cessie S, Vlieland TPMV. Comparison of high-grade and low-grade mobilization techniques

in the management of adhesive capsulitis of the shoulder: randomized controlled trial. Phys Ther. 2006;86(3):355–68.
65. Yang JL, Chang CW, Chen SY, Wang SF, Lin JJ. Mobilization techniques in subjects with frozen shoulder syndrome: randomized multiple-treatment trial. Phys Ther. 2007;87(10):1307–15.
66. Fayad F, Roby-Brami A, Yazbeck C, Hanneton S, Lefevre-Colau MM, Gautheron V, et al. Three-dimensional scapular kinematics and scapulohumeral rhythm in patients with glenohumeral osteoarthritis or frozen shoulder. J Biomech. 2008;41(2):326–32.
67. Roren A, Lefevre-Colau MM, Roby-Brami A, Revel M, Fermanian J, Gautheron V, et al. Modified 3D scapular kinematic patterns for activities of daily living in painful shoulders with restricted mobility: a comparison with contralateral unaffected shoulders. J Biomech. 2012;45(7):1305–11.
68. Lee SY, Lee KJ, Kim W, Chung SG. Relationships between capsular stiffness and clinical features in adhesive capsulitis of the shoulder. PM&R. 2015;7(12):1226–34.
69. Donatelli RA. Physical therapy of the shoulder. Netherlands: Elsevier Health Sciences; 2011.
70. Wyke B. The neurology of joints. Ann R Coll Surg Engl. 1967;41(1):25–50.
71. Watson L, Dalziel R, Story I. Frozen shoulder: a 12-month clinical outcome trial. J Shoulder Elb Surg. 2000;9(1):16–22.
72. Mueller MJ, Maluf KS. Tissue adaptation to physical stress: a proposed "physical stress theory" to guide physical therapist practice, education, and research. Phys Ther. 2002;82(4):383–403.
73. Kelley MJ, McClure PW, Leggin BG. Frozen shoulder: evidence and a proposed model guiding rehabilitation. J Orthop Sports Phys Ther. 2009;39(2):135–48.
74. Wilk KE, Macrina LC, Reinold MM. Non-operative rehabilitation for traumatic and atraumatic glenohumeral instability. N Am J Sports Phys Ther. 2006;1(1):16–31.
75. Streubel PN, Krych AJ, Simone JP, Dahm DL, Sperling JW, Steinmann SP, et al. Anterior glenohumeral instability: a pathology-based surgical treatment strategy. J Am Acad Orthop Surg. 2014;22(5):283–94.
76. Burkhart SS, De Beer JF. Traumatic glenohumeral bone defects and their relationship to failure of arthroscopic bankart repairs: significance of the inverted-pear glenoid and the humeral engaging hill-Sachs lesion. Arthroscopy. 2000;16(7):677–94.
77. Godin J, Sekiya JK. Systematic review of rehabilitation versus operative stabilization for the treatment of first-time anterior shoulder dislocations. Sports Health. 2010;2(2):156–65.
78. Merolla G, De Santis E, Cools AM, Porcellini G. Functional outcome and quality of life after rehabilitation for voluntary posterior shoulder dislocation: a prospective blinded cohort study. Eur J Orthop Surg Traumatol. 2015;25(2):263–72.
79. Leivadiotou D, Ahrens P. Arthroscopic treatment of posterior shoulder instability: a systematic review. Arthroscopy. 2015;31(3):555–60.
80. Knesek M, Skendzel JG, Dines JS, Altchek DW, Allen AA, Bedi A. Diagnosis and management of superior labral anterior posterior tears in throwing athletes. Am J Sports Med. 2013;41(2):444–60.
81. Jang SH, Seo JG, Jang HS, Jung JE, Kim JG. Predictive factors associated with failure of nonoperative treatment of superior labrum anterior-posterior tears. J Shoulder Elb Surg. 2016;25(3):428–34.
82. Gottschalk MB, Ghasem A, Todd D, Daruwalla J, Xerogeanes J, Karas S. Posterior shoulder instability: does glenoid retroversion predict recurrence and contralateral instability? Arthroscopy. 2015;31(3):488–93.
83. Duzgun I, Baltaci G, Turgut E, Atay OA. Effects of slow and accelerated rehabilitation protocols on range of motion after arthroscopic rotator cuff repair. Acta Orthop Traumatol Turc. 2014;48(6):642–8.
84. Singh H, Osbahr DC, Holovacs TF, Cawley PW, Speer KP. The efficacy of continuous cryotherapy on the postoperative shoulder: a prospective, randomized investigation. J Shoulder Elb Surg. 2001;10(6):522–5.
85. Cohen BB, Romeo AA, Bach B. Rehabilitation of the shoulder after rotator-cuff repair. Oper Tech Orthop. 2002;12(3):218–24.
86. Duzgun I, Baltaci G, Atay OA. Comparison of slow and accelerated rehabilitation protocol after arthroscopic rotator cuff repair: pain and functional activity. Acta Orthop Traumatol Turc. 2011;45(1):23–33.
87. Chang KV, Hung CY, Han DS, Chen WS, Wang TG, Chien KL. Early versus delayed passive range of motion exercise for arthroscopic rotator cuff repair: a meta-analysis of randomized controlled trials. Am J Sports Med. 2015;43(5):1265–73.
88. Kluczynski MA, Nayyar S, Marzo JM, Bisson LJ. Early versus delayed passive range of motion after rotator cuff repair: a systematic review and meta-analysis. Am J Sports Med. 2015;43(8):2057–63.
89. Hayes K, Ginn KA, Walton JR, Szomor ZL, Murrell GA. A randomised clinical trial evaluating the efficacy of physiotherapy after rotator cuff repair. Aust J Physiother. 2004;50(2):77–83.
90. Kellett J. Acute soft tissue injuries—a review of the literature. Med Sci Sports Exerc. 1986;18(5):489–500.
91. Arem AJ, Madden JW. Effects of stress on healing wounds. 1. Intermittent noncyclical tension. J Surg Res. 1976;20(2):93–102.
92. Kibler W, Livingston B, Bruce R. Current concepts in shoulder rehabilitation. In: Advances in operative orthopedics. Vol. 3; 1995. p. 249–300.
93. Long JL, Thiele RAR, Skendzel JG, Jeon J, Hughes RE, Miller BS, et al. Activation of the shoulder musculature during pendulum exercises and light activities. J Orthop Sports Phys Ther. 2010;40(4):230–7.

94. Poppen N, Walker P. Forces at the glenohumeral joint in abduction. Clin Orthop Relat Res. 1978;135:165–70.
95. Kibler WB. Shoulder rehabilitation: principles and practice. Med Sci Sports Exerc. 1998;30(4 Suppl):S40–50.
96. Gaunt BW, Shaffer MA, Sauers EL, Michener LA, McCluskey GM, Thigpen C, et al. The american society of shoulder and elbow therapists' consensus rehabilitation guideline for arthroscopic anterior capsulolabral repair of the shoulder. J Orthop Sports Phys Ther. 2010;40(3):155–68.
97. O'Connell PW, Nuber GW, Mileski RA, Lautenschlager E. The contribution of the glenohumeral ligaments to anterior stability of the shoulder joint. Am J Sports Med. 1990;18(6):579–84.
98. Turkel SJ, Panio MW, Marshall JL, Girgis FG. Stabilizing mechanisms preventing anterior dislocation of the glenohumeral joint. J Bone Joint Surg Am. 1981;63(8):1208–17.
99. Blasier RB, Guldberg RE, Rothman ED. Anterior shoulder stability: contributions of rotator cuff forces and the capsular ligaments in a cadaver model. J Shoulder Elb Surg. 1992;1(3):140–50.
100. Borsa PA, Dover GC, Wilk KE, Reinold MM. Glenohumeral range of motion and stiffness in professional baseball pitchers. Med Sci Sports Exerc. 2006;38(1):21–6.
101. Karduna AR, Williams GR, Williams JL, Iannotti JP. Kinematics of the glenohumeral joint: influences of muscle forces, ligamentous constraints, and articular geometry. J Orthop Res. 1996;14(6):986–93.
102. Labriola JE, Lee TQ, Debski RE, McMahon PJ. Stability and instability of the glenohumeral joint: the role of shoulder muscles. J Shoulder Elb Surg. 2005;14(1 Suppl S):32S–8S.
103. Louie JK, Mote CD. Contribution of the musculature to rotatory laxity and torsional stiffness at the knee. J Biomech. 1987;20(3):281–300.
104. Wilk KE, Macrina LC. Rehabilitation for patients with posterior instability and multidirectional instability. Oper Tech Sports Med. 2014;22(1):108–23.
105. Wilk KE, Reinold MM, Dugas JR, Arrigo CA, Moser MW, Andrews JR. Current concepts in the recognition and treatment of superior labral (SLAP) lesions. J Orthop Sports Phys Ther. 2005;35(5):273–91.
106. Manske R, Prohaska D. Superior labrum anterior to posterior (SLAP) rehabilitation in the overhead athlete. Phys Ther Sport. 2010;11(4):110–21.
107. Brems JJ. Rehabilitation after total shoulder arthroplasty: current concepts. Semin Arthroplast. 2007;18(1):55–65.
108. Wilcox III RB, Arslanian LE, Millett PJ. Rehabilitation following total shoulder arthroplasty. J Orthop Sports Phys Ther. 2005;35(12):821–36.
109. Seitz WH, Michaud EJ. Rehabilitation after shoulder replacement: be all you can be! Semin Arthroplast. 2012;23(2):106–13.
110. Boardman ND, Cofield RH, Bengtson KA, Little R, Jones MC, Rowland CM. Rehabilitation after total shoulder arthroplasty. J Arthroplast. 2001;16(4):483–6.
111. Jackins S. Postoperative shoulder rehabilitation. Phys Med Rehabil Clin N Am. 2004;15(3):643–82.
112. Lin TW, Cardenas L, Soslowsky LJ. Biomechanics of tendon injury and repair. J Biomech. 2004;37(6):865–77.
113. Harper D, Young A, McNaught C-E. The physiology of wound healing. Surgery (Oxford). 2014;32(9):445–50.
114. Bleakley CM, Davison G. Management of acute soft tissue injury using protection rest ice compression and elevation: recommendations from the Association of Chartered Physiotherapists in sports and exercise medicine (ACPSM) [executive summary]. Association of Chartered Physiotherapists in Sports and Exercise Medicine; 2010. p. 1–24.
115. Boudreau S, Boudreau E, Higgins LD, Wilcox III RB. Rehabilitation following reverse total shoulder arthroplasty. J Orthop Sports Phys Ther. 2007;37(12):734–43.
116. Grammont P, Baulot E. Delta shoulder prosthesis for rotator cuff rupture. Orthopedics. 1993;16(1):65.
117. Alta TD, de Toledo JM, Veeger H, Janssen TW, Willems WJ. The active and passive kinematic difference between primary reverse and total shoulder prostheses. J Shoulder Elb Surg. 2014;23(9):1395–402.
118. Millis D, Levine D. Canine rehabilitation and physical therapy. Netherlands: Elsevier Health Sciences; 2013.
119. Boileau P, Watkinson DJ, Hatzidakis AM, Balg F. Grammont reverse prosthesis: design, rationale, and biomechanics. J Shoulder Elb Surg. 2005;14(1):S147–S61.
120. Al-Hadithy N, Domos P, Sewell MD, Pandit R. Reverse shoulder arthroplasty in 41 patients with cuff tear arthropathy with a mean follow-up period of 5 years. J Shoulder Elb Surg. 2014;23(11):1662–8.

19 Injections

Filippo Familiari, Gazi Huri, Olimpio Galasso, Giorgio Gasparini, and Mahmut Nedim Doral

Background

Although the Authors advise against an indiscriminate use of injections at different sites of the shoulder, it has to be taken into account that injections are a powerful tool in selected cases and with precise indications.

Shoulder injections are used for a variety of conditions including osteoarthritis (OA), adhesive capsulitis (frozen shoulder), subacromial (SA) impingement, SA bursitis, rotator cuff disease, tenosynovitis or tendinitis of the long head of the biceps brachii tendon (LHBT), and labral pathology. Corticosteroids are the most commonly used injection medium; but, there is increasing evidence to support the use of hyaluronate (viscosupplementation) injections for the shoulder.

Studies have demonstrated that the degree of pain relief and functional improvement is greater when the injection is documented to be in the intended location [1, 2]. Accordingly, accurate placement of the injection is desirable in performing this procedure. In the glenohumeral (GH) joint, approaches include anterior and posterior. In the (SA) space, approaches include anterolateral, lateral, and posterior. In the acromioclavicular (AC) joint, only the superior approach is considered. For the LHBT, only the anterior approach is considered.

Moreover, studies have suggested that imaging modalities such as ultrasonography (US), magnetic resonance (MR) arthrography, and fluoroscopy can be used successfully to guide injections [2–6].

General Advice

Independently from the indication for injection, the site of the shoulder that has to be injected, the medium and the approach used, it is highly recommended (1) to follow a strict sterile technique and (2) that the solution should be injected out of the syringe only after excluding intravascular placement by performing drawback on the syringe itself.

Depending on the site of the shoulder that has to be injected, there are different sizes for the syringe and needle as well as for the injection medium (anesthetic or corticosteroid or both) that should be used [7]. The most frequently used drugs are anesthetics (1% lidocaine or 0.25–0.5% bupivacaine) and/or corticosteroids (betamethasone sodium phosphate and acetate or methylprednisolone, 40 mg/mL).

F. Familiari, M.D. (✉) • O. Galasso, M.D.
G. Gasparini, M.D.
Department of Orthopaedic and Trauma Surgery, Magna Græcia University, Catanzaro, Italy
e-mail: filippofamiliari@gmail.com

G. Huri, M.D. • M.N. Doral, M.D.
Department of Orthopaedics and Traumatology, Hacettepe University, Ankara, Turkey

G. Huri, N.K. Paschos (eds.), *The Shoulder*, Orthopaedic Study Guide Series,
DOI 10.1007/978-3-319-51979-1_19

Glenohumeral Joint

Indications

The main indications for intra-articular injections are OA, adhesive capsulitis, and rheumatoid arthritis; although, some physicians also use injections during diagnostic investigation in situations of suspected labral pathology.

Injection Technique

In the GH joint, the posterior approach avoids the subclavian artery, subclavian vein, and brachial plexus and offers the psychological advantage of hiding the needle completely from the patient's field of view. In contrast, the anterior approach offers the advantage of more reproducible bone landmarks to help guide the injection. Essential landmarks to palpate before performing the injection include the humeral head, the coracoid process, and the acromion. The joint is most easily accessible with the patient sitting, the patient's arm resting comfortably at the side, and the shoulder externally rotated. A 10 mL syringe with a 25 gauge needle is used to inject anesthetic (5–7 mL) and/or corticosteroid (1–2 mL).

Posterior Approach

The needle should be inserted 2 cm inferior to the posterolateral corner of the acromion and directed anteriorly in the direction of the coracoid process (Fig. 19.1).

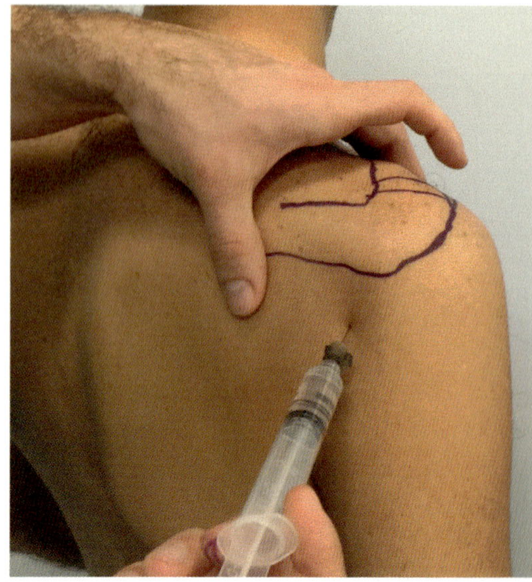

Fig. 19.1 Posterior approach to the glenohumeral joint.

Anterior Approach

The needle should be placed just medial to the head of the humerus and 1 cm lateral to the coracoid process (Fig. 19.2). The needle is directed posteriorly and slightly superiorly and laterally.

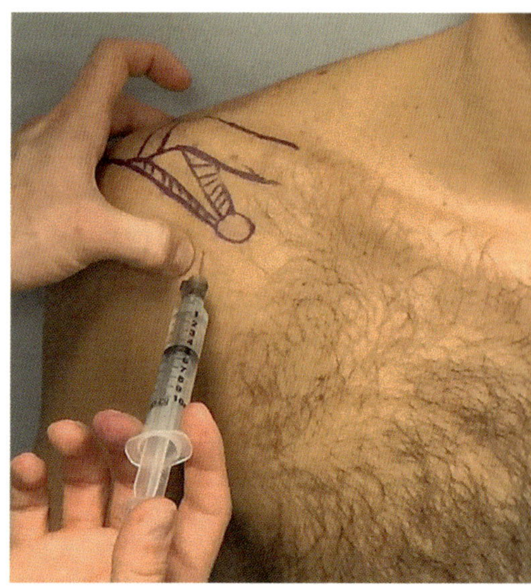

Fig. 19.2 Anterior approach to the glenohumeral joint.

Current Evidence

A recent systematic review [8] analyzed a total of 220 injections through two different approaches. There were 73 shoulders injected through an anterior approach, and the average of the reported accuracy rates of the included studies was 40% (range, 27–100%). There were 147 shoulders injected through a posterior approach with an average accuracy of 85% (no range because of only one posterior approach study). Gadolinium injections and MR arthrograms for accuracy were used in two studies [4, 6], MR arthrography with saline as a contrast agent in one study [5], and in one study [2] anteroposterior (AP) and axial shoulder radiographs were used to verify injection accuracy.

Subacromial Space

Indications

An injection is commonly performed within the SA space for different indications, including SA bursitis, rotator cuff impingement, and rotator cuff tendinosis; frequently local anesthetics are injected to differentiate antalgic impairment to impairment due to tendon(s) lesion.

Injection Technique

The distal, lateral, and posterior edges of the acromion are palpated. The patient is in a seated position with the arm resting comfortably at the side, and distracted by gravity. A 10 mL syringe with a 21–22 gauge needle is used to inject anesthetic (5–7 mL) and/or corticosteroid (1–2 mL).

Anterolateral Approach

The needle is initially inserted obliquely in relation to the axial plane, 1 cm inferior to the anterolateral corner of the acromion obliquely to the greater tuberosity (Fig. 19.3). When the bone is felt, the needle is slightly withdrawn and redirected in a more horizontal plane, and advanced posteriorly as a downward traction applied to the arm to widen the SA space.

Lateral Approach

Injection is performed just inferior to the midlateral aspect of the acromion, with the needle being angled slightly cephalad (Fig. 19.4).

Posterior Approach

The needle is inserted 2 cm caudal and 1 cm medial to the posterolateral corner of the acromion, with the needle being angled approximately 45° cephalad to follow the contour of the posterior acromion (Fig. 19.5).

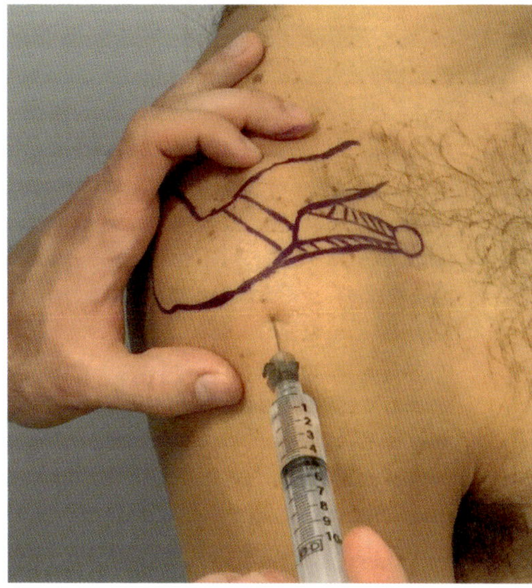

Fig. 19.3 Anterolateral approach to the subacromial space.

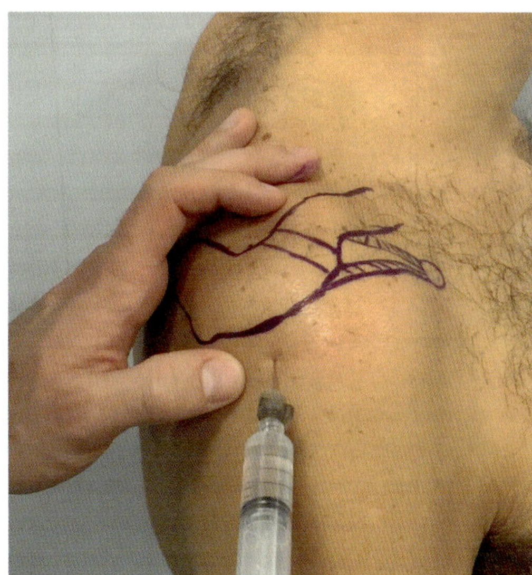

Fig. 19.4 Lateral approach to the subacromial space.

Current Evidence

Daley et al. [8] performed a systematic review on 281 injections performed in the SA space: 60 injections performed with imaging (average accuracy: 100%; no range), and 221 injections performed without imaging (average accuracy: 72%; range, 29–100%) [1, 2, 9–13]. The authors

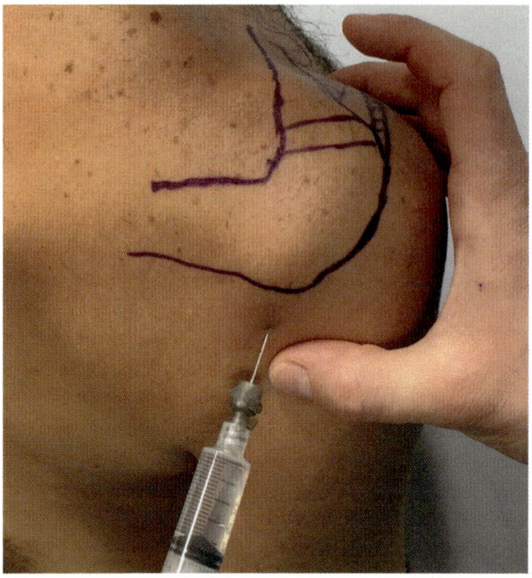

Fig. 19.5 Posterior approach to the subacromial space.

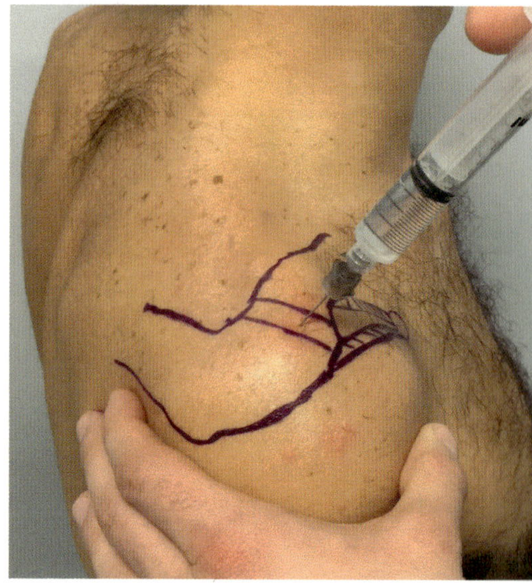

Fig. 19.6 Approach to the acromioclavicular joint.

reported a statistically significant difference ($P < .001$) in accuracy rates between imaging and non-imaging in the SA space, with imaging having a higher rate of injection accuracy.

Acromioclavicular Joint

Indications

Local anesthetics are injected as part of the diagnostic workup of the source of pain about the shoulder girdle and corticosteroid injections as part of the treatment for ACJ arthritis.

Injection Technique

Patients are placed in the supine or seated position with the affected arm resting comfortably at their side. A 3–5 mL syringe with a 25 gauge needle is used to inject anesthetic (0.5 mL) and/or corticosteroid (0.25–0.5 mL). To identify the AC joint, palpate the clavicle distally to its termination at which point a slight depression will be felt at the joint articulation. The needle is inserted from the superior and anterior approach into the AC joint and directed inferiorly (Fig. 19.6).

Current Evidence

A recent systematic review [8] evaluated 220 injections in the AC joint. There were 110 performed with imaging (average accuracy: 100%; no range), and 110 were performed without imaging (average accuracy: 45%; range, 39–55%) [3, 14]. The authors reported a statistically significant difference ($P < .001$) in accuracy rates between imaging and non-imaging in the AC joint, with imaging having a higher rate of injection accuracy.

Long Head of the Biceps Brachii Tendon

Indications

The LHBT is rarely involved without other concomitant shoulder pathology. Bicipital tendinitis generally is found along with rotator cuff tendinitis/SA bursitis as part of a more generalized shoulder impingement syndrome. These injections are needed uncommonly and often an injection is performed more logically into the SA space because this closer addresses the primary pathology.

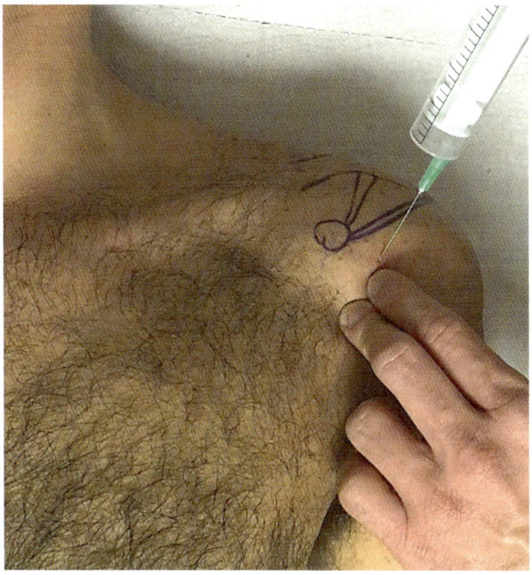

Fig. 19.7 Approach to the long head of the biceps brachii tendon.

Injection Technique

A 3–5 mL syringe with a 23 gauge needle is used to inject anesthetic (0.5 mL) and/or corticosteroid (0.25 mL). With the patient supine and with slight internal rotation of the shoulder, after the bicipital groove is placed at the front and identified by palpation, the needle is inserted at an angle of 30° and directed parallel to the groove (Fig. 19.7) [15].

Current Evidence

There is lack of data on the efficacy and accuracy of LHBT injections. A general statement appears throughout the literature that caution should be exercised with tendon sheath injections because inadvertent intratendinous injections have been associated with tendon rupture.

Hashiuchi et al. [16] compared the accuracy of US-guided biceps tendon sheath injection with unguided injection in 30 patients who had a primary diagnosis of tenosynovitis or tendinitis of the LHBT, or both. US-guided injection was performed in 15 shoulders and unguided injection was performed in 15 shoulders. Computed tomography imaging was performed immediately after a contrast agent was injected into the LHBT sheath. The locations of contrast seen on CT scan were classified into three types: type 1, only within the tendon sheath; type 2, inside the tendon, tendon sheath, and surrounding area; type 3, only the area outside the tendon sheath. US-guided injections resulted in 86.7% type 1 and 13.3% type 2 locations. Unguided injections resulted in 26.7% type 1, 40.0% type 2, and 33.3% type 3 locations. The difference for each location type was significant ($P < .05$). The authors concluded that injection into the tendon sheath of the LHBT can be more accurately performed using US guidance than by the blind method.

Questions

Landmarks that need to be identified before performing a shoulder injection include
- A Humeral head
- B Coracoid process
- C Posterior lateral acromion
- D Anterolateral acromion
- E A & B
- F All the above

The average reported accuracy for shoulder injections
- A Is higher with anterior approach
- B Is higher with posterior approach
- C Is similar regardless approach

Biceps tendon sheath injections
- A Are more accurate under U/S guidance
- B Are more accurate without U/S guidance
- C There is no difference between U/S guidance or not

References

1. Esenyel CZ, Esenyel M, Yeslitepe R, et al. The correlation between the accuracy of steroid injections and subsequent shoulder pain and function in subacromial impingement syndrome. Acta Orthop Traumatol Turc. 2003;37(1):41–5.
2. Eustace JA, Brophy DP, Gibney RP, Bresnihan B, FitzGerald O. Comparison of the accuracy of steroid placement with clinical outcome in patients with shoulder syndromes. Ann Rheum Dis. 1997;56(1):59–63.

3. Bisbinas I, Belthur M, Said HG, Green M, Learmoth DJ. Accuracy of needle placement in ACJ injections. Knee Surg Sports Traumatol Arthrosc. 2006;14(8):762–5.
4. Catalano OA, Manfredi R, Vanzulli A, et al. MR arthrography of the glenohumeral joint: modified posterior approach without imaging guidance. Radiology. 2007;242(2):550–4.
5. DeMouy EH, Menendez Jr CV, Bodin CJ. Palpation-directed (nonfluoroscopically guided) saline-enhanced MR arthrography of the shoulder. AJR Am J Roentgenol. 1997;169(1):229–31.
6. Sethi PM, Kingston S, Elattrache N. Accuracy of anterior intra-articular injection of the glenohumeral joint. Arthroscopy. 2005;21(1):77–80.
7. Tallia AF, Cardone DA. Diagnosis and therapeutic injection of the shoulder region. Am Fam Physician. 2003;15:1271–8.
8. Daley EL, Bajaj S, Bisson LJ, Cole BJ. Improving injection accuracy of the elbow, knee, and shoulder: does injection site and imaging make a difference? A systematic review. Am J Sports Med. 2011;39(3):656–62.
9. Henkus HE, Cobben LP, Coerkamp EG, Nelissen RG, van Arkel ER. The accuracy of subacromial injections: a prospective randomized magnetic resonance imaging study. Arthroscopy. 2006;22(3):277–82.
10. Kang MN, Rizio L, Prybicien M, Middlemas DA, Blacksin MF. The accuracy of subacromial corticosteroid injections: a comparison of multiple methods. J Shoulder Elb Surg. 2008;17(suppl):61S–6S.
11. Rutten M, Maresch B, Jager G, de Waal Malefijt MC. Injection of subacromial-subdeltoid bursa: blind or ultrasound guided? Acta Orthop. 2007;78(2):254–7.
12. Valls R, Melloni P. Sonographic guidance of needle position for MR arthrography of the shoulder. AJR Am J Roentgenol. 1997;169(3):845–7.
13. Yamakado K. The targeting accuracy of subacromial injection to the shoulder: an arthrographic evaluation. Arthroscopy. 2002;18(8):887–91.
14. Bain GI, Van Riet RT, Gooi C, Ashland N. The long term efficacy of corticosteroid injection into the acromioclavicular joint using a dynamic fluoroscopic method. Int J Shoulder Surg. 2007;1(4):104–7.
15. Churgay CA. Diagnosis and treatment of biceps tendonitis and tendinosis. Am Fam Physician. 2009;80:470–6.
16. Haschiuchi T, Sakurai G, Morimoto M, Komei T, Takakura Y, Tanaka Y. Accuracy of the biceps tendon sheath injection: ultrasound-guided or unguided injection? A randomized controlled trial. J Shoulder Elb Surg. 2011;20(7):1069–73. doi:10.1016/j.jse.2011.04.004. Epub 2011 Jul 22

Part VII

Operative Management of Shoulder Disorders

Arthroscopic Positioning: Beach Chair Versus Lateral

20

Kelly G. Kilcoyne and Uma Srikumaran

The Great Debate: Beach Chair Versus Lateral

The great debate amongst surgeon's about the 'best' position for shoulder arthroscopy continues. The surgeon's use and preference for positioning is often dictated by his or her training, and also commonly affected by geography. Historically, surgeon's who practice and or trained on the west coast typically use the lateral position, with those on the east coast preferring the beach chair position [1, 2]. The reality is there is a mixture of surgeons who prefer one position over the other in every location, and those who use a combination of both. However, even the most loyal to their preferred position would agree, there are certain advantages and disadvantages of both the beach chair and lateral position for shoulder arthroscopy.

The beach chair position is often easier for beginning arthroscopists to orient to as the arthroscopic anatomy matches that of the shoulder when it is examined (upright). This is in contrast to the typical orientation of the glenoid being parallel to the floor in the lateral position. Also, positioning the acromion parallel to the ground allows for easier access and orientation for the surgeon performing procedures like subacromial decompression and arthroscopic distal clavicle excision (Fig. 20.1). The view of the rotator cuff, and ease and familiarity with instrumentation, make beach chair a good option for rotator cuff repairs. Placement of anterior medial and superior portals can be somewhat challenging in this position as the head can block access and trajectory (i.e. subscapularis tears).

Just as the beach chair offers excellent visualization of the rotator cuff, the lateral position offers a great view of the entire glenoid, capsule, and labrum, making it an attractive option for instability procedures (Figs. 20.2 and 20.3). Additionally, many surgeons find the lateral position to be easier with no assistant (instruments can be left in place without risk of falling out or significant change in view).

As stated, both positions are reasonable and effective options for arthroscopic treatment of instability. The lateral position offers a more comprehensive and global look at the glenoid, labrum, and capsule. It also offers increased access and visualization of the posterior and inferior aspects of the glenohumeral joint [3]. Many proponents of the lateral position for instability argue that it allows more titration of capsular stitches. However, the trajectory when drilling for anchors can be flatter (parallel with glenoid) with more tendency to skive than with beach chair. Additionally, if a bump is placed in the axilla in the beach chair position, the glenohumeral space is widened affording increased access [1].

K.G. Kilcoyne, M.D. (✉) • U. Srikumaran, M.D., M.B.A.
Johns Hopkins Orthopaedic Surgery, Johns Hopkins University School of Medicine, Baltimore, MD, USA

G. Huri, N.K. Paschos (eds.), *The Shoulder*, Orthopaedic Study Guide Series,
DOI 10.1007/978-3-319-51979-1_20

A recent systematic review on outcomes of arthroscopic anterior shoulder instability compared lateral versus beach chair positioning [4]. After reviewing 64 studies, all with a minimum 2 year follow-up, the authors found that both arthroscopic methods led to a low rate of recurrence with excellent clinical outcomes. There was a statistically significant difference between the two with respect to instability recurrence, 14.65 ± 8.4% in the BC group compared with 8.5% ± 7.1% in the LD group (P = .002).

A slight disadvantage of the lateral position is conversion to open procedures [5]. This includes converting to an open bankart for example. This requires repositioning the patient at a minimum, with a frequent need to reposition and completely re-prep and drape. Similarly, performing an open sub pectoral tenodesis can be a bit inconvenient, requiring the nurse to deflate the bean bag and letting the patient into a 'sloppy' lateral, versus again re-prepping, position and draping. In contrast, if the patient is in the beach chair, little to no adjustments are needed to convert from an arthroscopic to open bankart, or to perform a sub pectoral biceps tenodesis.

While the beach chair may not offer the same visualization and access to the entire glenohumeral joint, it does not require any traction on the operative arm. Additionally, many anesthesia providers prefer its ease of access to the airway, and if the patient needs to be placed supine urgently or emergently, this is easier to accomplish in the beach chair compared with the lateral position.

Another important topic, especially in the anesthesia literature, is the topic of cerebral ischemia. It has been hypothesized that cerebral ischemic events could occur when the patient is sat up into beach chair position, under condition of controlled hypotension [6]. In a study assessing cerebral desaturation events in the beach chair and lateral positions, the incidence of these events was 80.3% in the beach chair position compared with 0% in the lateral group [7]. However, there is no evidence that cerebral desaturation events lead to any long term or permanent neurologic sequelae [1].

The optimal position is no doubt surgeon dependent. Some surgeons perform all procedures in one position, while others vary position according to the planned procedure. The surgeon should decide which position, or combination, works best for them, creating the most reproducible and best results.

Set-Up

Proponents of each position have claimed that set-up of one position is easier than the other. In our experience, the overall time to set the patient up in each position is fairly similar. Additionally, the key principles of positioning for safety of the patient, and for appropriate and efficacious performance of procedure are constant regardless of position. Care must be taken to pad all boney prominences, ensure the neck is in neutral alignment, and the patient is securely positioned on the bed, in both the beach chair and lateral position. In our practice, despite having trained residents and fellows, the primary surgeon is present for patient positioning to ensure it is done safely, appropriately, and in a timely manner.

Beach Chair

There are several beach chair bed attachments available (Fig. 20.4). Most have an adjustable head positioner, and removable side to allow access to the shoulder. The head holder attachment can be placed on the bed before the patient is transferred to the bed or after, depending on the design, as well as the comfort of the anesthesia provider. The head holder typically includes a foam pad or strap to be placed across the forehead and under the chin to hold the patients head and neck steady, and in a neutral position, during the procedure. The patient's waist should be placed just above the break in the bed. Two pillows, or a commercial foam block can be placed under the patients legs to prevent the patient from sliding down the table once positioned upright. Another option is to flex the bed to prevent sliding, but the former can save time. Once the patient is anesthetized and secured, they are placed upright. Sitting the patient up until the acromion is about parallel to the floor, typically about 70–90°, is advantageous as it makes the glenohumeral and subacromial anatomy reproducible and identifiable.

There are several operative arm holders to negate the need of additional assistants. Additionally, it allows for placement of the shoulder in specific positions depending upon the procedure, and for slight distraction of the humeral head for instability cases, or to open up the subacromial space. These pneumatic arm holders include the spider (Smith & Nephew, Inc.) and the trimano (Arthrex, Inc). Both use disposable arm attachments which are put on in the sterile field and subsequently attached to the main device attached to the table. Depending on the side and set-up of the operating room, the arm holder can be placed before or after the patient is transferred to the operating table. Some tables only allow for the arm positioner to be attached to the side, which necessitates switching the main attachment back and forth depending on the operative side. Tables that allow attachment of the holder to the back of the table do not need to be switched for right and left shoulders. The non operative arm is placed on a padded arm holder, ensuring the shoulder height is symmetric with the operative side, with no unnecessary traction on the extremity.

Prepping and draping are standard. There are commercially available beach chair drapes than include a clear pocket with a connection for suction. This serves as a catch for dropped instruments, and more importantly a collection point for leaked fluid.

The surgeon and assistant (if present) will stand on the operative side of the patient, with the surgical tech and mayo stand at the patients feet. The mayo stand will be organized with the most commonly used equipment and devices. A back table is used for additional and less commonly used equipment. The tower containing the pump, video equipment and power is placed so the surgeon can see it. Monitors (ideally two) are placed for easy visualization by the surgeon whether the camera is anterior or posterior. The operative bed is typically turned 45–90° once positioning is completed. This allows complete and free access to the operative shoulder for the surgeon and team.

Lateral

As stated, proponents of the lateral position often emphasize that time need for patient positioning is less than for beach chair [8]. However, there are many steps required to ensure appropriate and safe lateral patient positioning. A vacuum bean bag or peg board can be used for positioning, depending on preference. It is placed on the table prior to patient transfer. If a bean bag is being used, it should end at mid or superior scapula to ensure the shoulder remains stable throughout the procedure, and allow appropriate access for instrumentation. If the anesthesia provider is comfortable intubating in the lateral position, the patient can position themselves in a comfortable lateral position and then anesthesia can be induced. This ensures there is no undo pressure or traction on the patients down side, and also expedites the process of positioning. However, it does not allow an examination under anesthesia of the non operative shoulder, which should be taken into account when using this method. Alternatively, the patient is transferred to the table, intubated, and then positioned by the surgical team. Those in favor of the beach chair note that fewer people are needed to position the patient than are needed to roll the patient on their side, inflate bean bag etc. An axillary role is placed, under the non operative arm once the patient is on their side. Care should be taken to pad and slight flex the knee of the down leg, with specific focus to the peroneal nerve. One to two pillows are placed between the patients legs. The patient and the bean bag are secured to the bed with the padded bed strap, or tape, or a combination of both. We recommend placing tape as proximal as possible in the axilla, over a blue towel or other pad, to ensure the shoulder does not move too much during the case. If the shoulder is not secure it can make viewing and instrumentation throughout the case more challenging.

There are several commercially available lateral arm positioners (Fig. 20.5). One option is a traction tower, the most common in our experience being the lateral arm positioner made by Arthex (Fig. 20.6). It is attached at the foot of the bed, on the side opposite the operative arm. There are typically three cables that allow for traction, abduction and forward flexion. A 10 pound weight is typically used for traction. An additional 5 pound weight can be used on the abduction cable (Fig. 20.7). Alternatively, a large sterile bump can be used instead of attaching weight to the abduction cable. Both allow for excellent visualization and access to the entire glenoid by abducting the humeral head away from the glenoid articular surface.

Like the beach chair, there are lateral arm position packs that include a sterile arm sleeve, rope and cables to connect to the traction tower. Important aspects of placing this sleeve are ensuring a tight arm fit with the velcro fasteners (we reinforce by wrapping coban), ensuring the sleeve is as far proximal on the arm (level of axilla) as possible. Additionally, the abduction strap is used, ensure it is placed as proximal on the sleeve as possible. If placed too distal may put undo tension on the arm without adequately distraction the glenohumeral joint. The arm is placed in approximately 10–20° of forward flexion and 45–70° abduction depending on the procedure.

Many pneumatic beach chair positioners have attachments that allow for lateral positioning. The spider (Smith and Nephew) has available attachments for lateral positioning. One advantage of these devices is they do not require weights, and allow the arm to be placed (under traction) anywhere in space, as is afforded when device is used in beach chair position.

The surgeon must have access and the ability to use instruments on the anterior and posterior aspects of the shoulder. Thus, in the lateral position, we typically turn the bed 90° so anesthesia and equipment do not block or hinder access. The setup and positioning of the monitors and towers are the same as for the beach chair.

Portal Placement

Regardless of position, it is vital to be familiar with various portals according to procedure, and proper placement. Small deviations in placement of portals in both positions can lead to trouble with access and instrumentation during procedures.

Accurate portal placement begins with marking the surface anatomy. Starting posterior, the posterolateral acromial edge is a relatively identifiable landmark. Once palpated and marked, the scapular spine can be marked medially. Moving anterior from the posterior edge, the lateral acromial edge is palpated and marked. Then the anterolateral acromial edge is palpated and marked. From there the anterior and posterior edge of the clavicle can be marked medially. The supraspinatus fossa is a palpable depression on the superior aspect of the shoulder that can be marked. The AC joint, sometimes palpable, is typically at or near a 45° angle from this lateral aspect of this fossa. Finally, anteriorly, the coracoid process is palpated and marked.

A standard posterolateral portal is made with the posterolateral acromial edge as a reference. A spinal needle can be used prior to introducing the arthroscope into the joint to insufflate. There are differences in the location of portals between beach chair and lateral positions. In the beach chair, the posterolateral portal is typically placed 2 cm distal and 2 cm medial from the posterolateral acromial edge. In the lateral position, this portal is placed more lateral, no more medial the 1 cm from the posterolateral acromial edge. The tendency for new surgeons is to be too proximal and too medial when making portals in the lateral position. The subtle differences between positions, typically a little more lateral start point in the lateral position, are important for the surgeon to understand, especially if switching between positions according to surgical procedure.

Complications

As outlined in the setup section, the surgeon must take care to safely position the patients, ensure the head and neck are secure and in neutral alignment, and that all bony prominences all well padded. This will alleviate risk of injury and resultant complications.

In the lateral decubitus position the patient will be resting on their side, with pressure possible onto the brachial plexus. Placing an axillary role will help prevent direct pressure. Additionally, with weight on the down leg, the peroneal nerve is at risk, and must be protected and padded to avoid injury. Because the lateral position places the operative arm under traction, the brachial plexus is at risk for injury. The surgeon should avoid excess traction and used balanced suspension. Additionally, it has been reported that decreasing abduction (0°) and increasing forward flexion (90°) can decrease the amount of strain on the brachial plexus [8, 9]. The incidence of transient nerve injury reported in the literature for the lateral position ranges from 10 to 30% [1, 2, 5].

Neuropraxia of the injured limb is less common in the beach chair position. However, neuropraxia of the lesser occipital and greater auricular nerves and the hypoglossal nerve have been reported secondary to head positioning and inadequate padding [10, 11].

As discussed, one of the most serious potential complications in the beach chair is a combined decrease in heart rate and blood pressure when the patient is sat upright. While there is no direct correlation between cerebral desaturation events and permanent neurologic sequelae [1], the potential consequences of cerebral hypoperfusion include neurologic impairment, stroke, and death [6].

The risk of pulmonary embolism (PE) and deep vein thrombosis (DVT) are extremely low after shoulder arthroscopy, although there are reported cases in both the lateral and beach chair positions [12, 13]. The majority of patients in these reports have risk factors and or underlying heritable conditions that put them at increased risk for post operative clot. Thus, the surgeon must obtain a complete history in every patient prior to shoulder arthroscopy, and be aware of and potentially recognize the clinical symptoms (calf pain, chest pain, scapular pain, shortness of breath) in the postoperative period.

Images (*NEEDED*).

View of glenohumeral joint: (A) Beach chair (B) Lateral position.

View of posterior/inferior glenoid in lateral position.

View of rotator cuff insertion in beach chair position.

Commercially available arm holders for beach chair. (A) Spider (Smith & Nephew, Inc), (B) Trimano (Arthex, Inc).

Commercially available arm lateral arm positioner (Arthrex, Inc).

Completed patient positioning in the beach chair position.

Completed patient positioning in the lateral position.

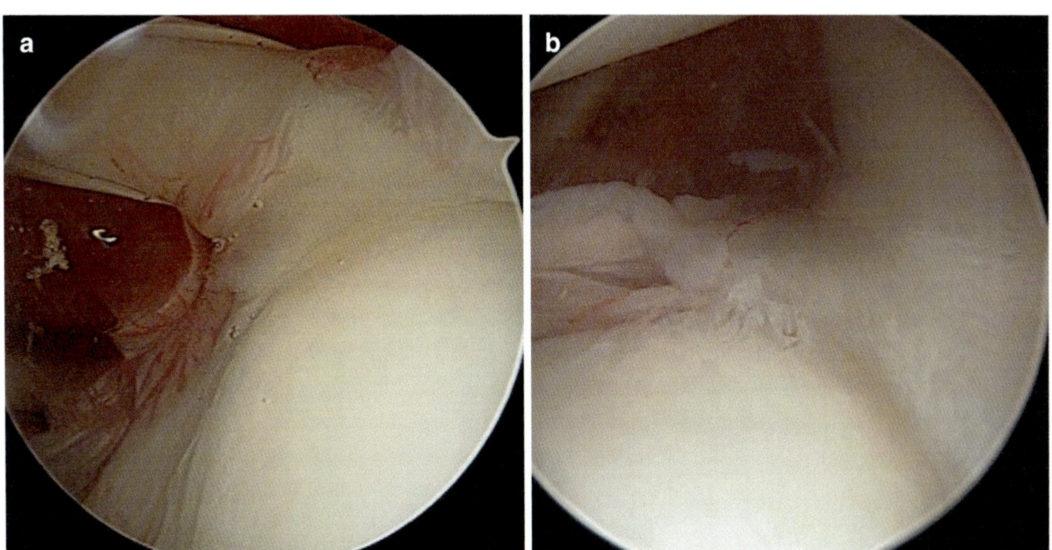

Fig. 20.1 Glenohumeral joint/Superior Labrum viewed from posterior portal. (**a**) Beach Chair (**b**) Lateral

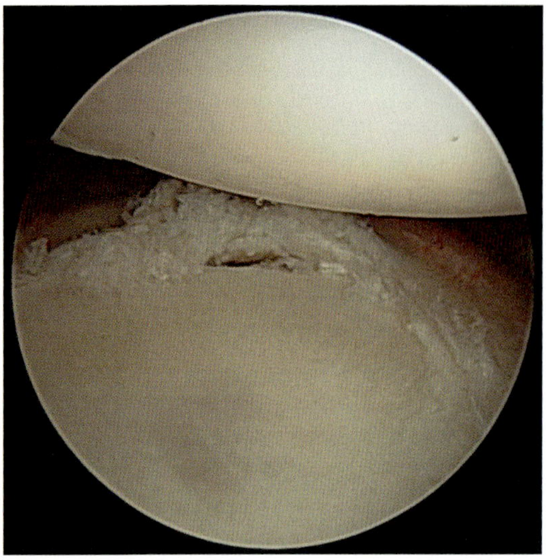

Fig. 20.2 Posterior inferior glenoid labrum viewed from anterior portal – lateral

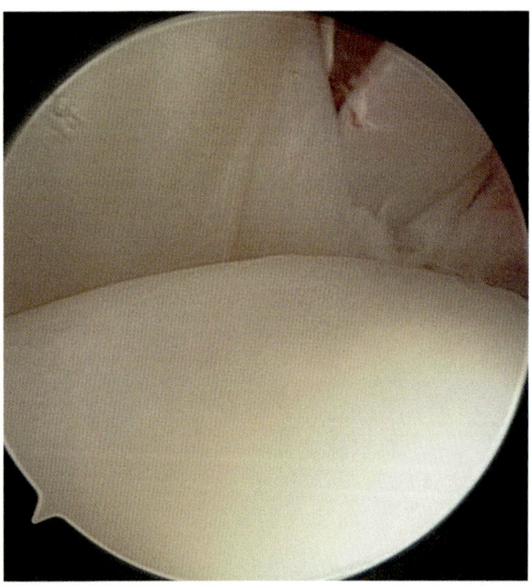

Fig. 20.3 RTC insertion from posterior portal – beach chair

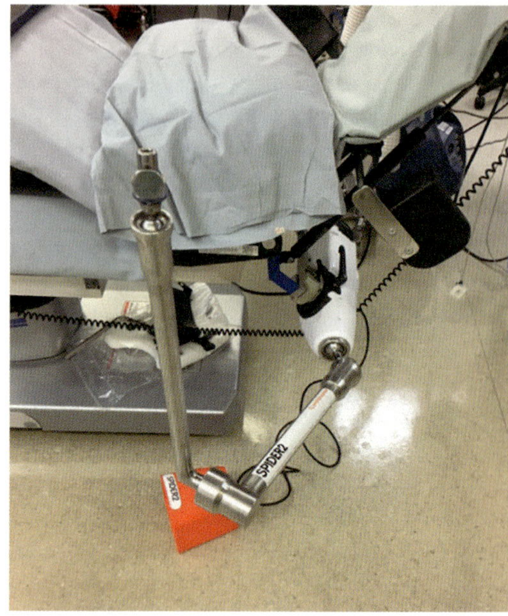

Fig. 20.4 Beach Chair Arm Holders – (**a**) spider

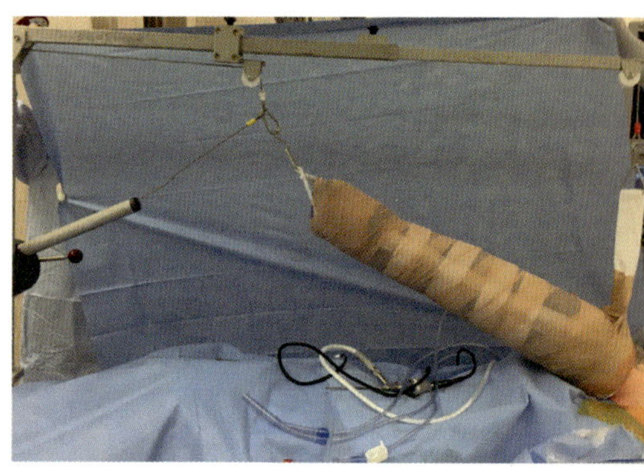

Fig. 20.5 Lateral Arm Holder

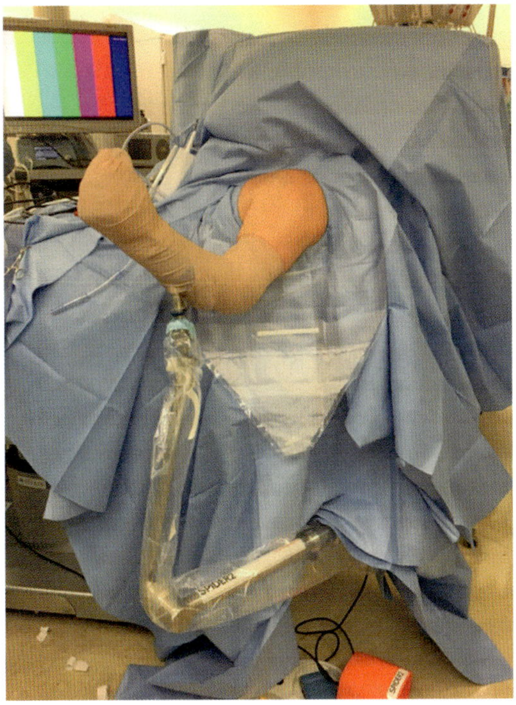

Fig. 20.6 Completed patient positioning Beach chair

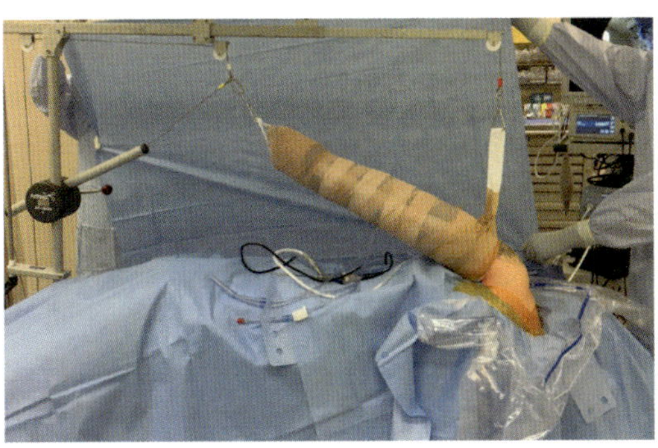

Fig. 20.7 Completed patient positioning Lateral (head is right, feet left in picture)

Questions

Match the condition with the preferred patient position for shoulder arthroscopy

A Subacromial decompression
B Rotator cuff repairs
C Lesions to the posterior and inferior glenohumeral joint
D Distal clavicle excision
E High possibility to convert to open procedure
F Complete labrum tear (entire labrum involved)
G Beach chair
H Lateral

Everything about lateral position for shoulder arthroscopy is correct except:

A Requires traction on the operative arm
B Associated with lower instability recurrence rate compared to beach chair position
C Is suggested to be easier when operating without an assistant
D Is hypothesized that predisposes more to cerebral ischemic events compared to beach chair position

Mark all landmarks that are usually marked for shoulder arthroscopy (select all that apply):

A Posterolateral acromial edge
B Lateral acromial edge
C Anterolateral acromial edge
D AC joint
E Coracoid process
F Great tuberosity
G Lesser tuberosity
H Supraspinatus fossa

Where is the posterolateral portal placed preferably?

A At the AP projection of the posterolateral acromial edge and 3 cm distally
B 2 cm distal and 2 cm medial from the posterolateral acromial edge
C 4 cm distal and 4 cm lateral from the posterolateral acromial edge
D 2 cm distal and 2 cm lateral from the posterolateral acromial edge

Which of the above nerves can be injured during shoulder arthroscopy?

A Axillary nerve
B Brachial plexus
C Peronial nerve
D A&B
E All the above

References

1. Li X, Eichinger JK, Hartshorn T, et al. A comparison of the lateral decubitus and beach-chair positions for shoulder surgery: advantages and complications. J Am Acad Orthop Surg. 2015;23:18–28.
2. Skyhar MJ, Altchek DW, Warren RF, et al. Shoulder arthroscopy with the patient in the beach-chair position. Arthroscopy. 1988;4:256–9.
3. Hewitt M, Getelman MH, Snyder SJ. Arthroscopic management of multidirectional instability: pancapsular plication. Orthop Clin North Am. 2003;34:549–57.
4. Frank RM, Saccomanno MF, McDonald LS, et al. Outcomes of arthroscopic anterior shoulder instability in the beach chair versus lateral decubitus position: a systematic review and meta-regression analysis. Arthroscopy. 2014;30:1349–65.
5. Peruto CM, Ciccotti MG, Cohen SB. Shoulder arthroscopy positioning: lateral decubitus versus beach chair. Arthroscopy. 2009;25:891–6.
6. Papadonikolakis A, Wiesler ER, Olympio MA, et al. Avoiding catastrophic complications of stroke and death related to shoulder surgery in the sitting position. Arthroscopy. 2008;24:481–2.
7. Murphy GS, Szokol JW, Marymont JH, et al. Cerebral oxygen desaturation events assessed by near-infrared spectroscopy during shoulder arthroscopy in the beach chair and lateral decubitus positions. Anesth Analg. 2010;111:496–505.
8. Angelo R, Esch J, Ryu R, editors. The shoulder. Philadelphia: Elsevier; 2010.
9. Klein AH, France JC, Mutschler TA, et al. Measurement of brachial plexus strain in arthroscopy of the shoulder. Arthroscopy. 1987;3:45–52.
10. Mullins RC, Drez Jr D, Cooper J. Hypoglossal nerve palsy after arthroscopy of the shoulder and open operation with the patient in the beach-chair position. A case report. J Bone Joint Surg Am. 1992;74:137–9.
11. Park TS, Kim YS. Neuropraxia of the cutaneous nerve of the cervical plexus after shoulder arthroscopy. Arthroscopy. 2005;21:631.
12. Burkhart SS. Deep venous thrombosis after shoulder arthroscopy. Arthroscopy. 1990;6:61–3.
13. Edgar R, Nagda S, Huffman R, et al. Pulmonary embolism after shoulder arthroscopy. Orthopedics. 2012;35:e1673–6.

Anatomic Shoulder Arthroplasty

21

Tsvieli Oren, Atoun Ehud, and Ofer Levy

The purpose of this chapter is to explore the new trends and horizons of shoulder arthroplasty. It will begin with a brief historical view of the development of shoulder arthroplasty, and evolution of indications. In general shoulder arthroplasty can be divided into several categories; by constrained/non-constrained/semi-constrained; by humeral resurfacing, stemmed humeral component; by hemiarthroplasty or as total shoulder arthroplasty with glenoid resurfacing; anatomical or reverse total shoulder arthroplasty; cemented or cementless technique.

History of the Procedure and Trends of Evolution

Key Points

- Shoulder arthroplasty developed from treatment of fracture-work in the USA and tumors in Europe. Later the use for arthritis developed and was primarily stemmed.
- The options are variable: resurfacing of humeral head, stemmed hemiarthroplasty, anatomical total shoulder replacement, and reverse total shoulder. Clinical judgement is needed to select the appropriate prosthesis.
- Today's trends are moving towards bone preserving (Fig. 21.1) modular prosthesis design, such as short or metaphyseal stems; designs are more anatomical.
- Unconstrained reverse prosthesis was designed for rotator cuff deficient shoulders.

Shoulder arthroplasty was first documented in 1891 when Themistocles Gluck published his report of the proximal humeral replacement with an ivory component. Two years later in 1893 Jules-Emiles Peans published his report about a shoulder replacement with a metal humeral component for tuberculosis osteomyelitis. The component had to be removed after two years due to persistence of the infection [1].

The stemmed cemented prostheses developed in Europe from tumor excision related replacement and in the USA from fracture work. Initially neither was specifically designed for the treatment of arthritis.

In the USA Neer [2–4] published his arthroplasty results as treatment for comminuted proximal humeral fractures. He first developed the humeral component and later added the plastic glenoid component. The first Neer type prostheses were made out of monoblock

T. Oren, M.D.
Ma'ayanei Hayeshua Medical Center, Bnei-Brak, Israel

A. Ehud, M.D.
Barzilai Medical Center, Ashkelon, Israel

O. Levy, M.D., M.Ch.(Orth), F.R.C.S. (✉)
Reading Shoulder Unit, Reading, UK
e-mail: oferlevy@readingshoulderunit.com; tsvieli@gmail.com

G. Huri, N.K. Paschos (eds.), *The Shoulder*, Orthopaedic Study Guide Series,
DOI 10.1007/978-3-319-51979-1_21

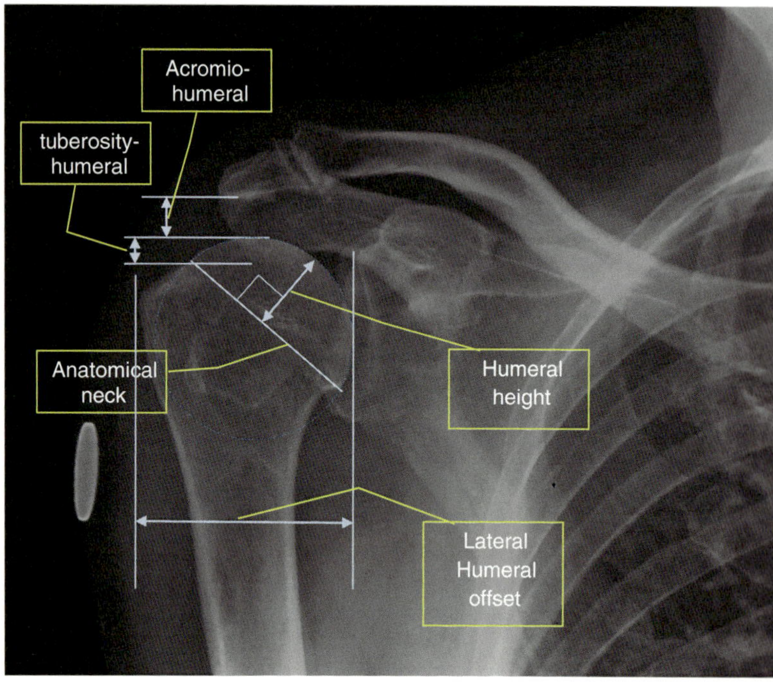

Fig. 21.1 The Copeland Humeral Resurfacing with biological glenoid Resurfacing (Drilling) preop (*left*) and post-op (*right*). The reference point for humeral size is the anatomical neck. This procedure respects the soft tissue as the rotator cuff, and is the reconstruction of the anatomy

stemmed humeral head. Several problems occurred using that design: due to limited variety of sizes often the non-flexible form of humeral head would overstuff the joint causing pain, limited abduction, flexion and rotation; medial glenoid wear was significant, and sometimes the components were unstable and dislocated. If the center of rotation lies too superiorly the subscapularis and infraspinatus become adductors, and by so doing oppose the abduction force of the supraspinatus [5, 6]. Moreover, some second generation prostheses were press-fit which gave less flexibility for correction of the head version. These problems in design changed the kinematics of the replaced shoulder and created imbalance and later eccentric wear of the glenoid and early degeneration of the rotator cuff. Neer set the goal for arthroplasty to strive to reconstruct the original anatomy of the glenohumeral joint. In the 1990s, the third generation of arthroplasties were developed [6, 7] following the work of Boileau & Walch [7] and Roberts [8]. These allow better accommodation to variable humeral head shapes, offset, version and inclination. Boileau and Walch [7] in their anatomical analysis found that the center of rotation of the articular head was offset posteriorly in relation to the humeral medullary axis, and in the sagittal plane it was offset medially. In order to find the correct version and offset the anatomical neck has to be defined. This is correct for stemmed arthroplasty as well as for resurfacing [9, 10].

In Europe in the 1950s shoulder replacement developed initially from the field of tumor resection surgery and the need for adequate spacers such as with the Stanmore shoulder arthroplasty [11]. The prostheses spanned over the excised gap of the tumor. One of the major problems was soft tissue deficiency following resections, or deficiency of the rotator cuff which caused a proximal migration of the humeral head. This was due to the unopposed deltoid muscle, and caused upper migration and anterior subluxation [10]. To prevent this subluxation the prostheses were initially constrained and the glenoid component lateralized. This created forces acting strongly on the glenoid-component interface and often it loosened and failed. Later reverse geometry shoulder replacement was developed to harness the deltoid to abduct the arm by Grammont [12].

In 1988 Franklin and associates [13] coined the term "rocking horse" phenomena for loosening of the glenoid component due to the unopposed deltoid muscle force to pulling upwards of the humeral head in cases of deficient or ruptured rotator cuff. Neer [14] described this entity previously in 1983 and suggested a large size head hemiarthroplasty and attempt at repair of the rotator cuff. Constrained reverse prostheses existed in the treatment of arthropathy of the glenohumeral joint but most of them failed due to lateralization of the center of rotation, thus creating an exaggerated lever arm on the glenoid causing it to loosen or dislocate. The fully-constrained or fixed-fulcrum prostheses included the designs of Neer [15], Bickel [15], Stanmore [16], Post [17], Kessel [18], Kolbel [19], Fenlin [20], Buechel [21]. Grammont [12] published in 1993 his "Delta" unconstrained reverse prosthesis. He devised it to be a prosthesis that functions with the deltoid muscle only, had to be stable and incapable of dislocation, and to eliminate the risk of loosening on the glenoid support. This design is nowadays the basis for surgical treatment for rotator cuff arthropathy with growing indications: massive, irreparable rotator cuff tears, primary treatment for comminuted proximal humeral fractures in the elderly, post extensive resection of soft tissue due to tumor or infection. The biomechanics of the Delta prosthesis led to less reaction forces on the glenoid due to medialization of the center of rotation as well as larger diameter glenosphere with a smaller unconstrained humeral cup; distalizing the glenosphere further down the glenoid. This allowed for better harnessing of the deltoid as well as improvement of range of movement. Thus better function is achieved. In recent years the Delta III has served as the mainstream of reverse total shoulder. Further developments have occurred in the understanding of shoulder replacement, since the target population is not only elderly, and even the elderly have higher demands and live longer. The understanding that revision surgery is likely brought about the notion of preserving bonestock and short stemmed such as the Aequalis Ascend™ (Aequalis® Shoulder and Aequalis® Total Shoulder, Tornier, St. Ismier Cedex, France) or metaphyseal stems were designed such as the Verso reverse prosthesis [22] (Innovative Design Orthopaedics, Worcestershire UK); Affinis® (Mathys AG, Bettlach, Switzerland) [23]; TESS shoulder system (Biomet® France) and the Eclipse™ (Arthrex® Naples, Florida USA). Another new trend expressed in the Verso as well as the Aequalis BIO-RSA™ is mild lateralization of the glenosphere. This change in design enables preventing one of the most common issues in reverse shoulder arthroplasty – notching. Notching is the wear of the inferior glenoid by the humeral component. It can cause particle disease, loosening and dislocation of the glenoid component and wear of the polyethylene insert. Lateralization of the glenosphere further enhances the deltoid muscle harnessing but without dramatically increasing the joint reaction force on the glenoid.

Etiology

Key Points

- Medical advancement brought higher life expectancy and quality demands for shoulder arthroplasty as a solution for different etiologies for arthritis when conservative treatment has been exhausted.
- Arthroplasty can be applied for primary osteoarthritis, inflammatory arthritis, rotator cuff arthropathy, humeral head avascular necrosis, trauma associated arthrosis and infection arthropathy. Conservative treatment should be the first option.

Average life expectancy has been improving during the last decades along with advances in medicine and medical technology. The development of solutions for shoulder problems has led to patients having higher expectations from medical and surgical treatment for shoulder pathologies as rotator cuff tears, and various kinds of arthritis.

Pathologies ultimately being the indication for shoulder arthroplasty involve shoulder dysfunction, malformation or pain. It is important to note that arthroplasty is not the first line of treatment and that conservative treatment modalities should be attempted before surgery. It should be stressed that function of the naturally shallow glenohumeral articulation depends on the soft tissue around it, the capsule, tendons, muscles and the coordination between them. Therefore success of any treatment depends in large on rehabilitating or recreating this soft tissue balance.

Osteoarthritis, Primary

This is a slow gradual degenerative process. It does not involve proximal migration of the humeral head and rotator cuff is usually preserved or only mildly damaged. Tightness of the capsule due to osteophytes may create imbalance of the gliding mechanism of the glenohumeral joint and posterior glenoid bone loss. Radiography usually demonstrates concentric or eccentric glenohumeral arthritis with inferior osteophytes. Conservative treatment should focus on preservation of range of movement and pain relief. Physiotherapy, NSAIDs and intraarticular steroid injections are common treatment options.

Inflammatory Arthritis

When discussing inflammatory arthritis it is most commonly rheumatoid arthritis, but also other kinds of inflammatory arthritis such as psoriatic arthritis. The rheumatoid pannus creates severe synovitis around the joint and dysfunction of the soft tissues, commonly the rotator cuff will be torn or dysfunctional. Patients with severe RA are younger population than osteoarthritis patients when showing up with shoulder arthritis. Radiography reveals osteopenia, subchondral bone cysts and erosions. Chronic steroid treatment may worsen the osteopenia. Characteristically symmetric and central wear of the glenoid are demonstrated.

Rotator Cuff Arthropathy

Long-standing rotator cuff tears or cuff insufficiency may cause the humeral head to migrate proximally. The imbalance of uncontained humeral head against the glenoid articular surface creates proximal wear. This in turn creates "acetabularisation" of the subacromial area and pseudo-articulation. The conservative treatment advised is strengthening of the deltoid muscle, specifically the anterior part. Rotator cuff arthropathy is a contraindication to anatomical shoulder replacement because of the proximal migration. The upwards directed forces on the glenoid component cause it to dislocate prematurely or if it is constrained be unstable and loosen. The surgical solution recommended today is reverse geometry total shoulder replacement. In some cases where the glenoid bonestock is insufficient, a hemiarthroplasty with large diameter head can be implanted as salvage procedure, although function is not expected to be optimal.

Avascular Necrosis

This uncommon etiology accounts for 3% of shoulder arthroplasties. Known causes or associated conditions are of variable etiologies: post-traumatic (fracture/dislocation), corticosteroid therapy, hemoglobinopathies, sickle cell disease, alcohol abuse/smoking, decompression sickness for divers, Gaucher disease, septic osteonecrosis, connective tissue disorders, hypercoagulable disease, chemotherapy, peripheral vascular disease, chronic dialysis, hyperlipidemia, SLE, Cushing's syndrome, pregnancy, hyperuricemia, myxedema, radiation therapy, pancreatitis, or idiopathic. It usually presents with pain and radiographic changes that follow the Cruess classification [24] modification of Ficat-Arlet. [Stage I no change detected on radiograph, only on MRI; stage II on radiograph sclerosis, osteopenia; stage III crescent sign, sphericity preserved, only subchondral bone collapse; stage IV collapse of joint surface, flattening; stage V involvement of the glenoid]. Conservative treatment includes unloading stresses from the shoulder joint, preservation of range of movement and management of pain, as well as treatment of underlying cause if possible. Salvage surgical technique before attempting arthroplasty, is core decompression or possibly vascularized strut graft. This procedure is believed to stimulate vascular neogenesis in the pre-collapse stage. Microfractures are principally a similar idea but more directed at stimulating fibrocartilage on affected bare bone in the joint.

Trauma Associated Arthritis

Deformation due to fracture malunion, post dislocation, and post capsular shift. The imbalance of soft tissue creates eccentric rather than concentric gliding of the humeral head on the glenoid causing eccentric wear. Conservative treatment is limited to stretching of the anterior capsule and attempt to preserve range of movement. Fracture sequelae such as malunion or non-union are among the most debilitating causes for shoulder pain and dysfunction. Often there is gross deformity of the humeral head creating mechanical blockage to movement, and some resultant muscle atrophy due to lengthy immobilization of the joint. Treating fracture sequelae is among the most challenging arthroplasties due to deformity, nonunion of the tuberosities, and collateral damage to the rotator cuff. Boileau and associates [25] in a multicenter study concluded that if prosthetic replacement is possible without an osteotomy of the tuberosities, surgeons should accept the distorted anatomy of the proximal humerus and adapt the prosthesis. Long term follow-up of anatomical shoulder arthroplasty by Jacobson [26] and associates registered good survivorship of prostheses as high as 90.1% at 10 and 15 years. Mean age was 65 (range 34–83). The conclusions were that anatomic shoulder arthroplasty improves pain and motion. Surgery is complex. Tuberosity osteotomies often heal. Postoperative instability is the most common complication leading to reoperation and is usually associated with rotator cuff and shoulder capsule injury. In the last decades reverse total shoulder arthroplasty for acute and delayed sequelae of proximal humeral fractures has become increasingly common, in agreement in the literature of being adequate for the elderly patients. This procedure usually requires a stemmed prosthesis due to bone loss or fracture at the surgical neck. All effort should be made to reconnect the tuberosities and the rotator cuff in order to allow range of movement and function.

Infection Arthropathy

Infection arthropathy such as in immunocompromised patients presents with swelling, pain, redness, warm skin, limitation of shoulder movements. Both aspirate cultures and blood inflammatory markers are necessary for diagnosis. Treatment should be prompt to try and prevent arthropathy. Multiple sick tissue debridement and lavage should ensue. If major debridement was performed and infection is thought to be resolved arthroplasty can be considered. Careful pre-planning of arthroplasty with pre-operative and intra-operative cultures can be planned. A bonestock sparing attitude is preferred. For cementation antibiotic cement should be used.

Neuropathic Arthropathy

Neuropathic Arthropathy of the Shoulder, also named Charcot shoulder; this rare condition is associated with cervical syringomyelia or with alcohol abuse. Joints become obliterated due to neuropathy. Usually at young age, must be differentiated from infection and tumor. This condition should be assessed well before deciding on arthroplasty because of the destructive nature of the disease. In real Charcot shoulders an arthrodesis is sometimes an option.

Indications and Contraindications

Key Points

- Arthroplasty is indicated for pain and disability of the shoulder which do not respond to conservative treatment due to arthropathy of the glenohumeral joint.
- In younger patients attempts to salvage by arthroscopic debridement, microfracture and rotator cuff repair should be trialed before decision to replace the affected joint.
- Contraindications are Charcot shoulders, active infection and neurologic instability. Relative contraindication is anatomic TSA for cuff deficient shoulders.

Indications for shoulder arthroplasty are pain and disability resulting from arthropathy of the glenohumeral joint, after conservative measures have been exhausted. In young active patients arthroscopic microfracture and debridement in early stages should be attempted. In pre-collapse stages of avascular necrosis core decompression should be attempted. For rotator cuff tears, physiotherapy and strengthening of the deltoid muscles should be offered, as well as an attempt to repair the tear, considering even augmentation with synthetic graft or allograft. Shoulder instability should be surgically repaired if not turned yet to be arthropathy.

Contraindications include active infection, neurologic conditions such as paralysis local or central because of fear of instability. Charcot shoulders are rare and considered unfit for arthroplasty if no proprioception exists. An irreparable rotator cuff tear is a contraindication for glenoid component with the anatomical prosthesis because of the proximal migration of the humerus which asserts the pressure on the proximal part of the glenoid component causing it to rock ("Rocking horse") and dislocate. A mega-head hemiarthroplasty is indicated or better, a reverse total shoulder arthroplasty. Contraindication to glenoid component is insufficient glenoid bonestock. In such cases a procedure of bone grafting can be done in one or two stages.

Patient History and Physical Examination

Key Points

- Rule out extrinsic conditions affecting shoulder pain. Accurately diagnose shoulder pathology before planning surgery.
- Create coordination of patient expectations before committing to the process.
- Utilize outcome measurement scores to monitor progress.

A thorough history of the disease and precipitating factors should be noted. The course of the pain and functional deficiency should be recorded and understood, as well as any previous treatments; full medical background of the patient including medications and medical conditions. Anticoagulation therapy should be stopped prior to surgery; if necessary consultation with a fellow cardiologist or internist should be sought. An anesthesiologist examination should be performed as preparation before surgery. Physical examination should begin by general examination, and should include any factors influencing the shoulder such as cervical spine conditions, cardiac pain affecting the shoulder, respiratory or abdominal findings. The shoulder examination should record range of movement, both active and passive, as well as painful range. Muscle power of each group of muscles should be noted. Muscle atrophy, scapular dyskinesia and neurological examination are necessary as well.

It is good practice to let the patient fill outcome measurements [27] such as the Constat-Murley [28] shoulder score, the Simple Shoulder Score [29], the Oxford Score [30], the UCLA [31] score, DASH [32] score or the ASES [33] score. The outcome measurement scores are important for understanding the success rates, failure points and pitfalls.

Imaging and diagnostic tests

Key Points

- Baseline high quality radiography is necessary, along with US and MRI or CT scans.
- Rule out active inflammation or infection with appropriate diagnostic tests.

Normal radiography: true anteroposterior scapular plane and axillary views along with size markers for templating; Ultrasound scan or MRI to assess the rotator cuff integrity; Computed tomography or MRI to assess humeral and glenoid bonestock and for measurement templating, as well as assessment of muscular fatty degeneration; joint aspiration, ESR, CRP, skin cultures and urinalysis, blood cultures to rule out infection; blood coagulation function, complete blood count and chemistry panel according to patient's comorbidities, as well as chest radiographs; electromyography and nerve conduction studies in case of suspected neuropathy or weakness. Relevant pre-operative consultations, as with cardiology or respiratory specialists should be reviewed.

Implant Choice

Key Points

- Implant choice must be tailored to the patient and specific patient needs. In anatomical TSA effort should be done to reproduce normal anatomy.
- Soft tissue around the shoulder is the main stabilizer, and provides the range of movement. Soft tissue must be respected when planning and engaging shoulder arthroplasty.
- For primary concentric osteoarthritis the literature is in favor of TSA, but long term results are unequivocal since there is variety of implants at hand.
- Glenoid treatment can be either biological or artificial components. As of today glenoid wear is a key issue in shoulder arthroplasty.
- We recommend bone preserving non cemented implants to the extent possible, in order to respect the soft tissue and for preservation of bonestock for future revision.
- For rotator cuff deficient arthropathy a reverse total shoulder is recommended. If glenoid bonestock cannot sustain a baseplate then either bone-grafting of the glenoid or mega-head hemiarthroplasty can be performed.
- Arthroplasty for comminuted proximal humeral fractures is a challenging issue mainly to restore anatomy due to missing landmarks. Osteosynthesis of the tuberosities is sometimes a challenge. A stemmed prosthesis is usually used.

The evolution of the debate between the indications for TSA (Total Shoulder Arthroplasty) and HSA (Hemiarthroplasty) dates back to the 1970s with Neer's [2, 34] historical indications for TSA: pain caused by glenoid incongruity that has failed to respond to nonoperative treatment in patients with adequate glenoid bonestock, good surgical risk and motivation, and no active infection, paralysis, or destruction of both the rotator cuff and deltoid muscles. Choices exist between stemmed, long and short or stemless resurfacing on the humeral side. On the glenoid side choices are to leave as is, to ream or burr asymmetric wear, to release capsule and drill for biological fibrocartilage formation, to apply different autograft or allograft interpositioning biological resurfacing, or to resurface the glenoid with an implant. Glenoid implant choices are full polyethylene pegged or keeled, metal backed polyethylene and various combinations of pegs or keels. Artificial components can either be cemented or cementless. It is therefore not just the simple choice between total shoulder arthroplasty and hemiarthroplasty.

Most of arthroplasty literature refers to stemmed humeral components. Pfhaler [35] and associates stated that stemmed TSA has had a proven superiority in chronic pathologic conditions, such as primary osteoarthritis, rheumatoid arthritis, and fracture sequelae. On the other hand, it seems preferable to perform stemmed HSA in the treatment of osteonecrosis and instability arthritis, as well as those conditions that are a result of neurologic or inflammatory damage. These results were followed up only up to 5 years, in which HSA group continued to show acceptable results. Sandow [36] in a randomized study of 33 shoulder arthroplasties reported better results with stemmed TSA in comparison with HSA after a decade, this included a 90% survivorship in both groups.

Burkhead [37, 38], with stemmed hemiarthroplasty, and Copeland [9, 39–41], with humeral head resurfacing, trialed biological resurfacing of the glenoid (Fig. 21.1). Krishnan and Burkead [38, 42] reported that long term glenoid resurfacing either with anterior capsule or with Achilles tendon allografts had favorable outcome. Strauss [43] reported inferior results with lateral meniscal allografts. Copeland [9] recommended that even when HSA was indicated, the glenoid should not be ignored. He recommended drilling the articular surface to encourage secondary formation of fibrocartilage. Levy and Copeland [41] in a long term review of cementless humeral resurfacing reported of better survivorship of hemiarthroplasty and biological glenoid resurfacing. Levy [41] and associates had also shown in a long term study up to 25 year's follow up of uncemented Copeland resurfacing arthroplasties that the survivorship of these prostheses with biological glenoid resurfacing was superior to the polyethylene and metal-backed glenoid resurfacing. The study included patients younger than 50 years old at the time of surgery. 49 patients (54 shoulders) with various indications including avascular necrosis, rheumatoid arthritis, instability arthropathy, primary osteoarthritis, fracture sequelae, post-infection arthritis, and psoriatic arthritis. 18.5% had revision surgery after more than 10 years. Functional outcome was favorable in terms of function and patient satisfaction. Survivorship of TSA was 71% at 14 years and 61% at 22 years, and of HSA 91% at 14 years and 85% at 22 years. Long-term results for humeral head resurfacing were published by Pritchett [44] who reported on 74 shoulders (41 total shoulder resurfacings and 33 humeral head resurfacings) in 61 patients. Mean age was 58 years, and follow-up was longer than 20 years in all patients (mean, 28 years). The survival rate of the humeral component at the time of final follow-up was 96%, and patient satisfaction was 95%. Of the 41 shoulders with glenoid resurfacing, 38 shoulders were available for radiographic follow-up. Three required revision because of loosening and 12 had radiographic evidence of loosening. Patients with total resurfacing fared slightly better at final follow-up.

Since the beginning of shoulder arthroplasty, much advancement has occurred with the humeral component. Nowadays third generation implants are available to mimic the humeral anatomy [7, 45]. Still, the glenoid poses a riddle. Although midterm reports are favorable, the development of artificial resurfacing of the glenoid has been less than successful in the long term follow up. There are reports of glenoid component loosening and catastrophic failure of the glenoid component for all-polyethylene and metal backed [46–50]. Glenoid components have the tendency to have radiolucent lines, but the clinical significance is not always expressed by outcome measures and not always correlates. Boileau [6] and others [10] dwelled on the subject, suggesting that part of the cause is in the surgical technique and humeral head component choice. Overstuffing or under-stuffing the joint, humeral head and glenoid resurfacing radii mismatch, non-anatomical version or neck-shaft angle are possible causes. Also Copeland [10] warranted the "pilot errors". It has been shown [51] that approximately 30% of the unsatisfactory results after shoulder replacements are due to humeral component malposition and, if version is incorrect by >15°, it can lead to a painful shoulder. Copeland had also suggested that the experience and long term follow-up had demonstrated favorable results with resurfacing hemiarthroplasty with biological resurfacing (drilling) of the glenoid.

Since the early nineties resurfacing hemiarthroplasty was not very well accepted, and most research was done with stemmed humeral arthroplasty. In 1996 Rodosky and Bigliani [52] advocated arthroplasty for patients who have glenohumeral arthritic pain which exhausted conservative treatment. Glenohumeral congruity, lack of active infection, exclusion of neuropathy, severe damage to the deltoid muscle or rotator cuff muscles and rehabilitation motivation were necessary criteria. Humeral hemiarthroplasty was recommended to younger and active patients, in cases of either intact glenoid cartilage or deficient glenoid bonestock. At the time hemiarthroplasty was also performed for rotator cuff tear arthropathy with repair of the remnants of the rotator cuff for preservation of anteroposterior stability. Glenoid resurfacing was advocated to the majority of arthritic cases in which minimal glenoid wear was mostly found. The common glenoid resurfacing components were all-polyethylene or metal backed polyethylene, cemented or press-fit, with suitable preparation of the glenoid. In cases of glenoid erosion reaming or burring the glenoid to achieve the correct version and in rare cases the glenoid erosion was bone-grafted. Secondary post traumatic arthritis often brings deformity of the tuberosities and eccentric loads on the glenoid, therefore not recommended glenoid resurfacing.

The potential advantages of glenoid resurfacing over proximal humeral replacement alone include a better fulcrum for improved strength and motion, increased stability, decreased friction, and elimination of glenoid socket pain. These advantages do not come without a price. The insertion of a glenoid component requires additional operating time and can result in additional blood loss. Also, the glenoid component has been associated with a higher incidence of radiolucencies and revisions. In the peer-reviewed literature for TSR and hemiarthroplasties, the overall glenoid revision rate is 3.2% compared with 1.8% for humeral components [52].

There are several comparative studies in the literature using stemmed implants. Sperling et al. [53] reported no significant difference in functional outcome between 74 shoulders treated with a hemiarthroplasty and 34 shoulders treated with a total shoulder arthroplasty using the Neer prosthesis. In a follow-up report on the same cohort of patients with a minimum of 15 years follow up [54] there was no significant difference between 29 total shoulder arthroplasties and 62 hemiarthroplasties with regard to pain relief or range of movement. The diagnoses in this cohort of patients differed markedly between the two groups with the majority of hemiarthroplasties performed for the sequelae of trauma and the majority of total shoulder arthroplasties performed for rheumatoid arthritis. Garstman [55] in a prospective trial in which 51 shoulders with osteoarthritis were randomized to be treated with either a hemiarthroplasty or a total shoulder arthroplasty using the Global™ prosthesis (DePuy, Warsaw, Indiana) observed better average functional scores with total shoulder arthroplasty but this difference was not significant because of the wide range of scores in both groups and the relatively small numbers in the study. Lo et al. [56] found no significant difference in functional outcome between 42 patients with osteoarthritis prospectively randomized to be treated with either a hemiarthroplasty or a total shoulder arthroplasty using the Neer Series-II modular prosthesis (3 M Canada, London, Ontario). However their study had a high risk of type I error for the same reasons (small numbers and wide confidence intervals).

In an attempt to overcome the problems of small numbers, Bryant et al. [57] performed a meta-analysis of three randomized controlled trials comparing hemiarthroplasty with total shoulder arthroplasty for the treatment of osteoarthritis. Fifty patients were managed with a hemiarthroplasty and sixty-two with a total shoulder arthroplasty. They reported a statistically significant difference of 1.5 points in the function domain of the UCLA shoulder score and a difference of 2.1 points in the pain domain of the UCLA score in favor of total shoulder arthroplasty. However there was a large degree of heterogeneity among the studies and the authors advised caution with interpretation of the significance of the pain data. It is important to note that there is a two-point difference between most of the categories of the function domain of the UCLA score and so an average difference of 1.5 points is of dubious clinical significance.

Edwards et al. [58] reported the results of the multicenter study comparing hemiarthroplasty with total shoulder arthroplasty for the treatment of osteoarthritis using the Aequalis® prosthesis (Tournier, Montbonot, France). This study had the advantages of large numbers (1542 primary shoulder arthroplasties) and a uniform method of assessment of outcome. Although it was a retrospective study and the indication for hemiarthroplasty was not clearly defined at the outset, the large numbers allowed comparison of subgroups of patients in order to minimize bias. At an average follow up of 43 months, they reported a statistically significant difference of 10.3 points in the adjusted Constant score ($p < 0.0005$) in favor of TSA. Gain in adjusted Constant score was better following TSA for the entire cohort and for the subgroup of shoulders with concentric glenoid morphology and for the subgroup of age, sex and follow-up matched shoulders. One may conclude that with the Aequalis® stemmed implant, TSA gives clinical and statistical significantly better functional results than HSA. However this comes at a price. 56% of TSA had radiolucent lines around the glenoid components. The estimated survival of TSA was much worse than HSA (from the diagram in the paper approximately 97% for HSA and 69% for TSA at 9 years; no figures given and no statistical analysis). The poor longevity of TSA was ascribed to the use of the metal-backed glenoid component which was subsequently shown to have an unacceptably high failure rate and its use was discontinued [59, 60]. However, in a follow up report using data from the same Aequalis multicenter group Pfahler et al. [35] found radiolucent lines around 67.9% of the cemented glenoid implants when metal-backed components were excluded. 50% of these radiolucent lines were progressive. Although the Constant score was significantly better in the TSA group even with the presence of radiolucent lines, the difference between the Constant score in the TSA group and the Constant score in the HSA group decreased over time due to an adverse effect on functional outcome by the presence of radiolucent lines.

Planning and Templating

Key Points

- Attempt to reconstruct anatomy in order to allow for correct soft tissue function.
- Use normal radiographs with calibration marking.
- Special attention should be given to glenoid asymmetric wear, humeral height, version and size.

The purpose is to achieve reconstruction that can mimic the original anatomy. This can be done using a true AP and an axillary view, along with a calibration mark. Templating has been found to be reliable for total shoulder arthroplasty [61]. In severe deformity of the humeral head the contralateral shoulder can sometimes be used for sizing, but with caution in order not to overstuff the already contracted joint. Commercial templates (digital or as hardware) are provided by the prosthesis manufacturer, to use with templating software. It is useful to have a CT scan with three dimensional volumetric reconstructions in order to assess the glenoid structure and bonestock. Boileau [7] and others [62, 63] emphasized the importance of the shape of the glenoid in terms of inclination (neck shaft angle) medial and posterior offset. It is important to realize the reference points, since an arthritic humeral head often does not preserve the round contour. Youderian and Iannotti [64] trialed inter-observer templating, concluding that using a circle in two plains utilizing the anatomical neck is reliable enough.

Humeral component size is appreciated by measuring humeral head diameter and height, the acromio-humeral interval, tuberosity-humeral interval and lateral humeral offset (Fig. 21.2).

Glenoid is assessed for version and wear (Fig. 21.3). The Walch [62] classification: type-A, concave (A1, moderate; A2, severe), type-B, biconcave (B1, moderate; B2, severe), and type-C, dysplastic (more than 25° of retroversion).

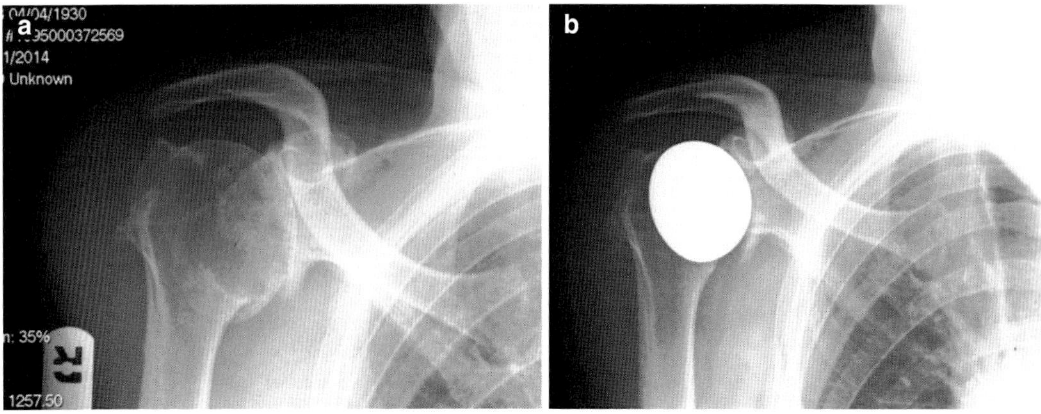

Fig. 21.2 Schematic templating

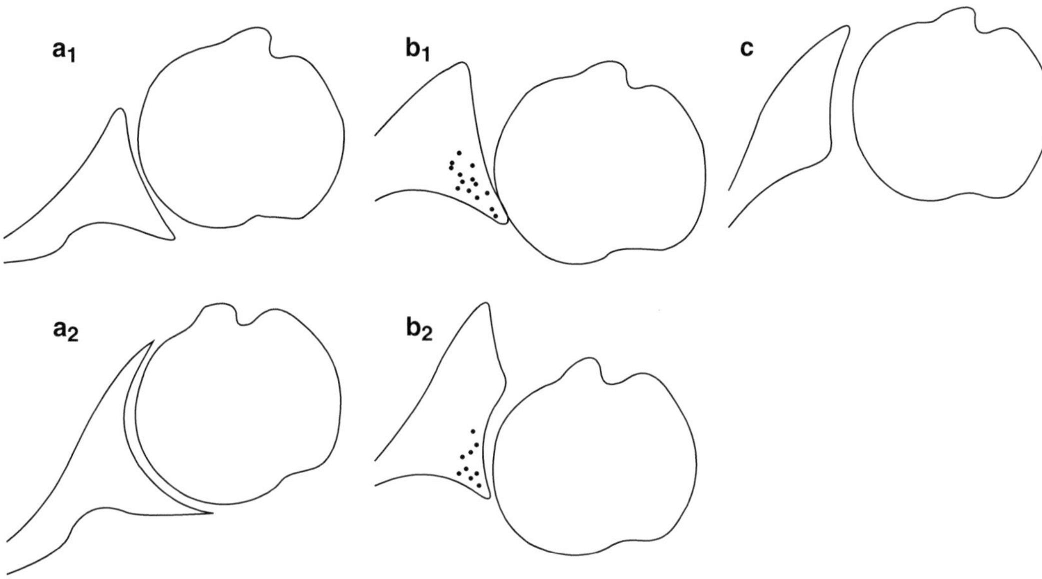

Fig. 21.3 The Walch62 classification: type-A, concave (A1, moderate; A2, severe), type-B, biconcave (B1, moderate; B2, severe), and type-C, dysplastic (more than 25° of retroversion). Reprinted with permission from [62]

Habermeyer [63] described an additional classification for assessment of glenoid vertical wear. Increased glenoid version or humeral head version have been discussed as causes of coronal decentralization of the humeral head in osteoarthritis. He stated that this radiographic classification system can facilitate the decision-making process to normalize glenoid inclination during glenoid replacement.

Patient Positioning

Key Points

- Patient positioning is usually in the beach chair position.
- "time-out" procedure should take place to verify patient and preparations.

A first "time-out" should include proper identification of the patient, presentation of the working team and coordination of requirements for the operation; also specific relevant patient details should be noted such as known allergies, operated side and prophylaxis. Preoperative prophylactic antibiotics should be given intravenously either one hour prior to surgery or at the time of anesthetic induction. Still, it is good practice to culture the glenohumeral joint during the approach, because of known prevalent infection with Propionibacterium acnes [65]. In that case prophylactic antibiotics should be given only after cultures have been taken.

It is good practice to induce both general anesthesia as well as an interscalene continuous block to allow for post-operative pain control.

Following anesthesia, he patient should be placed in a semi-sitting or beach chair position at about 45° of head-up tilt with the head on a headpiece and the arm on a short arm board attached to the side of the operating table. It is important to have the patient close to the edge of the table and the short arm board to permit hyperextension and adduction of the arm during surgery to allow delivery of the humeral head into the anterior wound and to facilitate insertion of the humeral component. A sandbag should be placed under the scapula to stabilize and elevate it for better access. The patient's head should be stabilized and any hair tucked away, eyes covered and protected from any antiseptic fluid while draping. Antiseptic preparation and draping should start at a high point in the neck, posteriorly to the scapula, and anteriorly to the midline of the chest.

Draping should include the arm and forearm which can be also covered by stockinet for free mobilization. Sterile drapes should overlap the draped borders and cover the head and body, leaving a curtain between the surgical field and the anesthetic team. A "time-out" procedure is necessary to confirm patient's identity, operation, operated side, any known allergies and anesthesia before proceeding with the approach.

Surgical Approaches

Deltopectoral Approach

Advantages

A true anatomic inter-nervous inter-muscular interval between the deltoid and pectoralis major. Amenable to extension of the approach. Deltoid muscle origin is preserved. Anterior dislocation of the humerus improves access to the inferior humeral and glenoid osteophytes, and inferior capsule for release in tight shoulders.

Disadvantages

Division of the Subscapularis, still controversial, can increase the risk of instability. Difficult access to posterior structures, specifically the greater tuberosity and posterior glenoid.Possible tendency to place glenoid component or baseplate anteriorly.

Approach

A 15 cm incision is made from the clavicle down across the tip of the coracoid and continued in a straight line to the anterior border of the insertion of the deltoid. The cephalic vein is mobilized lateral in the deltopectoral groove. The vein is retracted laterally with the deltoid. The arm is abducted 40° to 60°. The clavipectoral fascia is incised. The subacromial space is cleared and a broad elevator is placed beneath the acromion as a retractor. At this stage improved exposure will be obtained by dividing the proximal 2 cm of the insertion of pectoralis major. The shoulder is flexed and externally rotated to facilitate coagulation of the anterior circumflex humeral vessels. It is very important at this stage to insert stay sutures into the subscapularis muscle to control retraction. The tendon is divided 2 cm medial to the bicipital groove, some peel it with a fleck of bone from the lesser tuberosity. If the subscapularis appears tight it should be divided in an oblique or "Z" manner to allow repair with lengthening of the tendon. The joint capsule is then released anteriorly and inferiorly whilst taking care to protect the axillary nerve with a blunt elevator where it passes through the quadrilateral space. The glenohumeral joint may now be dislocated anteriorly by external rotation and extension, allowing a full exposure of the humeral head and neck.

Anterosuperior Approach (Described by Neviaser [66] and Mackenzie [67])

Advantages

Frontal exposure of the glenoid in the anteroposterior plane. Preservation of the subscapularis tendon. Neurologic injury to brachial plexus may be less likely. Improved access to the posterior aspect of the glenoidSimplicity.

Disadvantages

Difficult approach to inferior glenoid. For reverse TSA difficulty positioning the baseplate inferiorly and distally. Requires detachment and repair of the anterior deltoid, therefore some risk of deltoid dehiscence or weakening. This approach is not extensile, which limits exposure of the humerus.

Approach

The skin incision extends distally in a straight line from just posterior to the acromioclavicular joint, for a distance of 9 cm. The anterior deltoid fibres are split for a distance of not more than 6 cm, and a loose No. 1 stay suture is placed in the distal end of the split to prevent further extension and possible injury to the axillary nerve. The superior acromioclavicular ligament is elevated subperiosteally to expose the AC joint. The acromial attachment of the deltoid is lifted with an osteo-periosteal flap to expose the anterior acromion. The rotator interval is identified and longitudinally incised along the line of the long head of biceps to identify the exact insertion of subscapularis. Subscapularis is held by stay sutures and disinserted. The shoulder is dislocated anteriorly. Long head of biceps, if intact, is dislocated posteriorly over the humeral head.

Post-Operative Care

Key Points

- Post-operative care should start immediately following surgery.
- It is a mandatory part of the procedure and the patient should be aware of it and be prepared for it.
- As general rule early passive mobilization is followed by assisted range of movement, and after tuberosity healing strengthening and stretching program should continue.
- For each session co-ordination of expectation should take place.

Immediate Post-Operative Care

Immediate post-operative care should include a sling with body-belt. Interscalene block analgesia is used and gradually weaned off. Wound care should include daily inspection, and follow-up of vital signs and blood count. Post-operative radiography should confirm implant position and reveal any suspected fracture lines before mobilization.

Early Rehabilitation Post-Operation

The principle is to prevent from adhesions and joint contracture to occur. Appropriate analgesics should be given prior to physiotherapy. The success of the operation as well as rehabilitation depends on coordination of expectations and patient education in each of the treatment stages. It is important to set achievable goals and to build realistic expectations. Early passive motion is tailored to the surgical repair, whether subscapularis detachment was carried out, or tuberosity osteotomy for malunion rotational movements should be restricted or active motion should start only with proof of tuberosity healing. Huges and Neer [68] created a three phase rehabilitation program. Generally, passive mobilization is recommended for the first 48 hours. Gentle gravity-assisted pendulum exercises, passive elevation in the plane of the scapula as well as supine external rotation with a stick within defined limits are permitted with surgeon and therapist guidance. Elbow, wrist, and hand motion are also encouraged.

Healing Phase Rehabilitation

Once the patient has been discharged from hospital proper instructions concerning home exercises, use of analgesics, instruction of family members how to assist, and clear limits of range of movement must be given. At approximately 6–8 weeks after surgery with evidence of tuberosity healing assisted elevation with a pulley system and supine followed by erect isometric strengthening exercises are performed. Stretches to improve forward elevation, extension, abduction, external and internal rotation are done in addition to encouraging gradual use of the extremity in activities of daily living to promote strength and endurance.

Final Healing and Functional Phase Physiotherapy

Approximately 3 months after the operation progressive resistive exercises with light weights or bands are incorporated into the daily routine along with more aggressive stretching to improve range of motion. This phase should continue for a year or more until final strength and range of movement is achieved.

Evaluation and Follow Up

Key Points

- Clinical and radiographic follow-up should be consistent, detailed and thorough, and include outcome measures.
- Radiolucencies should be followed up closely to determine progress and extent.

Clinical Follow-Up

In the first weeks following surgery wound care and inspection are mandatory to make sure no occult infection develops. An evaluation by the surgeon as well as by the physiotherapist should take place at about 2–3 weeks post-operative, two to three months, six months and one year, as well as further follow-up if needed. Passive and active range of movement, as well as painful range should be recorded. Strength can be measured when applicable. Subjective patient pain, satisfaction, and function should be noted. As mentioned above it is of good practice to use outcome measures such as the Constat-Murley [28] shoulder score, the Simple Shoulder Score [29], the Oxford Score [30], the UCLA [31] score, DASH [32] score or the ASES [33] score.

Radiographic Evaluation

A radiographic evaluation at selected visits can include true scapular anteroposterior and axillary views. Scrutiny of the radiographs is necessary for documenting and decision making. Periprosthetic lucent lines or fracture lines; Cracks or fracture lines especially at the acromion due to loading of the deltoid muscle; this is more prevalent in reverse geometry total shoulder replacement; documentation of wear signs, subsidence of the components, stress shielding, notching, ossifications and osteophytes.

Evaluation of radiolucencies and of loosening have produced many classification schemes [69]. The importance and relevance of radiolucent lines (RLLs) has not yet been fully established. Sperling [70] defined specific 5 zones of the contact interface of the pegged glenoid component and bone in radiographs. Lucencies were measured by location and thickness. A glenoid component was "at risk" when a complete lucent line was present, some part of it being 1.5 mm or greater in width, or when at least 2 of 3 independent observers identified migration or tilt of the component. Mole [71] described a classification for keeled glenoid radiolucent lines using 6 zones around the cemented keel with 3 grades of lucencies. Multiplication of the number of lucent zones by the lucency grade produces a maximum score of 18, when 12 indicated loosening. Franklin [13] published a classification of radiolucent lines considering also the translation or dislocation of the glenoid component. Wilde [72] described a classification for assessment of radiolucency around the keel using axillary views: zone 1 is the interface of subchondral bone with the collar of the prosthesis, zone 2 is radiolucent lines in the lateral (superficial) part of the glenoid keel, and zone 3 is the medial (deeper) part of the interface of the keel with the subchondral bone. Lazarus [73] compared pegged and keeled glenoid components. He used Franklin's [13] classification for the keeled glenoid components and created a modification for pegged components. He concluded that radiolucencies and incomplete component seating occur more frequently in association with keeled components compared with pegged components. Mileti [74] and associates used a similar zonal representation of radiolucencies around the glenoid and the humeral components. They also stated that the glenoid component in total shoulder arthroplasty has been the focus of most radiographic scrutiny in the radiographic analysis of total shoulder arthroplasty.

Arthroplasty for Fractures

Key Points

- Arthroplasty for comminuted proximal humeral fractures is a challenging issue mainly to restore anatomy due to missing landmarks.
- Osteosynthesis of the tuberosities is sometimes a challenge.
- A stemmed prosthesis is usually used.

Boileau [25, 75] noted that hemiarthroplasty for fractures yielded unpredictable results. From sixty six consecutive patients 27% had initial tuberosity malposition, detachment and migration of the tuberosities was noticed in 23%; altogether 50% had malposition of tuberosities which correlated with subjective unsatisfactory results. His conclusion was that functional results after hemiarthroplasty for 3- and 4-part proximal humeral fractures appear to be directly associated with tuberosity osteosynthesis. Correctly establishing the height and retroversion of the humeral prosthesis is difficult in fracture cases because, except in rare cases, the proximal anatomic landmarks have disappeared as a result of bone loss. Lengthening of the humerus due to proud prosthesis caused the tuberosities to proximally migrate shortening the lever arm, causing failure in elevation and abduction. Shortening of the humerus was better tolerated clinically. In a later publication concerning management of fracture sequelae Boileau [25] recommends avoiding tuberosity osteotomy even in the price of accepting deformity. Mighell [76] noted also that the fracture pattern, type of implant, presence of neurologic injury, and patient's age and sex do not seem to affect outcome to the extent that timing of surgery and, most importantly, quality of tuberosity reconstruction do. Elderly people were a risk factor for failure of hemiarthroplasty and the trend today is moving towards offering reverse total shoulder arthroplasty for acute comminuted proximal humeral fractures in the elderly [77].

Conversion of Anatomic Shoulder Arthroplasty to Reverse Total Shoulder Arthroplasty

Key Points

- Revision is always an imminent option after arthroplasty.
- For elderly patients failed TSA or hemiarthroplasty can be converted to reverse total shoulder arthroplasty in the presence of massive or irreparable rotator cuff tear.
- This conversion created limb lengthening and sometimes tensioning or overtrmof the deltoid.

The frequency of total shoulder arthroplasty is constantly increasing. This increases revisions because of stem or glenoid component loosening, infection, instability or glenoid subsidence. Significant rotator cuff lesions necessitate reverse shoulder arthroplasty sometimes with bone reconstruction, which is a demanding procedure.

Reverse shoulder arthroplasty can be an efficacious salvage procedure in the management of failed arthroplasty due to rotator cuff-related instability or bone defects, or both [78]. Kiet [79] in a comparison between stemmed anatomical shoulder arthroplasty and reverse total shoulder replacement the two groups were similar in complication rate, pain and satisfaction scores, and most of ranges of movement except for greater external rotation in the anatomical arthroplasty group.

Recently new modular systems attempt to anticipate and minimize the intervention scale for revision, by allowing retention of the humeral stem or the glenoid baseplate, and by replacing only the hemisphere and inserts. Concerns are for limb lengthening and soft tissue imbalance due to overstuffing of the joint and over-tensioning the deltoid muscle. These might lead to pain and wear of the arthroplasty. Modular systems are constantly improving in effort to reduce these risks. Not always modular system can accommodate for surgeon's errors such as placing the humeral stem too proud or with the wrong version. Kany [80] reported good outcome with modular system still 25% of humeral stems had to be removed. Within these limits the literature finds that short and midterm results are on the positive side [81–84]. Yet limb lengthening is one concern but its clinical relevance is not entirely clear, and long term follow-up is still warranted. Teschner [83] experimented with six different modular systems by six manufacturers (DePuy Global Unite, Exactech™, Implantcast™, Mathys, Tornier and Zimmer). He measured the difference in height and offset when converting from hemiarthroplasty to reverse total shoulder arthroplasty. Results showed variable arm lengthening (smallest 11.6 ± 3.3 mm largest 33 ± 5.3 mm) and offsets (least of 1.5 ± 5.7 mm and most -21.7 ± 3.7 mm) with the Implantcast™ showing the least change in those parameters. Another solution offered by Matsoukis [85] is a custom adaptor to the well-fixed humeral stem in case of an older pre-modular type implant. Still, this was presented as a case report.

Another attitude is bonestock sparing strategies and implants. Humeral head resurfacing and metaphyseal implants can allow more revision options and are more anatomic. The Copeland humeral resurfacing is designed to cover an arthritic humeral head with minimal bone removal. Long term results [41] with this prosthesis and biological glenoid resurfacing in patients younger than 50 are satisfying with survivorship for hemiarthroplasty with biological glenoid resurfacing at 97% at 5 years, 97% at 11 years, 91% at 14 years, and 85% at 22 years. The estimated revision-free survival rate for cementless Copeland resurfacing total shoulder arthroplasty (TSA) was 100% at 5 years, 71% at 11 years, 71% at 14 years, and 61% at 22 years.

Outcome Predictors, Complication Rates and Risk Factors of Shoulder Arthroplasty

Key Points

- Main risk factors are obesity and young age
- Outcome is usually acceptable and shoulder arthroplasty is generally successful.
- The main complication is loosening

Singh [86], in an analysis of 1413 shoulders concluded that risk factors for TSR are obesity and young age. Aldinger [87] analyzed a prospective database of available 485 shoulder replacements including stemmed cemented and non-cemented hemiarthroplasties, humeral head resurfacing, cemented stemmed anatomical total shoulder arthroplasty for fractures and for arthritis, bipolar cemented stemmed humeral head, and cemented stemmed reverse total shoulder arthroplasty. Complications were classified into three categories: temporary complications not requiring intervention such as temporary nerve palsy, temporary dislocation, and cracks or fractures of humerus or glenoid; Soft tissue complications requiring soft tissue revision such as biceps tendonitis, recurrent dislocations, wound infection and joint contractures; Complications with implant revisions such as component malposition, painful glenoid erosion, loosening and deep infection. An overall complication rate of 11.6% was noted, of which 7% occurred in 1st category, 2.3% at the second category and 2.3% in the third category. For a median follow-up of 1.6 years (range 1–10) the survivorship rate was 90.5%, and patient satisfaction rate s were mostly positive. Bohsali [88] reviewed the literature of shoulder arthroplasty and found that complication rate was highly variable from 0% to 62%, mean range between 10% and 16%. The complication categories included component loosening, instability, periprosthetic fractures intra and postoperative, rotator cuff tears, neural injury, infection and deltoid detachment. Sperling [89] reviewed the literature and described shoulder arthroplasty complications: periprosthetic fractures 1.6–2.3%; Infection 0–4%; Instability with anatomic shoulder replacement – Anterior 0.9–1.8%, Posterior 1–1.3%; Instability with reverse total shoulder arthroplasty; Rotator cuff tears 1.3–7.8% specifically relating to the posterosuperior corner of the rotator cuff; Glenoid component loosening – although radiological lucent line are reported in 39% only 8% require revisions. In both primary and revisions tissue cultures must be obtained and specifically culture for Propionibacterium acnes. Levy [65] and associates cultured 41.8% positive Propionibacterium acnes in primary joint replacement.

Future Outlook

Shoulder arthroplasty is still evolving and the learning curve is steep, there is much to be explored. Glenoid treatment in shoulder arthroplasty is still controversial. Glenoid resurfacing has not yet been optimized and radiolucencies, loosening, wear and dislocation are still imminent issues. Copeland [10] said that "long-term glenoid loosening is a problem, and better materials and designs for the glenoid are required. There is no doubt that we have come a long way, and we are only just possibly reaching the surface". In general, our research should continue also to endeavor the more biological options such as optimizing biological resurfacing for better long term results. Since our candidates for arthroplasty are becoming younger we should seek to establish long lasting prosthetic designs, but keeping in mind that revision is inevitable, thus striving to use bone preserving techniques and designs, such as short or metaphyseal humeral stems, and using bone impaction techniques for prosthesis purchase rather than cement. Reverse total shoulder arthroplasty design is in extensive development, for more indications and for younger candidates. We are beginning to understand how to optimize the mechanics and materials. Shifting medially and distally of the glenosphere by Paul Grammont [12] were the first steps. Now we understand that some lateralization is necessary to achieve better range of movement, less notching and optimal deltoid muscle tensioning such as with the Verso reverse total shoulder and the BIO-RSA, what will be our next understanding?

Questions

Which of the following statements is correct?

A. Anatomical shoulder replacement is contraindicated in inflammatory arthropathy due to osteopenia
B. Reverse shoulder replacement is contraindicated in rotator cuff pathology due to proximal humeral migration
C. Anatomical shoulder replacement is contraindicated in rotator cuff pathology due to proximal humeral migration
D. Reverse shoulder replacement is preferred over anatomical shoulder replacement for Charcot shoulder joint

What is the most common complication that necessitates reoperation in shoulder arthroplasty for post-traumatic arthritis?

A. Infection
B. Avascular necrosis
C. Postoperative instability
D. Axillary nerve injury

Advantages of glenoid resurfacing over proximal humeral replacement are:

A. Better stability
B. Less operative time
C. Better strength
D. Minimal blood loss
E. Smaller revision rate for the glenoid component
F. Better range of motion,
G. Minimal glenoid socket pain
H. A & C & D & F
I. A & C & F & G
J. A & B & E & G

References

1. Bankes MJ, Emery RJ. Pioneers of shoulder replacement: Themistocles Gluck and Jules Emile Pean. J Shoulder Elb Surg. 1995;4(4):259–62.
2. Neer II CS. Replacement arthroplasty for glenohumeral osteoarthritis. J Bone Joint Surg Am. 1974;56(1):1–13.
3. Neer II CS. Articular replacement for the humeral head. J Bone Joint Surg Am. 1955;37-a(2):215.
4. Neer II CS. Follow-up notes on articles previously published in the journal: articular replacement for the humeral head. J Bone Joint Surg Am. 1964;46:1607–10.
5. Nyffeler RW, Sheikh R, Jacob HA, Gerber C. Influence of humeral prosthesis height on biomechanics of glenohumeral abduction. An in vitro study. J Bone Joint Surg Am. 2004;86-a(3):575–80.
6. Boileau P, Sinnerton RJ, Chuinard C, Walch G. Arthroplasty of the shoulder. J Bone Joint Surg Br. 2006;88(5):562–75.
7. Boileau P, Walch G. The three-dimensional geometry of the proximal humerus. Implications for surgical technique and prosthetic design. J Bone Joint Surg Br. 1997;79(5):857–65.
8. Roberts SN, Foley AP, Swallow HM, Wallace WA, Coughlan DP. The geometry of the humeral head and the design of prostheses. J Bone Joint Surg Br. 1991;73(4):647–50.
9. Copeland SA, Levy O, Brownlow HC. Resurfacing arthroplasty of the shoulder. Tech Should Elb Surg. 2003;4(4):199–210.
10. Copeland S. The continuing development of shoulder replacement: "reaching the surface". J Bone Joint Surg Am. 2006;88(4):900–5.

11. Lettin AW, Copeland SA, Scales JT. The Stanmore total shoulder replacement. J Bone Joint Surg Br. 1982;64(1):47–51.
12. Grammont PM, Baulot E. Delta shoulder prosthesis for rotator cuff rupture. Orthopedics. 1993;16(1):65–8.
13. Franklin JL, Barrett WP, Jackins SE, Matsen FA. Glenoid loosening in total shoulder arthroplasty. Association with rotator cuff deficiency. J Arthroplast. 1988;3(1):39–46.
14. Neer CS, Craig EV, Fukuda H. Cuff-tear arthropathy. J Bone Joint Surg Am. 1983;65(9):1232–44.
15. Flatow EL, Harrison AK. A history of reverse total shoulder arthroplasty. Clin Orthop Relat Res. 2011;469(9):2432–9.
16. Coughlin MJ, Morris JM, West WF. The semiconstrained total shoulder arthroplasty. J Bone Joint Surg Am. 1979;61(4):574–81.
17. Post M, Jablon M, Miller H, Singh M. Constrained total shoulder joint replacement: a critical review. Clin Orthop Relat Res. 1979;144:135–50.
18. Kessel L, Bayley I. Prosthetic replacement of shoulder joint: preliminary communication. J R Soc Med. 1979;72(10):748–52.
19. Kolbel R, Friedebold G. Shoulder joint replacement. Arch Orthop Unfallchir. 1973;76(1):31–9.
20. Fenlin Jr JM. Total glenohumeral joint replacement. Orthop Clin North Am. 1975;6(2):565–83.
21. Buechel FF, Pappas MJ, DePalma AF. "Floating-socket" total shoulder replacement: anatomical, biomechanical, and surgical rationale. J Biomed Mater Res. 1978;12(1):89–114.
22. Atoun E, Funk L, Copland SA, Even T, Levy O, Rath E. The effect of shoulder manipulation on rotator cuff integrity. Acta Orthop Belg. 2013;79(3):255–9.
23. Bell SN, Coghlan JA. Short stem shoulder replacement. Int J Shoulder Surg. 2014;8(3):72–5.
24. Cruess RL. The current status of avascular necrosis of the femoral head. Clin Orthop Relat Res. 1978;131:309–11.
25. Boileau P, Trojani C, Walch G, Krishnan SG, Romeo A, Sinnerton R. Shoulder arthroplasty for the treatment of the sequelae of fractures of the proximal humerus. J Shoulder Elb Surg. 2001;10(4):299–308.
26. Jacobson JA, Duquin TR, Sanchez-Sotelo J, Schleck CD, Sperling JW, Cofield RH. Anatomic shoulder arthroplasty for treatment of proximal humerus malunions. J Shoulder Elb Surg. 2014;23(8):1232–9.
27. Kirkley A, Griffin S, Dainty K. Scoring systems for the functional assessment of the shoulder. Arthroscopy. 2003;19(10):1109–20.
28. Constant CR, Murley AH. A clinical method of functional assessment of the shoulder. Clin Orthop Relat Res. 1987;214:160–4.
29. Godfrey J, Hamman R, Lowenstein S, Briggs K, Kocher M. Reliability, validity, and responsiveness of the simple shoulder test: psychometric properties by age and injury type. J Shoulder Elb Surg. 2007;16(3):260–7.
30. Dawson J, Fitzpatrick R, Carr A. Questionnaire on the perceptions of patients about shoulder surgery. J Bone Joint Surg Br. 1996;78(4):593–600.
31. Amstutz HC, Sew Hoy AL, Clarke IC. UCLA anatomic total shoulder arthroplasty. Clin Orthop Relat Res. 1981;155:7–20.
32. Kennedy CA, Beaton DE, Solway S, McConnell S, Bombardier C. Disabilities of the Arm, Shoulder and Hand (DASH). The DASH and QuickDASH Outcome Measure User's Manual 2011. http://dash.iwh.on.ca/
33. Richards RR, An KN, Bigliani LU, et al. A standardized method for the assessment of shoulder function. J Shoulder Elb Surg. 1994;3(6):347–52.
34. Neer II CS, Watson KC, Stanton FJ. Recent experience in total shoulder replacement. J Bone Joint Surg Am. 1982;64(3):319–37.
35. Pfahler M, Jena F, Neyton L, Sirveaux F, Mole D. Hemiarthroplasty versus total shoulder prosthesis: results of cemented glenoid components. J Shoulder Elb Surg. 2006;15(2):154–63.
36. Sandow MJ, David H, Bentall SJ. Hemiarthroplasty vs total shoulder replacement for rotator cuff intact osteoarthritis: how do they fare after a decade? J Shoulder Elb Surg. 2013;22(7):877–85.
37. Burkhead Jr WZ, Hutton KS. Biologic resurfacing of the glenoid with hemiarthroplasty of the shoulder. J Shoulder Elb Surg. 1995;4(4):263–70.
38. Krishnan SG, Reineck JR, Nowinski RJ, Harrison D, Burkhead WZ. Humeral hemiarthroplasty with biologic resurfacing of the glenoid for glenohumeral arthritis. Surgical technique. J Bone Joint Surg Am. 2008;90(Suppl 2 Pt 1):9–19.
39. Levy O, Copeland SA. Cementless surface replacement arthroplasty of the shoulder. 5- to 10-year results with the Copeland mark-2 prosthesis. J Bone Joint Surg Br. 2001;83(2):213–21.
40. Levy O, Copeland SA. Cementless surface replacement arthroplasty (Copeland CSRA) for osteoarthritis of the shoulder. J Shoulder Elb Surg. 2004;13(3):266–71.
41. Levy O, Tsvieli O, Merchant J, et al. Surface replacement arthroplasty for glenohumeral arthropathy in patients aged younger than fifty years: results after a minimum ten-year follow-up. J Shoulder Elb Surg. 2015;24(7):1049–60.
42. Krishnan SG, Nowinski RJ, Harrison D, Burkhead WZ. Humeral hemiarthroplasty with biologic resurfacing of the glenoid for glenohumeral arthritis. Two to fifteen-year outcomes. J Bone Joint Surg Am. 2007;89(4):727–34.
43. Strauss EJ, Verma NN, Salata MJ, et al. The high failure rate of biologic resurfacing of the glenoid in young patients with glenohumeral arthritis. J Shoulder Elb Surg. 2014;23(3):409–19.
44. Pritchett JW. Long-term results and patient satisfaction after shoulder resurfacing. J Shoulder Elb Surg. 2011;20(5):771–7.

45. Walch G, Boileau P, Noel E. Shoulder arthroplasty: evolving techniques and indications. Joint Bone Spine. 2010;77(6):501–5.
46. Papadonikolakis A, Matsen III. FA. Metal-backed glenoid components have a higher rate of failure and fail by different modes in comparison with all-polyethylene components: a systematic review. J Bone Joint Surg Am. 2014;96(12):1041–7.
47. Skirving AP. Total shoulder arthroplasty—current problems and possible solutions. J Orthop Sci. 1999;4(1):42–53.
48. Feldman AY, Bunker TD. Rotational dissociation of glenoid components in a total shoulder prosthesis: an indication that sagittal torque forces may be important in glenoid component design. J Shoulder Elb Surg. 1999;8(3):279–80.
49. Levy O, Copeland SA. Rotational dissociation of glenoid components in a total shoulder prosthesis: an indication that sagittal torque forces may be important in glenoid component design. J Shoulder Elb Surg. 2001;10:197.
50. Burkhead Jr WZ, Krishnan SG, Lin KC. Biologic resurfacing of the arthritic glenohumeral joint: historical review and current applications. J Shoulder Elb Surg. 2007;16(5 Suppl):S248–53.
51. Hasan SS, Leith JM, Campbell B, Kapil R, Smith KL, Matsen III. FA. Characteristics of unsatisfactory shoulder arthroplasties. J Shoulder Elb Surg. 2002;11(5):431–41.
52. Rodosky MW, Bigliani LU. Indications for glenoid resurfacing in shoulder arthroplasty. J Shoulder Elb Surg. 1996;5(3):231–48.
53. Sperling JW, Cofield RH, Rowland CM. Neer hemiarthroplasty and Neer total shoulder arthroplasty in patients fifty years old or less. Long-term results. J Bone Joint Surg Am. 1998;80(4):464–73.
54. Sperling JW, Cofield RH, Rowland CM. Minimum fifteen-year follow-up of Neer hemiarthroplasty and total shoulder arthroplasty in patients aged fifty years or younger. J Shoulder Elb Surg. 2004;13(6):604–13.
55. Gartsman GM, Roddey TS, Hammerman SM. Shoulder arthroplasty with or without resurfacing of the glenoid in patients who have osteoarthritis. J Bone Joint Surg Am. 2000;82(1):26–34.
56. Lo IK, Litchfield RB, Griffin S, Faber K, Patterson SD, Kirkley A. Quality-of-life outcome following hemiarthroplasty or total shoulder arthroplasty in patients with osteoarthritis. A prospective, randomized trial. J Bone Joint Surg Am. 2005;87(10):2178–85.
57. Bryant D, Litchfield R, Sandow M, Gartsman GM, Guyatt G, Kirkley A. A comparison of pain, strength, range of motion, and functional outcomes after hemiarthroplasty and total shoulder arthroplasty in patients with osteoarthritis of the shoulder. A systematic review and meta-analysis. J Bone Joint Surg Am. 2005;87(9):1947–56.
58. Edwards TB, Kadakia NR, Boulahia A, et al. A comparison of hemiarthroplasty and total shoulder arthroplasty in the treatment of primary glenohumeral osteoarthritis: results of a multicenter study. J Shoulder Elb Surg. 2003;12(3):207–13.
59. Boileau P, Avidor C, Krishnan SG, Walch G, Kempf JF, Mole D. Cemented polyethylene versus uncemented metal-backed glenoid components in total shoulder arthroplasty: a prospective, double-blind, randomized study. J Shoulder Elb Surg. 2002;11(4):351–9.
60. Boileau P, Moineau G, Morin-Salvo N, et al. Metal-backed glenoid implant with polyethylene insert is not a viable long-term therapeutic option. J Shoulder Elb Surg. 2015;24(10):1534–43.
61. Buzzell JE, Lutton DM, Shyr Y, Neviaser RJ, Lee DH. Reliability and accuracy of templating the proximal humeral component for shoulder arthroplasty. J Shoulder Elb Surg. 2009;18(5):728–33.
62. Walch G, Badet R, Boulahia A, Khoury A. Morphologic study of the glenoid in primary glenohumeral osteoarthritis. J Arthroplast. 1999;14(6):756–60.
63. Habermeyer P, Magosch P, Luz V, Lichtenberg S. Three-dimensional glenoid deformity in patients with osteoarthritis: a radiographic analysis. J Bone Joint Surg Am. 2006;88(6):1301–7.
64. Youderian AR, Ricchetti ET, Drews M, Iannotti JP. Determination of humeral head size in anatomic shoulder replacement for glenohumeral osteoarthritis. J Shoulder Elb Surg. 2014;23(7):955–63.
65. Levy O, Iyer S, Atoun E, et al. Propionibacterium acnes: an underestimated etiology in the pathogenesis of osteoarthritis? J Shoulder Elb Surg. 2013;22(4):505–11.
66. Neviaser JS. Surgical approaches to the shoulder. Clin Orthop Relat Res. 1973;91:34–40.
67. Mackenzie D. The antero-superior exposure for total shoulder replacement. Orthop Traumatol. 1993;2(2):71–7.
68. Hughes M, Neer II. CS. Glenohumeral joint replacement and postoperative rehabilitation. Phys Ther. 1975;55(8):850–8.
69. Jean K. Classifications of glenoid dysplasia, glenoid bone loss and glenoid loosening: a review of the literature. Eur J Orthop Surg Traumatol. 2013;23(3):301–10.
70. Sperling JW, Cofield RH, O'Driscoll SW, Torchia ME, Rowland CM. Radiographic assessment of ingrowth total shoulder arthroplasty. J Shoulder Elb Surg. 2000;9(6):507–13.
71. Molé D, Roche O, Riand N, Lévigne C, Walch G. Cemented glenoid component: results in osteoarthritis and rheumatoidarthritis. In: Walch G, Boileau P, editors. Shoulder arthroplasty. Berlin: Springer; 1999. p. 163–71.
72. Wilde AH, Borden LS, Brems JJ. Experience with Neer total shoulder replacement. In: Bateman JE, Welsh RP, editors. Surgery of the shoulder. Philadelphia: B.C. Decker; 1984. p. 224–8.
73. Lazarus MD, Jensen KL, Southworth C, Matsen III. FA. The radiographic evaluation of keeled and pegged glenoid component insertion. J Bone Joint Surg Am. 2002;84-a(7):1174–82.
74. Mileti J, Boardman III ND, Sperling JW, et al. Radiographic analysis of polyethylene glenoid components using modern cementing techniques. J Shoulder Elb Surg. 2004;13(5):492–8.

75. Boileau P, Krishnan SG, Tinsi L, Walch G, Coste JS, Mole D. Tuberosity malposition and migration: reasons for poor outcomes after hemiarthroplasty for displaced fractures of the proximal humerus. J Shoulder Elb Surg. 2002;11(5):401–12.
76. Mighell MA, Kolm GP, Collinge CA, Frankle MA. Outcomes of hemiarthroplasty for fractures of the proximal humerus. J Shoulder Elb Surg. 2003;12(6):569–77.
77. Routman HD. Indications, technique, and pitfalls of reverse total shoulder arthroplasty for proximal humerus fractures. Bull Hosp Jt Dis (2013). 2013;71(Suppl 2):64–7.
78. Kelly II JD, Zhao JX, Hobgood ER, Norris TR. Clinical results of revision shoulder arthroplasty using the reverse prosthesis. J Shoulder Elb Surg. 2012;21(11):1516–25.
79. Kiet TK, Feeley BT, Naimark M, et al. Outcomes after shoulder replacement: comparison between reverse and anatomic total shoulder arthroplasty. J Shoulder Elb Surg. 2015;24(2):179–85.
80. Kany J, Amouyel T, Flamand O, Katz D, Valenti P. A convertible shoulder system: is it useful in total shoulder arthroplasty revisions? Int Orthop. 2015;39(2):299–304.
81. Castagna A, Delcogliano M, de Caro F, et al. Conversion of shoulder arthroplasty to reverse implants: clinical and radiological results using a modular system. Int Orthop. 2013;37(7):1297–305.
82. Wieser K, Borbas P, Ek ET, Meyer DC, Gerber C. Conversion of stemmed hemi- or total to reverse total shoulder arthroplasty: advantages of a modular stem design. Clin Orthop Relat Res. 2015;473(2):651–60.
83. Teschner H, Albrecht UV, Meller R, et al. Conversion of hemi into reverse shoulder arthroplasty: implant design limitations. Arch Orthop Trauma Surg. 2014;134(12):1683–9.
84. Dilisio MF, Miller LR, Siegel EJ, Higgins LD. Conversion to reverse shoulder arthroplasty: humeral stem retention versus revision. Orthopedics. 2015;38(9):e773–9.
85. Matsoukis J, Billuart F, Houssam K, Dujardin F, Walch G. Conversion of total shoulder arthroplasty to reverse shoulder arthroplasty made possible by custom humeral adapter. Orthop Traumatol Surg Res. 2015;101(6):759–61.
86. Singh JA, Sperling JW, Cofield RH. Risk factors for revision surgery after humeral head replacement: 1,431 shoulders over 3 decades. J Shoulder Elb Surg. 2012;21(8):1039–44.
87. Aldinger PR, Raiss P, Rickert M, Loew M. Complications in shoulder arthroplasty: an analysis of 485 cases. Int Orthop. 2010;34(4):517–24.
88. Bohsali KI, Wirth MA, Rockwood Jr CA. Complications of total shoulder arthroplasty. J Bone Joint Surg Am. 2006;88(10):2279–92.
89. Sperling JW, Hawkins RJ, Walch G, Zuckerman JD. Complications in total shoulder arthroplasty. J Bone Joint Surg Am. 2013;95(6):563–9.

22 Reverse Shoulder Arthroplasty

Matthew Baker, Kyubo Choi, Seyedali R. Ghasemi, and Edward G. McFarland

Introduction, History, and Biomechanics

When Neer introduced his proximal humerus prosthesis in the 1950s, there was renewed interest in shoulder arthroplasty. In his original paper describing hemiarthroplasty, five of 12 patients had good or excellent range of motion, and one of 12 had pain with use [1]. As the use of hemiarthroplasty and eventually total shoulder arthroplasty (TSA) increased, it became apparent that this procedure was not a panacea for all degenerative shoulder conditions. This was especially true for arthritis and massive rotator cuff tears. Early failures using an anatomic prosthesis were characterized by a disappointing restoration of active motion and functional ability. "Limited goals rehab" was implemented for patients with cuff tear arthropathy because of the anticipated inability to regain full motion and strength [2].

M. Baker, M.D. • K. Choi, M.D. • S.R. Ghasemi, M.D.
E.G. McFarland, M.D. (✉)
Department of Orthopaedic Surgery, The Johns Hopkins University, 10753 Falls Rd, Suite 215, Lutherville, MD 21093, USA
e-mail: editorialservices@jhmi.edu

Cuff Tear Arthropathy

Neer et al. [3] first coined the term "cuff tear arthropathy" in 1983 to describe joint changes associated with massive rotator cuff tears and accompanying shoulder joint degeneration. They found three issues that were unique to patients with cuff tear arthropathy.

First, the tendon tissue in massive tears often does not hold sutures well, especially if placed under tension when repaired. Therefore, rotator cuff repair alone or with shoulder arthroplasty often would result in failure of the repair. Second, with large to massive rotator cuff tears, there can be an alteration of the glenohumeral joint congruity, which contributes to pain. Third, as the humeral head migrated superiorly, there was contact of the greater tuberosity with the acromion.

When discussing biomechanics of the shoulder, a key concept is concavity-compression [4]. If one uses the analogy of a golf ball on a tee when thinking of the glenohumeral joint, the deeper the cup of the tee (the glenoid), the more force is needed to move the ball (humeral head) off the tee. The rotator cuff compresses the humeral head into the glenoid. With loss of the rotator cuff, the ball does not stay centered in the socket with certain motions, and the center of rotation (COR) of the ball on the center of the socket is altered. This alteration of the COR of

G. Huri, N.K. Paschos (eds.), *The Shoulder*, Orthopaedic Study Guide Series,
DOI 10.1007/978-3-319-51979-1_22

the ball on the tee leads to abnormal wear of the tee (or socket in this case). It also makes the shoulder work harder mechanically for the same motion or activity.

With motion, there is a considerable amount of stress across the glenoid. At 90° of arm elevation, the pressure against the glenoid is at least ten times the weight of the extremity. If you consider that the arm makes up approximately 5% of the body's weight, the resultant pressure/friction is equal to half of a person's body weight [5].

With a loss of the normal force couples about the shoulder with massive rotator cuff tears, there is an alteration of the compressive forces that leads to loss of the concentric arc of motion. With the loss of the rotator cuff, the humeral head starts to subluxate superiorly. When the deltoid fires to elevate the arm, the mechanical advantage is gone and, instead of the arm elevating with muscle activity, it becomes more of a translational movement.

Superior subluxation can be seen on physical examination (Fig. 22.1). When attempting to elevate the arm, the humeral head elevates with respect to the anatomic COR of the glenoid. This is seen by observing the humeral head producing a mass or bump in the anterior and superior area of the shoulder.

Although not all patients with massive rotator cuff tears experience pain and loss of motion, certain patients developed a spectrum of changes seen radiographically, which are often associated with symptoms. These changes include superior movement of the COR of the humeral head away from the COR of the glenoid. This then causes eccentric load on the glenoid, which eventually can produce bone loss in the superior glenoid. Simultaneously, the greater tuberosity has increased contact with the acromion, causing wear of the greater tuberosity and the acromion. These sequential changes seen in cuff tear arthropathy were described by Hamada et al. [6] (Fig. 22.2).

The movement of the COR of the humeral head also is seen in patients with rotator cuff tears in whom an anatomical total shoulder replacement has been performed. If the rotator cuff tear is large enough, the humeral head of an anatomical TSA will also begin to slide superiorly over time. This causes the proximal

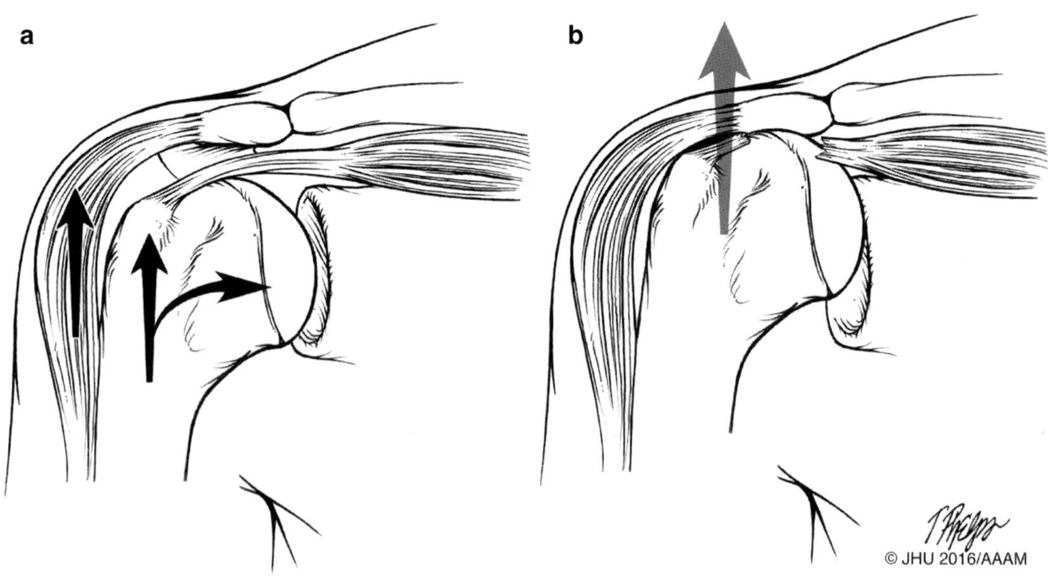

Fig. 22.1 Superior subluxation of the humeral head caused by loss of force couples associated with massive rotator cuff tear. (**a**) The intact rotator cuff keeps the humeral head compressed against the glenoid allowing for elevation of the arm. (**b**) When there is a massive tear, the humeral head subluxes superiorly because of a disruption of the force couples

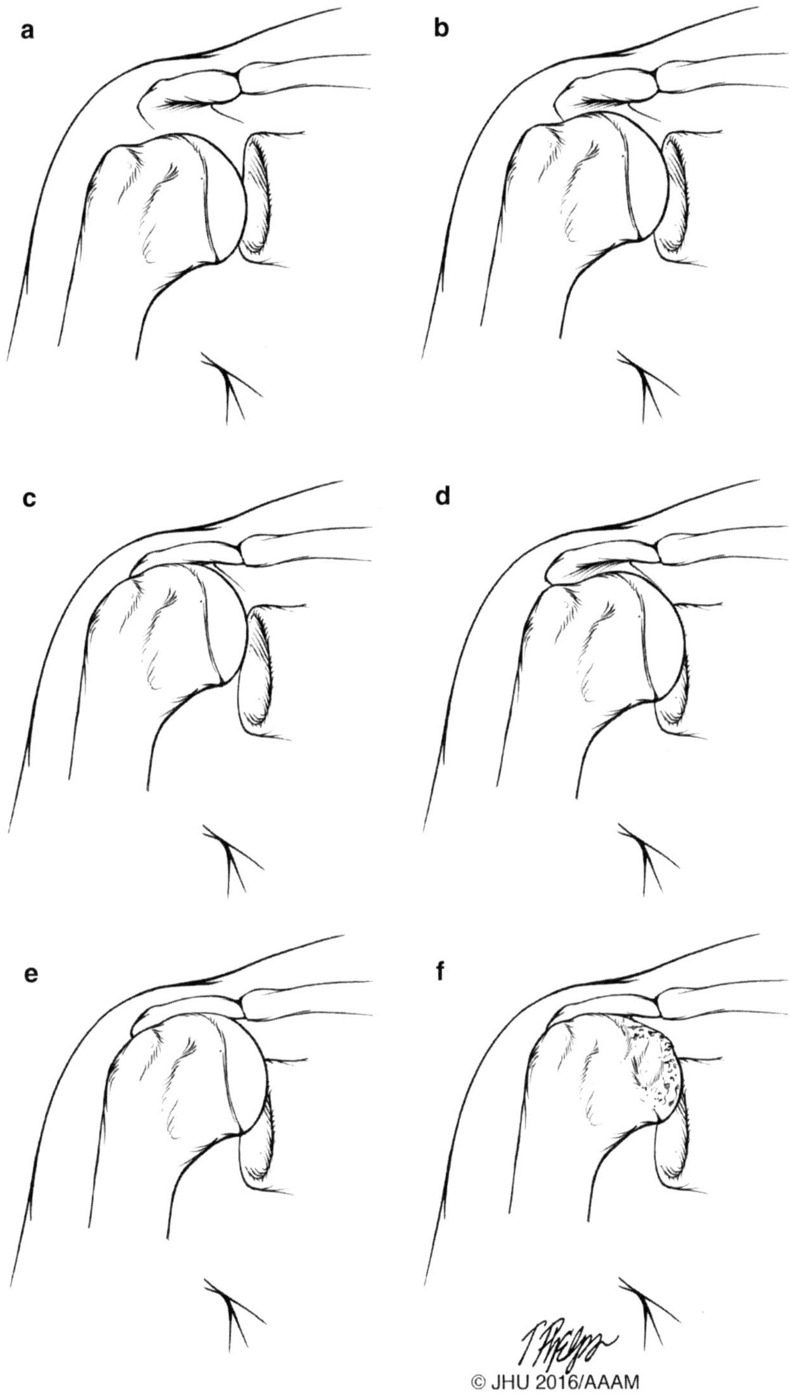

Fig. 22.2 The Hamada Classification. (**a**) Grade 1-AHI >6 mm. (**b**) Grade 2-AHI < 5 mm. (**c**) Grade 3-Acetabularization of the acromion. (**d**) Grade 4A-Glenohumeral joint space narrowing without acetabularization of the acromion. (**e**) Grade 4B-Glenohumeral joint space narrowing with acetabularization of the acromion. (**f**) Grade 5-End-stage disease with collapse of the humeral head. (**g**) Radiograph showing Grade 3 changes. (**h**) Radiograph showing Grade 4B changes. (**i**) Radiograph showing Grade 5 changes

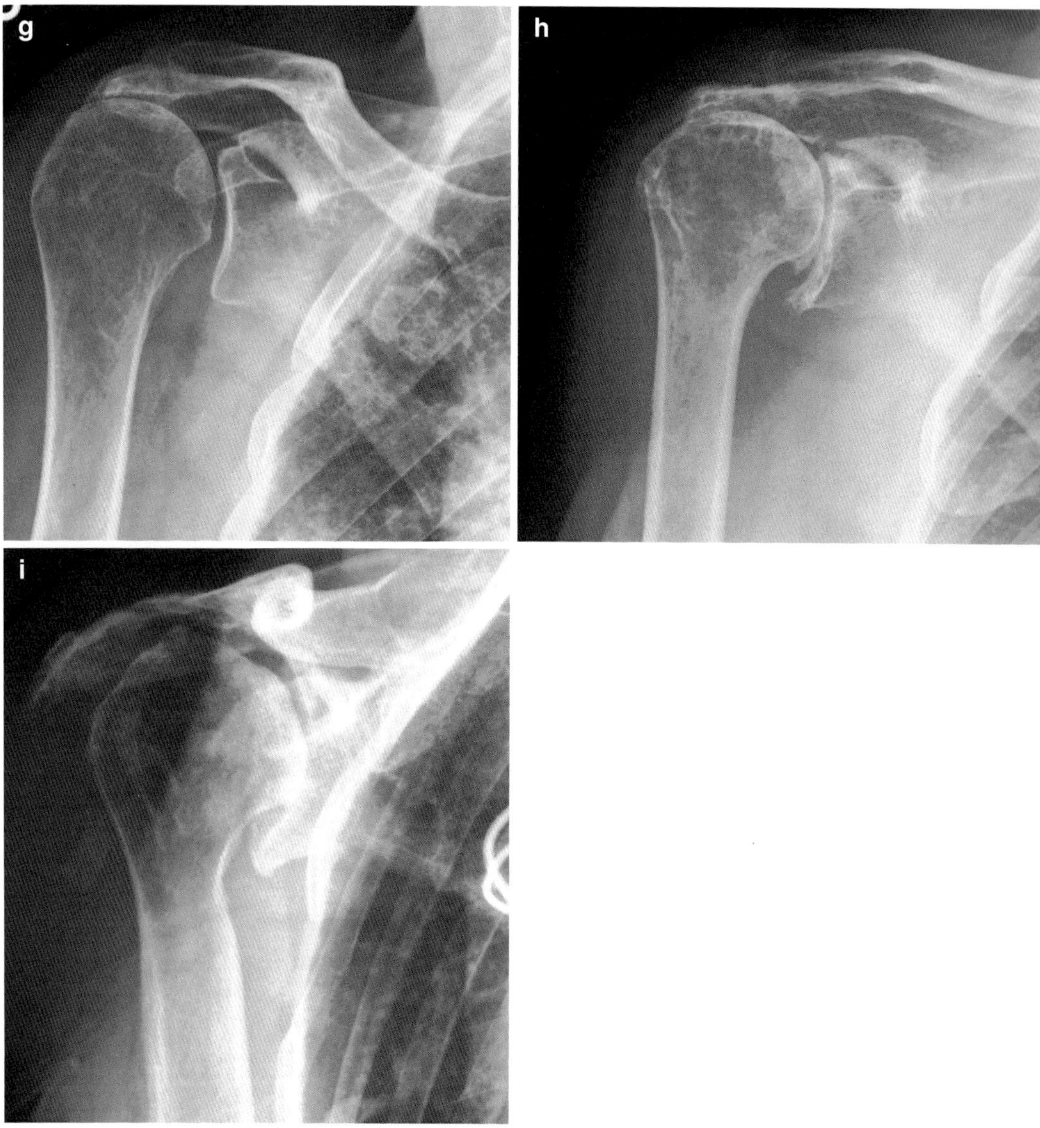

Fig. 22.2 (continued)

humerus to move superiorly with arm elevation, resulting in eccentric forces putting extreme stress on the glenoid component. With loss of the rotator cuff, the deltoid forces become translational. This can lead to abnormal movement or translation. The abnormal motion in the setting of anatomic TSA can lead to early failure caused by the "rocking horse phenomenon" (Fig. 22.3), which results in accelerated loosening of the glenoid prosthesis [7].

Development of Reverse Shoulder Arthroplasty

Between 1970 and 1973, Neer developed the first TSA in the United States in which the components were reversed. Designated the Mark 1, this was an attempt to use a more constrained shoulder implant to address the poor functional and radiological outcomes of patients with deficient rotator cuffs (Fig. 22.4). The purpose of a

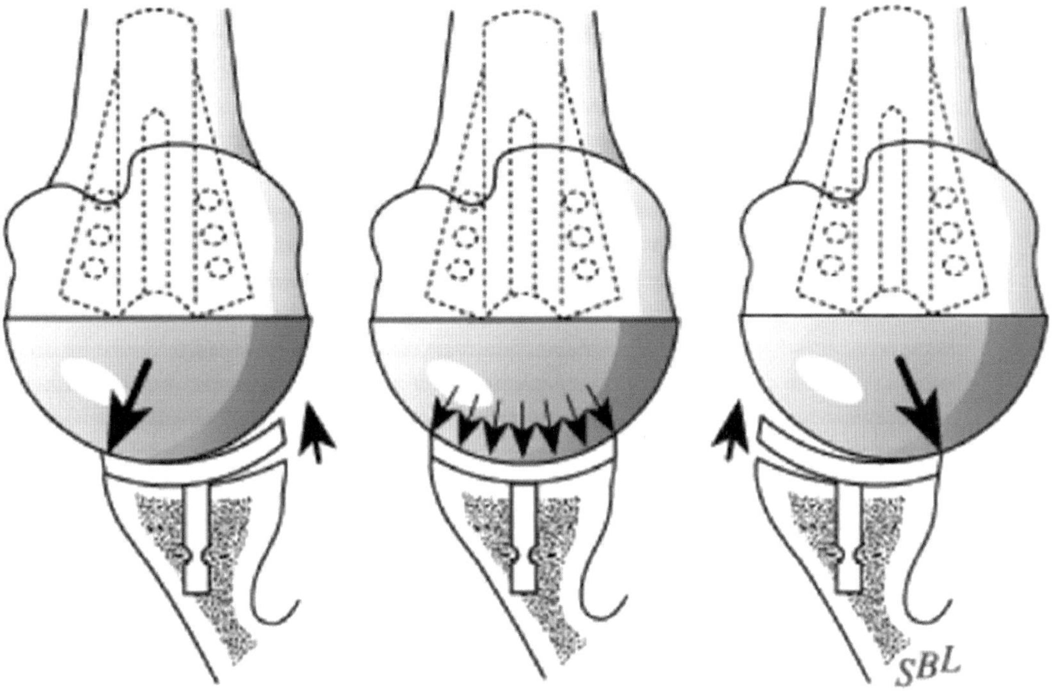

Fig. 22.3 Rocking-horse loosening. Although the glenoid component is stable when the load applied by the humeral head is centered (*middle*), anterior (*left*), or posterior (*right*) translation of the head of the glenoid causes eccentric loading and lifting up of the opposite, unloaded glenoid rim. (Reprinted with permission from: Matsen FA III, Lippitt SB. Shoulder surgery: principles and procedures. Philadelphia: Saunders; 2004. Principles of glenoid arthroplasty: p. 508.)

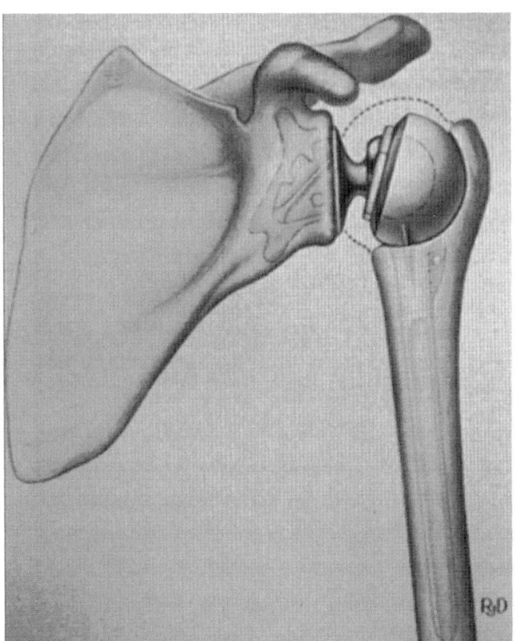

Fig. 22.4 Neer Mark 1 reverse shoulder prosthesis

constrained (fixed-fulcrum) implant was to prevent the need for rotator cuff repair and subsequently to simplify the procedure while maintaining the motion and function needed. Neer ultimately abandoned three iterations of the prosthesis because of unsatisfactory results.

In 1974, Kessel developed his version of the reversed shoulder implant based on the idea that "the scapular bone is unsuitable for holding a prosthesis with acrylic cement" [8, p. 749] (Fig. 22.5). Instead of a cemented keel as in the Neer device, his used a central screw to fix the glenosphere to the scapula, and the humeral component was cemented in. In his study of 23 patients, most of whom were treated for rheumatoid arthritis, there was an overall success rate of 72% [8]. After an average of just more than 3 years of follow-up, he found sufficient justification for continued use of the technique. Unfortunately, his optimism was tempered over the long term by a high failure rate, and the device was removed from the market.

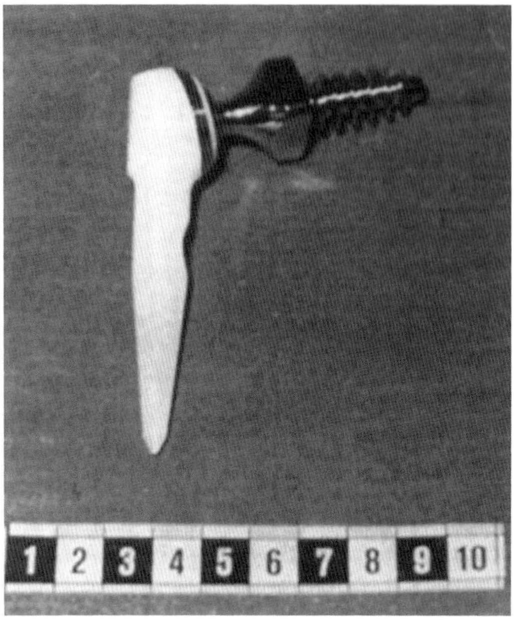

Fig. 22.5 Kessel reverse shoulder prosthesis. This design had a screw in the glenoid component

In 1975, Fenlin released a reverse design that was a fixed-fulcrum system (Fig. 22.6). It was engineered to allow the deltoid to compensate for the deficient rotator cuff, creating a system that was designed for patients with rotator cuff tear arthropathy. Although early results were promising, long-term follow-up identified instability, implant breakage, and loosening of the prosthesis [9]. There were nearly a dozen subsequent designs in which the components were reversed during that period (Table 22.1). Unfortunately, most failed because of being over-constrained, which led to glenoid component failure.

In 1985, Dr. Paul Grammont introduced a prosthesis with a reversed design. This prosthesis fixed a "glenosphere" to the scapular neck replacing the anatomic socket [10]. This system differed from the others in several important ways. The key concepts were that the components must be inherently stable or constrained because of the loss of the rotator cuff; the

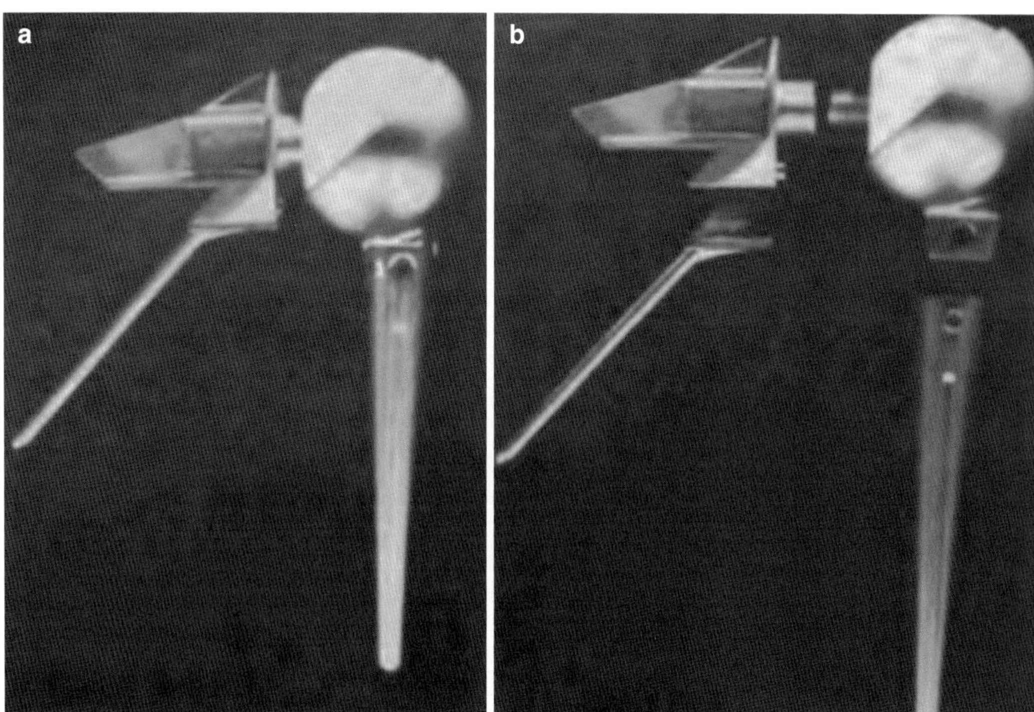

Fig. 22.6 Fenlin reverse shoulder prosthesis designed with a fixed fulcrum system. (**a**) Fully assembled. (**b**) Unassembled components. (Reprinted with permission from: Fenlin JM, Jr. Total glenohumeral joint replacement. Orthop Clin North Am. 1975;6(2):565–83.)

Table 22.1 Reverse shoulder prosthesis designs

Prosthesis	Designer	Year introduced	Key features
Mark 1–3 shoulder	Neer [130]	1970	Constrained component to address rotator cuff deficiency
Leeds shoulder	Reeves et al. [131]	1972	Glenoid component with divergent threaded peg; anatomic COR
Kessel	Brostrom [132]	1973	Single central glenoid screw; lateral COR
Kobel prosthesis	Köbel and Friedebold [133]	1973	Flange bolted glenoid component to scapular spine; designed to allow dislocation at lower forces
Bayley-Walker reverse shoulder	Bayley-Walker [134]	1973	Large hydroxyapatite-coated screw; moved COR distal and medial
Fenlin reverse shoulder	Fenlin [135]	1975	Larger glenosphere to increase deltoid lever arm
Liverpool	Beddow and Elloy [136]	1975	Glenoid component included a stem fixed into the scapular pillar to improve fixation
Floating socket	Buechel et al. [137]	1978	"Floating socket"; smaller glenosphere to increase shoulder motion
Trispherical	Gristina and Webb [138]	1978	Glenosphere and small sphere on the humerus, both articulating in a larger polyethylene cup
Grammont version 1	Grammont et al. [139]	1985	COR medialized but remained lateral to native glenoid surface; glenoid baseplate with press-fit central peg
Delta III	Grammont [140]	1991	COR further medialized to native glenoid face; hydroxyapatite-coated glenoid baseplate to improve fixation
SMR	Randelli [141]	1994	Modular system; metal-backed glenoid
RSP	Frankle [142]	1998	More lateral offset than Delta III
Aequalis	Walch et al. [143]	2002	Lateralized humeral component
Equinoxe	Wright and Zuckerman	2006	Baseplate shifted inferior; lateralized humerus

COR center of rotation, *RSP* reverse shoulder prosthesis

weight-bearing surface (the glenoid) must be convex, whereas the supported part (humeral side) should be concave, providing stability in the presence of altered mechanics; the COR of the joint must be at or within the glenoid neck to decrease the shear forces on the glenoid component; and the COR must be distal and medial to increase the function of the deltoid (Fig. 22.7). This medialization compared with the anatomic COR in a reverse shoulder prostheses was an important step in addressing implant loosening, which was the main cause of failure in earlier designs [11].

The pioneering work of Grammont (Fig. 22.8) and the development of his prosthesis have been key to all subsequent reverse shoulder arthroplasty devices. Grammont proposed two solutions to improve the deltoid muscle vector as an arm elevator when there was an absent rotator cuff. The first was lateralization of the acromion. From comparative anatomic studies, Grammont hypothesized that there was a relationship between the position of the acromion and the function of the rotator cuff. The concept was that a more lateral position of the acromion to the joint's COR would create an increase in the abductor component of the deltoid. This would also lower the ascending force component, the combination of which would facilitate the function of the intact rotator cuff [11].

The second solution to rotator cuff deficiency was Grammont's concept of medialization of the COR of the prosthesis. Following the principles

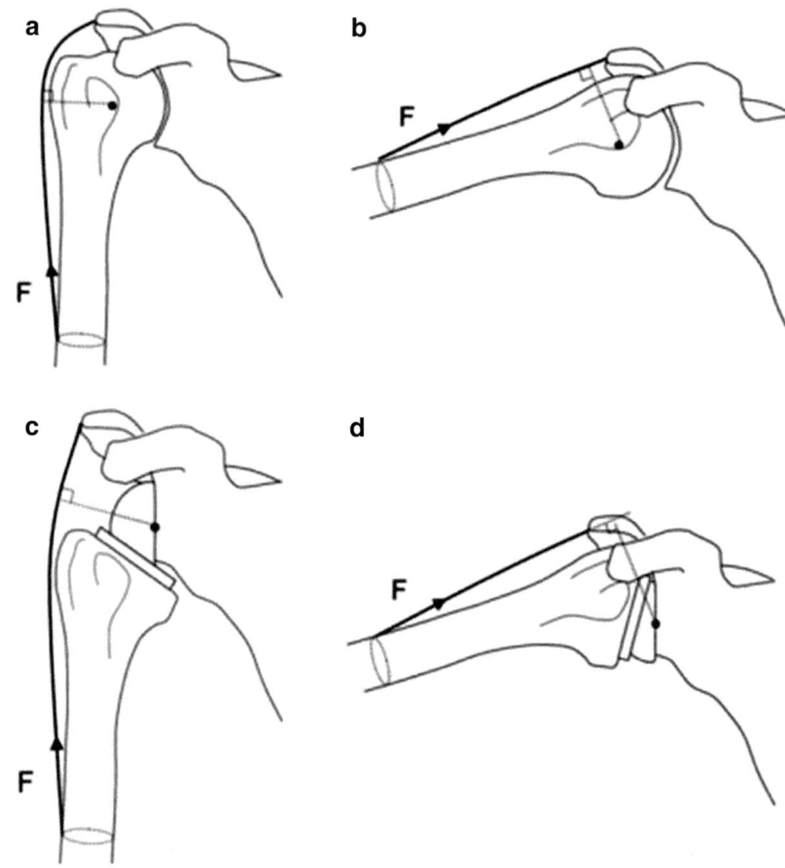

Fig. 22.7 Center of rotation and position of the humerus and the deltoid muscle with the arm at the side (**a**) and in abduction (**b**) in normal shoulder anatomy. (**c** and **d**) Reverse total shoulder arthroplasty medializes the center of rotation, distalizes the humerus, and elongates the deltoid. The lever arm of the deltoid muscle (*dotted line*) is lengthened so that for any given angular displacement of the humerus, shortening of the deltoid is greater than in total shoulder arthroplasty (F indicates force). (Reprinted with permission from: Gerber C, Pennington SD, Nyffeler RW. Reverse total shoulder arthroplasty. J Am Acad Orthop Surg. 2009 May;17(5):284–95.)

of hip arthroplasty, first it was attempted to medialize the prosthetic head relative to the diaphyseal axis. This prosthesis had a small head attached to a neck component that was inserted into the humerus. He soon realized that using a constrained prosthesis was impractical because of the high shear forces placed on the construct. The initial version of the Grammont prosthesis was called the Ovoide prosthesis and was the first step toward a "nonanatomic" solution for rotator cuff–deficient shoulders [11].

Grammont hypothesized that medialization of the COR leads to more concentric forces at the prosthesis-bone junction in the early degrees of elevation. This was expected to decrease the shear forces at the baseplate and glenoid-bone interface, thereby preventing baseplate failure, which had hampered previous designs of the reverse prosthesis.

The power exerted by the deltoid is increased by the restoration of muscle tension. This can be accomplished by bringing the humerus more inferior. By increasing the power of the deltoid, the incompetent rotator cuff is addressed allowing for more range of motion of the upper extremity.

The Grammont prosthesis continued to evolve until it was approved for use in Europe in 1991 (Fig. 22.9). Grammont died in March 2013 after contributing numerous advances in the field of orthopaedics.

Biomechanics

The glenoid offset is the distance between the base of the coracoid and the deepest portion of the glenoid articular surface. This offset sets the

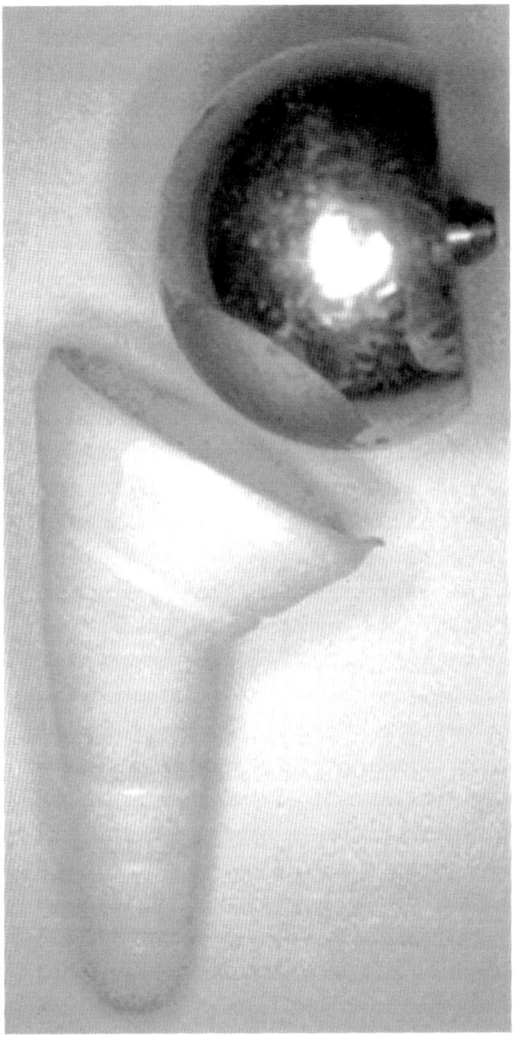

Fig. 22.8 Original Grammont reverse shoulder prosthesis. The glenosphere has no neck and is attached directly to the glenoid bone. This effectively shifts the center of rotation to the bone/implant interface. (Reprinted with permission from: Boileau P, Watkinson DJ, Hatzidakis AM, Balg F. Grammont reverse prosthesis: design, rationale, and biomechanics. J. Shoulder Elb Surg. 2005; 14(1):147S–161S.)

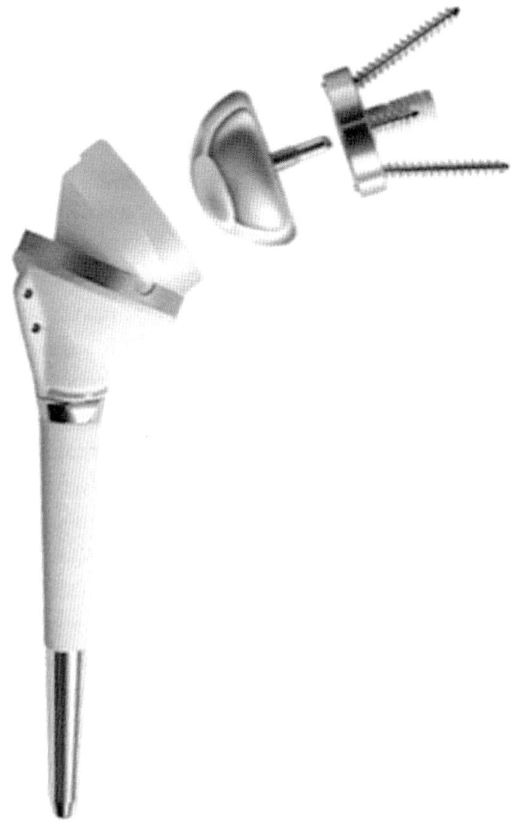

Fig. 22.9 Modern Delta III reverse shoulder prosthesis. (Reprinted with permission from: Boileau P, Watkinson DJ, Hatzidakis AM, Balg F. Grammont reverse prosthesis: design, rationale, and biomechanics. J Shoulder Elb Surg. 2005;14(1):147S–161S.)

location of the glenohumeral joint line and is not related to the size of the patient. The resting tension of the rotator cuff, as well as the moment arm of the deltoid, is set by the lateral glenohumeral offset, the distance between the base of the coracoid, and the most lateral aspect of the greater tuberosity [12]. The reverse shoulder prosthesis medializes this COR. The extent to which this medialization occurs depends on the prosthesis being used. This results in decreased shear forces and forces that are more compressive in nature.

Articular Geometry of the Glenohumeral Joint

When considering a reverse shoulder prosthesis, "medialized" and "lateralized" components are relative terms. Both types of implant move the COR medial to the anatomic location; one is just less medial.

There are benefits to both designs. With medialized implants, the COR is at the glenoid component–bone interface. This places less shear stress at the glenoid bone–prosthesis interface. However, there is encroachment on the glenoid, less mechanical advantage, and laxity of the remaining cuff. Lateralized implants address the issues associated with medialized components but result in more force across the glenoid bone–implant interface.

With medial encroachment, the risk of scapular notching is increased. Sirveaux first described scapular notching in 1997 [13, 14]. Notching is a divot in the scapular neck attributed to the impact of the medial border of the humeral prosthesis against the upper portion of the scapular pillar when the arm is brought into an adducted position. It has also been suggested that polyethylene wear particles can contribute to the progression of notching. Implants with a more lateral COR offset have been shown to reduce scapular notching [15].

Humeral Neck Shaft Angle

The humeral neck shaft angle (Figs. 22.10 and 22.11) is the angle between the central intramedullary axis of the humeral shaft and the anatomical neck of the humerus. The mean neck shaft angle is 40° but variation occurs between individuals, ranging from 30 to 55° [16]. The humeral component of a reverse prosthesis has a nonanatomical orientation with neck shaft angles ranging from 125 to 155°. The design of the prosthesis

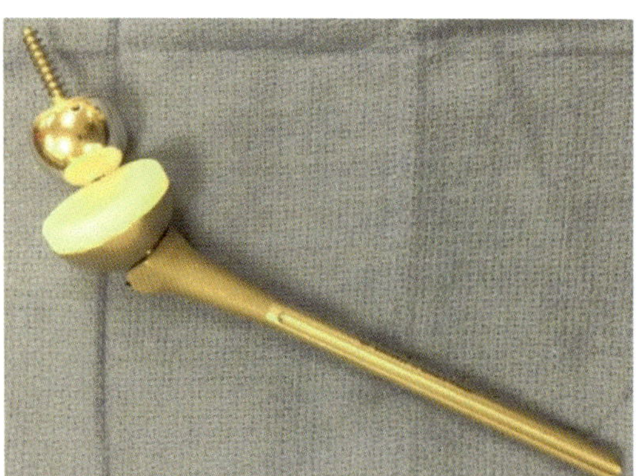

Fig. 22.10 Reverse shoulder prosthesis showing a 135-degree neck shaft angle

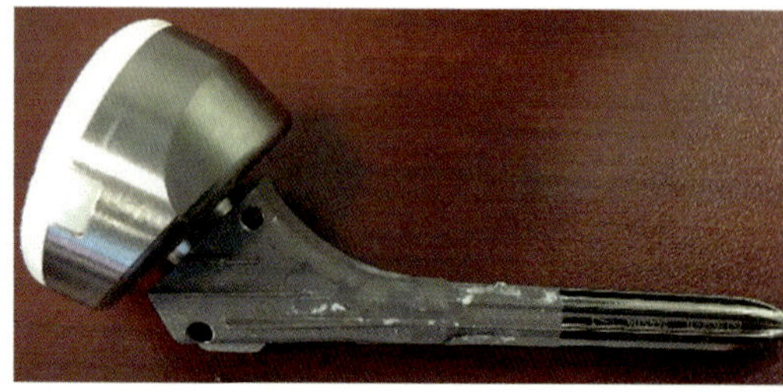

Fig. 22.11 Modern reverse shoulder prosthesis with a 150-degree neck shaft angle

can alter the mechanics. Implants with a more horizontal neck shaft angle have been shown to reduce scapular notching [15]. Decreasing the neck shaft angle has also been shown to reduce the contact area of the glenosphere, which in turn, increases the contact stress [17]. This suggests that although decreasing the neck shaft angle can increase the impingement-free range of motion, it can also increase contact stress, which can potentiate wear.

Humeral Component Positioning

The native humeral head is retroverted approximately 30° (range, −8 to 46°) relative to the shaft of the humerus [18]. Implant position varies from neutral to 30° of retroversion for the humeral component. The position of the humeral and glenoid components affects the overall range of motion, and it can also affect the resting position of the extremity. This contributes to the stability of the implant. There is evidence that neutral version provides better outcomes in activities of daily life, Constant-Murley scores, strength, and radiographic loosening. When evaluating the adduction deficit, 10° of retroversion has been associated with increased deficit [19]. New evidence points to a lower neck shaft angle increasing abduction motion with increased retroversion, resulting in loss of internal rotation up the back [20].

Humeral offset (Fig. 22.12) is also a system-specific characteristic that can alter range of motion and impingement [21]. There are advantages and disadvantages to any alteration. By increasing the humeral offset, abduction can be

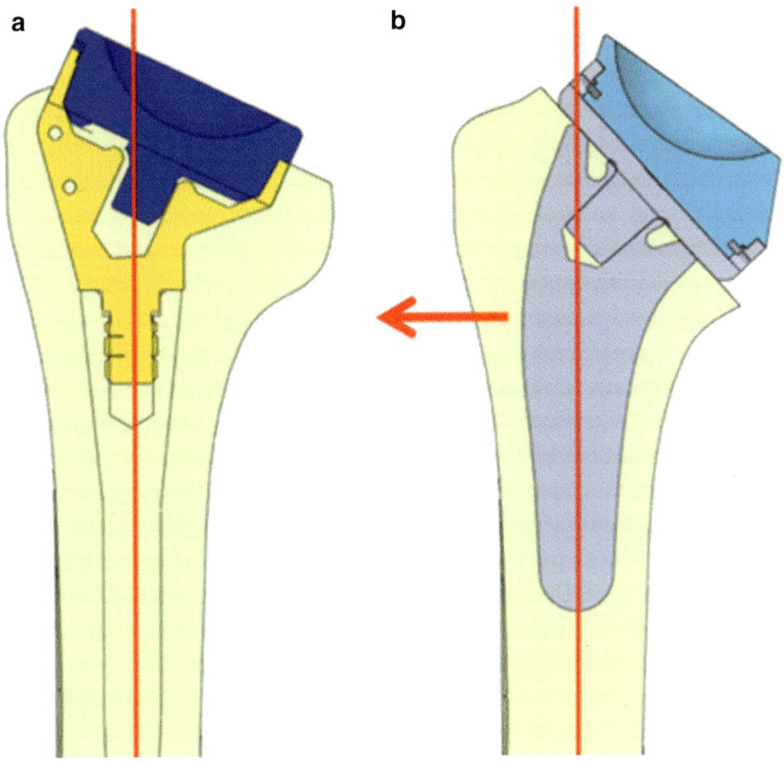

Fig. 22.12 (**a**) Traditional inlay Grammont reverse shoulder prosthesis with a straight stem. (**b**) Example of a new design with a curved stem and an onlay humeral tray. The *red* line passes through the center of the stem. Note that the center of the polyethylene is more medial with the curved stem, which results in lateralization of the humerus (*red arrow*). (Reprinted with permission from: Ladermann A, Denard PJ, Boileau P, Farron A, Deransart P, Terrier A, Ston J, Walch G. Effect of humeral stem design on humeral position and range of motion in reverse shoulder arthroplasty. Int Orthop. 2015;39(11):2205–13.)

decreased with a subsequent increase in external rotation, extension, and adduction.

Positioning of the Metaglene/ Glenosphere

It is accepted that superior tilt of the glenosphere is deleterious because it increases shear forces between the baseplate and the bone, which can lead to early failure [22]. When comparing 15°, neutral, and −15° of glenoid tilt in a laboratory environment, inferior tilt was associated with decreased overall magnitude of force, more evenly distributed force at the baseplate, and decreased micromotion [23]. However, it has not been proven that tilting the glenoid baseplate 10° inferiorly, as recommended by some researchers, decreases the incidence or severity of scapular notching [15].

Guitierrez et al. [24] proposed several factors that can be altered to minimize scapular impingement and increase range of motion of a reverse shoulder. Lateral offset of the implant influenced impingement-free range of motion the most. Inferior positioning of the glenoid was the second most influential factor with respect to increasing range of motion. Inferior glenoid tilt was also found to increase range of motion. The angle at which scapular impingement occurs is called the adduction deficit. When the humeral neck shaft angle is increased from 130 to 155° (more vertical), abduction motion increases but the adduction deficit also increases. When

Guitierrez et al. evaluated factors that increased the adduction deficit, the primary factor was increasing the humeral neck shaft angle. In decreasing order of magnitude, the factors leading to increased adduction deficit were superior positioning of the glenosphere, superior tilting of the glenosphere, and decreased lateral offset of the COR.

One study [25] reported no difference when comparing inferior tilt of the baseplate to a neutral position, whereas another study [26] suggested that greater inferior tilt increased the incidence of notching.

Kelly et al. [27] and Poon et al. [28] have suggested that placing the glenoid baseplate inferiorly on the glenoid vault can reduce impingement and therefore decrease notching. Kowalsky et al. [29] compared glenoid component position below versus at the glenoid rim. They found lower incidence and less severe notching in those with the implant below the glenoid rim, but the difference was not statistically significant. Care must be taken when positioning the baseplate to ensure that the inferior screw has adequate purchase and is not compromised by positioning the component too inferior.

Glenoid Design

Fixation of the glenoid implant relies on various factors. Preservation of bone stock through precise reaming is important. Reduction of micromotion through secure initial screw fixation, maximization of bone-implant contact, and ultimately, bone ingrowth can help prevent glenoid loosening. A study comparing two baseplate designs (curved versus flat-backed) showed that using a curved baseplate can increase the contact area between the implant and bone. However, this can increase the amount of bone removed and decrease screw fixation. When adequate contact between the implant and bone cannot be obtained, a flat-back baseplate can provide better screw engagement [30].

Another consideration in the design of a reverse shoulder prosthesis is the size and shape of the glenosphere. Although the size of the glenosphere has not been shown to increase stability or have as major an impact on range of motion as other factors previously discussed, there are several important factors to consider regarding how the size and shape affects the biomechanical and clinical performance of reverse prostheses. Glenospheres come in multiple sizes and may be eccentric or concentric (Fig. 22.13). In theory, a larger glenosphere gives more excursion for the socket around the sphere. This increases impingement-free range of motion, which should decrease notching. Increasing the size of the glenosphere can increase the contact area with the humeral component but only minimally affects the contact stress [17]. Increasing the diameter has been shown to increase joint load and deltoid force; however, the clinical implications of this are unknown [31]. Use of a concentric (versus eccentric) glenosphere has also been an area of interest. Eccentric glenospheres are intended to decrease the incidence of scapular notching by moving the COR more inferior compared with concentric glenospheres [32]. There has been no definitive evidence that one size or shape of glenosphere is significantly better than any other in terms of function or long-term clinical success.

Finally, there is evidence that lateralizing the COR can lower the incidence of scapular notching (Figs. 22.14 and 22.15) [33]. The tradeoff is the potential increase of shear forces at the glenoid bone–component interface.

Indications for RTSA

Initially, the main indication for reverse total shoulder arthroplasty (RTSA) was cuff tear arthropathy (Fig. 22.16). The prosthesis was designed to restore the biomechanical COR and allow the deltoid muscle vector to abduct the

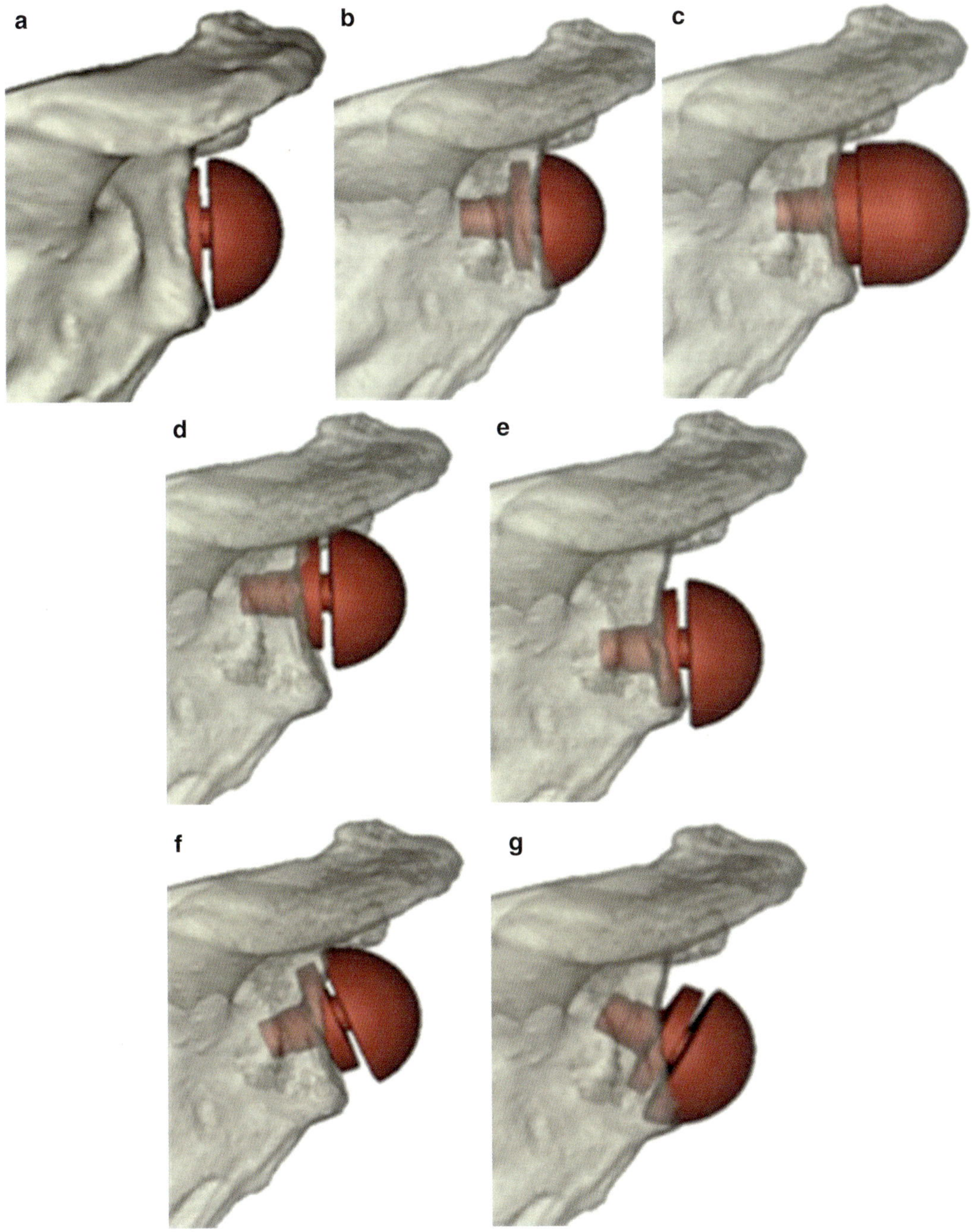

Fig. 22.13 Baseplate/glenosphere positioning. (**a**) Neutral position, (**b**) medialized position, (**c**) lateralized position, (**d**) superior translation, (**e**) inferior translation, (**f**) superior tilt, and (**g**) inferior tilt. (Reprinted with permission from: Li X, et al. Effects of glenosphere positioning on impingement-free internal and external rotation after reverse total shoulder arthroplasty. J Shoulder Elb Surg. 2013;22(6):807–13.)

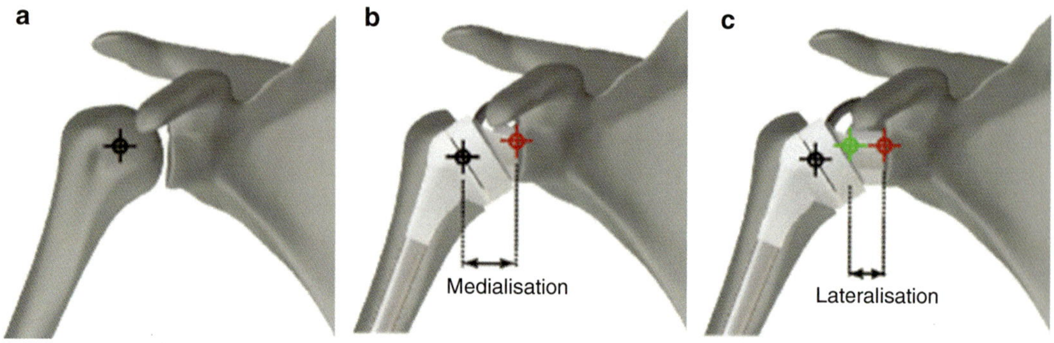

Fig. 22.14 Diagram illustrating joint center of rotation location for the anatomical shoulder (**a**), reverse shoulder (**b**), and reverse shoulder with a lateral-offset glenoid component (**c**). Medialization after reverse total shoulder arthroplasty is shown, as well as lateralization caused by a lateral-offset glenoid component. *Black*, *red*, and *green* bull's-eyes indicate joint center of rotation position for the anatomical shoulder, reverse shoulder, and reverse shoulder with a lateral-offset glenoid component, respectively. (Reprinted with permission from: Ackland DC, Patel M, Knox D. Prosthesis design and placement in reverse total shoulder arthroplasty. 2015;10(101). Open access through Creative Commons license)

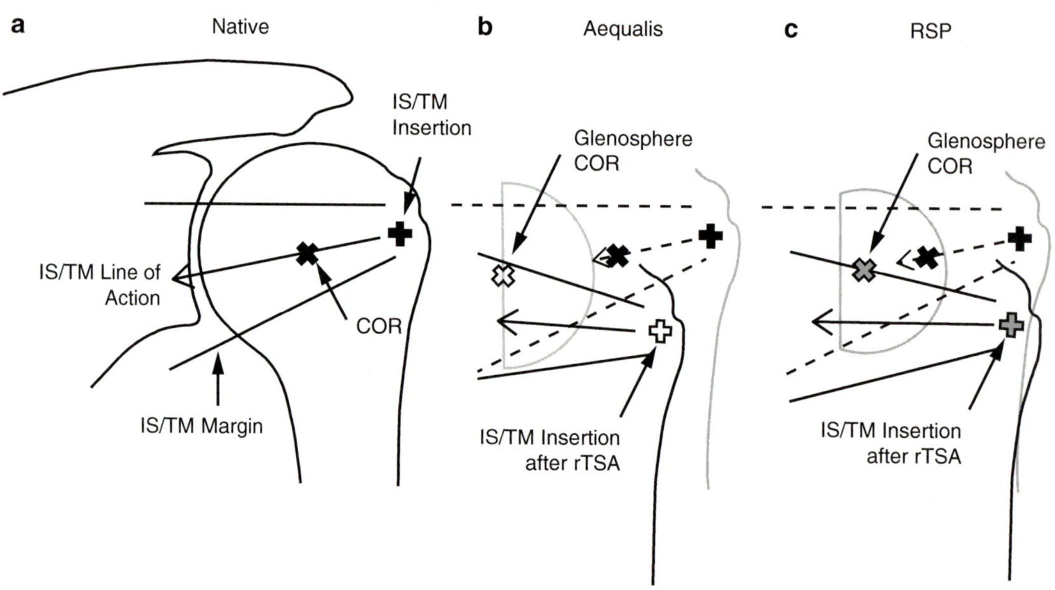

Fig. 22.15 Schematic of humeral position before and after reverse total shoulder arthroplasty (rTSA). (**a**) In native arms, the midline of the infraspinatus/teres minor (IS/TM) line of action passes through the joint center of rotation (COR), shown as the bisector of the IS/TM margins. (**b**) With the Aequalis (Tornier, France), the IS/TM line of action passes below the COR, and the IS/TM is shortened when the humerus is shifted inferior and medial, respectively. (**c**) With the Reverse Shoulder Prosthesis (RSP) (DJO, Texas), the line of action passes below the joint COR because of inferior humeral shift, but nearly anatomic IS/TM length is likely to be maintained because the humerus does not translate significantly medial to the native after rTSA. (Reprinted with permission from: Henninger HB, King FK, Tashjian RZ, Burks RT. Biomechanical comparison of reverse total shoulder arthroplasty systems in soft tissue-constrained shoulders. 2013;23(5):e108–117.)

arm, thereby eliminating superior subluxation, which impairs the patient's ability to lift the arm. Because failure rates of the early designs were high, there was initial caution in the use of RTSA for other indications. However, with further research and changes in RTSA design, the clinical results improved enough to allow expansion for a much wider spectrum of shoulder disorders and conditions previously not treated successfully with anatomical shoulder arthroplasty.

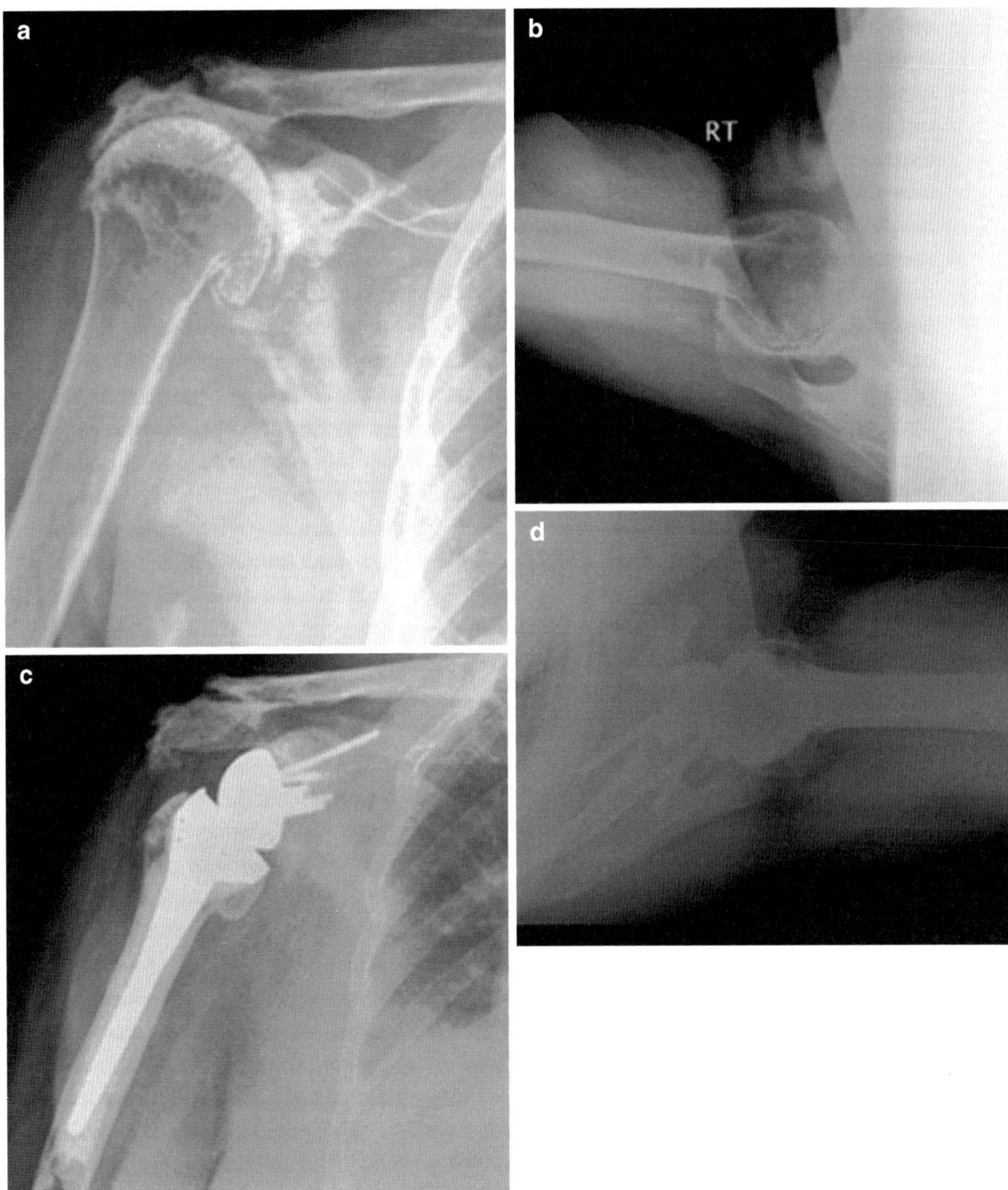

Fig. 22.16 (**a**) Anteroposterior and (**b**) axillary preoperative radiographs showing cuff-tear arthropathy. Note the characteristic radiographic findings, including joint space narrowing, diminished acromiohumeral interval, acetabulization of the undersurface of the acromion, and a femoralized and subacromial position of the humeral head. (**c**) Anteroposterior and (**d**) axillary postoperative radiographs

Disorders successfully treated with RTSA include conditions that, when treated with anatomic total shoulder arthroplasty, have been associated with poor outcomes. These conditions include shoulders with failed previous rotator cuff or arthroplasty surgery. The primary indications are cuff tear arthropathy, failed rotator cuff repair, osteoarthritis with rotator cuff tears, osteoarthritis with severe glenoid bone loss, pseudoparalysis without arthritis, immunological arthritis such as rheumatoid arthritis, dislocation arthropathy, chronic fixed shoulder dislocations, shoulder dysplasias, acute proximal humerus fractures, malunited proximal humerus fractures, bone tumors, and primary shoulder infections. For failed arthroplasty, RTSA can effectively treat failed proximal humeral head replacements, including failed hemiarthroplasty, cup arthroplasty, and head cap replacements. RTSA has also been effective for failed TSA, including failed RTSA.

All of these conditions have in common one or more combinations of rotator cuff deficiency and glenoid bone loss. The assumption in some cases is that RTSA should be performed to preempt complications of anatomical shoulder arthroplasty. However, results are mixed regarding this assumption, and further research is needed to determine which type of implant is best for which indication. For example, RTSA has been successful for patients with cuff tear arthropathy (for which anatomical TSA is not predictably successful), whereas patients with osteoarthritis and rotator cuff tears have been successfully treated with anatomical TSA [34]. Although RTSA might prevent future complications in patients with osteoarthritis and cuff tears, no studies have compared these two treatments over the long term.

Similarly, when the indication for RTSA is glenoid bone loss, the extent of bone loss that is better treated with RTSA than anatomical TSA is poorly defined. Studies have shown that lower levels of glenoid bone loss (e.g., Walch types A1 and B1) can be treated successfully with anatomical TSA [35–37], but for higher grades of glenoid bone loss (e.g., Walch types A2, B2, and C) the best treatment is unclear. Similarly, there have been no direct comparisons of the performance of anatomical TSA versus RTSA when the glenoid must be bone grafted for implant stability. Further study and longer-term follow-up will allow clinicians to make decisions based on well-defined criteria about the use of RTSA in patients with severe glenoid bone loss.

Patient Evaluation

Patients undergoing RTSA should be approached similarly to any patient considering treatment options for painful or debilitating shoulder conditions. Because many patients have complex histories, a careful and complete history should be obtained (Chap. 10). This should include how the pain began, including traumatic or atraumatic causes. Signs of neurological involvement should be ascertained such as paresthesias or upper extremity weakness. Painless weakness with no trauma should be considered a neurological condition until proven otherwise. We have seen several patients with shoulder replacements for cuff tears and no arthritis who had amyotrophic neuropathy because no clinician had taken a complete history or performed a thorough examination. Cervical spondylolysis should be considered if there is bilateral weakness, pain, and paresthesias. In patients with previous surgery, it is important to determine why the surgery might have failed, and any previous wound drainage or swelling should be ascertained. Lastly, patients with a painful arthroplasty should be considered infected until proven otherwise.

The thorough examination of the shoulder should include observation, range-of-motion testing, strength testing, palpation, and assessment of the rotator cuff. The posterior thorax should be evaluated for atrophy of the musculature and winging of the scapula. Because of stiffness of the glenohumeral joint, many patients compensate with more motion of the scapular-thoracic articulation; this represents a form of scapular dyskinesis and does not reflect true winging. The deltoid muscle should be evaluated specifically for atrophy or detachment from previous surgery. The rotator cuff should be tested using strength testing but also with lag signs (Chap. 10).

One factor found to influence the success of RTSA is the status of the shoulder external rotators, including the infraspinatus and teres minor tendons [14]. If a patient has weakness in external rotation with the arm at the side, then the supraspinatus and perhaps the infraspinatus maybe be torn or weak. If the patient has a positive external rotation lag sign with the arm at the side, then the patient most likely has torn the supraspinatus, infraspinatus, and teres minor [38]. If the patient has a positive "dropping sign," which is a lag sign performed with the arm abducted to 90° and externally rotated to 90°, then all of the external rotators are torn. These are important findings because the loss of these tendons makes the arm fall into internal rotation, which is called a "hornblower's sign." If a patient has these findings, the patient will have difficulty reaching full elevation and with reaching the mouth in some instances. RTSA alone will not compensate for these deficiencies, and if patients expect these deficits to be solved, they will likely be disappointed [39]. The use of latissimus dorsi transfer with or without the teres major at the time of RTSA to restore external rotation has been reported [40–43] with favorable results [40, 42, 43]. However, this procedure adds a level of complexity to the operation and prolongs recovery.

The workup for a patient considering RTSA should include plain radiographs of the shoulder, including Grashey [44, 45] and axillary views. If the patient cannot tolerate positioning for an axillary view, a computed tomography (CT) scan of the shoulder should be obtained to determine the humeral head relationship to the glenoid and the amount of glenoid bone loss.

In patients undergoing RTSA, the routine use of CT scanning remains controversial. If a high-quality axillary radiograph shows little bone loss, then CT scanning is probably not necessary. Some surgeons recommend a CT scan in all patients, and some decide whether to obtain a CT scan on the basis of the axillary radiograph quality. The use of 3-dimensional CT scanning has been advocated by some surgeons [46]. The use of scapular models made from the CT scans has been used by some surgeons to assist in assessing glenoid morphology and bone loss (Fig. 22.17).

Patients with previous surgery, including open reduction and fixation for proximal humerus fractures and patients with any form of previous arthroplasty should be evaluated for infection. The major symptom of infected hardware is the presence of pain, but because pain can have many causes such as implant loosening, infection should be ruled out. The basic workup for infection should include blood tests for C-reactive protein and sedimentation rate and aspiration of the shoulder. A reliable and accurate test to diagnose infection has not been established. Although it is beyond the scope of this chapter, the future of detecting infection may involve additional immunological markers from blood or joint aspiration fluid testing [47, 48].

Cuff Tear Arthropathy

Cuff tear arthropathy typically is defined as arthritis caused by abnormal biomechanics of the rotator cuff–deficient shoulder [49]. Because of the lack of a supraspinatus and often other rotator cuff tendons, the glenohumeral joint is subject to abnormal forces that lead to cartilage wear. This wear pattern can be highly variable, and the variations were classified by Hamada et al. [6]. According to this system, grade 1 shows minimal radiographic changes; grade 2 shows narrowing of the subacromial space to less than 5 mm; grade 3 shows erosion or "acetabulization" of the acromion; grade 4 is associated with glenohumeral arthritis; and grade 5 is associated with humeral head osteonecrosis. Grade 4 is subdivided into two groups: grade 4A is without acetabulization, and grade 4B is associated with humeral head avascular necrosis. In this condition, as the space between the acromion and the tuberosity becomes narrower (by superior migration of the head because of a rotator cuff tear), the greater tuberosity and the acromion become worn. Eventually, wear of the greater tuberosity on the undersurface of the acromion leads to its

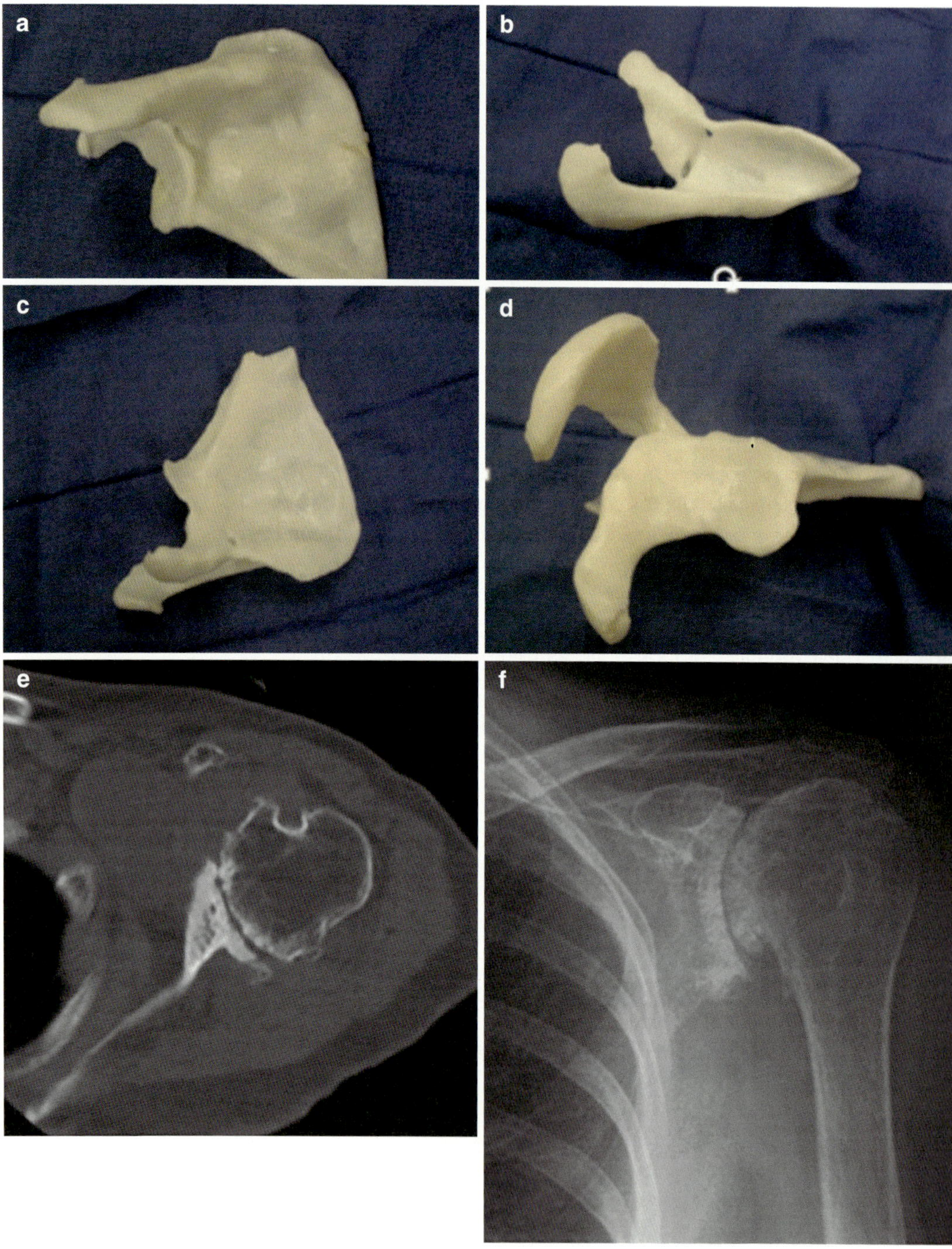

Fig. 22.17 Three-dimensional model in (**a**) posterior view, (**b**) superior view, (**c**) anterior view, and (**d**) enface view. (**e**) CT scan and (**f**) anteroposterior radiograph of a patient with glenoid bone loss

acetabulization, and the humeral head takes on an "ice cream cone" appearance (Fig. 22.16). In its extreme form, the humeral head can migrate superiorly and medially, eroding the acromion to the point that it fractures, and wearing away the acromioclavicular joint. This degree of superior migration can make successful RTSA difficult because a stable acromion is needed for the deltoid muscle to function properly. Also, the degree of bone loss of the glenoid can affect the amount of bone available for secure placement of the RTSA baseplate.

Generally, the results of RTSA for cuff tear arthropathy have been good, and they serve as the benchmark for other indications for RTSA (Tables 22.2 and 22.3). The reasons for this success are that RTSA relieves pain and restores the deltoid vector to allow the arm to elevate above shoulder level. Wall et al. [50] reviewed the results of RTSA performed for various diagnoses and found that the best results were in patients with cuff tear arthropathy, osteoarthritis with a cuff tear, and massive rotator cuff tears without arthritis.

Failed Previous Rotator Cuff Surgery

These patients are similar in presentation and required treatment to patients with rotator cuff tear arthropathy (Fig. 22.18). Both groups have torn rotator cuff tendons and various degrees of glenoid bone loss. The major difference between these two groups is that patients with previous surgery may have failed labrum lesions, failed hardware, more scar formation, or even the

Table 22.2 Results of RTSA in patients with rotator cuff tear arthropathy

Study	No. of patients	Mean age, years	Mean (range) follow-up, months	CM score		ASES score		Complication rate, %	Reoperation rate, %
				Initial	Final	Initial	Final		
Boulahia et al. [144]	16	72	35 (24–65)	22	59	NR	NR	25	12
Sirveaux et al. [14]	74	73	44 (24–97)	23	66	NR	NR	NR	NR
Werner et al. [65]	17	68	38 (min 24)	35%[a]	72%[a]			53	18
Frankle et al. [142]	60	71	33 (24–68)	NR	NR	34	68	22	13
Seebauer et al. [145]	57	70	18 (3–44)	NR	67	NR	NR	9	NR
Boileau et al. [101]	21	77	40 (24–72)	18	66	NR	76	19	5
Wall et al. [50]	59	73	40 (24–86)	22	65	NR	NR	NR	NR
Cuff et al. [97]	94	72	28 (24–88)	NR	NR	30	86	9.5	5
Cuff et al. [146]	74	70	62 (60–79)	NR	NR	32	75	13.5	NR

ASES American Shoulder and Elbow Surgeons, *CM* Constant-Murley, *min* minimum, *NR* not reported
[a]Relative Constant-Murley score

Table 22.3 Range of motion before and after RTSA

Study	Active elevation		Active abduction		Active external rotation, arm at side		Active external rotation with 90° abduction		Active external rotation	
	Initial	Final	Initial	Final	Initial	Final	Initial	Final	Initial	Final
Boulahia et al. [144]	70	138	NR	NR	6	3	NR	NR	NR	NR
Sirveaux et al. [14]	73	138	NR	NR	3.5	11	17	40	NR	NR
Werner et al. [65]	43	103	39	84	NR	NR	NR	NR	NR	NR
Frankle et al. [142]	55	105	41	102	NR	NR	NR	NR	12	41
Seebauer et al. [145]	NR	145	NR	140	NR	NR	NR	NR	NR	NR
Boileau et al. [101]	53	123	NR	NR	NR	NR	NR	NR	9	14
Wall et al. [50]	76	142	NR	NR	5	7	29	43	NR	NR
Cuff et al. [97]	74	130	70	123	NR	NR	NR	NR	20	36
Cuff et al. [146]	64	118	61	110	NR	NR	NR	NR	15	28

NR not reported

presence of an occult infection. Previous surgery can affect the results of RTSA in rotator cuff arthropathy patients. Boileau et al. [51] compared a group of patients who underwent RTSA for cuff tear arthropathy with a group who had failed previous rotator cuff surgery. They found that the group with no previous surgery had better Constant-Murley scores and range of motion

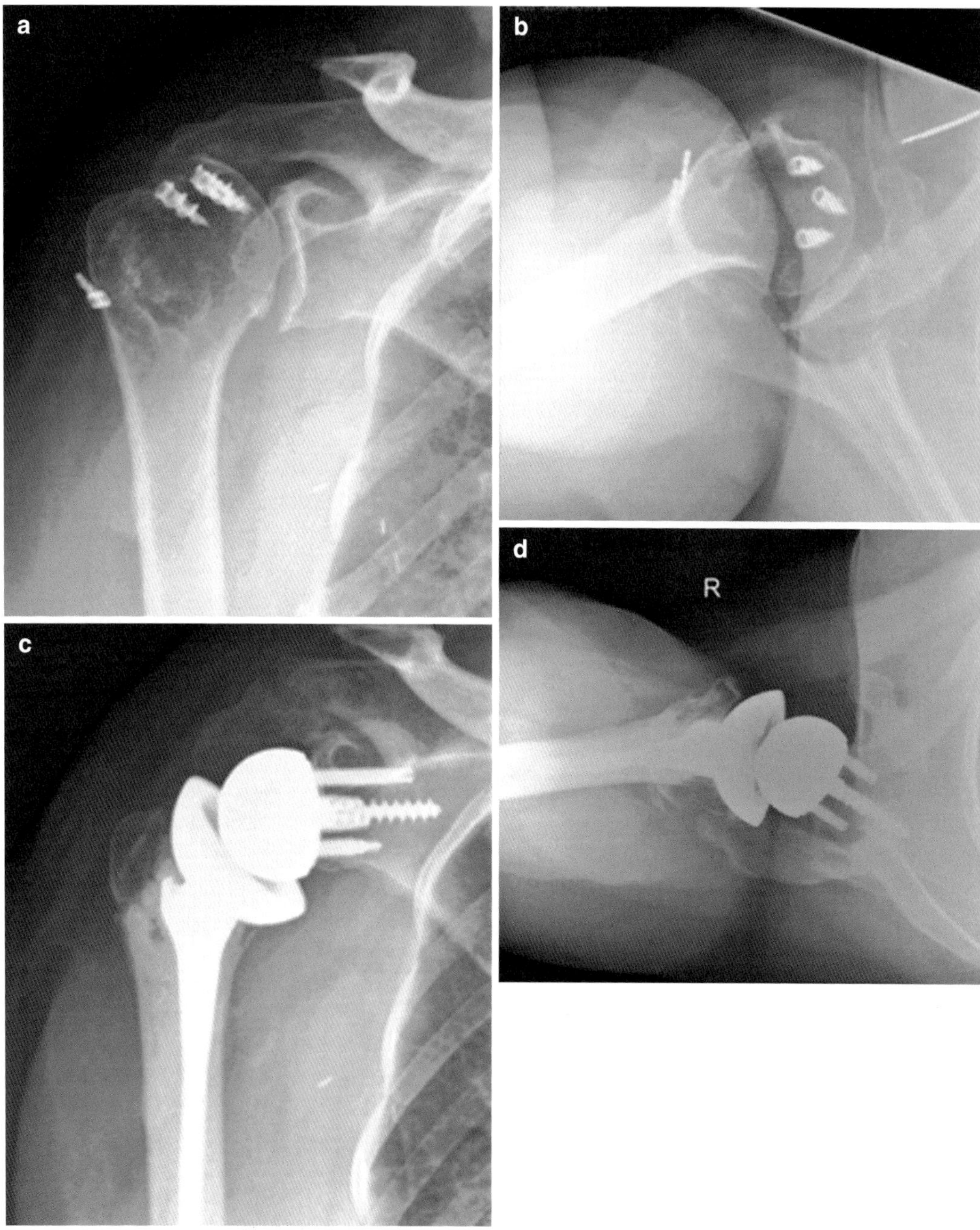

Fig. 22.18 (**a**) Anteroposterior and (**b**) axillary radiographs of a patient with failed rotator cuff repair and radiographic changes associated with cuff-tear arthropathy. (**c**) Anteroposterior and (**d**) axillary radiographs after the patient underwent reverse total shoulder arthroplasty

than the group with previous surgery. They speculated that the previous surgery was responsible for more postoperative scar tissue, and they concluded that previous rotator cuff repair surgery was a relative contraindication for RTSA.

Osteoarthritis with Cuff Tears

Another group of patients who may benefit from RTSA is those with osteoarthritis and concomitant rotator cuff tears (Fig. 22.19). Studies of the results of anatomical TSA in this patient population have shown excellent results [52, 53]. These studies suggest that small tears can be repaired or ignored when performing anatomical TSA, but the follow-up in both studies was short.

As the natural history of rotator cuff tears becomes better understood, there is increasing concern that, over time, rotator cuff tears become larger and result in glenoid component loosening or superior escape of the humeral implant. Because no studies have compared the use of RTSA with anatomical TSA in this population, no definitive conclusions can be made about the size of the tear or the physical findings that can guide treatment. In some cases, such as in patients older than 75 years who are unhealthy and can tolerate only one operation, RTSA might be a better choice if future cuff tearing is a concern. Wall et al. [50] reported that patients with primary osteoarthritis and rotator cuff tears treated with RTSA had results as good as those in patients who underwent RTSA for cuff tear arthropathy.

Osteoarthritis with Bone Loss

The rationale for RTSA in patients with no rotator cuff tear and severe bone loss (Fig. 22.20) is primarily to avoid the high failure rate associated with bone grafting of the glenoid. The options for treating glenoid bone loss in this population are (1) hemiarthroplasty or cup arthroplasty with or without "ream and run," (2) anatomical TSA with reaming the glenoid only, (3) augmented glenoid components, (4) bone grafting of the glenoid with anatomical TSA, and (5) RTSA with or without bone grafting. For anatomical TSA bone grafting, biomechanical studies [54–56] indicate that glenoid component fixation decreases when placed into a glenoid with more than 15° of retroversion [57]. Similarly, retroversion of the glenoid more than 25° (a Walch type C or "dysplastic" glenoid) would typically require bone grafting for a standard anatomical TSA. Although they have been used successfully in type C glenoids, augmented glenoid components have not been studied long enough to make definitive conclusions about their effectiveness for these glenoids [58].

Another option is to bone graft the glenoid and place an anatomical TSA. Unfortunately, the failure rates with this approach can be high. Walch et al. [59] reported using glenoid bone grafting and anatomical TSA in patients with osteoarthritis and biconcave glenoids. They subsequently had to revise 16% (15/92) of the patients, and another 21% (19/92) had glenoid component loosening. Hill and Norris [60] used bone grafting during anatomical TSA to compensate for glenoid defiency. In their cohort, 30% (5/17) had to be revised, some as early as 2 years postoperatively.

The results of RTSA in patients with intact rotator cuffs and severe glenoid bone loss have been encouraging. Mizuno et al. [61] reported on 27 shoulders with Walch type B2 glenoids, 17 of which were treated without bone grafting and ten with bone grafting. They reported excellent clinical outcomes with significant improvement in Constant-Murley scores and shoulder range of motion. A similar study by Steen et al. [62] compared patients with glenoid bone loss who underwent RTSA with patients who underwent anatomical TSA. Their results were similar for RTSA and TSA without bone grafting for patients with intact rotator cuffs and type A2, B2, or C glenoids. McFarland et al. [63] used RTSA without bone grafting in 34 patients with type A2, B2, or C glenoids. There was only one baseplate failure (2%) at a minimum follow-up of 2 years.

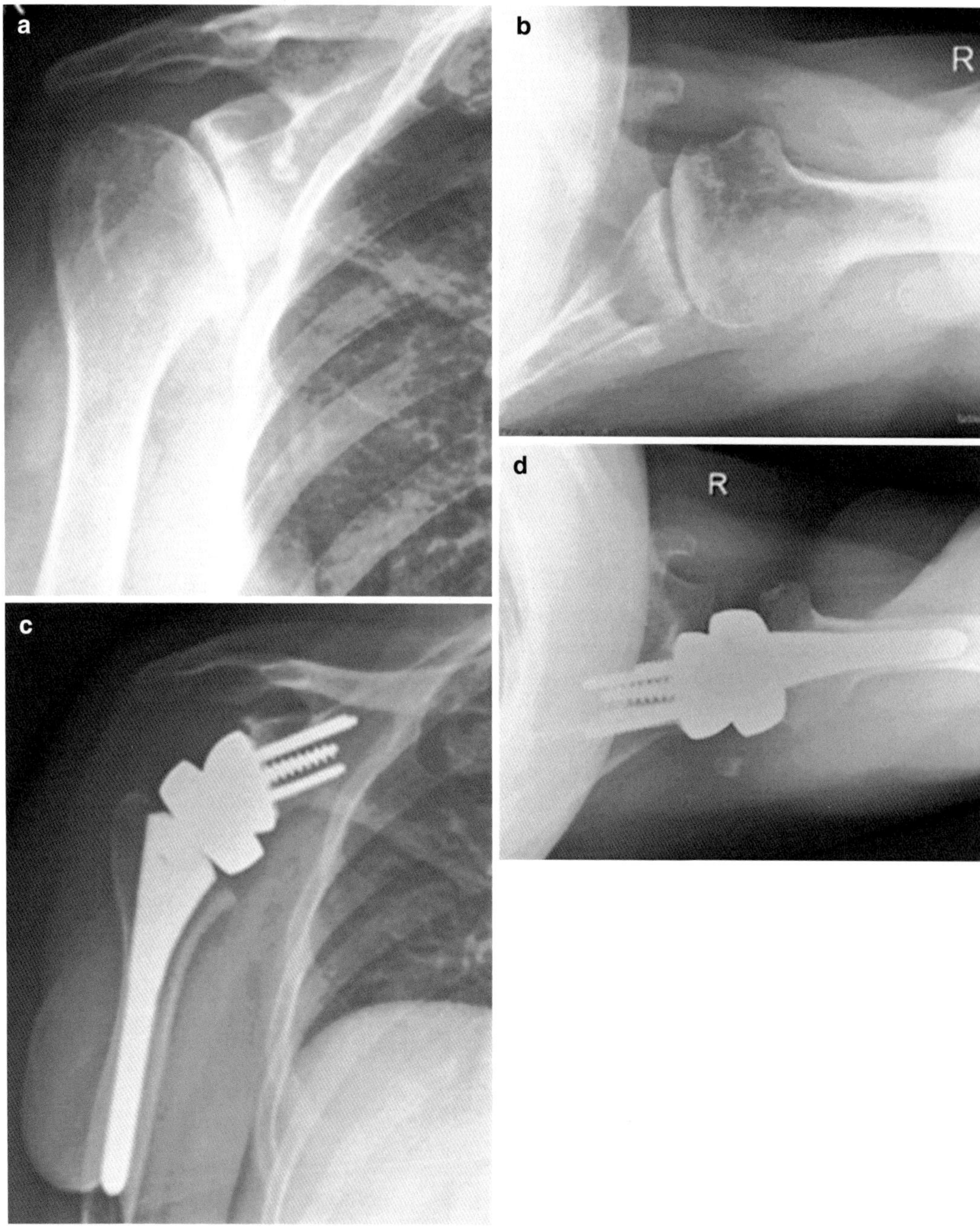

Fig. 22.19 Preoperative (**a**) anteroposterior and (**b**) axillary radiographs of a patient with shoulder osteoarthritis with rotator cuff tear. Postoperative (**c**) anteroposterior and (**d**) axillary radiographs after reverse total shoulder arthroplasty

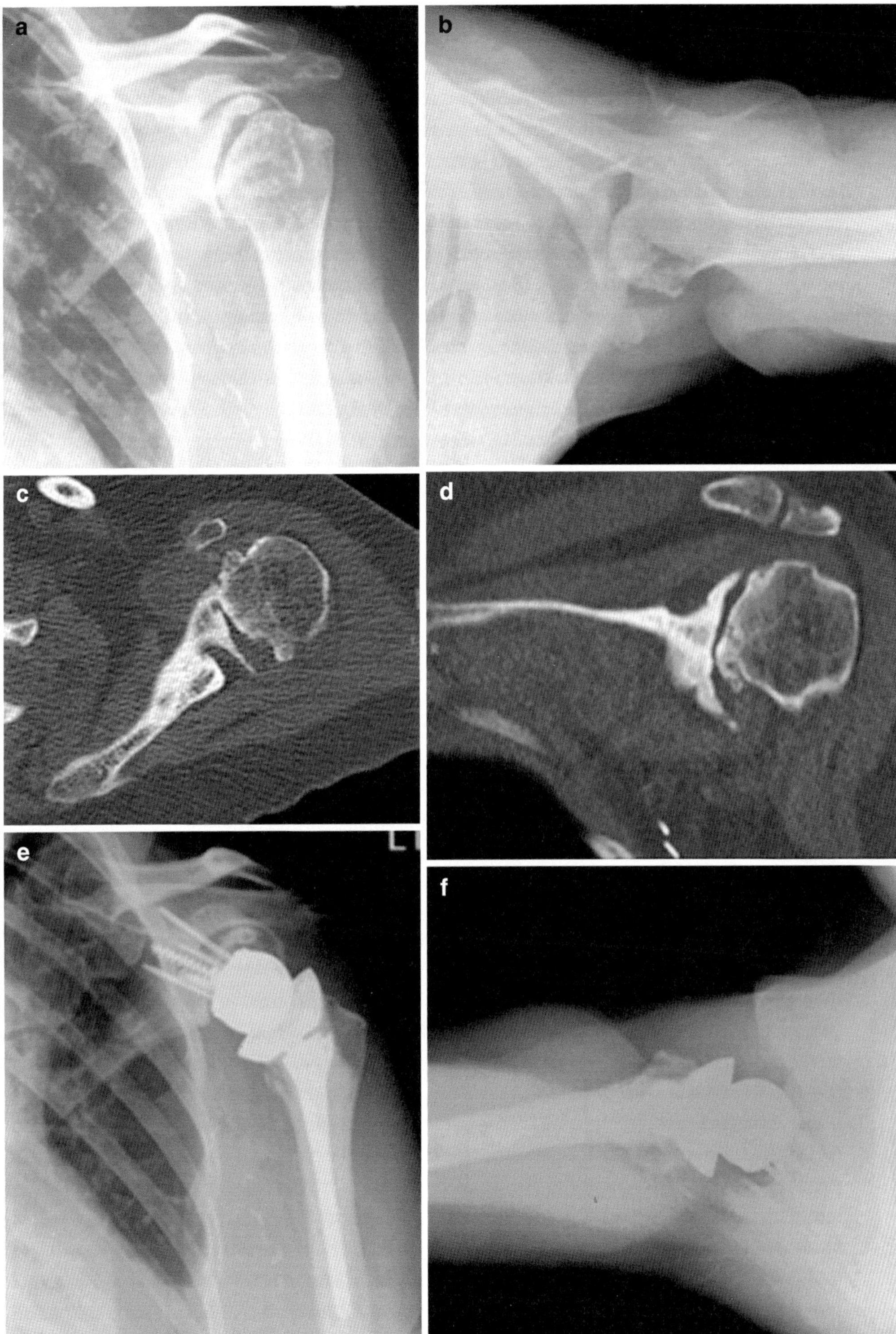

Fig. 22.20 (**a**) Anteroposterior and (**b**) axillary radiographs and (**c**, **d**) CT scans of a patient with glenoid bone loss. (**e**) Anteroposterior and (**f**) axillary postoperative radiographs

Although these studies show that RTSA can be successful in the short term, the long-term results of this approach to glenoid bone loss are unknown.

Pseudoparalysis Without Arthritis

A unique group of patients are those who have "pseudoparalysis" from superior escape of the shoulder but who do not have shoulder pain. It is important in such patients to be sure that the painless loss of motion is not caused by an underlying neurological disorder. The most common cause is a massive rotator cuff tear, which includes the subscapularis, supraspinatus, and infraspinatus tendons. This can be caused by trauma or, occasionally, failed rotator cuff repairs in which the coracoacromial ligament has been cut with or without concomitant partial acromioplasty. Typically, these patients have full passive range of motion, reasonable function with their arms below shoulder level, and no pain. In these patients, the major goal of surgery is not pain relief but rather increased range of motion.

Two studies have addressed the use of RTSA in this population. Mulieri et al. [64] reported on 72 shoulders with Hamada stage 1, 2, or 3 without glenohumeral arthritis, some of which had pseudoparalysis. Werner et al. [65] reported on a series of 58 patients with pain, pseudoparalysis, and irreparable cuff tears treated with RTSA. They found improvement in range of motion, subjective shoulder value, and Constant-Murley scores; however, they found a significant decrease in the degree of active external rotation. Regardless of whether the patients had previous surgery, all patients had improved visual analog scale scores for pain, improved range of motion, and improved outcome scores.

When considering this patient population, a critical factor is the status of the external rotators and the deltoid muscle. If the patient lacks external rotation strength and has a positive external rotation lag sign, then performance of a concomitant latissimus dorsi transfer at the time of RTSA should be considered. Although some patients with deltoid dysfunction may experience pain relief with RTSA [66, 67], Ladermann et al. [68] suggest that performing this procedure will only moderately improve range of motion, especially if the entire deltoid is dysfunctional.

Immunological Arthritis

Immunological causes of arthritis include rheumatoid arthritis (RA) (Fig. 22.21), juvenile RA, and arthritis associated with psoriasis, ulcerative colitis, Crohn's disease, and ankylosing spondylitis. The major issues in these populations as they relate to shoulder replacements typically are glenoid bone loss caused by the disease or steroid use, rotator cuff tears, and immunological suppression leading to infection. Soft bone is particularly a concern on the glenoid side, where over-reaming of the glenoid can occur during surgery, or baseplate fixation may be compromised leading to loosening and baseplate failure.

Young et al. [69] reported on 18 shoulders in patients with RA treated with RTSA with a mean follow-up of 3.8 years. Patients with an intact teres minor had better results than those without a functioning teres minor. There were four cases of proximal humerus fracture either intraoperatively or postoperatively. The authors recommended consideration of cementing the humeral component in such patients. Rittmeister and Kerschbaumer [70] reported on eight patients with RA who also had torn rotator cuff tendons. There were three baseplate failures caused by sepsis in one and aseptic loosening in two. Although sepsis is a concern in these patients, a review of the RTSA literature does not show a higher infection rate in this population.

Dislocation Arthropathy

Dislocation arthropathy can result from arthritis caused by multiple episodes of shoulder instability, or it can be caused by surgical procedures. The most obvious surgical cause of dislo-

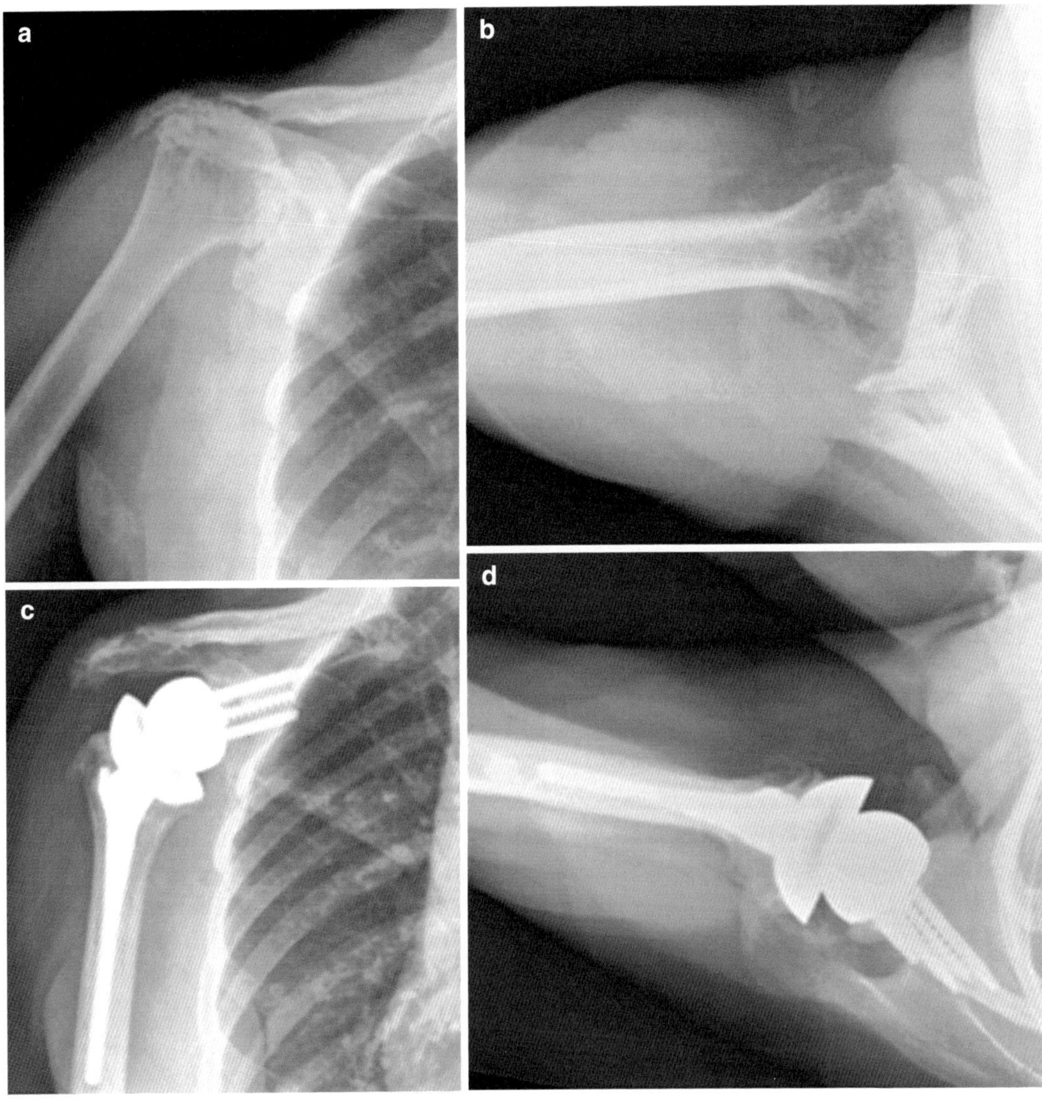

Fig. 22.21 (**a**) Anteroposterior and (**b**) axillary radiographs showing shoulder of a patient with rheumatoid arthritis. (**c**) Anteroposterior and (**d**) axillary postoperative radiographs after reverse total shoulder arthroplasty

cation arthropathy is screws or anchors penetrating the articular cartilage. The second cause is overtightening of the shoulder in internal rotation associated with posterior humeral head subluxation and posterior glenoid wear. Many of these patients have substantial glenoid wear and deformity from these causes (Fig. 22.22). However, many patients also have subscapularis tendon dysfunction from the subscapularis tendon detachment and reattachment to the lesser tuberosity. The rationale for RTSA in these patients is to address not only the severe bony glenoid deformity but also the subscapularis dysfunction [71].

Lastly, many of these patients have fixed internal rotation contractures, making failure of anatomical TSA likely. Studies of anatomical TSA show that patients who undergo TSA for dislocation arthropathy have the worst outcomes [72].

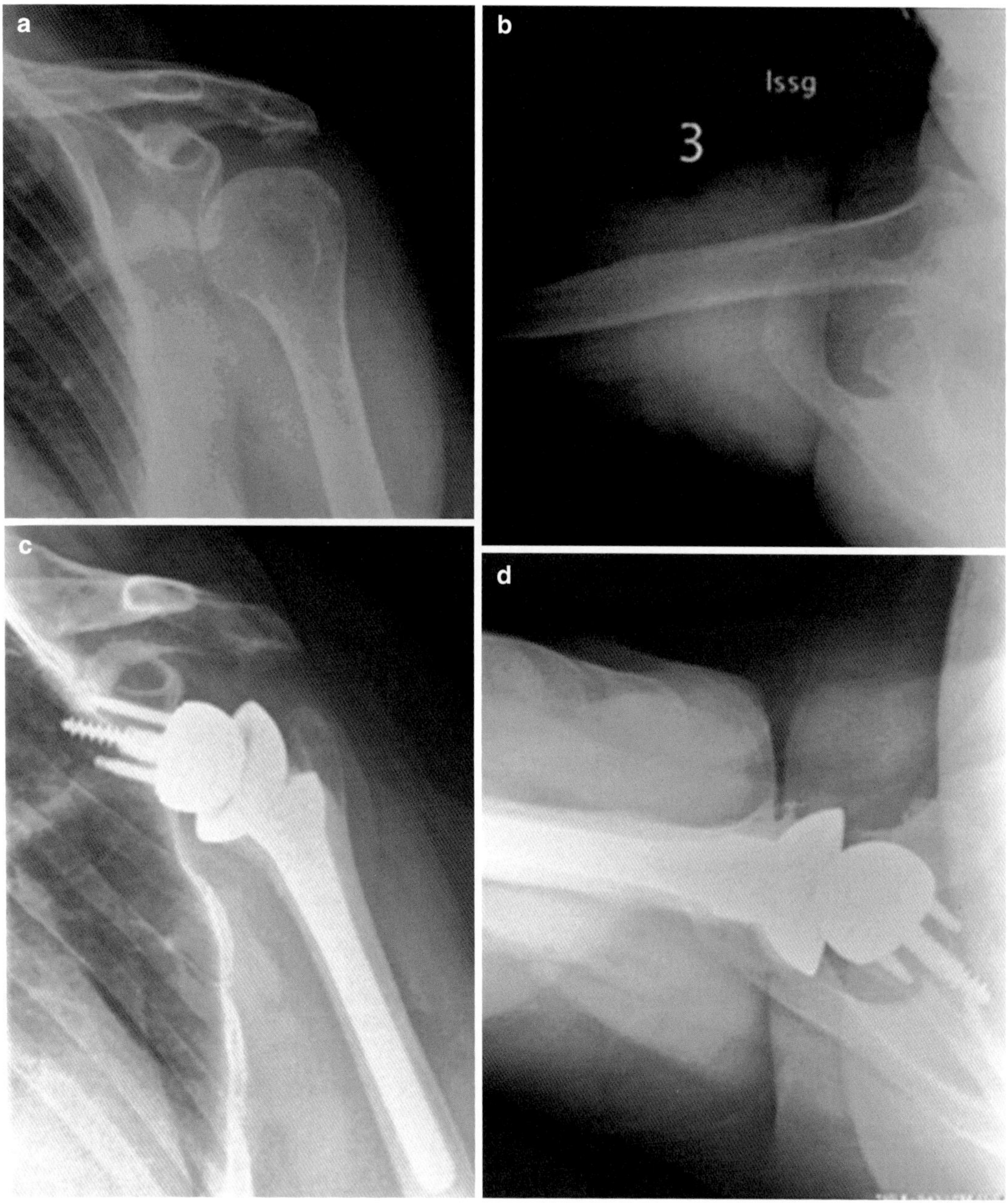

Fig. 22.22 (**a**) Anteroposterior and (**b**) axillary preoperative radiographs of a patient with chronic anterior dislocation. (**c**) Anteroposterior and (**d**) axillary postoperative radiographs after reverse total shoulder arthroplasty

Chronic Fixed Dislocations

Although fixed dislocations of the glenohumeral joint are uncommon, they can present substantial challenges when associated with rotator cuff tearing, glenoid bone loss, and humeral head impaction fractures (Fig. 22.23). In fixed posterior dislocations, the patient has a substantial internal rotation contracture. In fixed anterior dislocations, the patient has similar loss of abduction and shoulder rotation. In both instances, glenoid bone loss can be substantial and should be evaluated

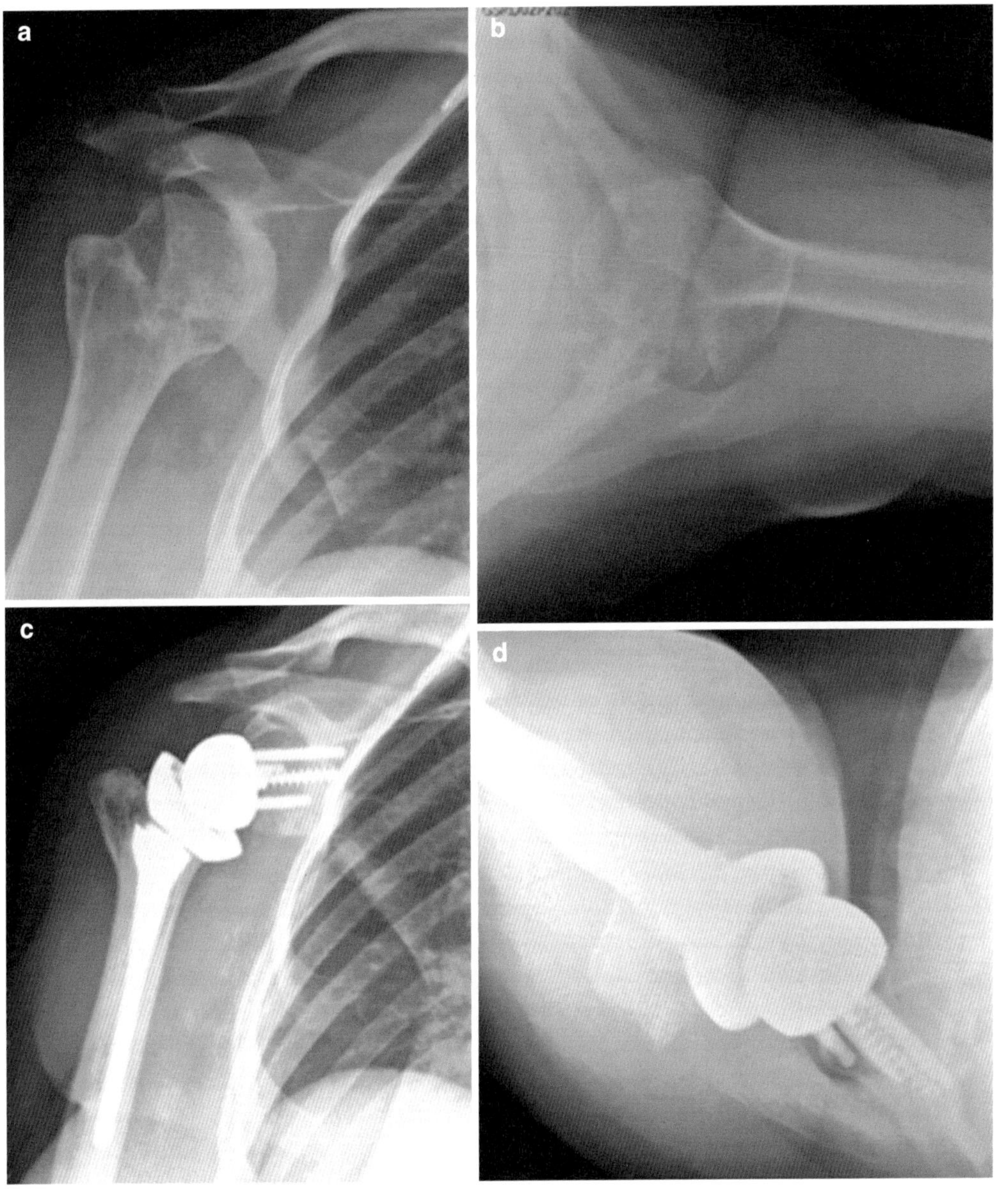

Fig. 22.23 (**a**) Anteroposterior and (**b**) axillary preoperative radiographs of a patient with fixed shoulder dislocation. (**c**) Anteroposterior and (**d**) axillary radiographs after reverse total shoulder arthroplasty

with CT scanning [73]. In our experience, RTSA has produced excellent pain relief but return of range of motion is unpredictable.

Shoulder Dysplasias

Although rare, shoulder dysplasias with arthritis and pain can be treated successfully with RTSA. These conditions include epiphyseal dysplasia, congenital shoulder dislocation–associated glenoid dysplasia, and Kneist syndrome [73] (Fig. 22.24). The main reason to use RTSA in these patients is to address bone loss in the glenoid. The major goal is pain relief because the longstanding tissue contractures may make increases in range of motion difficult.

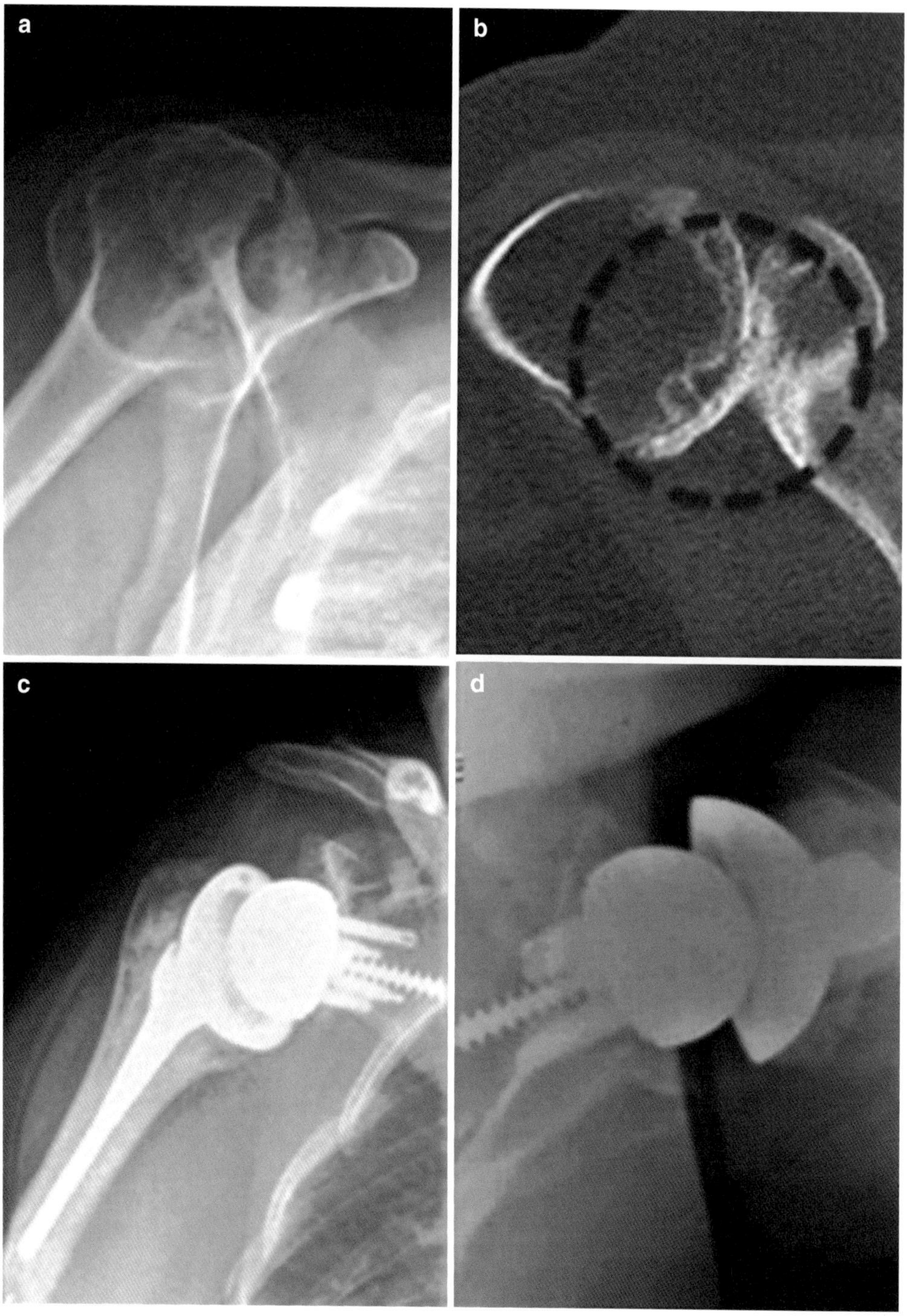

Fig. 22.24 A 44-year-old woman with glenoid dysplasia. (**a**) Preoperative conventional anteroposterior radiograph of the shoulder showing the altered glenoid anatomy, consistent with dysplasia. (**b**) Preoperative computed tomography scan, axial cut, shows narrowed joint space and severely distorted articular surfaces of head and glenoid (*dotted circle*). Conventional radiographs of the shoulder at 6-month follow-up show a well-fixed prosthesis: (**c**) anteroposterior view, and (**d**) axillary view. (Reprinted with permission from: Hyun YS, Huri G, Garbis NG, McFarland EG. Uncommon indications for reverse total shoulder arthroplasty. Clin Orthop Surg. 2013;5(4):243–55. Open access through Creative Commons license.)

Acute Proximal Humerus Fractures

The treatment of proximal humerus fractures continues to evolve because of the development of custom proximal humerus plates and the use of RTSA in select patients (Fig. 22.25). In patients with good bone, who are younger and who have fragments capable of fixation, the standard of care for displaced fracture is open reduction and internal fixation. For patients with poor bone, comminution, and lower expectations for function, hemiarthroplasty has been the traditional treatment. However, the failure rate of hemiarthroplasty is high because of tuberosity failure and pain from bone wear by the humeral component on the glenoid. Pain and loss of motion from failed hemiarthroplasty have led some to advocate for RTSA as the first-line of treatment rather than hemiarthroplasty [74].

Several studies have compared the results of RTSA to hemiarthroplasty for acute proximal

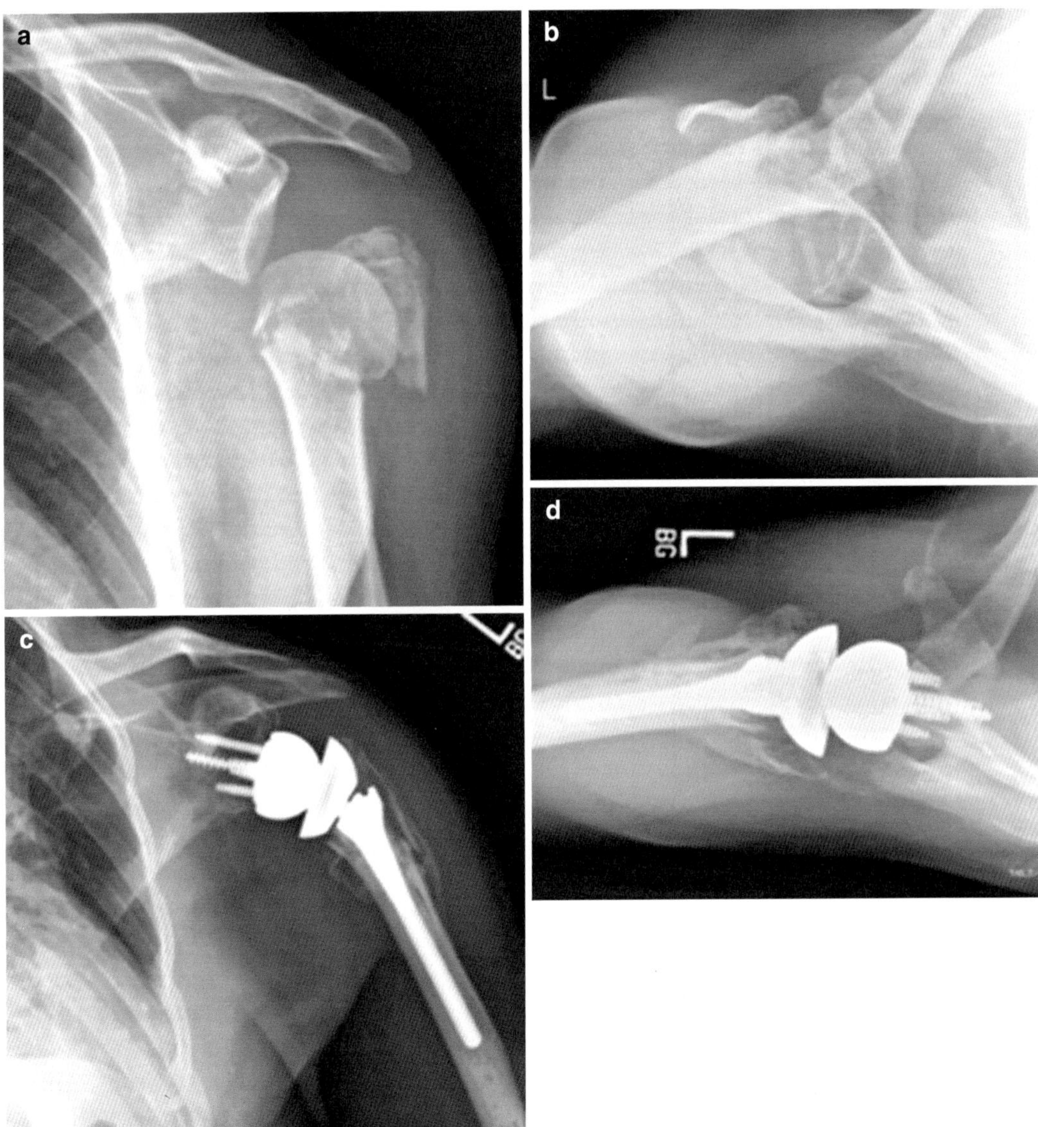

Fig. 22.25 (**a**) Anteroposterior and (**b**) axillary radiographs of a patient with comminuted fracture of the proximal humerus. (**c**) Anteroposterior and (**d**) axillary radiographs after reverse total shoulder arthroplasty

humerus fractures [75]. A systematic review of these level-1 and -2 studies found that although the range of motion between the two treatments was similar, RTSA provided better pain relief than hemiarthroplasty [76]. However, neither treatment method restored range of motion to normal, so patients should be advised that the goal of treatment is the ability to reach to the top of their heads without pain.

Malunited Proximal Humerus Fractures

Although RTSA has proven successful in treating acute proximal humeral fractures, the results of RTSA for treating malunited proximal humerus fractures (Fig. 22.26) have not been encouraging [77]. In a study of the various indications for RTSA, Wall et al. [50] found that the group with

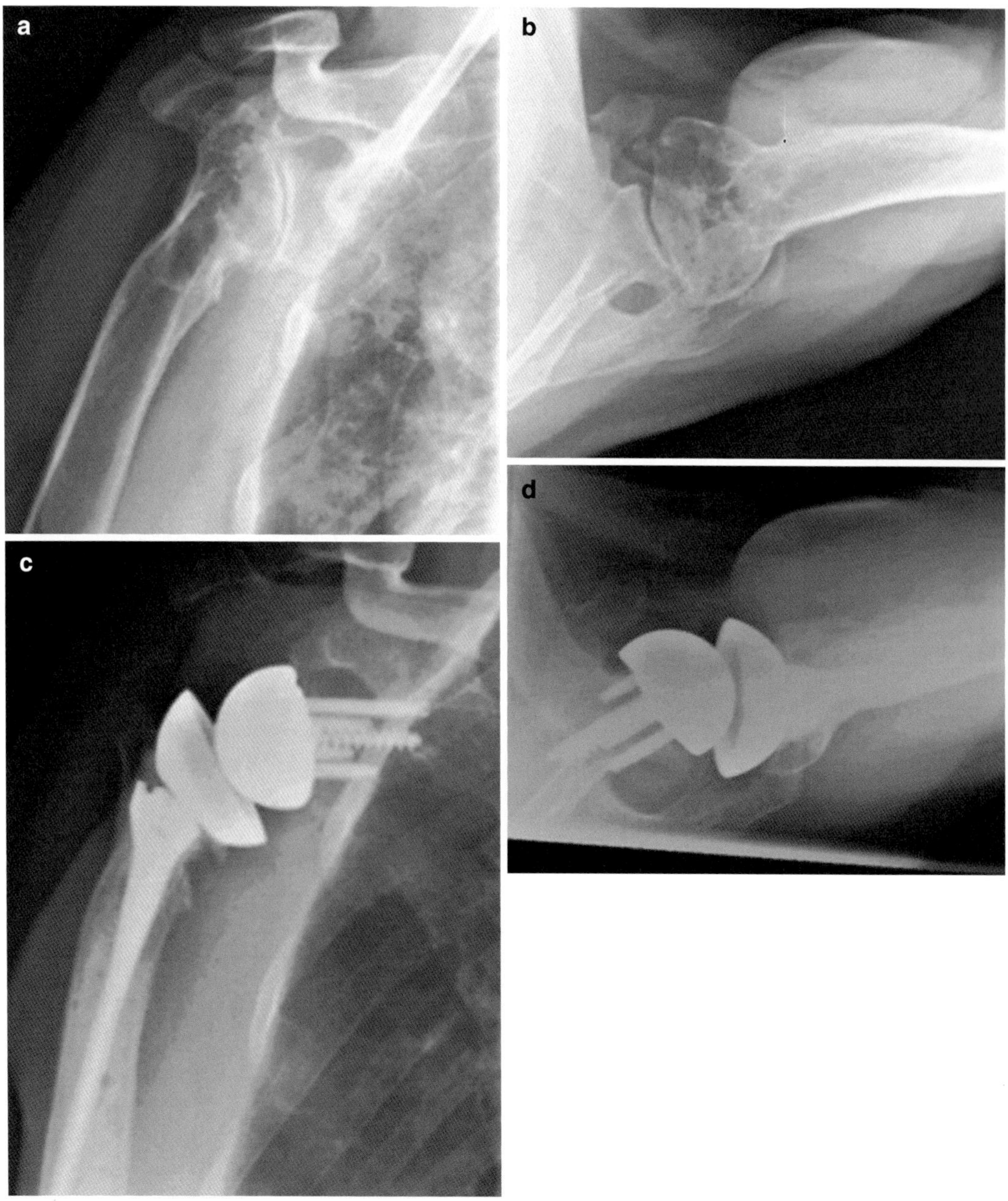

Fig. 22.26 (**a**) Anteroposterior and (**b**) axillary radiographs of a patient with posttraumatic sequelae. (**c**) Anteroposterior and (**d**) axillary radiographs after reverse total shoulder arthroplasty

the least satisfaction were patients with malunited proximal humerus fractures. This has been attributed to the difficulty of correcting posterior subluxation of the greater tuberosity with shortening of the infraspinatus and teres minor tendons. Because of soft tissue contracture, the fragment cannot be reduced back to the proximal humerus to restore external rotation. Also, the retention of that fragment can contribute to instability by pushing the implant anteriorly and superiorly when the arm is adducted and externally rotated. Lastly, extensive scar formation from the healing of the fracture makes improvements in range of motion difficult.

Bone Tumors

The use of RTSA for tumors of the proximal humerus (Fig. 22.27) has been reported but there are no extensive case series documenting its use [78]. The use of RTSA for this purpose is challenging because of the loss of bone support for the prosthesis and the loss of soft tissue to maintain reduction. Infection and instability are common and difficult to manage [79].

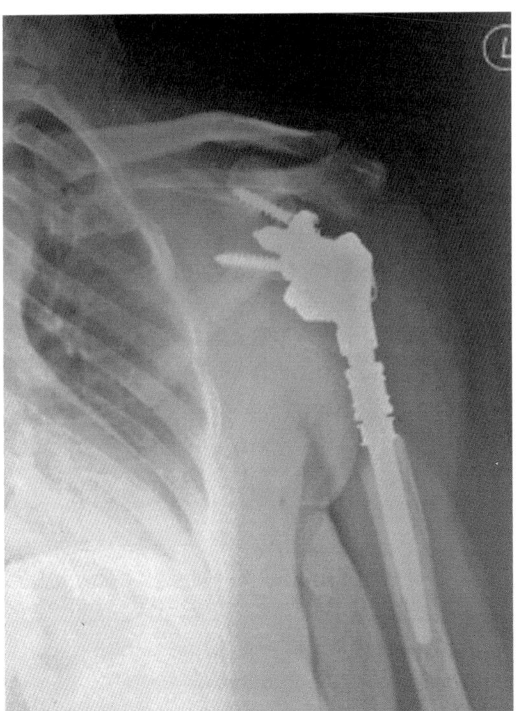

Fig. 22.27 Reverse shoulder tumor resection prosthesis reconstruction after excision of chondrosarcoma located in proximal humerus of a 47-year-old woman. (Reprinted with permission from: Guven MF, Aslan L, Botanlioglu H, Kaynak G, Kesmezacar H, Babacan M. Functional outcome of reverse shoulder tumor prosthesis in the treatment of proximal humerus tumors. J. Shoulder Elb Surg. 2016;25(1):e1–6.)

Primary Shoulder Infections

Although primary shoulder infections are rare, they can result in extensive bone and rotator cuff destruction [80]. After the infection is controlled with debridement and intravenous antibiotics, a 1-stage implantation of RTSA or a 2-stage reconstruction with an antibiotic spacer followed at a later date by RTSA can be performed (Fig. 22.28). Although anatomical TSA can be considered in these cases, in our practice, RTSA with cementless components is the treatment of choice.

Failed Hemiarthroplasty

Unfortunately, not all shoulder arthroplasties provide immediate or even long-term pain relief (Fig. 22.29). The use of humeral-sided hemiarthroplasty for younger and active patients with osteoarthritis of the shoulder has been shown to relieve pain and increase function [81]. However, the long-term results are not encouraging, as a large percent will fail in the first 5 years [82]. The failures are caused by various factors such as eccentrically eroded glenoids, the development of glenoid bone wear over time, and subscapularis failure [83]. One study showed that hemiarthroplasty for this population has a 5-year patient satisfaction rate of 72% and a 5-year implant survival rate of 89% [82].

Similar issues are seen with cup arthroplasty and partial humeral head replacements or "caps" [84]. In any of these partial replacements, the glenoid must be reamed flat to eliminate posterior erosions. Also, the metal surface of the implants has contact with the glenoid bone and can result in erosion of the glenoid over time. The results of RTSA for failed

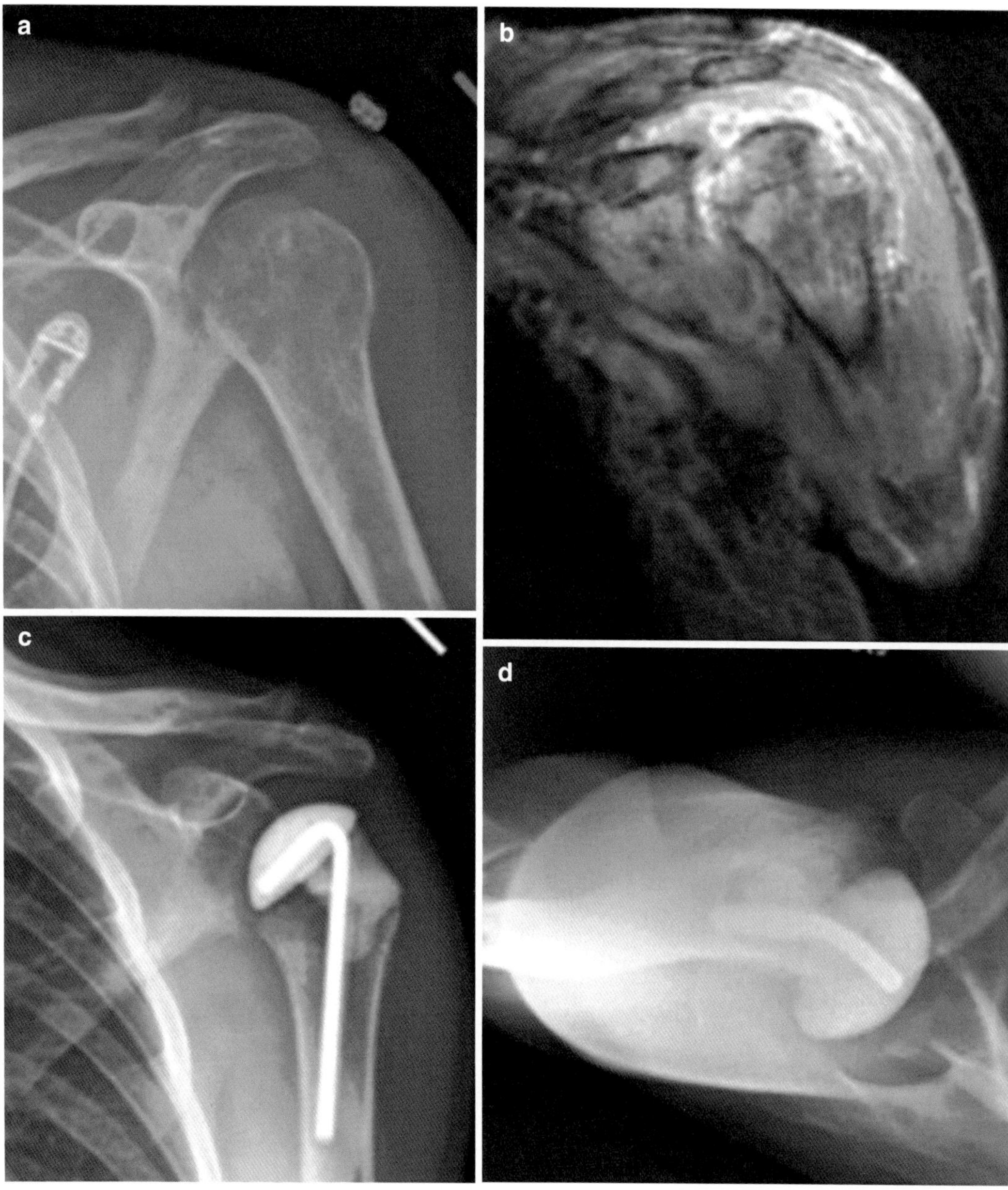

Fig. 22.28 (**a**) Radiograph and (**b**) MRI of septic shoulder and osteomyelitis of the glenoid and humeral head. (**c**) Anteroposterior and (**d**) axillary radiographs after first-stage operation, antibiotic spacer insertion. (**e**) Anteroposterior and (**f**) axillary radiographs after second-stage operation

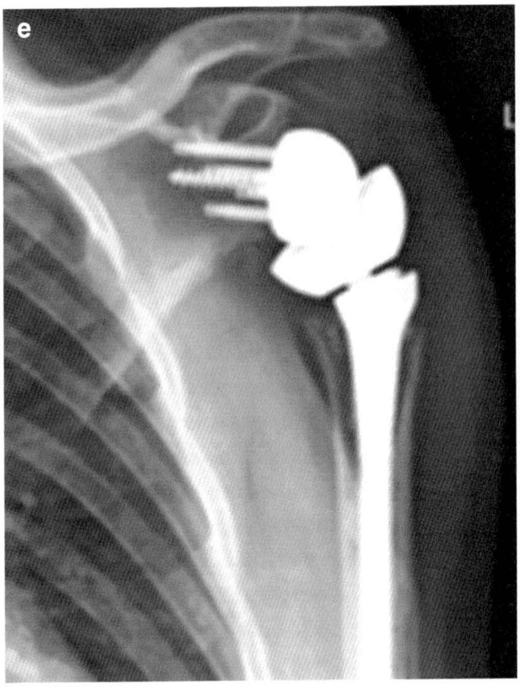

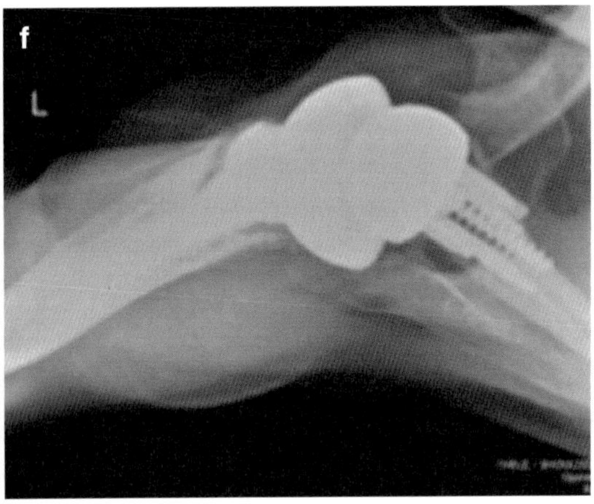

Fig. 22.28 (continued)

hemiarthroplasty show that pain relief can be achieved, and that range of motion improvements are modest [85, 86].

Failed Anatomical TSA

Failed anatomical TSA (Fig. 22.30) presents special challenges for revision surgery. The major cause for the revision largely determines the success. Infected TSA presents challenges of eradicating the infection along with substantial bone loss on the glenoid side and potential bone loss on the humeral side. Glenoid loosening without infection can be difficult, especially when a keeled glenoid component with cement has worn away the glenoid to produce a cavitary defect in the glenoid. Removal of the humeral component can result in fractures requiring bone grafting or allograft reconstruction. Intense scar formation can make the exposure difficult and contribute to decreased range of motion postoperatively. Despite these challenges, revision of a failed TSA to RTSA can produce satisfactory results, especially in pain relief [87, 88].

Revision of Failed RTSA

Since the approval of RTSA by the US Food and Drug Administration in 2004, its use has increased steadily, with a corresponding increase in the number of RTSA revisions. The major causes of revision of RTSA are instability and infection [89]. Other causes of failure (but less commonly for revision) are glenoid notching, implant disassociation, and nerve injury.

Revision of a failed RTSA (Fig. 22.31) presents the same challenges as revision of a TSA to RTSA. Infection can result in bone loss on both the glenoid and humeral side of the joint. Instability is often multifactorial and includes causes such as a poor or loose soft tissue envelope, component design, lack of deltoid compressive force from loss of the tuberosities, and posterior-inferior capsular contracture forcing the adducted shoulder anteriorly and superiorly. Each of these issues must be considered when revising a failed RTSA. There are few studies on the results of revision of RTSA [90, 91].

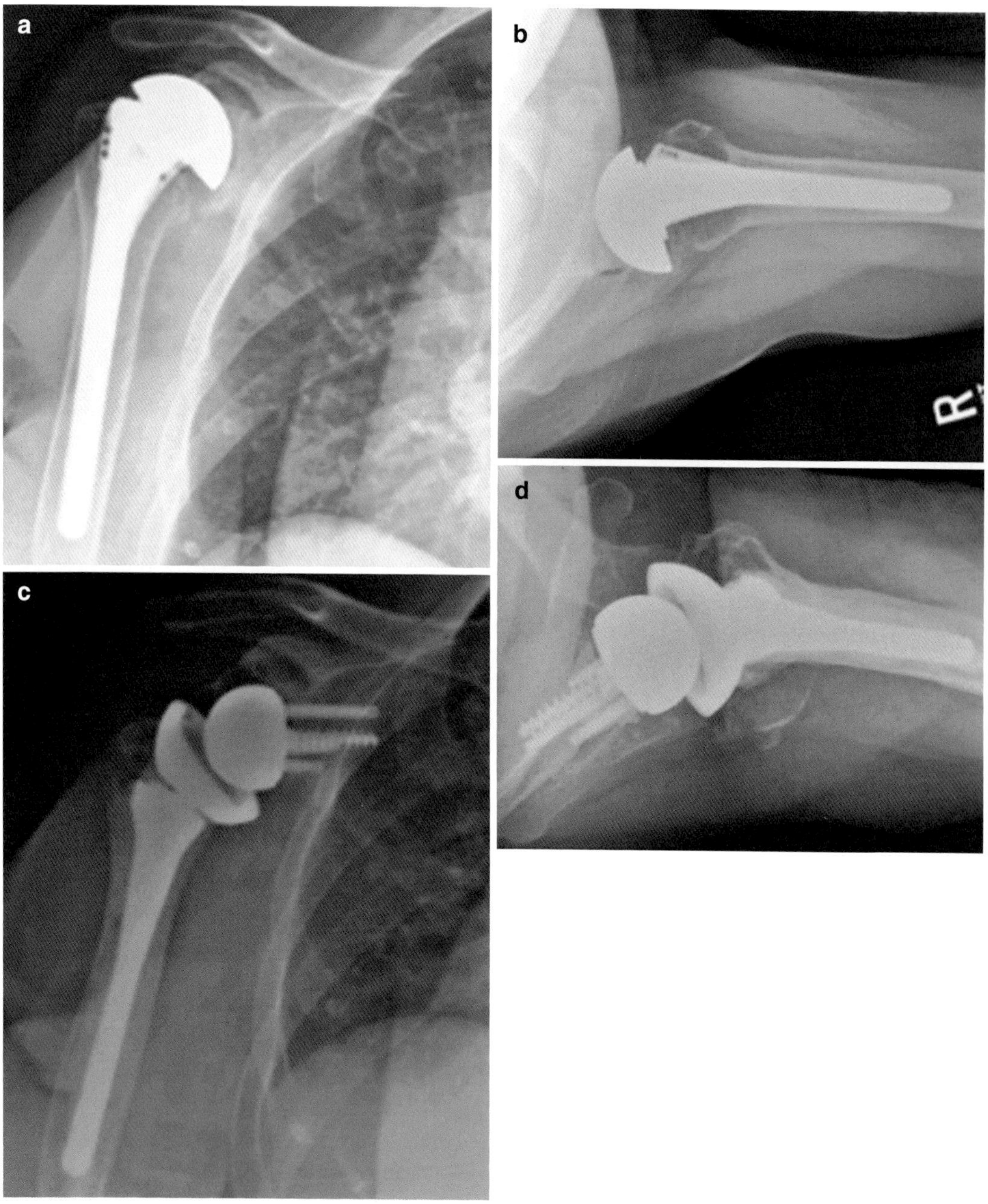

Fig. 22.29 (**a**) Anteroposterior and (**b**) axillary preoperative radiographs of a patient with failed hemiarthroplasty at 62 months after primary operation. (**c**) Anteroposterior and (**d**) axillary radiographs after revision reverse total shoulder arthroplasty

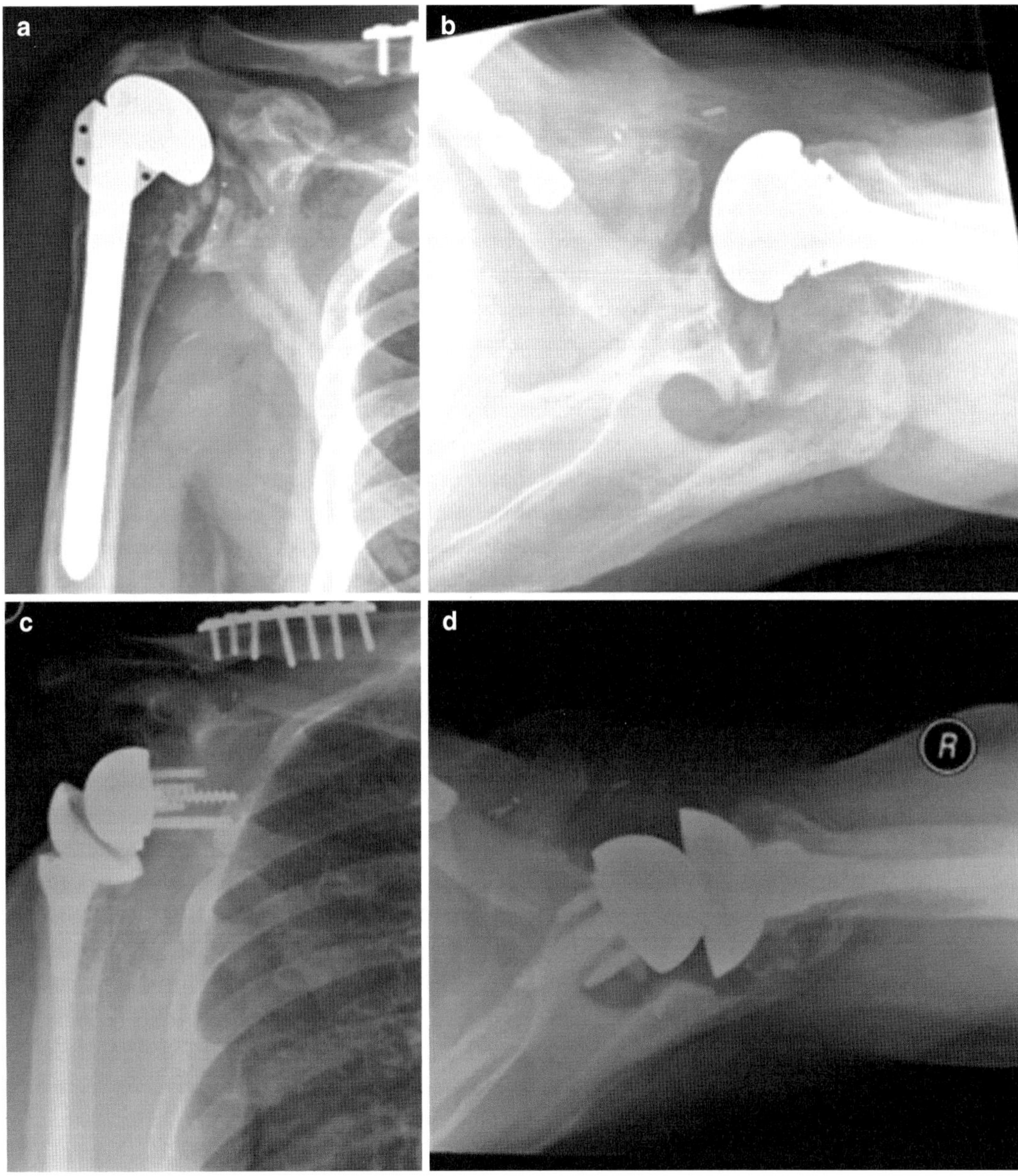

Fig. 22.30 (**a**) Anteroposterior and (**b**) axillary radiographs of a patient with failed total shoulder arthroplasty 1 year after primary operation. (**c**) Anteroposterior and (**d**) axillary radiographs after revision reverse total shoulder arthroplasty

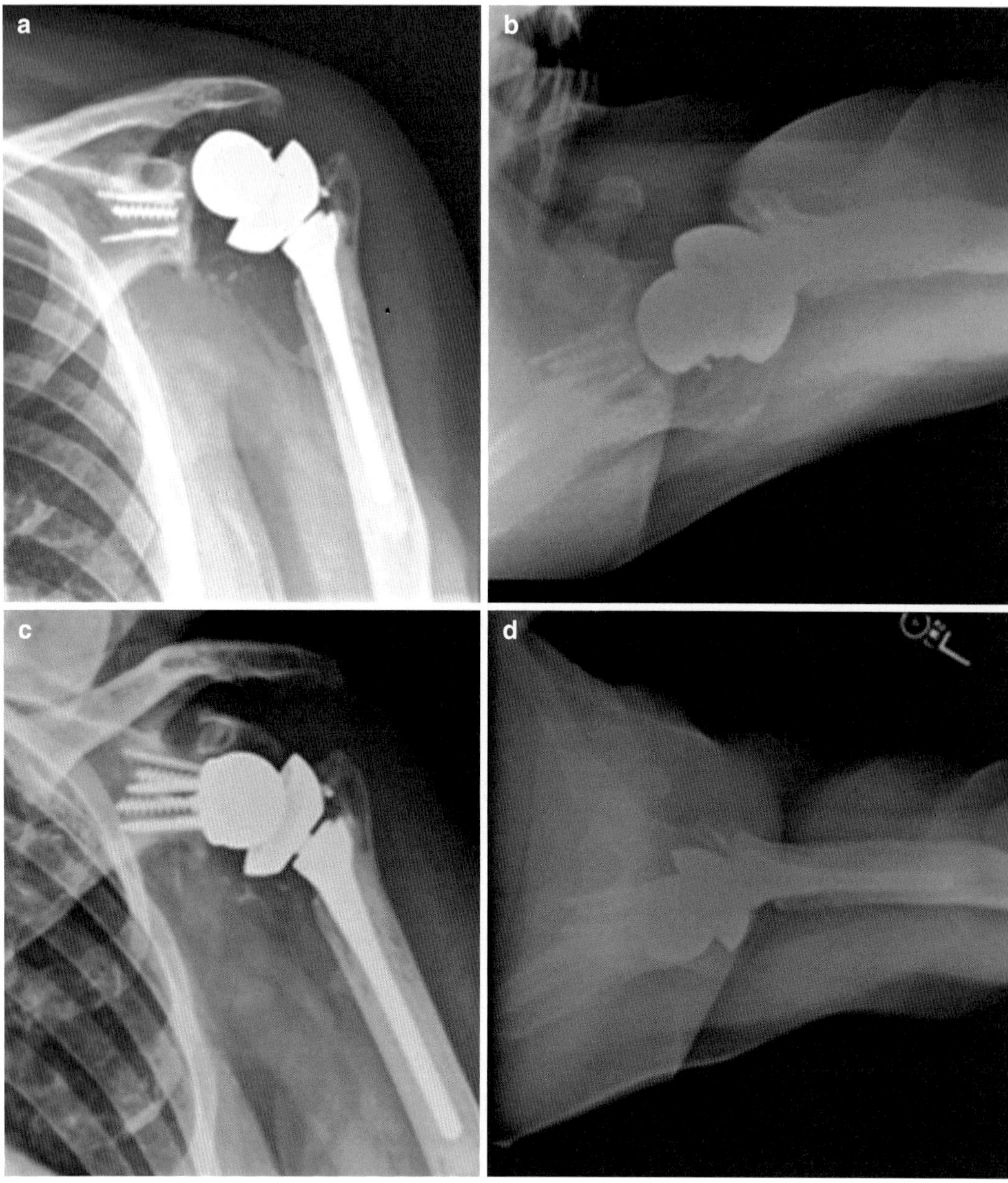

Fig. 22.31 (**a**) Anteroposterior and (**b**) axillary radiographs showing failed RTSA with baseplate loosening at 19 months after RTSA. (**c**) Anteroposterior and (**d**) axillary radiographs after revision reverse total shoulder arthroplasty

Complications

As indications for the use of the RTSA have expanded to include failed TSA and other conditions previously not amenable to successful anatomic arthroplasty, the number and spectrum of complications of RTSA have increased. Reported complication rates range from 0% to 75% (Table 22.4). This high variation is related not only to range of follow-up but also to unclear definitions of what is considered a complication. For example, some studies reported all

Table 22.4 Summary of complications after RTSA

Study	No. of patients	Mean (range) age, years	Diagnosis (no.)	Mean (range) follow-up, months	Prosthesis (manufacturer)	Complications (no.)	Complication rate, %
Werner et al. [65]	58	68 (44–84)	CTA	38 (minimum 24)	Delta III (Dupuy, Warsaw, IN)	Hematoma (12); dislocation (5); aseptic baseplate loosening (3); scapular fracture (4); infection (6); nerve injury, humeral stem loosening, polyethylene dissociation (1 each)	50
Frankle et al. [142]	60	71 (34–86)	CTA	33 (24–68)	RSP (DJO Surgical, Austin, TX)	Baseplate loosening (7); infection, acromial fracture (2 each); scapular fracture, humeral dissociation (1 each)	17
Wall et al. [50]	186 (191 shoulders)	73 (23–86)	CTA (115); revision (54); primary OA (33); posttraumatic arthritis (33); tumor (2); acute fracture (2); RA(1)	40 (24–118)	Delta III; Aequalis (Tornier, Montbonnot, France)	Dislocation (15); infection (8); glenoid fracture, postoperative humeral fracture, symptomatic hardware, nerve injury, aseptic baseplate loosening (<5 each)	19
Cuff et al. [97]	94 (96 shoulders)	72 (52–88)	CTA (70); revision (23), humeral nonunion (3)	28 (24–38)	RSP (Encore Medical, Austin, TX)	Dislocation, traumatic dislocation, infection (2 each); hematoma, baseplate loosening, acromial fracture (1 each)	9.3
Mulieri et al. [64]	58 (60 shoulders)	71(52–88)	Irreparable RC tear	52 (24–101)	RSP (DJO Surgical)	Baseplate failure (4); acromial fracture (2); infection, dislocation, hematoma, traumatic proximal humerus fracture (1 each)	20
Holcomb et al. [115]	21	70 (53–86)	RA	36 (24–73)	RSP (DJO Surgical)	Infection (2); periprosthetic fracture, aseptic baseplate loosening, scapular fracture, intraoperative glenoid fracture (1 each)	28
Klein et al. [147]	141 (143 shoulders)	72 (42–87)	CTA (141); posttraumatic arthritis (2)	31 (24–51)	RSP (DJO Surgical)	Infection, acromial fracture (2 each); traumatic periprosthetic fracture (1)	3.5
Kempton et al. [148]	192	71 (48–92)	Various	19 (6–49)	Trabecular metal (Zimmer, Warsaw, IN); Delta III; Aequalis	Transient neuropathy (5); intraoperative fracture (4); dislocation (3); chronic subluxation (2); acromial fracture (1)	9.8

(continued)

Table 22.4 (continued)

Study	No. of patients	Mean (range) age, years	Diagnosis (no.)	Mean (range) follow-up, months	Prosthesis (manufacturer)	Complications (no.)	Complication rate, %
Muh et al. [149]	66 (67 shoulders)	52 (23–60)	RC insufficiency (29); CTA (11); revision (9); RA (6); posttraumatic arthritis (4); other (8)	36 (24–77)	Aequalis	Dislocation (5); infection (3); neurologic injury, humeral stress fracture (1 each)	15
Ortmaier et al. [150]	50	64 (44–84)	Revision	54 (24–101)	Delta III; Delta Xtend (Dupuy, Warsaw, IN)	Instability (5); infection, periprosthetic fracture (2 each); aseptic glenoid loosening, hematoma (1 each)	24
Ek et al. [151]	35 (40 shoulders)	50 (46–64)	Irreparable RC tear	93 (60–171)	Delta III; anatomic shoulder reverse (Zimmer, Winterthur, Switzerland)	Dislocation (7); infection (5); glenoid component loosening, scapular fracture (3 each); neurologic injury (2); periprosthetic fracture, soft tissue impingement, PE wear (1 each)	38
Groh et al. [152]	112 (114 shoulders)	64 (53–86)	Irreparable RC tear (73); proximal humerus fracture (20); revision (21)	26 (12–48)	RSP (DJO, Austin, TX); Delta Xtend; Delta III	Periprosthetic fracture, hematoma (3 each); infection, acromial fracture (1 each)	20 (revision) and 4.3 (primary)
Wagner et al. [153]	40	68	Revision	37 (24–72)	Comprehensive reverse shoulder (Biomet, Warsaw, IN); Encore RSP (DJO); Delta Xtend; Aequalis	Aseptic glenoid loosening (4); dislocation (2); infection (1)	18
Ross et al. [154]	20 (21 shoulders)	79 (67–90)	Proximal humerus fracture	55 (25–107)	SMR modular shoulder system (Lima Corp, Udine, Italy)	Nerve injury (1)	5
Irlenbusch et al. [155]	113	75	CTA (80); revision (12); posttraumatic arthritis (14); other (7)	27 (minimum 24)	Affinis Inverse (Mathys, Bettlack, Switzerland)	Dislocation (3); periprosthetic fracture, traumatic avulsion of the metaglene (1 each)	4.4

CTA cuff tear arthropathy, *OA* osteoarthritis, *PE* polyethylene, *RA* rheumatoid arthritis, *RC* rotator cuff, *RSP* reverse shoulder prosthesis complications, ranging from infection to suture abscess postoperatively. Some included scapular notching as a complication. Others reported only complications that resulted in revision surgery.

The incidence of complications after RTSA is greater than after anatomic TSA. The reasons for this are related to patient factors unique to the population undergoing RTSA, including relatively old age, high number of previous operations, and poor bone and soft tissue quality. The main complications after RTSA are scapular notching, instability, aseptic baseplate loosening, infection, nerve injury, intraoperative fracture, and component disassociation.

Scapular Notching

Scapular notching is a complication unique to RTSA and is the most common complication of RTSA (Table 22.5). Scapular notching is defined as the erosion of the lateral pillar of the scapula (Fig. 22.32). Although it is believed to be caused by mechanical impingement of the inferior medial humeral implant on the inferior scapular neck with adduction of the upper extremity, the role of direct contact or possible particle disease is unknown. Notching tends to appear during the first year after implantation of the prosthesis, sometimes as early as a few months after implantation. The presence of notching can be identified with a true anteroposterior view or Grashey view of the shoulder. Sirveaux et al. [14] classified scapular notching according to the extent of scapular neck erosion seen on the postoperative radiographs. In their classification, grade 1 is confined to the pillar, grade 2 extends to the lower screw, grade 3 encompasses the screw, and grade 4 extends under the baseplate (Fig. 22.33).

The relationship between scapular notching and symptoms is unclear. Sirveaux et al. [14] found that inferior scapular notching is associated with worse clinical outcomes. Higher grades of notching (grades 3 and 4) were associated with lower Constant-Murley scores. Similarly, Simovich et al. [26] found decreased range of motion and increased pain scores in patients with the presence of notching. Conversely, Levigne et al. [92] reported no correlation between the presence of scapular notching and clinical outcomes such as range of motion or the Constant-Murley score. Furthermore, Sadoghi et al. [93]

Table 22.5 Incidence of scapular notching after reverse total shoulder arthroplasty

Study	No. of patients	Scapular notching, %	Mean (range) follow-up, months	Prosthesis (manufacturer)	Sirveaux classification, %				Baseplate failure
					1	2	3	4	
Sirveaux et al. [14]	80	64	44 (24–97)	Delta III (Dupuy, Warsaw, IN)	33	12	8.7	7.5	NR
Werner et al. [65]	48	96	48	Delta III	54		46		NR
Boileau et al. [101]	38	68	40 (24–72)	Delta III	47	13	13	0	0
Simovitch et al. [26]	77	44	44 (24–96)	Delta III	7.8	18	16	2.6	NR
Cuff et al. [97]	96	0	28 (24–38)	RSP (DJO Surgical, Austin, TX)	NR	NR	NR	NR	NR
Levigne et al. [92]	337	62	47 (24–120)	Delta III; Aequalis (Tornier, Montbonnot, France)	22	18	14	8	1 at 112 months
Melis et al. [95]	68	88	114 (96–144)	Delta III	7	19	13	49	0
Levigne et al. [94]	461	68	51 (24–206)	Delta III; Aequalis	22	23	13	10	NR

NR not reported, *RSP* reverse shoulder prosthesis

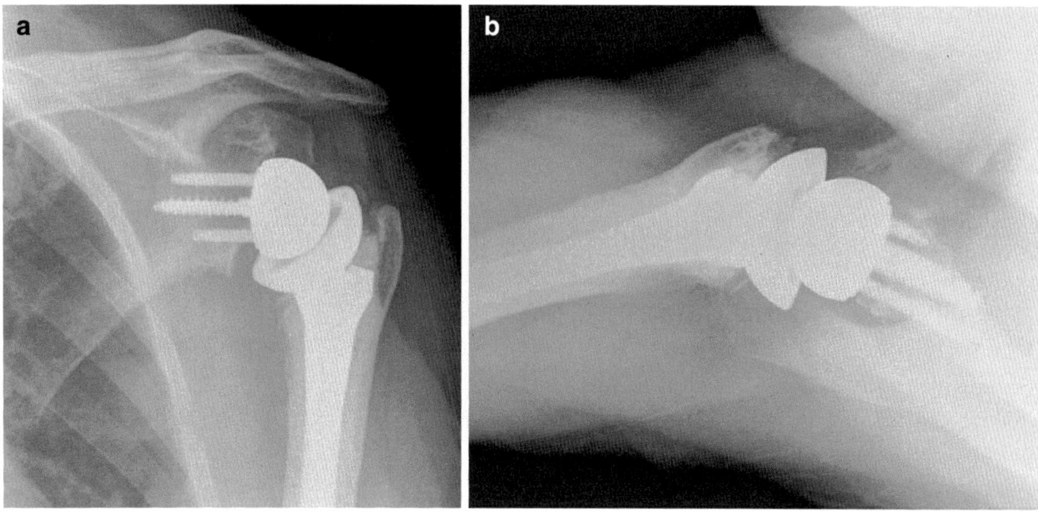

Fig. 22.32 (**a**) Anteroposterior and (**b**) axillary radiographs showing scapular neck erosion extending to the lower screw (grade-2 notching according to Nerot-Sirveaux)

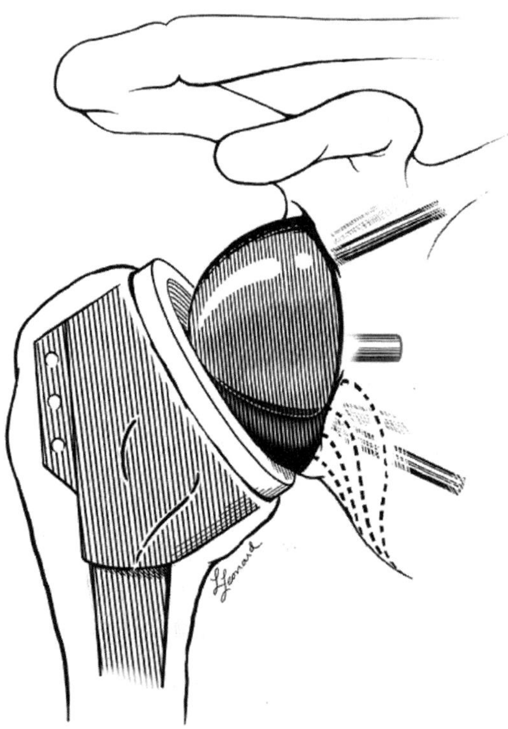

Fig. 22.33 The Nerot-Sirveaux classification of scapular notching is shown. Grade 1 (*lowest dotted line*), confined to the pillar; grade 2 (*lower middle dotted line*), extending to the lower screw; grade 3 (*upper middle dotted line*), encompassing the screw; grade 4 (*top dotted line*), notching extending under the baseplate. (Reprinted with permission from: Wierks C, Skolasky RL, Ji JH, McFarland EG. Reverse total shoulder replacement: intraoperative and early postoperative complications. Clin Orthop Relat Res. 2009;467(1):225–34.)

reported that during follow-up ranging from 2 to 5 years, there was no correlation between infraglenoid notching and clinical outcomes as measured by Constant-Murley score, DASH score, Oxford instability score, Rowe score, and active range of motion. When follow-up extended longer than 5 years, there was a significant correlation between the presence of notching and declines in Constant-Murley pain score, active elevation, and active external rotation. However, there were no correlations with the total Constant-Murley score, DASH score, or active abduction.

The timing of the appearance of scapular notching and the rate of progression have been topics of interest. Early clinical studies reported that scapular notching seemed to stabilize and did not progress in most patients [65]. However, recent studies have shown that the frequency of notching increases significantly with follow-up time, and the grade typically increases over time, as well. In a series of 448 patients, Levigne et al. [94] found notching in 48% of cases at 1 year postoperatively, 60% at 2 years, and 68% at 3 years. Melis et al. [95] studied a cohort with a mean of 9.5 years of follow-up (range 8–12 years) and showed that the incidence of notching increased with time. Nyffeler et al. [96] suggested that repetitive contact between the polyethylene of the humeral component and the opposing scapular bone may result in wear debris, chronic inflammation, and osteolysis. Although some of the notching observed on radiographs may be caused in part by osteolysis from particle debris, this has not been established in RTSA. However, no study has shown that scapular notching is associated with eventual glenoid loosening.

The reported incidence of scapular notching varies from 0 to 96% (Table 22.5). Notching has been found to be caused by various factors. Levigne et al. [92] noted that postoperative scapular notching was seen more frequently in patients who had rotator cuff arthropathy, fatty infiltration of the infraspinatus, narrowed acromiohumeral distance, and superior glenoid erosion, as well as those who underwent an anterosuperior surgical approach. Superior inclination of the glenosphere was identified as a factor that can lead to high shear forces between the baseplate and the glenoid surface. Preoperatively, it is important to determine whether the glenoid has superior tilt using a coronal CT scan or to evaluate the glenoid morphology with 3-dimensional imaging or 3-dimensional plastic scapular models. If there is a neutral orientation or inferior tilt to the glenoid surface, it should be reamed to create up to 10° of inferior tilt. However, if there is a superior tilt to the glenoid, the glenoid should be reamed to at least a neutral position to correct the superior inclination. Nyffeler et al. [96] found that inferior tilt of the glenoid component can reduce the incidence of scapular notching. Although several technical considerations have been proposed to help address the issue of scapular notching, including tilting the baseplate inferiorly, allowing the baseplate to hang over the inferior lip of the glenoid, and using an asymmetric glenosphere, none of these modifications has been definitively proven to alter scapular notching.

Changes in the design of RTSA components may have influenced frequency of scapular notching. One area of controversy has been the relationship of the COR of the prosthesis as it relates to the COR of the normal shoulder. The use of a less medial COR has been suggested to produce less scapular notching. Cuff et al. [97] felt that the more lateral COR helped prevent contact of the humeral prosthesis.

Another factor believed to be related to less notching is the head-neck angle of the humeral prosthesis [98]. Nicholson et al. [99] used a prosthesis with a head-neck angle of 150° and reported a decreased incidence of scapular notching at 6 months (0%) and at 14 months (8%) versus those with a more horizontal component. Gutierrez et al. [24] found that reducing the humeral component neck-shaft angle had the largest effect on inferior scapular impingement allowed by inferior placement of the glenosphere baseplate relative to the native glenoid in a laboratory RTSA model. In addition, Kempton et al. [15] reported that a prosthesis with a neck-shaft angle of 143° and a 2.5-mm COR offset had a lower incidence of scapular notching (16%) than another prosthesis with a neck-shaft angle of 155° and no COR offset (61%).

Instability

Instability or dislocation of the RTSA components is a common complication of RTSA. Usually, these are not subluxations but rather dislocations of the humeral component off the glenosphere. Instability of RTSA has been reported to occur at rates of 0 to 31% (Table 22.6). Dislocation typically occurs when the humeral component comes out anteriorly and laterally (Fig. 22.34). The arm often is obviously deformed as it falls into extension, adduction, and internal rotation.

There are several possible reasons for instability of RTSA. Instability can result from inadequate tension of the soft tissue envelope around the shoulder. This is a concern in patients with previous surgery and those who have failed previous arthroplasty. A second contributing factor is believed to be impingement of the humeral component on the glenoid with the arm in adduction. The last factor is that tight inferior capsular structures such as those seen with posterior displaced greater tuberosities after a fracture can lever the component out of the socket laterally. Chalmers et al. [100] reported that the variables that increased risk of dislocation in RTSA included a body mass index higher than 30, male sex, subscapularis deficiency, and previous surgery.

Table 22.6 Instability rates and risk factors from the literature on RTSA

Study	No. of patients	Instability rate, %	Prosthesis (manufacturer)	Primary, %	Revision, %	Risk factors
Werner et al. [65]	58	8.6	Delta III (DePuy, Warsaw, IN)	5	14	NR
Boileau et al. [101]	45	6.7	Delta III	4	10	Insufficient tension of deltoid
Wall et al. [50]	191	7.5	Delta III; Aequalis (Tornier, Montbonnot, France)	NR	NR	NR
Gallo et al. [103]	57	16	Delta III; Encore RSP (Encore Medical, Austin, TX)	10	28	Revision; infection; subscapularis abnormality
Trappey et al. [111]	284	6	Aequalis	5	8	Subscapularis deficiency; fracture sequelae
Clark et al. [106]	120	4	RSP (DonJoy Surgical, Austin, TX)	NR	NR	NR
Muh et al. [149]	67	7.5	Aequalis	NR	NR	NR
Ortmaier et al. [150]	50	10	Delta III; Delta Xtend (Depuy)	0	10	Insufficient tension of deltoid
Chalmers et al. [100][a]	385	2.9	Trabecular metal (Zimmer, Warsaw, IN); Aequalis; Delta III	NR	NR	BMI >30; male sex; subscapularis deficiency; previous surgery

NR not reported, *RSP* reverse shoulder prosthesis
[a]Reported on dislocations occurring in the first 3 months

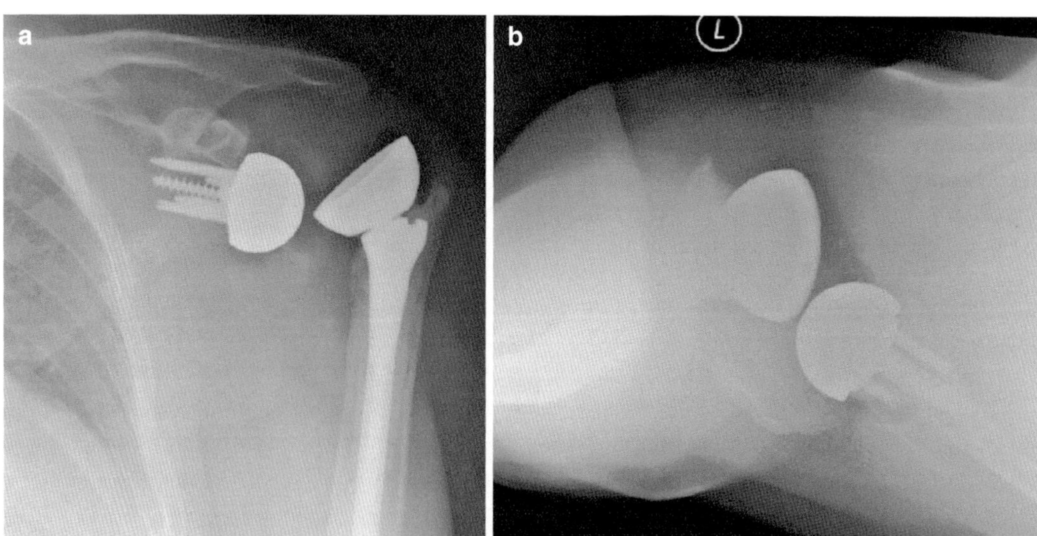

Fig. 22.34 (**a**) Anteroposterior and (**b**) axillary radiographs showing anterior dislocation of prosthesis after reverse total shoulder arthroplasty

Surgical factors have also been implicated as a cause of instability. These include decisions the surgeon makes about soft tissue tension and position. Prosthetic choices such as the glenosphere offsets and sizes, version of the humeral prosthesis, thickness of the humeral insert, bony deficiency, and axillary nerve/deltoid dysfunction can influence instability. Patients who have a lax soft tissue envelope may require a larger sphere or thicker humeral polyethylene to achieve proper tensioning. Gutierrez et al. [24] recommended a humeral neck shaft angle of 130°, lateral offset of 19 mm, and glenosphere with a 42-mm diameter to increase the range of impingement-free adduction.

Soft tissue tension during the implantation of RTSA can be helpful in preventing instability. Boileau et al. [101] suggested that proper tensioning of the prosthesis can be determined by palpating the tension generated within the conjoined tendon after reduction of the implant. Ladermann et al. [102] described a radiographic method of determining optimal deltoid tension on the basis of humeral length, comparing the operative side and using the distance from the acromion to the epicondyle on scaled radiographs. Instability also may be caused by loosening and infection. Therefore, patients who present with instability after RTSA should be evaluated for infection, especially if there is component loosening. Instability accompanied infection in 44% of cases reported in the literature [103].

The role of subscapularis repair to the lesser tuberosity in the development of postoperative instability of RTSA is controversial. Edwards et al. [104] suggested that subscapularis reattachment may be beneficial in reducing the rate of dislocation. Boileau et al. [101] suggested that an anterosuperior transdeltoid approach without damage of the subscapularis contributes to a lower incidence of instability. Ackland et al. [105] suggested that in RTSA, the anterior and middle deltoid subregion, along with the superior aspect of the pectoralis major muscle subregion, acts as an abductor, whereas the latissimus dorsi, the teres major, and the inferior aspect of the pectoralis major muscle subregion act like an adductor, leading to increased tension and stability. However, Clark et al. [106] reported that subscapularis repair had no significant effect on dislocation rates. The role of the subscapularis with respect to instability is likely related to the design of the prosthesis used.

Before reduction of a dislocated RTSA, the patient should undergo radiography to rule out fractures, component loosening, and disassociation. A complete neurological and vascular examination should also be performed. After completing a thorough evaluation, first-line management of a dislocation typically consists of closed reduction, which is best performed with fluoroscopic guidance and intravenous sedation. If the reduction is unsuccessful, the shoulder can be reduced under general anesthesia at a later time. The reduced shoulder should be checked through a range of motion to determine which position produces instability. After closed reduction, the arm can be braced in a stable position for 6 weeks or more.

Gerber et al. [107] suggested that dislocations in the first 3 months after surgery are most likely secondary to surgical error and less likely to be successfully treated with closed reduction compared with late dislocations. Conversely, Chalmers et al. [100] reported on early dislocation (within 3 months) after RTSA and found that four of nine patients remained stable at a mean follow-up of 2.5 years. Teusink et al. [108] showed that an initial dislocation episode after RTSA can be treated successfully with closed reduction and temporary immobilization regardless of the time since dislocation. If instability persists despite closed reduction, attention should be directed to correcting any soft tissue or component positioning that might be contributing to the instability. Malposition of implants and inadequate soft tissue tensioning should be considered indications for revision surgery when the instability is recurrent. Treatment options include placement of a larger glenosphere or use of a more constrained humeral polyethylene implant.

Aseptic Baseplate Loosening

Baseplate loosening can be aseptic or septic. In a review of the Norwegian Arthroplasty Register from 1994 to 2005, the authors found the aseptic baseplate loosening (Fig. 22.35) rate from 1994 to 2005 in Grammont-type RTSA to be 5% [109]. A systematic review of the literature reported that the rate of aseptic loosening in 782 patients with RTSA was 3.5% [89]. The most common cause of baseplate loosening was poor initial fixation of the baseplate. Because the reverse shoulder baseplate is fixed without cement, sufficient initial fixation is critical.

The more recent designs of baseplate components may have reduced the incidence of aseptic baseplate loosening. The use of multiple or large-diameter locking screws, as well as variable-angle locking screws, is designed to improve initial fixation of the baseplate until bone ingrowth occurs. Guides for reaming the glenoid in a slight inferior tilt have been theorized to decrease the shear forces that can cause baseplate failure [23].

The relationship between scapular notching and subsequent baseplate loosening and failure continues to be debated. The longest clinical study of RTSA, with follow-up of more than 9 years, reported a 32% rate of glenoid loosening [110]. Longer clinical follow-up is needed to better understand the relationship between scapular notching and glenoid loosening. In the previous study, the notching rate after 9 years of follow-up was 90%. If radiographs show baseplate screw failure alone without other signs of movement of the baseplate, early removal of the implant can be considered. Other factors can also influence baseplate failure (Table 22.7).

Infection

Periprosthetic infection after RTSA is difficult to treat for several reasons. Infection after RTSA (Fig. 22.36; Table 22.8) can lead to severe bone loss and poor functional outcome because of destruction of rotator cuff tendons that were previously functioning. Therefore, early diagnosis and proper treatment are important to prevent severe bone and soft tissue damage. Infection rates after RTSA have been reported to range from 1 to 15% [111]. According to a systematic review of 21 studies including 782 patients, the rate of deep infection after RTSA was 3.8% [89]. A case series of 301 patients with minimum 1-year follow-up reported a 5% infection rate

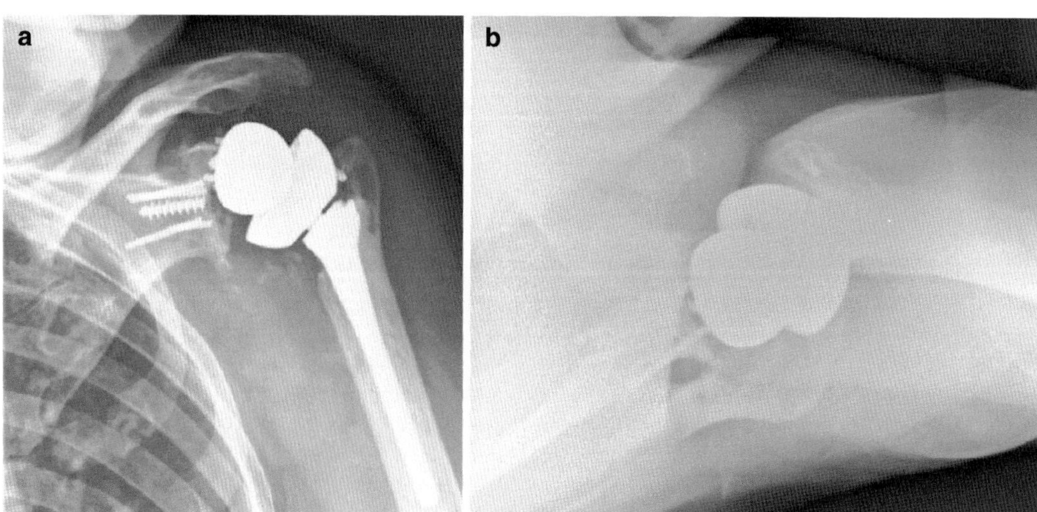

Fig. 22.35 (**a**) Anteroposterior and (**b**) axillary radiographs 19 months after reverse total shoulder arthroplasty showing an aseptic baseplate loosening with broken screw

Table 22.7 Baseplate failure after RTSA

Study	No. of shoulders	Mean (range) follow-up, months	Prosthesis (manufacturer)	Failure rate, %	Mean months to loosening	Treatment (no.)	Cause
Frankle et al. [142]	60	33 (24–68)	RSP (DJO Surgical, Austin, TX)	8.3	21	Revision to another RSA (5)	Metal fatigue in screws
Werner et al. [65]	58	38 (minimum 24)	Delta III (DePuy, Warsaw, IN)	5.1	NR	Conversion to hemiarthroplasty (3)	NR
Guery et al. [156]	80	70 (60–121)	Delta III	2.5	NR	Conversion to hemiarthroplasty (1)	Baseplate malposition
Wall et al. [50]	191	40 (24–118)	Delta III; Aequalis (Tornier, Montbonnot, France)	1.0	NR	NR	Surgical error (superior tilt, peg of baseplate too short)
Cuff et al. [97]	96	28 (24–38)	RSP (Encore Medical, Austin, TX)	1.0	12	Revision to another RSA (1)	NR
Mulieri et al. [64]	60	52 (24–101)	RSP (DJO Surgical)	6.7	36	Revision to another RSA (4)	3.5-mm nonlocking peripheral screws (4)
Melis et al. [157]	37	47 (24–104)	Delta III; Aequalis	8.1	NR	Glenoid revision, graft and long peg (2); conversion to hemiarthroplasty (1)	Peg of baseplate too short (3)
Ek et al. [151]	40	93 (60–171)	Delta III; Anatomic shoulder reverse (Zimmer, Winterthur, Switzerland)	7.5	NR	Conversion to hemiarthroplasty (3)	Glenoid fracture (1), infection (1), unknown (1)
Wagner et al. [153]	40	37 (24–72)	Comprehensive reverse shoulder (Biomet, Warsaw, IN); Encore RSP (DJO Surgical); Delta Xtend (DePuy); Aequalis	10	14	Conversion to hemiarthroplasty (3); revision to another RSA (1)	Smoker

NR not reported, *RSA* reverse shoulder arthroplasty, *RSP* reverse shoulder prosthesis

[112]. In comparison, the prevalence of deep infection after anatomical TSA has been reported to range from 0.7 to 3.9% [113, 114].

The reason for the higher infection rate in RTSA versus TSA is multifactorial. These include the large dead space caused by the reverse prosthesis configuration and soft tissue loss, the relatively older age of patients who undergo RTSA, and history of previous shoulder surgeries. The risk of infection after revision to RTSA is 7% compared with an infection rate of 1% in patients who have not had previous surgery [111]. Hematoma formation is a known risk factor for deep infection, and Gerber et al. [35] reported hematoma formation was a risk for reoperation in the period immediately after RTSA. Patients with rheumatoid arthritis have been reported to have a higher infection rate, upwards of 9.5%, after RTSA [115]. Morris et al. [112] reported history of a prior failed arthroplasty and age younger than 65 years as independent risk factors for infection after RTSA.

Infection of RTSA should be considered to be present in a patient with persistent pain. Pain is the most reliable evidence of infection. Most patients have no constitutional signs of infection or physical signs such as redness, warmth, swelling, or drainage. Laboratory blood test results may or may not be abnormal but there are many false-negative results [116, 117] for erythrocyte sedimentation rate and C-reactive protein. Aspiration can be of some benefit but the accuracy of identifying the presence of infection and isolating pathogens continues to be debated [118]. Loosening of the components, especially the humeral component, is nearly diagnostic for infection.

The most common organisms isolated from culture have changed over the last decade. Initially, *Staphylococcus* species were the most common organisms causing infections after shoulder arthroplasty. However, recently most shoulder arthroplasty infections have been caused by *Propionibacterium acnes*. These organisms typically cause chronic, low-grade infections with bone erosion and subsequent loosening of the prosthesis. This species may require 10–14 days of incubation in the laboratory to ensure proper identification. It is important that the laboratory incubate these specimens for at least 15 days after aspiration or tissue culturing (Fig. 22.36).

The guidelines for treatment of deep infection after RTSA are similar to those for other joint arthroplasties. Acute infection occurring less than 6 weeks after surgery can be treated with thorough irrigation, debridement, and polyethylene exchange. If an infection presents later than 6 weeks after surgery, which meets the definition of a chronic infection, a 2-stage revision is recommended. The first stage includes prosthesis removal, irrigation and debridement, and antibiotic spacer insertion, followed by a minimum 6-week course of parenteral, culture-specific antibiotics (Fig. 22.37). The second stage involves removal of the spacer and RTSA prosthesis reimplantation. At the time of surgery, microscopic evaluation of the joint tissue should confirm the absence of infection before implantation of the revision prosthesis. After confirming the infection has been eliminated by joint aspiration, inflammatory marker trends, and intraoperative frozen sections, revision surgery can proceed.

Nerve Injury

The incidence of nerve injury after RTSA has been reported to be 1.5 to 24% (Table 22.9). This is comparable to the reported nerve injury rate for TSA of between 2.2 and 20% [119]. Ladermann et al. [120] compared patients who underwent TSA with a group who underwent RTSA. They found that, compared with TSA, the relative risk of nerve injury for RTSA was 11 with an odds ratio of 17 after adjusting for patient age. The most common involvement is a partial brachial plexus lesion, followed by individual nerve injuries. Similar to anatomical TSA, the most commonly injured nerve is the axillary nerve. Most nerve injuries are neuropraxia and fully resolve with no residual symptoms.

Nerve injury may be caused by several intraoperative factors: direct nerve injury by surgical

Category	Criteria
No evidence for infection	All negative cultures (tissue or aspirate) and no preoperative or intraoperative findings of infection*
Possible infection	Negative preoperative or intraoperative finding and one positive intraoprative culture
Probable infection	More than one positive intraoperative culture and negative preoperative or intraoperative findings
	OR
	At least one positive preoperative or intraoperative finding and one positive culture
Definite infection	At least one positive preoperative or intraoperative finding of infection and more than one positive intraoperative culture
	OR
	One positive preoperative (aspirate) culture† and one positive intraoperative culture

* Preoperative or intraoperative findings of infection include preoperative clinical signs (swelling, sinus tract, redness, drainage), positive erythrocyte sedimentation rate or C-reactive protein, positive frozen section, and intraoperative gross findings (pus, drainage, necrosis).

† Positive preoperative aspirate has its own category, because it is more definitive then these findings.

Fig. 22.36 Criteria for infection categories. (Reprinted with permission from: Grosso MJ, Frangiamore SJ, Ricchetti ET, Bauer TW, Iannotti JP. Sensitivity of frozen section histology for identifying *Propionibacterium acnes* infections in revision shoulder arthroplasty. J Bone Joint Surg Am. 2014;96:442–7.)

Table 22.8 Infection rate after RTSA

Study	No. of shoulders	Mean (range) follow-up, months	Infection rate, %	Organisms (no. of cases)	Result of surgery (no.)
Boileau et al. [101]	45	40 (24–72)	7	NR	Resection arthroplasty (2); 1-stage humeral stem revision (1)
Wall et al. [50]	191	40 (24–118)	4	NR	NR
Zavala et al. [158]	137	44 (minimum 12)	6	*Propionibacterium*, no growth (2 each); MSSA, MRSA (1 each)	Poly exchange (3); resection arthroplasty, irrigation and debridement (2 each)
Ortmaier et al. [159]	192	74 (24–115)	10	Mixed organisms (7); *Propionibacterium* (6); *Staphylococcus epidermidis* (4); *Corynebacterium* (3)	Two-stage revision (13); resection arthroplasty (4); irrigation and debridement (2); prolonged spacer implantation (1)[a]
Morris et al. [112]	301	Minimum 12	5	No growth (5); MSSA (3); MRSA, *Propionibacterium* (2); *S. epidermidis*, coagulase-negative *Staphylococcus*, *Enterobacter* (1 each)	Resection arthroplasty (11); 2-stage revision (4)

MRSA methicillin-resistant *Staphylococcus aureus*, *MSSA* methicillin-susceptible *S. aureus*, *NR* not reported
[a]Outcomes were reported as good or excellent (30%), satisfying (40%), or dissatisfying (30%)

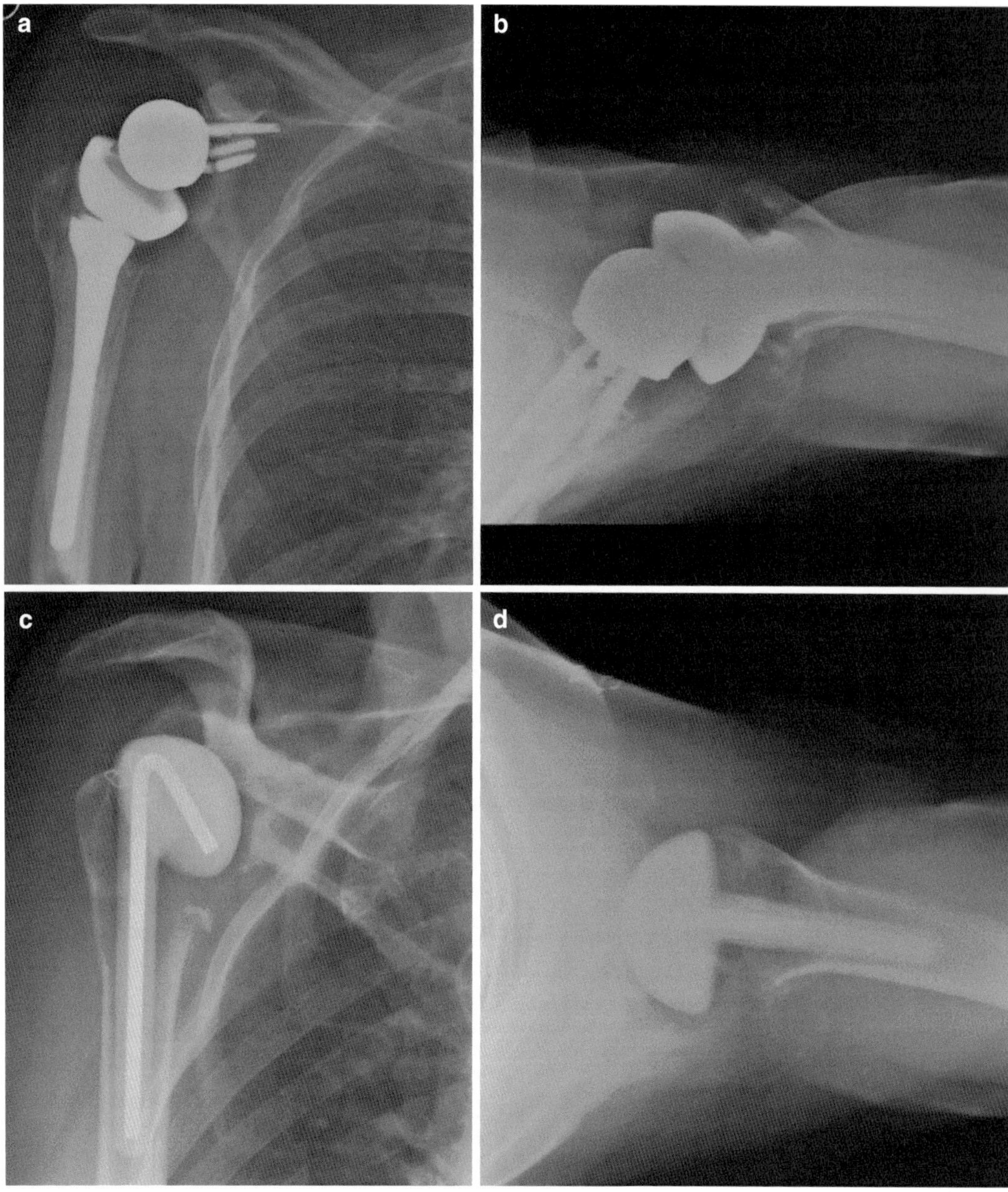

Fig. 22.37 (**a**) Anteroposterior and (**b**) axillary radiographs showing gross baseplate loosening caused by infection. (**c**) Anteroposterior and (**d**) axillary radiographs after first-stage revision with a temporary antibiotic spacer

dissection or nerve stretch by traction on the arm, manipulation of the arm in adduction and external rotation, and exuberant retractor placement [121]. Arm lengthening with RTSA may also contribute to nerve injury. Van Hoof et al. [122] showed that the RTSA prosthesis can place the brachial plexus under tension in a cadaver study using a 3D computer model. They found that their model estimated strains up to 15% greater than anatomic conditions for the lateral root and 19% for the medial root of the median nerve when implanting RTSA components.

Table 22.9 Summary of neurologic injury after RTSA

Study	No. of patients	Mean (range) follow-up, months	Neurologic injury rate, %	Nerve	Mean time to recovery, months	Recovery
Werner et al. [65]	58	48	1.7	Axillary	NR	Complete
Boileau et al. [101]	45	40 (24–72)	2.2	Axillary	36	Limited
Levy et al. [85]	29	NR	3.4	Radial	NR	Complete
Kempton et al. [148]	192	19 (6–49)	3.6	NR	Several weeks	Complete
Ek et al. [151]	40	93 (60–171)	5	Radial; brachial plexus	6 (radial nerve) and 12 (brachial plexus nerve)	Complete
Muh et al. [149]	67	36 (24–77)	1.5	Radial	30 (most recent follow-up)	Limited
Ball et al. [160]	116	NR	24	Median	24 (maximum)	Slow (most by 6 months)

NR not reported

Intraoperative Fracture

Intraoperative fractures are uncommon, and although they occur mainly on the humeral side, glenoid fractures can also occur. Zumstein et al. [89] reported 16 intraoperative humeral fractures (2%) and seven glenoid fractures (0.9%) in a systematic review of 782 cases of RTSA.

Intraoperative glenoid fractures typically are caused by the reaming process or during implantation of the glenoid baseplate [89]. Preoperative CT scanning is helpful to know the glenoid morphology. It also helps the surgeon know preoperatively where the glenoid bone is the thinnest and whether bone grafting might be needed. The surgeon should ensure that the reamer is started before contacting the glenoid and should not ream beyond the subchondral bone. It is important to ream cautiously to prevent the reamer from catching on the edge of unreamed subchondral bone, causing the reamer to torque off and fracture the glenoid [121].

Treatment of an intraoperative glenoid fracture primarily depends on the location and extent of the fracture. The major consideration is that stability of the baseplate not be compromised. If the fracture is into the central hole of the baseplate, then stability of the baseplate may be compromised. In some cases, bone grafting and reliance on peripheral screw fixation may be sufficient. In rare instances, the central fixation of the baseplate may be moved to a portion of the glenoid not fractured. If there are grossly unstable fragments, then consideration should be given to bone grafting and performing hemiarthroplasty with RTSA as a second stage. Fracture fragment fixation in such cases can be technically demanding, and unless secure fixation can be obtained, 2-stage reconstruction should be considered [123].

The major risk factor for humerus fracture is previous surgery, especially a previous arthroplasty with either a cemented or cementless humeral stem [124]. The proximal humerus is frequently osteopenic, especially if cemented humeral stems are implanted. Avoiding excessive torque while placing the arm in adduction or extension during preparation and reaming of the humeral canal and reaming the canal by hand are recommended [121].

As in anatomical TSA, the management of humeral fractures in RTSA depends on the location and extent of the fracture. If the humeral fracture occurs at the metaphysis or tuberosities, it can be treated with cerclage fixation or reattachment of the fragment. Repair of the external rotators and greater tuberosity should be attempted to avoid weakness in external rotation. Fragment excision is discouraged unless the fragments are too comminuted to repair. Lesser tuberosity fractures are important mainly if they are large enough to affect the stability of the humeral implant. If fracture of the humeral diaphysis occurs before humeral implantation, there are several options. The first is to use cerclage wires around the shaft proximally. If necessary, these can be augmented with autograft from the humeral head or with allograft either as morselized bone or strut augmentation. Plate-and-screw fixation may be needed if the fracture is extensive and at the tip of the prosthesis. Lastly, the use of a longer stem to bypass the fracture site can be considered. Cementing the stem can also ensure that the prosthesis is stable after fracture fixation. A fracture after humeral stem implantation should be treated according to its location. Proximal fractures can be treated with a combination of cerclage wires or plates and screws. More distal fractures may need to be repaired with plates and screws or conversion to a long-stem prosthesis [121, 123].

Component Disassociation

Component disassociation can be a devastating complication, but fortunately it is rare. There are three types of disassociation. The glenosphere can come off, the polyethylene can come out of the component, or the humeral component can become unscrewed. Displacement of the glenosphere from the baseplate occurred in prosthetic designs used before 1995. It led to a change in the prosthetic design using a Morse taper between the glenosphere and baseplate. Despite using a Morse taper, Middernacht et al. [125] reported glenosphere disengagement in 16 of 479 patients (3.3%) with RTSA. The authors found 13 cases of partial disengagement, in which the central screw was intact and the glenosphere remained seated on the baseplate but with a clear step-off on radiographs, and three cases of total disengagement of the glenosphere from the baseplate. Cusick et al. [126] reported 13 glenosphere dissociations (total disengagement), which was less than 1% of their 1800 patients. They concluded that glenosphere dissociation was caused by trauma, improper taper engagement, or larger diameter glenospheres (40 or 44 mm).

Disassociation of the implant also can occur with the unscrewing of the metaphysis-diaphysis (Fig. 22.38) joint in the modular humeral component [113, 127–129]. Unscrewing of the humeral component typically occurred in patients with proximal humeral bone deficiency treated with a modular humeral component. Two of three cases of humeral component unscrewing reported by De Wilde and Walch [128] suggested that the mechanism of unscrewing can be explained by blockage of the epiphysis against the anterior wall of the glenoid in maximal internal rotation during forearm flexion. Ansari et al. [127] found extensive metallosis in two cases that had unscrewing of the humeral component at the time of removal. They proposed that metal debris released from fretting wear at the unstable screw joint can cause major tissue damage. Also, the authors reported one fracture that occurred at the metaphysis-diaphysis screw junction. They suggested that three factors (lack of proximal bone support, reduction of the cross-sectional diameter, and stress concentration provided by the through-hole) contributed to a weaker metaphysis-diaphysis interface in this case. Both studies suggested that unscrewing of the humeral

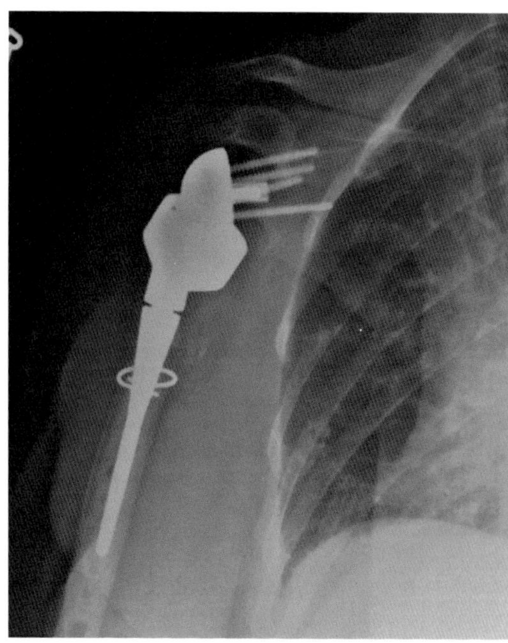

Fig. 22.38 Radiograph showing unscrewing of the metaphysis-diaphysis joint

prosthesis can be prevented by improved prosthetic design.

Questions

Common complications seen with RTSA for three- and four-part humeral fractures are:

A. *Complex regional pain syndrome*
B. *Scapular notching*
C. *Tuberosity malunion*
D. *All of the above*

Commonly found micro-organisms are (select all that apply):

A. *Staphylococci*
B. *Propionibacterium acnes*
C. *Streptococci*
D. *Escherichia coli*

According to level-1 studies, there is strong evidence to support that four-part fractures of the proximal humerus in elderly patients should be treated with:

A. *Hemiarthroplasty rather than reverse shoulder arthroplasty*
B. *Reverse shoulder arthroplasty rather than hemiarthroplasty*
C. *Both techniques are equally effective*
D. *No high-level studies exist to support this yet*

References

1. Neer II CS. Articular replacement for the humeral head. J Bone Joint Surg Am. 1955;37-A(2):215–28.
2. Neer II CS, Watson KC, Stanton FJ. Recent experience in total shoulder replacement. J Bone Joint Surg Am. 1982;64(3):319–37.
3. Neer II CS, Craig EV, Fukuda H. Cuff-tear arthropathy. J Bone Joint Surg Am. 1983;65(9):1232–44.
4. Halder AM, Kuhl SG, Zobitz ME, Larson D, An KN. Effects of the glenoid labrum and glenohumeral abduction on stability of the shoulder joint through concavity-compression: an in vitro study. J Bone Joint Surg Am. 2001;83-A(7):1062–9.
5. Inman VT, Saunders JB, Abbott LC. Observations of the function of the shoulder joint. 1944. Clin Orthop. 1996;330:3–12.
6. Hamada K, Fukuda H, Mikasa M, Kobayashi Y. Roentgenographic findings in massive rotator cuff tears. A long-term observation. Clin Orthop. 1990;254:92–6.
7. Matsen III FA, Clinton J, Lynch J, Bertelsen A, Richardson ML. Glenoid component failure in total shoulder arthroplasty. J Bone Joint Surg Am. 2008;90(4):885–96. doi:10.2106/jbjs.g.01263.
8. Kessel L, Bayley I. Prosthetic replacement of shoulder joint: preliminary communication. J R Soc Med. 1979;72(10):748–52.
9. Fenlin Jr JM. Total glenohumeral joint replacement. Orthop Clin North Am. 1975;6(2):565–83.
10. Grammont P, Laffay JP, Deries X. Concept study and realization of a new total shoulder prosthesis [French]. Rhumatologie. 1987;39:407–18.
11. Baulot E, Sirveaux F, Boileau P. Grammont's idea: the story of Paul Grammont's functional surgery concept and the development of the reverse principle. Clin Orthop. 2011;469(9):2425–31. doi:10.1007/s11999-010-1757-y.
12. Howell SM, Galinat BJ. The glenoid-labral socket. A constrained articular surface. Clin Orthop. 1989;243:122–5.
13. Sirveaux F. Grammont prosthesis in the treatment of shoulder arthropathies with massive cuff tear. Multicenter series of 42 cases [in French]. Medical Doctor Thesis. Nancy I University (France), 1997.
14. Sirveaux F, Favard L, Oudet D, Huquet D, Walch G, Mole D. Grammont inverted total shoulder arthroplasty in the treatment of glenohumeral osteoarthritis with massive rupture of the cuff. Results of a multicentre study of 80 shoulders. J Bone Joint Surg Br. 2004;86(3):388–95. doi:10.1302/0301-620X.86B3.
15. Kempton LB, Balasubramaniam M, Ankerson E, Wiater JM. A radiographic analysis of the effects of prosthesis design on scapular notching following reverse total shoulder arthroplasty. J Shoulder Elb Surg. 2011;20(4):571–6. doi:10.1016/j.jse.2010.08.024.
16. Williams GR, Iannotti JP. Biomechanics of the glenohumeral joint: influence on shoulder arthroplasty. In: Iannotti JP, Williams GR, editors. Disorders of the shoulder: diagnosis and management. 1st ed. Philadelphia: Lippincott Williams and Wilkins; 1999. p. 471–83.
17. Langohr GD, Willing R, Medley JB, Athwal GS, Johnson JA. Contact mechanics of reverse total shoulder arthroplasty during abduction: the effect of neck-shaft angle, humeral cup depth, and glenosphere diameter. J Shoulder Elb Surg. 2015; doi:10.1016/j.jse.2015.09.024.
18. Edelson G. Variations in the retroversion of the humeral head. J Shoulder Elb Surg. 1999;8(2):142–5.
19. Henninger HB, Barg A, Anderson AE, Bachus KN, Tashjian RZ, Burks RT. Effect of deltoid tension and humeral version in reverse total shoulder arthroplasty: a biomechanical study. J Shoulder Elb Surg. 2012;21(4):483–90. doi:10.1016/j.jse.2011.01.040.

20. Jeon BK, Panchal KA, Ji JH, Xin YZ, Park SR, Kim JH, Yang SJ. Combined effect of change in humeral neck-shaft angle and retroversion on shoulder range of motion in reverse total shoulder arthroplasty—a simulation study. Clin Biomech (Bristol, Avon). 2016;31:12–9. doi:10.1016/j.clinbiomech.2015.06.022.
21. Ladermann A, Denard PJ, Boileau P, Farron A, Deransart P, Terrier A, Ston J, Walch G. Effect of humeral stem design on humeral position and range of motion in reverse shoulder arthroplasty. Int Orthop. 2015;39(11):2205–13. doi:10.1007/s00264-015-2984-3.
22. Frankle MA, Siegal S, Pupello DR, Gutierrez S, Griewe M, Mighell MA, Hart R. Coronal plane tilt angle affects the risk of catastrophic failure in patients treated with a reverse shoulder prosthesis [abstr]. J Shoulder Elb Surg. 2007;16(2):e46.
23. Gutierrez S, Greiwe RM, Frankle MA, Siegal S, Lee III WE. Biomechanical comparison of component position and hardware failure in the reverse shoulder prosthesis. J Shoulder Elb Surg. 2007;16(3 Suppl):9S–12S. doi:10.1016/j.jse.2005.11.008.
24. Gutierrez S, Comiskey IV CA, Luo ZP, Pupello DR, Frankle MA. Range of impingement-free abduction and adduction deficit after reverse shoulder arthroplasty. Hierarchy of surgical and implant-design-related factors. J Bone Joint Surg Am. 2008;90(12):2606–15. doi:10.2106/jbjs.h.00012.
25. Edwards TB, Trappey GJ, Riley C, O'Connor DP, Elkousy HA, Gartsman GM. Inferior tilt of the glenoid component does not decrease scapular notching in reverse shoulder arthroplasty: results of a prospective randomized study. J Shoulder Elb Surg. 2012;21(5):641–6. doi:10.1016/j.jse.2011.08.057.
26. Simovitch RW, Zumstein MA, Lohri E, Helmy N, Gerber C. Predictors of scapular notching in patients managed with the Delta III reverse total shoulder replacement. J Bone Joint Surg Am. 2007;89(3):588–600.
27. Kelly 2nd JD, Humphrey CS, Norris TR. Optimizing glenosphere position and fixation in reverse shoulder arthroplasty, Part One: the twelve-mm rule. J Shoulder Elb Surg. 2008;17(4):589–94. doi:10.1016/j.jse.2007.08.013.
28. Poon PC, Chou J, Young SW, Astley T. A comparison of concentric and eccentric glenospheres in reverse shoulder arthroplasty: a randomized controlled trial. J Bone Joint Surg Am. 2014;96(16):e138. doi:10.2106/jbjs.m.00941.
29. Kowalsky MS, Galatz LM, Shia DS, Steger-May K, Keener JD. The relationship between scapular notching and reverse shoulder arthroplasty prosthesis design. J Shoulder Elb Surg. 2012;21(10):1430–41. doi:10.1016/j.jse.2011.08.051.
30. James J, Huffman KR, Werner FW, Sutton LG, Nanavati VN. Does glenoid baseplate geometry affect its fixation in reverse shoulder arthroplasty? J Shoulder Elb Surg. 2012;21(7):917–24. doi:10.1016/j.jse.2011.04.017.
31. Langohr GD, Giles JW, Athwal GS, Johnson JA. The effect of glenosphere diameter in reverse shoulder arthroplasty on muscle force, joint load, and range of motion. J Shoulder Elb Surg. 2015;24(6):972–9. doi:10.1016/j.jse.2014.10.018.
32. Chou J, Malak SF, Anderson IA, Astley T, Poon PC. Biomechanical evaluation of different designs of glenospheres in the SMR reverse total shoulder prosthesis: range of motion and risk of scapular notching. J Shoulder Elb Surg. 2009;18(3):354–9. doi:10.1016/j.jse.2009.01.015.
33. Katz D, Valenti P, Kany J, Elkholti K, Werthel JD. Does lateralisation of the centre of rotation in reverse shoulder arthroplasty avoid scapular notching? Clinical and radiological review of one hundred and forty cases with forty five months of follow-up. Int Orthop. 2016;40(1):99–108. doi:10.1007/s00264-015-2976-3.
34. Iannotti JP, Norris TR. Influence of preoperative factors on outcome of shoulder arthroplasty for glenohumeral osteoarthritis. J Bone Joint Surg Am. 2003;85(2):251–8.
35. Gerber C, Costouros JG, Sukthankar A, Fucentese SF. Static posterior humeral head subluxation and total shoulder arthroplasty. J Shoulder Elb Surg. 2009;18(4):505–10. doi:10.1016/j.jse.2009.03.003.
36. Habermeyer P, Magosch P, Lichtenberg S. Recentering the humeral head for glenoid deficiency in total shoulder arthroplasty. Clin Orthop. 2007;457:124–32. doi:10.1097/BLO.0b013e31802ff03c.
37. Walch G, Badet R, Boulahia A, Khoury A. Morphologic study of the glenoid in primary glenohumeral osteoarthritis. J Arthroplast. 1999;14(6):756–60. doi:10.1016/S0883-5403(99)90232-2.
38. Collin P, Treseder T, Denard PJ, Neyton L, Walch G, Ladermann A. What is the best clinical test for assessment of the teres minor in massive rotator cuff tears? Clin Orthop. 2015;473(9):2959–66. doi:10.1007/s11999-015-4392-9.
39. Namdari S, Voleti P, Baldwin K, Glaser D, Huffman GR. Latissimus dorsi tendon transfer for irreparable rotator cuff tears: a systematic review. J Bone Joint Surg Am. 2012;94(10):891–8. doi:10.2106/jbjs.k.00841.
40. Gerber C, Pennington SD, Lingenfelter EJ, Sukthankar A. Reverse Delta-III total shoulder replacement combined with latissimus dorsi transfer. A preliminary report. J Bone Joint Surg Am. 2007;89(5):940–7. doi:10.2106/jbjs.f.00955.
41. Boileau P, Chuinard C, Roussanne Y, Bicknell RT, Rochet N, Trojani C. Reverse shoulder arthroplasty combined with a modified latissimus dorsi and teres major tendon transfer for shoulder pseudoparalysis associated with dropping arm. Clin Orthop. 2008;466(3):584–93. doi:10.1007/s11999-008-0114-x.
42. Boileau P, Rumian AP, Zumstein MA. Reversed shoulder arthroplasty with modified L'Episcopo for combined loss of active elevation and external rota-

tion. J Shoulder Elb Surg. 2010;19(2 Suppl):20–30. doi:10.1016/j.jse.2009.12.011.
43. Ortmaier R, Resch H, Hitzl W, Mayer M, Blocher M, Vasvary I, Mattiassich G, Stundner O, Tauber M. Reverse shoulder arthroplasty combined with latissimus dorsi transfer using the bone-chip technique. Int Orthop. 2014;38(3):553–9. doi:10.1007/s00264-013-2139-3.
44. Sanders TG, Jersey SL. Conventional radiography of the shoulder. Semin Roentgenol. 2005;40(3): 207–22.
45. Koh KH, Han KY, Yoon YC, Lee SW, Yoo JC. True anteroposterior (Grashey) view as a screening radiograph for further imaging study in rotator cuff tear. J Shoulder Elb Surg. 2013;22(7):901–7. doi:10.1016/j.jse.2012.09.015.
46. Frankle MA, Teramoto A, Luo ZP, Levy JC, Pupello D. Glenoid morphology in reverse shoulder arthroplasty: classification and surgical implications. J Shoulder Elb Surg. 2009;18(6):874–85. doi:10.1016/j.jse.2009.02.013.
47. Frangiamore SJ, Saleh A, Grosso MJ, Kovac MF, Higuera CA, Iannotti JP, Ricchetti ET. alpha-Defensin as a predictor of periprosthetic shoulder infection. J Shoulder Elb Surg. 2015;24(7):1021–7. doi:10.1016/j.jse.2014.12.021.
48. Villacis D, Merriman JA, Yalamanchili R, Omid R, Itamura J, Rick Hatch III GF. Serum interleukin-6 as a marker of periprosthetic shoulder infection. J Bone Joint Surg Am. 2014;96(1):41–5. doi:10.2106/jbjs.l.01634.
49. Eajazi A, Kussman S, LeBedis C, Guermazi A, Kompel A, Jawa A, Murakami AM. Rotator cuff tear arthropathy: pathophysiology, imaging characteristics, and treatment options. Am J Roentgenol. 2015;205(5):W502–11. doi:10.2214/ajr.14.13815.
50. Wall B, Nove-Josserand L, O'Connor DP, Edwards TB, Walch G. Reverse total shoulder arthroplasty: a review of results according to etiology. J Bone Joint Surg Am. 2007;89(7):1476–85. doi:10.2106/JBJS.F.00666.
51. Boileau P, Gonzalez JF, Chuinard C, Bicknell R, Walch G. Reverse total shoulder arthroplasty after failed rotator cuff surgery. J Shoulder Elb Surg. 2009;18(4):600–6. doi:10.1016/j.jse.2009.03.011.
52. Ahearn N, McCann PA, Tasker A, Sarangi PP. The influence of rotator cuff pathology on functional outcome in total shoulder replacement. Int J Shoulder Surg. 2013;7(4):127–31. doi:10.4103/0973-6042.123509.
53. Simone JP, Streubel PH, Sperling JW, Schleck CD, Cofield RH, Athwal GS. Anatomical total shoulder replacement with rotator cuff repair for osteoarthritis of the shoulder. Bone Joint J. 2014;96-B(2):224–8. doi:10.1302/0301-620x.96b.32890.
54. Clavert P, Millett PJ, Warner JJ. Glenoid resurfacing: what are the limits to asymmetric reaming for posterior erosion? J Shoulder Elb Surg. 2007;16(6):843–8. doi:10.1016/j.jse.2007.03.015.
55. Gillespie R, Lyons R, Lazarus M. Eccentric reaming in total shoulder arthroplasty: a cadaveric study. Orthopedics. 2009;32(1):21.
56. Nowak DD, Bahu MJ, Gardner TR, Dyrszka MD, Levine WN, Bigliani LU, Ahmad CS. Simulation of surgical glenoid resurfacing using three-dimensional computed tomography of the arthritic glenohumeral joint: the amount of glenoid retroversion that can be corrected. J Shoulder Elb Surg. 2009;18(5):680–8. doi:10.1016/j.jse.2009.03.019.
57. Mori D, Abboud JA, Namdari S, Williams GR. Glenoid bone loss in anatomic shoulder arthroplasty: literature review and surgical technique. Orthop Clin North Am. 2015;46(3):389–97. x doi:10.1016/j.ocl.2015.02.007.
58. Sabesan V, Callanan M, Sharma V, Iannotti JP. Correction of acquired glenoid bone loss in osteoarthritis with a standard versus an augmented glenoid component. J Shoulder Elb Surg. 2014;23(7):964–73. doi:10.1016/j.jse.2013.09.019.
59. Walch G, Moraga C, Young A, Castellanos-Rosas J. Results of anatomic nonconstrained prosthesis in primary osteoarthritis with biconcave glenoid. J Shoulder Elb Surg. 2012;21(11):1526–33. doi:10.1016/j.jse.2011.11.030.
60. Hill JM, Norris TR. Long-term results of total shoulder arthroplasty following bone-grafting of the glenoid. J Bone Joint Surg Am. 2001;83(6):877–83.
61. Mizuno N, Denard PJ, Raiss P, Walch G. Reverse total shoulder arthroplasty for primary glenohumeral osteoarthritis in patients with a biconcave glenoid. J Bone Joint Surg Am. 2013;95(14):1297–304. doi:10.2106/jbjs.l.00820.
62. Steen BM, Cabezas AF, Santoni BG, Hussey MM, Cusick MC, Kumar AG, Frankle MA. Outcome and value of reverse shoulder arthroplasty for treatment of glenohumeral osteoarthritis: a matched cohort. J Shoulder Elb Surg. 2015;24(9):1433–41. doi:10.1016/j.jse.2015.01.005.
63. McFarland EG, Familiari F, Gonzalez-Zapata A. Intact rotator cuff. In: Frankle MA, Marberry S, Pupello D, editors. Reverse shoulder arthroplasty: biomechanics, clinical techniques, and current technologies. 1st ed. New York: Springer; 2016. p. 159–62.
64. Mulieri P, Dunning P, Klein S, Pupello D, Frankle M. Reverse shoulder arthroplasty for the treatment of irreparable rotator cuff tear without glenohumeral arthritis. J Bone Joint Surg Am. 2010;92(15):2544–56. doi:10.2106/jbjs.i.00912.
65. Werner CM, Steinmann PA, Gilbart M, Gerber C. Treatment of painful pseudoparesis due to irreparable rotator cuff dysfunction with the Delta III reverse-ball-and-socket total shoulder prosthesis. J Bone Joint Surg Am. 2005;87(7):1476–86. doi:10.2106/jbjs.d.02342.
66. Schneeberger AG, Muller TM, Steens W, Thur C. Reverse total shoulder arthroplasty after failed deltoid flap reconstruction. Arch Orthop

Trauma Surg. 2014;134(3):317–23. doi:10.1007/s00402-013-1908-1.
67. Warner JJ, Parsons IM. Latissimus dorsi tendon transfer: a comparative analysis of primary and salvage reconstruction of massive, irreparable rotator cuff tears. J Shoulder Elb Surg. 2001;10(6):514–21. doi:10.1067/mse.2001.118629.
68. Ladermann A, Walch G, Denard PJ, Collin P, Sirveaux F, Favard L, Edwards TB, Kherad O, Boileau P. Reverse shoulder arthroplasty in patients with pre-operative impairment of the deltoid muscle. Bone Joint J. 2013;95-B(8):1106–13. doi:10.1302/0301-620x.95b8.31173.
69. Young AA, Smith MM, Bacle G, Moraga C, Walch G. Early results of reverse shoulder arthroplasty in patients with rheumatoid arthritis. J Bone Joint Surg Am. 2011;93(20):1915–23. doi:10.2106/jbjs.j.00300.
70. Rittmeister M, Kerschbaumer F. Grammont reverse total shoulder arthroplasty in patients with rheumatoid arthritis and nonreconstructible rotator cuff lesions. J Shoulder Elb Surg. 2001;10(1):17–22. doi:10.1067/mse.2001.110515.
71. Raiss P, Zeifang F, Pons-Villanueva J, Smithers CJ, Loew M, Walch G. Reverse arthroplasty for osteoarthritis and rotator cuff deficiency after previous surgery for recurrent anterior shoulder instability. Int Orthop. 2014;38(7):1407–13. doi:10.1007/s00264-014-2325-y.
72. Lehmann L, Magosch P, Mauermann E, Lichtenberg S, Habermeyer P. Total shoulder arthroplasty in dislocation arthropathy. Int Orthop. 2010;34(8):1219–25. doi:10.1007/s00264-009-0928-5.
73. Hyun YS, Huri G, Garbis NG, McFarland EG. Uncommon indications for reverse total shoulder arthroplasty. Clin Orthop Surg. 2013;5(4):243–55. doi:10.4055/cios.2013.5.4.243.
74. Gallinet D, Adam A, Gasse N, Rochet S, Obert L. Improvement in shoulder rotation in complex shoulder fractures treated by reverse shoulder arthroplasty. J Shoulder Elb Surg. 2013;22(1):38–44. doi:10.1016/j.jse.2012.03.011.
75. Boyle MJ, Youn SM, Frampton CMA, Ball CM. Functional outcomes of reverse shoulder arthroplasty compared with hemiarthroplasty for acute proximal humeral fractures. J Shoulder Elb Surg. 2013;22(1):32–7. doi:10.1016/j.jse.2012.03.006.
76. Borade AU, Familiari F, Choi K, Joseph J, McFarland EG. Comparison of reverse total shoulder arthroplasty to hemiarthroplasty for acute fractures of the proximal humerus: systematic review. Punjab J Orthop. 2016 in press.
77. Alentorn-Geli E, Guirro P, Santana F, Torrens C. Treatment of fracture sequelae of the proximal humerus: comparison of hemiarthroplasty and reverse total shoulder arthroplasty. Arch Orthop Trauma Surg. 2014;134(11):1545–50. doi:10.1007/s00402-014-2074-9.
78. De Wilde L, Boileau P, Van der Bracht H. Does reverse shoulder arthroplasty for tumors of the proximal humerus reduce impairment? Clin Orthop. 2011;469(9):2489–95. doi:10.1007/s11999-010-1758-x.
79. Kaa AK, Jorgensen PH, Sojbjerg JO, Johannsen HV. Reverse shoulder replacement after resection of the proximal humerus for bone tumours. Bone Joint J. 2013;95-B(11):1551–5. doi:10.1302/0301-620x.95b11.31545.
80. Saltzman MD, Marecek GS, Edwards SL, Kalainov DM. Infection after shoulder surgery. J Am Acad Orthop Surg. 2011;19(4):208–18.
81. Burroughs PL, Gearen PF, Petty WR, Wright TW. Shoulder arthroplasty in the young patient. J Arthroplast. 2003;18(6):792–8.
82. Eichinger JK, Miller LR, Hartshorn T, Li X, Warner JJ, Higgins LD. Evaluation of satisfaction and durability after hemiarthroplasty and total shoulder arthroplasty in a cohort of patients aged 50 years or younger: an analysis of discordance of patient satisfaction and implant survival. J Shoulder Elb Surg. 2015; doi:10.1016/j.jse.2015.09.028.
83. Rispoli DM, Sperling JW, Athwal GS, Schleck CD, Cofield RH. Humeral head replacement for the treatment of osteoarthritis. J Bone Joint Surg Am. 2006;88(12):2637–44. doi:10.2106/jbjs.e.01383.
84. Rasmussen JV, Polk A, Sorensen AK, Olsen BS, Brorson S. Outcome, revision rate and indication for revision following resurfacing hemiarthroplasty for osteoarthritis of the shoulder: 837 operations reported to the Danish Shoulder Arthroplasty Registry. Bone Joint J. 2014;96-B(4):519–25. doi:10.1302/0301-620x.96b4.31850.
85. Levy J, Frankle M, Mighell M, Pupello D. The use of the reverse shoulder prosthesis for the treatment of failed hemiarthroplasty for proximal humeral fracture. J Bone Joint Surg Am. 2007;89(2):292–300. doi:10.2106/JBJS.E.01310.
86. Levy JC, Virani N, Pupello D, Frankle M. Use of the reverse shoulder prosthesis for the treatment of failed hemiarthroplasty in patients with glenohumeral arthritis and rotator cuff deficiency. J Bone Joint Surg Br. 2007;89(2):189–95. doi:10.1302/0301-620X.89B2.18161.
87. Valenti P, Kilinc AS, Sauzieres P, Katz D. Results of 30 reverse shoulder prostheses for revision of failed hemi- or total shoulder arthroplasty. Eur J Orthop Surg Traumatol. 2014;24(8):1375–82. doi:10.1007/s00590-013-1332-9.
88. Walker M, Willis MP, Brooks JP, Pupello D, Mulieri PJ, Frankle MA. The use of the reverse shoulder arthroplasty for treatment of failed total shoulder arthroplasty. J Shoulder Elb Surg. 2012;21(4):514–22. doi:10.1016/j.jse.2011.03.006.
89. Zumstein MA, Pinedo M, Old J, Boileau P. Problems, complications, reoperations, and revisions in reverse total shoulder arthroplasty: a systematic review. J Shoulder Elb Surg. 2011;20(1):146–57. doi:10.1016/j.jse.2010.08.001.

90. Boileau P. Complications and revision of reverse total shoulder arthroplasty. Orthop Traumatol Surgery Res. 2016; doi:10.1016/j.otsr.2015.06.031.
91. Boileau P, Melis B, Duperron D, Moineau G, Rumian AP, Han Y. Revision surgery of reverse shoulder arthroplasty. J Shoulder Elb Surg. 2013;22(10):1359–70. doi:10.1016/j.jse.2013.02.004.
92. Levigne C, Boileau P, Favard L, Garaud P, Mole D, Sirveaux F, Walch G. Scapular notching in reverse shoulder arthroplasty. J Shoulder Elb Surg. 2008;17(6):925–35. doi:10.1016/j.jse.2008.02.010.
93. Sadoghi P, Leithner A, Vavken P, Holzer A, Hochreiter J, Weber G, Pietschmann MF, Muller PE. Infraglenoidal scapular notching in reverse total shoulder replacement: a prospective series of 60 cases and systematic review of the literature. BMC Musculoskelet Disord. 2011;12:101. doi:10.1186/1471-2474-12-101.
94. Levigne C, Garret J, Boileau P, Alami G, Favard L, Walch G. Scapular notching in reverse shoulder arthroplasty: is it important to avoid it and how? Clin Orthop. 2011;469(9):2512–20. doi:10.1007/s11999-010-1695-8.
95. Melis B, DeFranco M, Ladermann A, Mole D, Favard L, Nerot C, Maynou C, Walch G. An evaluation of the radiological changes around the Grammont reverse geometry shoulder arthroplasty after eight to 12 years. J Bone Joint Surg Br. 2011;93(9):1240–6. doi:10.1302/0301-620x.93b9.25926.
96. Nyffeler RW, Werner CML, Gerber C. Biomechanical relevance of glenoid component positioning in the reverse Delta III total shoulder prosthesis. J Shoulder Elb Surg. 2005;14(5):524–8. doi:10.1016/j.jse.2004.09.010.
97. Cuff D, Pupello D, Virani N, Levy J, Frankle M. Reverse shoulder arthroplasty for the treatment of rotator cuff deficiency. J Bone Joint Surg Am. 2008;90(6):1244–51. doi:10.2106/JBJS.G.00775.
98. Erickson BJ, Frank RM, Harris JD, Mall N, Romeo AA. The influence of humeral head inclination in reverse total shoulder arthroplasty: a systematic review. J Shoulder Elb Surg. 2015;24(6):988–93. doi:10.1016/j.jse.2015.01.001.
99. Nicholson GP, Strauss EJ, Sherman SL. Scapular notching: recognition and strategies to minimize clinical impact. Clin Orthop. 2011;469:2521–30.
100. Chalmers PN, Rahman Z, Romeo AA, Nicholson GP. Early dislocation after reverse total shoulder arthroplasty. J Shoulder Elb Surg. 2014;23(5):737–44. doi:10.1016/j.jse.2013.08.015.
101. Boileau P, Watkinson D, Hatzidakis AM, Hovorka I. Neer Award 2005: the Grammont reverse shoulder prosthesis: results in cuff tear arthritis, fracture sequelae, and revision arthroplasty. J Shoulder Elb Surg. 2006;15(5):527–40. doi:10.1016/j.jse.2006.01.003.
102. Ladermann A, Williams MD, Melis B, Hoffmeyer P, Walch G. Objective evaluation of lengthening in reverse shoulder arthroplasty. J Shoulder Elb Surg. 2009;18(4):588–95. doi:10.1016/j.jse.2009.03.012.
103. Gallo RA, Gamradt SC, Mattern CJ, Cordasco FA, Craig EV, Dines DM, Warren RF, Sports Medicine and Shoulder Service at the Hospital for Special Surgery. Instability after reverse total shoulder replacement. J Shoulder Elb Surg. 2011;20(4):584–90. doi:10.1016/j.jse.2010.08.028.
104. Edwards TB, Williams MD, Labriola JE, Elkousy HA, Gartsman GM, O'Connor DP. Subscapularis insufficiency and the risk of shoulder dislocation after reverse shoulder arthroplasty. J Shoulder Elb Surg. 2009;18(6):892–6. doi:10.1016/j.jse.2008.12.013.
105. Ackland DC, Roshan-Zamir S, Richardson M, Pandy MG. Moment arms of the shoulder musculature after reverse total shoulder arthroplasty. J Bone Joint Surg Am. 2010;92(5):1221–30. doi:10.2106/jbjs.i.00001.
106. Clark JC, Ritchie J, Song FS, Kissenberth MJ, Tolan SJ, Hart ND, Hawkins RJ. Complication rates, dislocation, pain, and postoperative range of motion after reverse shoulder arthroplasty in patients with and without repair of the subscapularis. J Shoulder Elb Surg. 2012;21(1):36–41. doi:10.1016/j.jse.2011.04.009.
107. Gerber C, Pennington SD, Nyffeler RW. Reverse total shoulder arthroplasty. J Am Acad Orthop Surg. 2009;17(5):284–95.
108. Teusink MJ, Pappou IP, Schwartz DG, Cottrell BJ, Frankle MA. Results of closed management of acute dislocation after reverse shoulder arthroplasty. J Shoulder Elb Surg. 2015;24(4):621–7. doi:10.1016/j.jse.2014.07.015.
109. Fevang BT, Lie SA, Havelin LI, Skredderstuen A, Furnes O. Risk factors for revision after shoulder arthroplasty: 1,825 shoulder arthroplasties from the Norwegian Arthroplasty Register. Acta Orthop. 2009;80(1):83–91.
110. Favard L, Levigne C, Nerot C, Gerber C, De Wilde L, Mole D. Reverse prostheses in arthropathies with cuff tear: are survivorship and function maintained over time? Clin Orthop. 2011;469(9):2469–75. doi:10.1007/s11999-011-1833-y.
111. Trappey IV GJ, O'Connor DP, Edwards TB. What are the instability and infection rates after reverse shoulder arthroplasty? Clin Orthop. 2011;469(9):2505–11. doi:10.1007/s11999-010-1686-9.
112. Morris BJ, O'Connor DP, Torres D, Elkousy HA, Gartsman GM, Edwards TB. Risk factors for periprosthetic infection after reverse shoulder arthroplasty. J Shoulder Elb Surg. 2015;24(2):161–6. doi:10.1016/j.jse.2014.05.020.
113. Bohsali KI, Wirth MA, Rockwood Jr CA. Complications of total shoulder arthroplasty. J Bone Joint Surg Am. 2006;88(10):2279–92. doi:10.2106/jbjs.f.00125.
114. Braman JP, Sprague M, Bishop J, Lo IK, Lee EW, Flatow EL. The outcome of resection shoulder arthroplasty for recalcitrant shoulder infections. J Shoulder

Elb Surg. 2006;15(5):549–53. doi:10.1016/j.jse.2005.11.001.
115. Holcomb JO, Hebert DJ, Mighell MA, Dunning PE, Pupello DR, Pliner MD, Frankle MA. Reverse shoulder arthroplasty in patients with rheumatoid arthritis. J Shoulder Elb Surg. 2010;19(7):1076–84. doi:10.1016/j.jse.2009.11.049.
116. Del Pozo JL, Patel R. Clinical practice. Infection associated with prosthetic joints. N Engl J Med. 2009;361(8):787–94. doi:10.1056/NEJMcp0905029.
117. Piper KE, Fernandez-Sampedro M, Steckelberg KE, Mandrekar JN, Karau MJ, Steckelberg JM, Berbari EF, Osmon DR, Hanssen AD, Lewallen DG, Cofield RH, Sperling JW, Sanchez-Sotelo J, Huddleston PM, Dekutoski MB, Yaszemski M, Currier B, Patel R. C-reactive protein, erythrocyte sedimentation rate and orthopedic implant infection. PLoS One. 2010;5(2):e9358. doi:10.1371/journal.pone.0009358.
118. Updegrove GF, Armstrong AD, Kim HM. Preoperative and intraoperative infection workup in apparently aseptic revision shoulder arthroplasty. J Shoulder Elb Surg. 2015;24(3):491–500. doi:10.1016/j.jse.2014.10.005.
119. Lynch NM, Cofield RH, Silbert PL, Hermann RC. Neurologic complications after total shoulder arthroplasty. J Shoulder Elb Surg. 1996;5(1):53–61.
120. Ladermann A, Lubbeke A, Melis B, Stern R, Christofilopoulos P, Bacle G, Walch G. Prevalence of neurologic lesions after total shoulder arthroplasty. J Bone Joint Surg Am. 2011;93(14):1288–93. doi:10.2106/jbjs.j.00369.
121. Cheung E, Willis M, Walker M, Clark R, Frankle MA. Complications in reverse total shoulder arthroplasty. J Am Acad Orthop Surg. 2011;19(7):439–49.
122. Van Hoof T, Gomes GT, Audenaert E, Verstraete K, Kerckaert I, D'Herde K. 3D computerized model for measuring strain and displacement of the brachial plexus following placement of reverse shoulder prosthesis. Anat Rec. 2008;291(9):1173–85. doi:10.1002/ar.20735.
123. Jarrett CD, Brown BT, Schmidt CC. Reverse shoulder arthroplasty. Orthop Clin North Am. 2013;44(3):389–408. x doi:10.1016/j.ocl.2013.03.010.
124. Zhou HS, Chung JS, Yi PH, Li X, Price MD. Management of complications after reverse shoulder arthroplasty. Curr Rev Muscoskelet Med. 2015;8(1):92–7. doi:10.1007/s12178-014-9252-9.
125. Middernacht B, De Wilde L, Mole D, Favard L, Debeer P. Glenosphere disengagement: a potentially serious default in reverse shoulder surgery. Clin Orthop. 2008;466(4):892–8. doi:10.1007/s11999-007-0090-6.
126. Cusick MC, Hussey MM, Steen BM, Hartzler RU, Clark RE, Cuff DJ, Cabezas AF, Santoni BG, Frankle MA. Glenosphere dissociation after reverse shoulder arthroplasty. J Shoulder Elb Surg. 2015;24(7):1061–8. doi:10.1016/j.jse.2014.12.019.
127. Ansari F, Major C, Norris TR, Gunther SB, Ries M, Pruitt L. Unscrewing instability of modular reverse shoulder prosthesis increases propensity for in vivo fracture: a report of two cases. J Shoulder Elb Surg. 2014;23(2):e40–5. doi:10.1016/j.jse.2013.11.001.
128. De Wilde L, Walch G. Humeral prosthetic failure of reversed total shoulder arthroplasty: a report of three cases. J Shoulder Elb Surg. 2006;15(2):260–4. doi:10.1016/j.jse.2005.07.014.
129. Scarlat MM. Complications with reverse total shoulder arthroplasty and recent evolutions. Int Orthop. 2013;37(5):843–51. doi:10.1007/s00264-013-1832-6.
130. Neer II CS. Shoulder reconstruction. Philadelphia: WB Saunders; 1990.
131. Reeves B, Jobbins B, Dowson D, Wright V. A total shoulder endoprosthesis. Eng Med. 1974;1:64–7.
132. Brostrom LA, Wallensten R, Olsson E, Anderson D. The Kessel prosthesis in total shoulder arthroplasty. A five-year experience. Clin Orthop. 1992;277:155–60.
133. Kolbel R, Friedebold G. Shoulder joint replacement. Arch Orthop Unfallchir. 1973;76(1):31–9.
134. Ahir SP, Walker PS, Squire-Taylor CJ, Blunn GW, Bayley JI. Analysis of glenoid fixation for a reversed anatomy fixed-fulcrum shoulder replacement. J Biomech. 2004;37(11):1699–708. doi:10.1016/j.jbiomech.2004.01.031.
135. Fenlin Jr JM. Semi-constrained prosthesis for the rotator cuff deficient patient. Orthop Trans. 1985;9:55.
136. Blauth W, Donner K. Notes on the history of arthroplasty (author's transl). Z Orthop Ihre Grenzgeb. 1979;117(6):997–1006.
137. Buechel FF, Pappas MJ, DePalma AF. "Floating-socket" total shoulder replacement: anatomical, biomechanical, and surgical rationale. J Biomed Mater Res. 1978;12(1):89–114. doi:10.1002/jbm.820120109.
138. Gristina AG, Webb LX. The trispherical total shoulder replacement. In: Bayley I, Kessel L, editors. Shoulder surgery. New York, NY: Springer; 1982. p. 153–7.
139. Grammont P, Trouilloud P, Laffay J, Deries X. Concept study and realization of a new total shoulder prosthesis [in French]. Rhumatologie. 1987;39:407–18.
140. Grammont PM, Baulot E. Delta shoulder prosthesis for rotator cuff rupture. Orthopedics. 1993;16(1):65–8.
141. Young SW, Everts NM, Ball CM, Astley TM, Poon PC. The SMR reverse shoulder prosthesis in the treatment of cuff-deficient shoulder conditions. J Shoulder Elb Surg. 2009;18(4):622–6. doi:10.1016/j.jse.2009.01.017.
142. Frankle M, Siegal S, Pupello D, Saleem A, Mighell M, Vasey M. The Reverse Shoulder Prosthesis for glenohumeral arthritis associated with severe rotator cuff deficiency. A minimum two-year follow-up study of sixty patients. J Bone Joint Surg Am. 2005;87(8):1697–705. doi:10.2106/JBJS.D.02813.

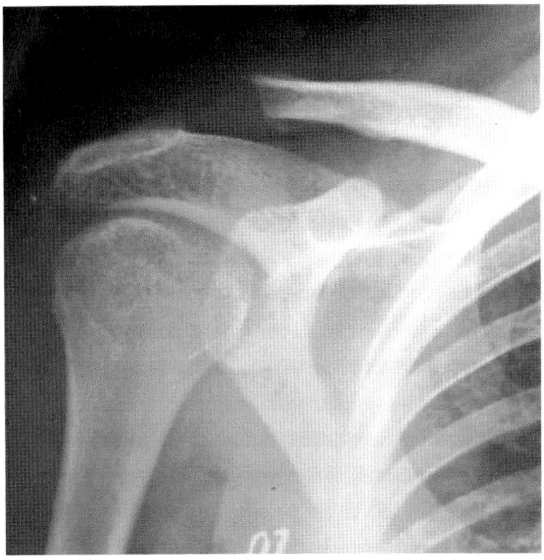

Fig. 23.2 Anteroposterior radiograph showing a resection of distal clavicle

[33]. There exist two approaches being used in arthroscopy which are named as direct and indirect approaches. While an intra-articular resection is being performed in the direct approach, acromioclavicular joint is viewed inferiorly by a subacromial approach in the indirect approach. The most important advantage of the indirect approach is the convenience to perform additional procedures by this access. In the arthroscopic technique, joint instability can be avoided by virtue of preservation of the acromioclavicular joint capsule. The distal clavicle resection is indicated in degenerative joint disease and osteolysis and relatively contraindicated in acromioclavicular joint instability. A failure after the resection procedure could be attributed to insufficient resection, bony impingement, or instability caused by over-resection.

Surgical treatment of acromioclavicular joint degeneration should be planned after considering the potential copathologies. Acromioclavicular joint type, acromion type, osteophytes, the existence of os acromiale, and subchondral cysts also should be assessed with radiographs. The conditions related with poor outcomes are a persistent pain, heterotypic ossification, instability caused by over-resection, and bony impingement caused by incomplete resection [34].

Surgical Technique

The distal clavicle resection can be performed in lateral decubitus or beach-chair position considering the copathologies to be intervened and surgeon's experience. The standard shoulder equipment is adequate for this procedure. Firstly, osseous landmarks are designated with a surgical skin marker (anterolateral and posterolateral corners of the acromion, lateral edge of acromion, spine of scapula, posterior aspect of clavicle, and acromioclavicular joint).

Indirect approach; Shoulder arthroscopy is initiated by the standard posterior portal. After intervening to subacromial pathologies by the virtue of anterior portal constituted through the rotator interval, the subacromial space is then viewed. The pathologies in this region are intervened through the lateral portal. Then, the anterior working portal is constituted after determining with a spinal needle at the inferior aspect of the acromioclavicular joint. If the posterior portal is being used as a viewing portal, posterior aspect of the acromioclavicular joint should be debrided towards the medial aspect of it by a radiofrequency probe or an arthroscopic shaver to view the cite clearly that the procedure to be performed. The soft tissue at the inferior aspect of the acromioclavicular joint and inferior joint capsule is removed by a radiofrequency probe or an arthroscopic shaver to expose the inferior aspect of the joint beforehand. The bleeding tissues should be seared to sustain the clear view during the resection. The resection amount and borders are determined by decorticating the inferior aspect of the planned resection cite by an arthroscopic burr inserted through the anterior working portal. The resection of the inferior aspect of the joint is pursued from anterior to posterior considering the determined resection amount. The posterior capsular ligament should be protected to sustain the acromioclavicular joint stability. The surgeon should be careful and meticulous during the resection of the posterior cortex, and he/she must separate the bony tissue off of the ligamentous tissue. The superior acromioclavicular ligament and joint capsule are the mainstays of the joint stability after the resection.

The most important advantage of the arthroscopic surgery is its superiority over the open surgery in the preservation of the joint capsule and superior acromioclavicular ligament. Eight to ten millimeters resection is efficient for an appropriately performed procedure. After completing the procedure, the posterior-superior cite of the joint should be reassessed because of being the most associated cite with a potential insufficient resection. After being assured of a symmetric and a sufficient resection and removal of the osteophytes, the procedure can be ended.

Direct approach; This can be performed in select young patient groups with an isolated acromioclavicular joint pathology like osteolysis of the distal clavicle. It can be a rational choice because of not traumatising the subacromial space and bursa in isolated cases. However, assessment of the intra-articular pathologies before the resection is crucial because of being the gold standard for the diagnosis of pathologies accompanying to acromioclavicular joint disorders. In the direct approach, 2.7 mm diameter arthroscope is used. The portals are constituted on the fictitious line lying anteroposteriorly constant with the acromioclavicular joint. The posterior viewing portal is constituted through the posterior aspect of the acromioclavicular joint. The anterior portal is constituted following the spinal needle insertion and determining the exact entry point of the portal. The soft tissue at the inferior aspect of the acromioclavicular joint and inferior joint capsule is removed by a radiofrequency probe or an arthroscopic shaver to expose the inferior aspect of the joint beforehand. Then, the anterior aspect of the joint is exposed meticulously as the superior acromioclavicular ligament and capsule are protected. The resection amount and borders are determined by decorticating the inferior aspect of the planned resection cite by an arthroscopic burr inserted through the anterior working portal. The resection process is then initiated from anteroinferior to anterosuperior considering the determined resection amount and kept on resecting towards the posterior aspect. Then, the arthroscope is inserted through the anterior portal and the burr to the posterior portal in order to resect the posterior aspect of the joint properly. Eight to ten millimeter resection is preferred for an appropriate distal clavicle resection. After completing the procedure, the posterior-superior cite of the joint should be reassessed because of being the most associated cite with a potential insufficient resection. Assuring a symmetric and a sufficient resection and removal of the osteophytes, the procedure can be ended.

Postoperative Rehabilitation

Patients who underwent isolated distal clavicle resection are prescribed immobilisation with a sling postoperatively for the pain control. Postoperative active and passive range of motion exercises are begun on the postoperative first day to preclude postoperative shoulder stiffness. After the sixth week, overhead activities are begun under the control of the range of shoulder motion. Lifting heavy objects is not allowed first 3 months because of the weakening of the acromioclavicular ligamentous structures which are crucial in joint stability. Returning back to sports is allowed after the third month.

Literature

Arthroscopic distal clavicle resection for acromioclavicular degenerative arthritis is reported to have 88–100% good or excellent outcomes [33, 35, 36]. Satisfactory results in returning to physical activity after an arthroscopic distal clavicle resection were reported also in athletes [37]. Snyder et al. [38] found that 16% of patients developed calcification in the rotator interval following the arthroscopic distal clavicle resection, but this finding was not associated with outcomes. Flatow et al. [39] found a mild acromioclavicular joint instability after an arthroscopic distal clavicle resection, which affected the outcomes negatively. In the literature, the recommended resection amount is 5 mm–2 cm [40–42]. However, there is no consensus yet in resection amount necessary for preserving the contact between the acromion and the clavicle.

Sternoclavicular Joint Resection Arthroplasty (Proximal Clavicle Resection)

As very rare conditions, sternoclavicular degenerative arthritis (SDA) and sternoclavicular septic arthritis (SSA) could be treated also by the sternoclavicular joint resection (SJR). The sternoclavicular joint involvement is seen only 0.5–1% of the septic arthritis cases [43]. In SDA, pain and disability may occur, but fortunately, most of the symptoms regress spontaneously. Persistent pain and shoulder disability despite the conservative and palliative treatment can be managed by surgical interventions like resection arthroplasty. There exist studies reporting good or excellent outcomes with open resection technique [44, 45]. In open resection, there are the risks of postoperative instability caused by joint capsule opening and vital structure injury caused during the posterior resection. Tayakkolizadeh et al. [46] described the advantages of the arthroscopic SJR as less surgical trauma, less vital structure injury risk, less postoperative instability, and less cosmetic problems. Arthroscopic SJR is reported as an appropriate option for selected patients with symptomatic SDA [47, 48].

Surgical Technique

Arthroscopic SJR is executed in the supine position. The joint stability is assessed following the anaesthesia induction. Bony landmarks are designated (medial clavicle and lateral sternum). The joint is perforated by a spinal needle inserted anteroinferiorly, and the joint capsule is inflated by injecting physiologic sodium chloride solution. Then, 2.7 mm diameter arthroscope is inserted bluntly through the inferior viewing portal, which is at the anteroinferior aspect of the joint, in a superior direction and in a careful way not to penetrate the posterior aspect of the joint. The sternoclavicular ligament and capsule are protected as possible. The superior portal, also used as the working portal, is constituted after determining the appropriate angle with a spinal needle at the anterosuperior aspect of the joint. The posterior joint capsule should be preserved because of being crucial for the joint stability and adjacent to vital structures [49]. The resection amount should be 5–10 mm [50, 51]. Firstly, the joint cavity debridement is performed protecting the joint capsule and ligamentous structures for a clear view. Then, 7–8 mm diameter portion of the medial clavicle is resected by a burr inserted through the superior portal. Subsequently, the joint surface of the sternum is debrided, and the remnant intra-articular disk is excised. After completing the resection procedure, stability and a potential impingement owing to a bony tissue should be controlled by moving the shoulder as the arthroscope is still in the joint.

Postoperative Rehabilitation

Patients are prescribed immobilisation with a sling postoperatively for the pain control. Postoperative active and passive range of motion exercises are begun on the postoperative first day to preclude postoperative shoulder stiffness. After the sixth week, overhead activities are begun under the control of the range of shoulder motion. Lifting heavy objects is not allowed first 3 months because of the weakening of the sternoclavicular ligamentous structures.

Literature

There exist fair results with resection arthroplasty for the SDA in the literature [44, 45]. The superiority of arthroscopic SJR over open SJR are the feasibility of assessment of intra-articular disks and joint surfaces thoroughly, less surgical risks thanks to the appropriate instruments placed into the joint, rapid healing, and less cosmetic problems [47]. In a study evaluating ten patients followed-up for a mean of 28 months who underwent arthroscopic medial clavicle resection for a sternoclavicular osteoarthritis reported satisfactory outcomes with no complication [48].

Questions

What are reasonable expectations after resection arthroplasty of the shoulder?

A. Pain relief
B. Return to sports activities
C. Full range of motion
D. All the above

Indications for resection arthroplasty can be all the above except:

A. 65 yo male with chronic not-controlled infection
B. 75 yo male with disabling shoulder pain
C. 69 yo female with inadequate bone reserve for revision
D. 52 yo male with a failed reverse total shoulder arthroplasty that want to retain
E. 50 yo female with insufficient soft tissue and muscle support
F. 85 yo male not demanding additional surgery
G. 80 yo female unable to handle an additional surgery
H. 72 yo male with morbidity risk because of recurrent surgeries

Most common reason for failure after distal clavicle resection procedure are (select all that apply):

A. Insufficient resection
B. Nerve injury
C. Bony impingement
D. AC-joint instability caused by over-resection
E. Infection

References

1. Cheung EV, Sperling JW, Cofield RH. Infection associated with hematoma formation after shoulder arthroplasty. Clin Orthop Relat Res. 2008;466:1363–7.
2. Coste JS, Reig S, Trojani C, Berg M, Walch G, Boileau P. The management of infection in arthroplasty of the shoulder. J Bone Joint Surg Br. 2004;86:65–9.
3. Jerosch J, Schneppenheim M. Management of infected shoulder replacement. Arch Orthop Trauma Surg. 2003;123:209–14.
4. Piper KE, Fernandez-Sampedro M, Steckelberg KE, Mandrekar JN, Karau MJ, Steckelberg JM, et al. C-reactive protein, erythrocyte sedimentation rate and orthopedic implant infection. PLoS One. 2010;5:e9358.
5. Kelly JD, Hobgood ER. Positive culture rate in revision shoulder arthroplasty. Clin Orthop Relat Res. 2009;467:2343–8.
6. Dodson CC, Craig EV, Cordasco FA, Dines DM, Dines JS, Dicarlo E, et al. Propionibacterium acnes infection after shoulder arthroplasty: a diagnostic challenge. J Shoulder Elb Surg. 2010;19:303–7.
7. Grosso MJ, Sabesan VJ, Ho JC, Ricchetti ET, Iannotti JP. Reinfection rates after 1-stage revision shoulder arthroplasty for patients with unexpected positive intraoperative cultures. J Shoulder Elb Surg. 2012;21:754–8.
8. Sperling JW, Kozak TK, Hanssen AD, Cofield RH. Infection after shoulder arthroplasty. Clin Orthop Relat Res. 2001;382:206–16.
9. Mileti J, Sperling JW, Cofield RH. Shoulder arthroplasty for the treatment of postinfectious glenohumeral arthritis. J Bone Joint Surg Am. 2003;85:609–14.
10. Strickland JP, Sperling JW, Cofield RH. The results of two-stage reimplantation for infected shoulder replacement. J Bone Joint Surg Br. 2008;90:460–5.
11. Debeer P, Plasschaert H, Stuyck J. Resection arthroplasty of the infected shoulder: a salvage procedure for the elderly patient. Acta Orthop Belg. 2006;72:126–30.
12. Jones L. Reconstructive operation for non-reducible fractures of the head of the humerus. Ann Surg. 1933;97:217–25.
13. Milbrink J, Wigren A. Resection arthroplasty of the shoulder. Scand J Rheumatol. 1990;19:432–6.
14. Gariepy R. Glenoidectomy in the repair of the rheuroatoid shoulder. J Bone Joint Surg Br. 1977;59:122.
15. Singh JA, Sperling JW, Schleck C, Harmsen W, Cofield RH. Periprosthetic infections after shoulder hemiarthroplasty. J Shoulder Elb Surg. 2012;21:1304–9.
16. Singh JA, Sperling JW, Schleck C, Harmsen WS, Cofield RH. Periprosthetic infections after total shoulder arthroplasty: a 33-year perspective. J Shoulder Elb Surg. 2012;21:1534–41.
17. Jacquot N, Chuinard CH, Boileau P. Results of deep infection after a reverse shoulder arthroplasty. In: Walch G, Boileau P, Mole D, et al., editors. Reverse shoulder arthroplasty: clinical results, complications, revision. Montpellier: Sauramps Medical; 2006. p. 307–12.
18. Seebauer L. Total reverse shoulder arthroplasty: European lessons and future trends. Am J Orthop (Belle Mead NJ). 2007;36(Suppl 1):22–8.
19. Ortmaier R, Resch H, Hitzl W, Mayer M, Stundner O, Tauber M. Treatment strategies for infection after reverse shoulder arthroplasty. Eur J Orthop Surg Traumatol. 2014;24:723–31.
20. Cofield RH. Shoulder arthrodesis and resection arthroplasty. Instr Course Lect. 1985;34:268–77.
21. Braman JP, Sprague M, Bishop J, Lo IK, Lee EW, Flatow EL. The outcome of resection shoulder arthroplasty for recalcitrant shoulder infections. J Shoulder Elb Surg. 2006;15:549–53.

22. Weber P, Utzschneider S, Sadoghi P, Andress HJ, Jansson V, Muller PE. Management of the infected shoulder prosthesis: a retrospective analysis and review of literature. Int Orthop. 2011;35:365–73.
23. Rispoli DM, Sperling JW, Athwal GS, Schleck CD, Cofield RH. Pain relief and functional results after resection arthroplasty of the shoulder. J Bone Joint Surg Br. 2007;80:1184–7.
24. Stevens N, Kim HM, Armstrong AD. Functional outcomes after shoulder resection: the patient's perspective. J Shoulder Elb Surg. 2015;24:247–54.
25. Muh S, Streit JJ, Leranz CJ, et al. Resection arthroplasty for failed shoulder arthroplasty. J Shoulder Elb Surg. 2013;22:247–52.
26. Verhelst L, Stuyck J, Bellemans J, Debeer P. Resection arthroplasty of the shoulder as a salvage procedure for deep shoulder infection: does the use of a cement spacer improve outcome? J Shoulder Elb Surg. 2011;20:1224–33.
27. Themistocleous G, Zalavras C, Stine I, Zachos V, Itamura J. Prolonged implantation of an antibiotic cement spacer for management of shoulder sepsis in compromised patients. J Shoulder Elb Surg. 2007;16:701–5.
28. Marculescu CE, Berbari EF, Hanssen AD, et al. Outcome of prosthetic joint infections treated with debridement and retention of components. Clin Infect Dis. 2006;42:471–8.
29. Codd TP, Yamaguchi K, Pollock RG, Flatow EL, Bigliani LU. Infected shoulder arthroplasties: treatment with staged reimplantation vs. resection arthroplasty. J Shoulder Elbow Surg. 1996;5:S5.
30. Jonsson E, Brattström M, Lidgren L. Evaluation of the rheumatoid shoulder function after hemiarthroplasty and arthrodesis. Scand J Rheumatol. 1988;17:17–26.
31. Rowe CR, Zarins B. Chronic unreduced dislocations of the shoulder. J Bone Joint Surg Am. 1982;64:494–505.
32. Worcester JN, Green DP. Osteoarthritis of the acromioclavicular joint. Clin Orthop Relat Res. 1968;58:69–73.
33. Kay SP, Dragoo JL, Lee R. Long-term results of arthroscopic resection of the distal clavicle with concomitant subacromial decompression. Arthroscopy. 2003;19:805–9.
34. Strauss EJ, Barker JU, McGill K, et al. The evaluation and management of failed distal clavicle excision. Sports Med Arthrosc. 2010;18(3):213–9.
35. Levine WN, Barron OA, Yamaguchi K, et al. Arthroscopic distal clavicle resection from a bursal approach. Arthroscopy. 1998;14:52–6.
36. Martin SD, Baumgarten TE, Andrews JR. Arthroscopic resection of the distal aspect of the clavicle with concomitant subacromial decompression. J Bone Joint Surg Am. 2001;83:328–35.
37. Charron KM, Schepss AA, Voloshin L. Arthroscopic distal clavicle resection in athletes. A prospective comparison of the direct and indirect approach. Am J Sports Med. 2007;35(1):53–8.
38. Snyder SJ, Banas MP, Karzel RP. The arthroscopic Mumford procedure: an analysis of results. Arthroscopy. 1995;11:157–64.
39. Flatow EL, Duralde XA, Nicholson GP, et al. Arthroscopic resection of the distal clavicle with a superior approach. J Shoulder Elb Surg. 1995;4(1):39–50.
40. Branch TP, Burdette HL, Shahriari AS, Carter II FM, Hutton WC. The role of the acromioclavicular ligaments and the effect of distal clavicle resection. Am J Sports Med. 1996;24:293–7.
41. Edwards SL, Wilson NA, Flores SE, Koh JL, Zhang LQ. Arthroscopic distal clavicle resection: a biomechanical analysis of resection length and joint compliance in a cadaveric model. Arthroscopy. 2007;23:1278–84.
42. Matthews LS, Parks BG, Pavlovich Jr LJ, Giudice MA. Arthroscopic versus open distal clavicle resection: a biomechanical analysis on a cadaveric model. Arthroscopy. 1999;15:237–40.
43. Ross JJ, Shamsuddin H. Sternoclavicular septic arthritis: review of 180 cases. Medicine (Baltimore). 2004;83:139–48.
44. Pingsmann A, Patsalis T, Michiels I. Resection arthroplasty of the sternoclavicular joint for the treatment of primary degenerative sternoclavicular arthritis. J Bone Joint Surg Br. 2002;84:513–7.
45. Panzica M, Zeichen J, Hankemeier S, Gaulke R, Krettek C, Jagodzinski M. Long-term outcome after joint reconstruction or medical resection arthroplasty for anterior SCJ instability. Arch Orthop Trauma Surg. 2010;130:657–65.
46. Tavakkolizadeh A, Hales PF, Janes GC. Arthroscopic excision of sternoclavicular joint. Knee Surg Sports Traumatol Arthrosc. 2009;17:405–8.
47. Warth RJ, Lee JT, Campbell KJ, Millett PJ. Arthroscopic sternoclavicular joint resection arthroplasty: a technical note and illustrated case report. Arthrosc Tech. 2014;3(1):165–73.
48. Tytherleigh-Strong G, Griffith D. Arthroscopic excision of the sternoclavicular joint for the treatment of sternoclavicular osteoarthritis. Arthroscopy. 2013;29:1487–91.
49. Spencer EE, Kuhn JE, Huston LJ, Carpenter JE, Hughes RE. Ligamentous restraints to anterior and posterior translation of the sternoclavicular joint. J Shoulder Elb Surg. 2002;11:43–7.
50. Bisson LJ, Dauphin N, Marzo JM. A safe zone for resection of the medial end of the clavicle. J Shoulder Elb Surg. 2003;12:592–4.
51. Tytherleigh-Strong G, Getgood AM, Griffiths DE. Arthroscopic intra-articular disk excision of the sternoclavicular joint. Am J Sports Med. 2012;40:1172–5.

Revision Shoulder Arthroplasty 24

Ulunay Kanatlı, M. Baybars Ataoğlu,
and Mehmet Cetinkaya

With the development of technology and improvement in implant options and quality, implantation of the shoulder prosthesis (SA) has increased as the other surgical implants. Thus, the rate of shoulder prosthesis procedures has also increased. A study conducted to evaluate the increment in the rate of arthroplasties performed between 2006 and 2010 found 29% for the shoulder while that was 10% for the knee and 1% for the hip. This was attributed to the increase in usage of shoulder prostheses compared to other prosthesis types and especially expansion of the indications because of the coming into use of the reverse shoulder prosthesis designs [1]. Shoulder prostheses were found to have 90% 10-year and 80% 15-year survival rates [2, 3]. In another study, the 15-year survival rate of the SA is given as 87% with 15% of complication rate [4]. Sing et al. found 20-year survival rate of the anatomic SA as 81% and stated risk factors for revision surgery [5] of which those leading are; accompanying rotator cuff tears, male sex, and an accompanying tumours [5]. In a recent compilation, complication rate following the SA was reported as 39%, and most common complication was reported as loosening [6]. To avoid an early revision following the SA, a meticulous surgical execution, and soft tissue balance is crucial [7].

Reasons for total shoulder prosthesis revision:

Infection

The infection rate of SA is not high in comparison with the hip and knee prosthesis procedures. This rate is reported as 1–10% in SA [8]. Usual infection symptoms, wound inflammation, and fistulization are the most explicit findings of infection. The existence of infection should be investigated systematically. Pain persisting after the surgery, elevated blood levels of erythrocyte sedimentation rate (ESR), white blood cell (WBC), c-reactive protein (CRP), interleukin-6 (IL-6), and loosening of the both components should remind infection in patients having immunodeficiency, diabetes mellitus, radiotherapy and in patients who underwent shoulder arthroplasty for inflammatory arthritis [1, 9]. The agent is typically *Staphylococcus aureus* or Propionibacterium acnes [8]. A joint puncture is recommended in suspicious cases. In a multicenter study, it was reported that out of the patients presented with

U. Kanatlı, M.D. (✉) • M.B. Ataoğlu, M.D.
Faculty of Medicine, Department of Orthopaedics and Traumatology, Gazi University, Ankara, Turkey
e-mail: ulunayk@hotmail.com

M. Cetinkaya, M.D.
Department of Orthopaedics and Traumatology, Erzincan University Mengücek Gazi Training and Research Hospital, Erzincan, Turkey

G. Huri, N.K. Paschos (eds.), *The Shoulder*, Orthopaedic Study Guide Series,
DOI 10.1007/978-3-319-51979-1_24

infection after an SA, 97.7% were having pain, 54.5% flowing fistula, 47.7% warmness and reddishness, and 61.4% osteolysis and loosening [8]. In the same study, culture results were positive in 77%, the agent was a Gram-positive cocci in 70%, and early infections were caused by S. aureus in 34.1%. However, in that study, no bacteria was isolated preoperatively in 65.9% of patients, and neither intraoperatively in 22.7%. Therefore, the authors pronounced the importance of gathering the materials during the surgery for microbiologic examination [8]. The mediums must be observed at least 3 weeks to isolate P. acnes of which awareness have increased recently. Whether on the ground of glenoid or humeral component, the success rate of revisions for infection is inferior to that for loosening [7].

Instability

The rate of instability is 30% in the usual SA complications [6]. It can be avoided during the initial surgery. Therefore, this step should be executed meticulously. It occurs as a result of multifactorial reasons. However, instability commonly develops because of the three reasons described below.

1. Malposition of the prosthesis components (alignment, height);
   (a) Excessive retroversion causes posterior instability and excessive anteversion anterior instability. A too small head or a short humeral component compromises the soft tissue tension and pave the way for the instability [6].
   (b) A glenoid component placed to a posteriorly defective glenoid surface may cause posterior instability.
2. Capsule; Posterior capsulorrhaphy or a loose posterior capsule may give birth to instability
3. Rotator cuff; Absence of the rotator cuff in patients who underwent non-constrained anatomic prostheses may cause static and dynamic instability, commonly the former with accompanying superior humeral head migration. The dynamic instability is commonly encountered in anterior instability, and the most common reason for soft tissue imbalance is subscapularis insufficiency [10] (Figs. 24.1 and 24.2)

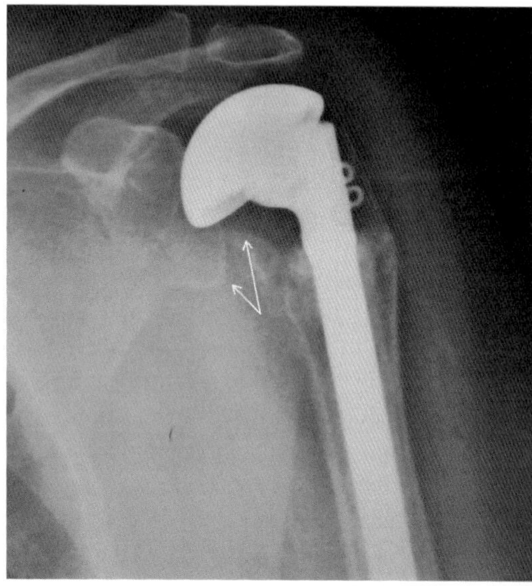

Fig. 24.1 Superior migration of the humeral component on the glenoid fossa because of the rotator cuff insufficiency developed following the hemiarthroplasty which was performed for a proximal humeral fracture

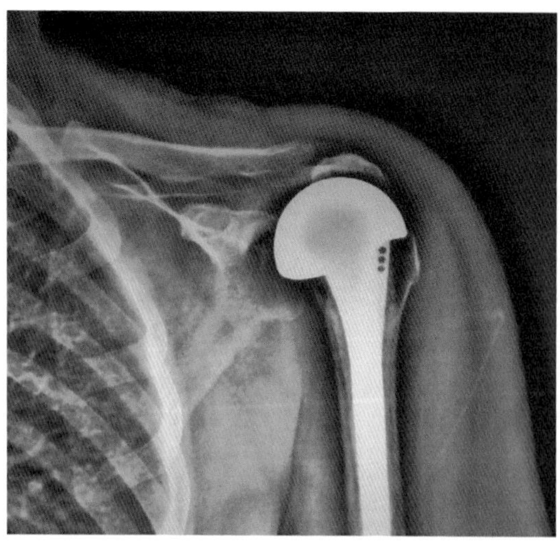

Fig. 24.2 Coracoacromial arc insufficiency following a partial shoulder prosthesis with a CTA head performed for a rotator cuff arhtropathy

The patient may present with dislocation of the humeral head, or an insidiously developing decentralisation and subluxation [11]. Instability problem varies according to the performed prosthesis design.

Instability in Anatomic Total Shoulder Prosthesis

Instability may develop in anterior, posterior, superior, or inferior direction.

Anterior Instability

Typically, the patient presents with shoulder pain. The subscapularis test reveals insufficiency, and the external rotation is increased both actively and passively [10]. The diagnosis of instability is made with magnetic resonance imaging (MRI), computerised tomography (CT), and ultrasonography (USG). Early diagnosis, thus immediate initiation of treatment is crucial for successful outcomes. The axillary radiograph taken within the routine radiographs is pretty helpful for revealing any potential dislocation or subluxation [10].

Reasons for anterior instability are stated below;

1. Implant placement fault; it usually occurs after inaccurately placed glenoid component caused by posterior glenoid insufficiency.
2. Small glenoid component
3. Excessively slack posterior capsule
4. Malposition or retroversion of humeral head or small head.

Superior Instability

It is not rare as assumed. The instability is in superior direction in 20% of total SA cases, and this problem develops in years [6, 10]. Reasons are stated below;

1. The imbalance between deltoid and rotator cuff muscles causes superior migration of humeral head by deltoid muscle when the rotator cuff is feeble.
2. Coracohumeral arc insufficiency
3. Rotator cuff injuries

Superior instability management is best done by avoiding aforementioned issues. Reverse shoulder prostheses may be more appropriate in these patient group (Fig. 24.3).

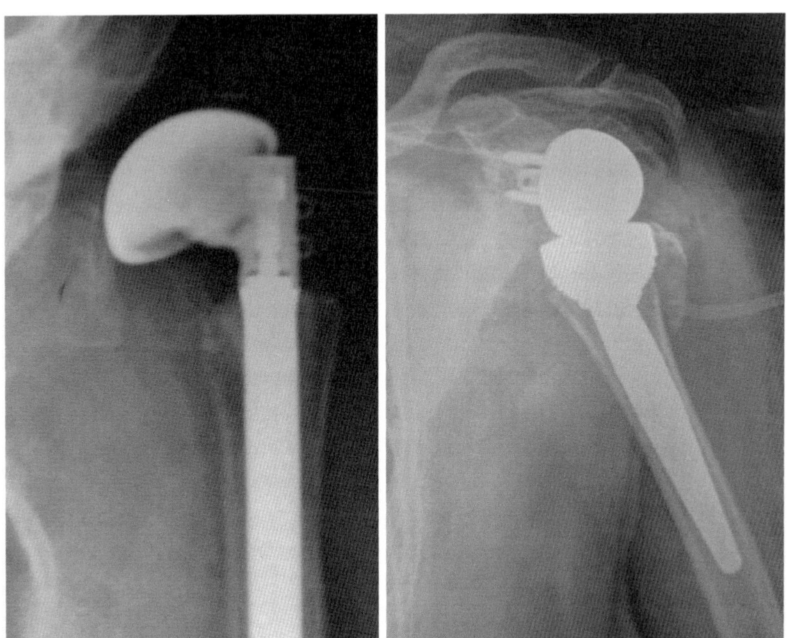

Fig. 24.3 There exist a superior instability in a patient who underwent partial SA for a proximal humeral fracture. The patient underwent reverse SA who also had rotator cuff insufficiency

Inferior Instability

Subscapularis insufficiency.
Use of small diameter glenospheres.
Unadjusted humeral length.

Loosening

Humeral Loosening

Loosening occurs in the humeral component in 6% of prostheses [12].

1. The amount of bony stock after the loosening, the region where the bony stock is copious, and the region where the loosening is abundant.
2. Using cement is critical in both development and treatment of loosening. Especially, the technique for using cement and the quality of the cement in the primary procedure is very important.
3. Taking the advantage of cement plug placement prevents migration of cement to the distal humerus, thus providing convenience for revision procedures.
4. The cortical thickness, especially the osteoporosis level of patients are noteworthy for determining the treatment options.

Glenoid Loosening

According to a meta-analysis, glenoid loosening is encountered in 14.3% of cases [12]. On radiographs, the medially migrated implant and radiolucent lines over 2 mm are assumed as glenoid loosening findings. (Fig. 24.4) CT is recommended in all loosening cases during the planning of the revision surgery to take the advantage of it in giving information about the location of the loosening area and bony stock [14]. Antoine et al. defines three types of glenoid bone loss [13];

- Partial bone loss. Bone loss usually occurs in anterior aspect of the glenoid.
- Central bone loss. It is characterised by bone loss in the centre of the glenoid and causes significant difficulty during the placement of the glenoid component.
- Mix bone loss occurs in every region of glenoid in variable amounts, and in this type of bone loss, revision surgery may turn into a very challenging procedure.

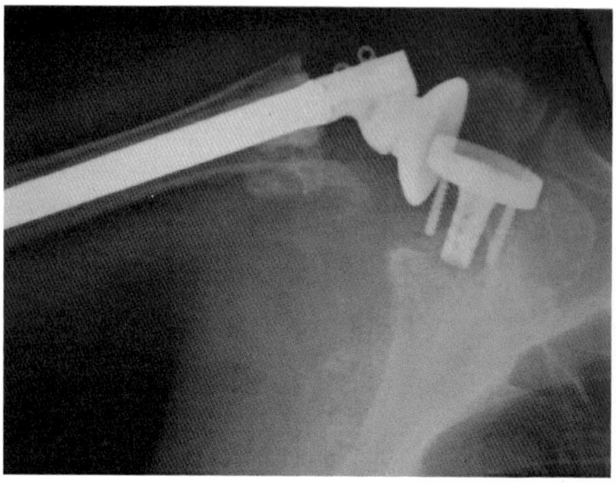

Fig. 24.4 Glenoid component loosening in a patient with reverse SA

Walch et al. defined the glenoid loosening in three types according to the location that the glenoid migrated towards.

1. Superior tilt of the glenoid component (41%)
2. Collapse of glenoid cavity (32.5%)
3. Posterior tilt of the glenoid component (26.5%)

Attrition

The polyethylene insert of the glenoid component may develop attrition [1].

Rotator Cuff Problem

In patients with SA, the imaging of the rotator cuff is difficult because of the artifacts. Superior migration of the humeral head gives information about the condition of the rotator cuff. However, Young et al. reported humeral head superior migration in 46.5% of patients already who underwent total SA [15].

Problems Other Than Loosening Which Could be Developed After SA

- Problems regarding the acromioclavicular joint.
- Problems regarding the long head of biceps.
- Stress fractures of the scapular spine (during the implementation of reverse prostheses). The preoperative disorders of acromion are reported to be inefficacious in reverse SA, but upcoming fractures of it bring forth poor outcomes [16].
- Complex regional pain syndrome. Stiffness may occur even in the absence of any reason lying behind [1].

Treatment Options

Revision Without Changing the Implants

This treatment option is rarely performed. The reasons for revision performed without changing the implants are;

1. Hematoma drainage caused by dead-space
2. Tenotomy for painful long head of biceps tendon
3. Distal clavicle resection for painful acromioclavicular degenerative arthritis
4. Internal fixation for humeral shaft fractures without prosthesis loosening
5. In some infection cases
6. In some loosening cases

Revision With Changing the Implants

The most common reason for this procedure is the defective glenoid components. Problems of implants can be evaluated in four parts: Instability, infection, glenoid component problems, humeral component problems.

Instability

Revisions performed for instability may offer some differences between anatomic and reverse total SA designs.

Anatomic Total SA

Reduction and physical examination are substantial steps after acute dislocations of the shoulder. After the reduction, the patient is observed in a sling with her/his shoulder in 30° of external rotation for 4 weeks, and the reason for instability is determined in this period of time. If there exist an anterior instability depending on the subscapularis insufficiency, then primary repair may be considered in the first 4 weeks [10]. In the subscapularis repairs to be performed after the first month, augmentation process has to be added to the repair procedure. These augmentation techniques include pectoralis major tendon transfer and Achilles tendon allograft applications. The chronic posterior instability is treated by intervention to the tight anterior structures, slack posterior capsule, and malpositioned components. By this means, appropriate glenoid version, humeral alignment, and appropriate soft tissue balance are procured. For this purpose, anterior releasing, subscapularis lengthening, anterior inferior capsulectomy or posterior capsulorrhaphy, and correction of the malpositioned implants are performed. The subscapularis repair, pectoralis major tendon transfer, and capsule strengthening procedures result in 50% of unsatisfactory outcomes either in both anterior and posterior instability. It seems like the best choice for the instability in anatomic total SA is the reverse SA [17].

Reverse Total SA

Dislocations following the first month after the surgery are reduced and immobilised for 45 days. Recurrence rate is higher in dislocations after the first month with conservative treatment [1]. The reason for instability in reverse SA is the defect in length adjustment of the extremity. This problem can be solved by a thicker insert, a bigger glenosphere, or if the length deficiency is more than 2 cm, then exchange of the humeral stem [1].

Infection

In early stage (3 weeks), the infection may occur in the form of haematogenous or late infection. In the elderly patients without systemic infection findings and poor general condition, implants can be left and the patient can be observed, even if there exist a flowing fistula. In patients with haematogenous or early stage infections, debridement lavage, or polyethylene component exchange can be performed. While one-stage revision provides more favourable outcomes, if a two-stage revision is planned, some authors advocate that antibiotic-loaded cement spacers are obligatory in these cases [1, 8]. Total SA infection treatments are still under debate. It is recommended to choose the antibiotic agent according to the culture results and to prescribe at least two separate antibiotics. Surgical intervention options;

a. Antibiotic suppression without surgical intervention:

    This option can be carried out in low-demand elderly patients without systemic infection findings [1].

b. Debridement:

    Recurrence rate following the surgery with the only debridement is high.

c. Two-stage revision:

    There are successful outcome reports with antibiotic-loaded cement spacer applications [18] (Fig. 24.5). In a study, it was reported only a one recurrent infection in 17 patients revised with reverse SA following the application of antibiotic-loaded polymethylmethacrylate (PMMA) [19].

d. One-stage revision:

    Although the two-stage revisions are accepted as a gold standard, one-stage revisions are also considered to be successful options [18]. Out of few studies investigating this issue, Klatte et al. reported only two recurrences out of 35 patients and found the one-stage revision associated with shorter treatment durations, lower treatment costs, and preventing from a second surgery [20]. Ince et al. reported no recurrent infection after one-stage revision prosthesis placement with antibiotic-loaded cement in nine patients [21].

e. Observing with permanent antibiotic-loaded cement spacer following the resection:

    A permanent antibiotic-loaded cement spacer can be performed for patients who could not deal with a second surgery. For this purpose, spacers prepared on the operating table or maquette derived antibiotic-loaded cement spacers can be used [9]. It is recommended to perform this method in low-demand patients with poor general condition [9, 22]

f. Resection arthroplasty:

    This method is recommended for patients who are not appropriate candidates for a second implantation or have recurrent infection. Also, it can be performed in elderly patients with low-demand as an alternative option. Braman et al. reported satisfactory results in seven patients that they performed resection arthroplasty for infected SA [23].

Glenoid Component Problems

Glenoid component revision is usually more challenging than humeral component revision. Therefore, the patients should be evaluated thoroughly and a detailed planning should be made preoperatively for a successful surgery. The structures to be evaluated before the revision of glenoid

1. Humeral head, whether centralised or not; stable/instable
2. The condition of the rotator cuff
3. Glenoid bone stock

Considering the aforementioned factors, different revision options emerge. Thus, three options can be stated which are the removal of the glenoid component, removal of glenoid component with corticocancellous grafting, and the glenoid reimplantation [24]. Although Cofield and Edgerton propose revision with grafting and without reimplantation in glenoid revisions with over bony loss, biomechanical problems develop in these patients. Medially migration of humeral head because of the absence of glenoid component affects on the moment arms of the rotator cuff and deltoid muscle and disrupts the elevation of the arm [24]. The graft choice is still under debate, but tricortical corticocancellous grafts are found to be more appropriate [24]. The methods that glenoid reimplantation not to be added are assumed as salvage procedures, and

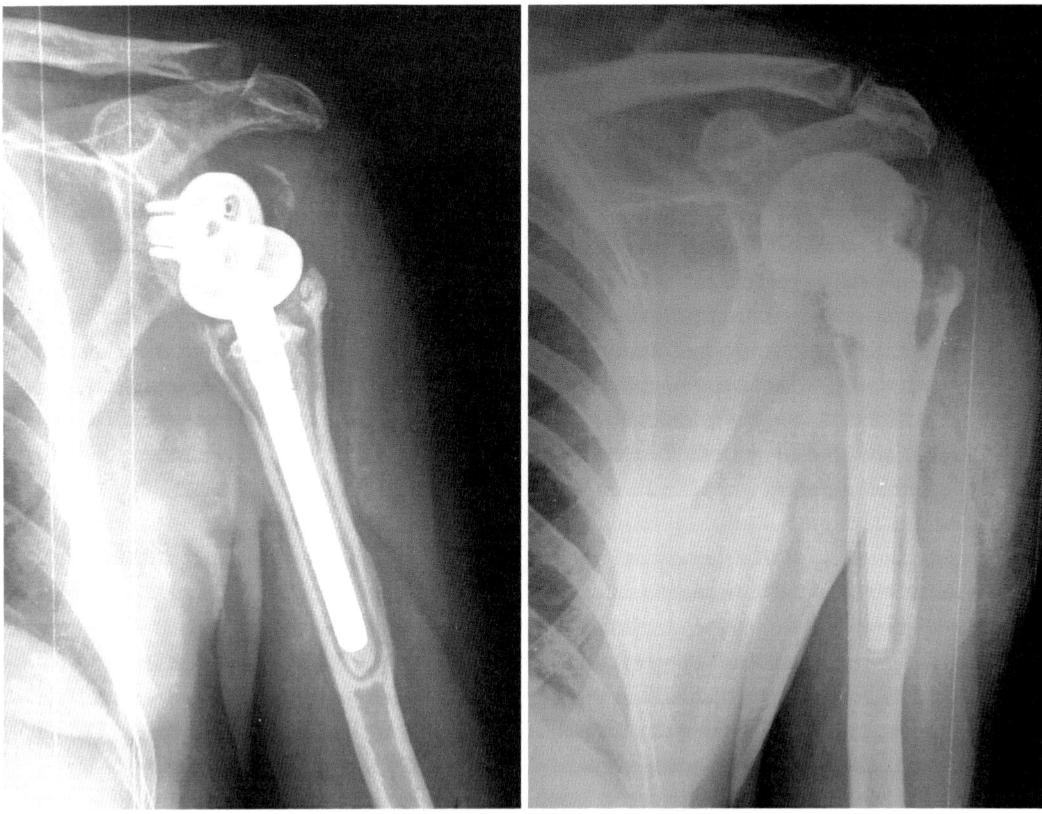

Fig. 24.5 Infected reverse SA. (**a**) Loosening in the cemented humeral component. (**b**) An antibiotic-loaded cement spacer was performed after the removal of the components

these procedures should be performed whenever enough bone stock does not exist [24]. The implanted component varies in terms of anatomic, reverse, and whether an instability developed or not in the revision surgery.

Anatomic Glenoid Component

The exchange of the glenoid component when the bone stock is enough results in better outcomes than grafting-only procedures (Fig. 24.6). The indications for anatomic glenoid component implantation;

Young patient

Intact rotator cuff

Centralised humeral head

Revision of anatomic glenoid component with the reverse glenoid component is a more favourable option in elderly patients with damaged rotator cuff and decentralised humeral head.

If the bone stock of the glenoid is not ample for a glenoid component implantation, tricortical grafting, leaving as pulsied shoulder, and hemiarthroplasty are the recommended options. Melissa et al. found the exchange of glenoid component with reverse total SA as a promising method [25]. This method has both some advantages and disadvantages. The advantages are being suitable for graft fixation and correcting the instability or a soft tissue insufficiency by its constrained design. The disadvantages are having higher complication rate and the higher risk of recurrent surgery [25].

Reverse Glenoid Component

Revisions with reverse prosthesis designs are associated with better outcomes [1]. However, what really matters is the bone stock amount when performing the revision surgery.

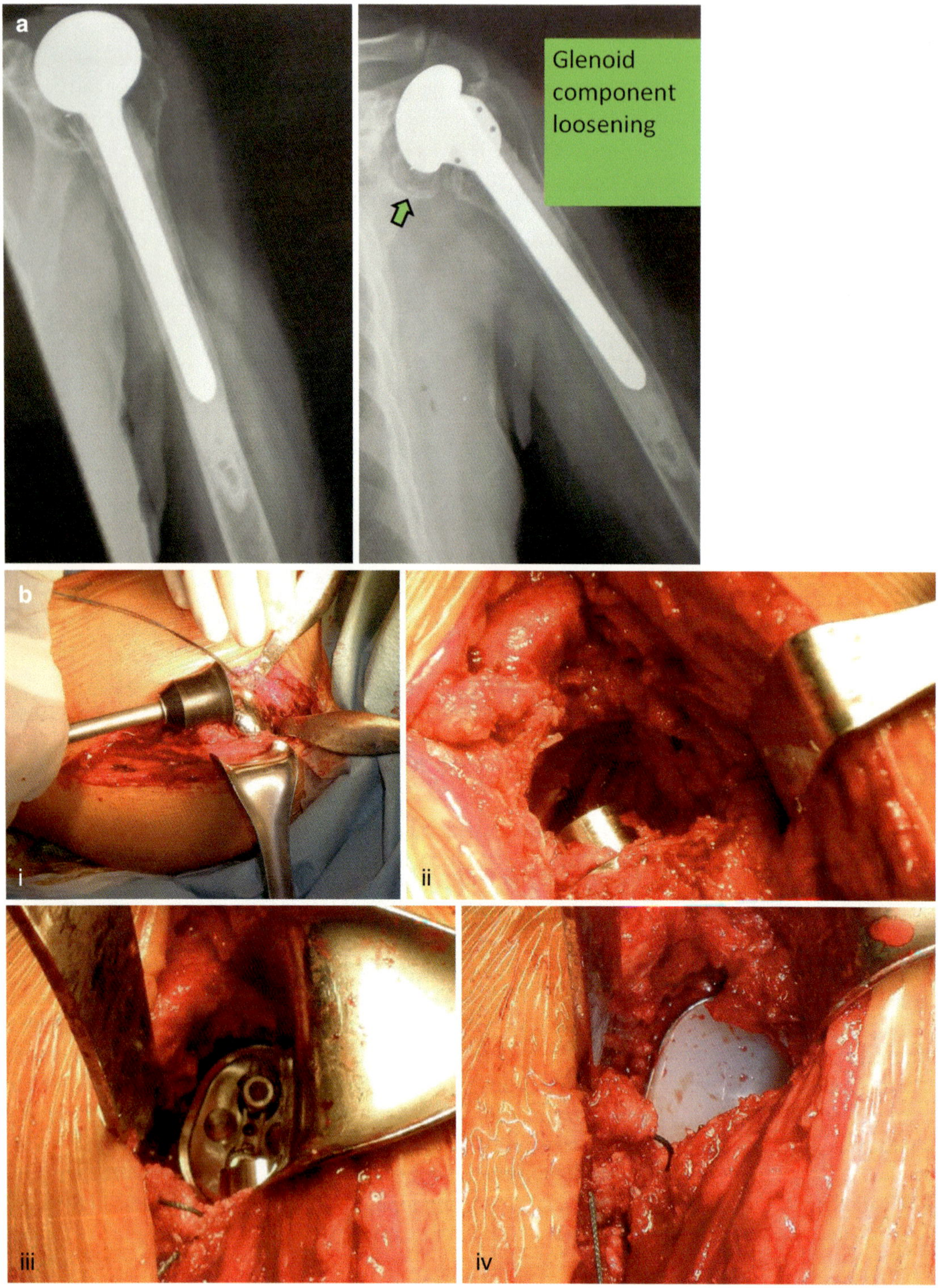

Fig. 24.6 (**a**) Loose glenoid component developed after a total SA. (**b**): Revision of the glenoid component; *i.* Removal of the humeral head, *ii.* Minimal central bony defect after the removal of the glenoid component, *iii.* Placement of the uncemented metal-based glenoid component after filling the defect with spongious bone graft. (**c**): Direct radiographic appearance of the metal-based glenoid component after the procedure

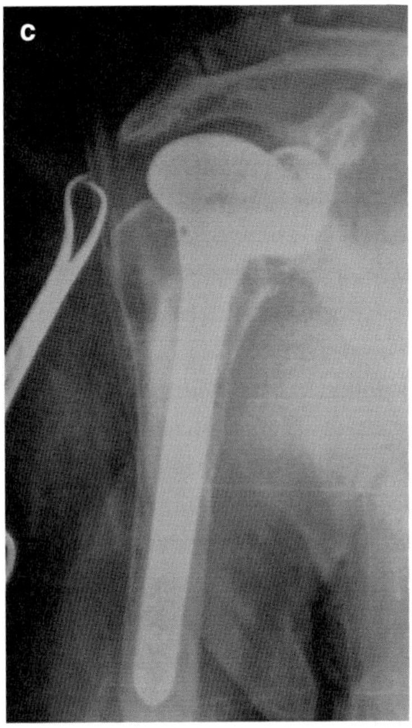

Fig. 24.6 (continued)

Glenoid Component With No Loosening

Revision prostheses in these patient group are made for an instability, infection, or an attrition.

The cemented glenoid component; removal of this implant is easier than uncemented components.

The uncemented glenoid component; removal of these components, if there is no loosening, can be quite difficult, and there can be some bone loss during the removal process. If there is no loosening, only an exchange of the polyethylene insert can be sufficient in these patients.

Humeral Component Problems

Periprosthetic Fractures

Studies including the periprosthetic fractures following total SAs does not have a vast number in the literature [26]. Gonzalez et al. stated the rate of humeral shaft fractures following shoulder prostheses as 2.2% of all complications [12]. Lots of authors recommend conservative treatment, but some pronounce that consolidation speed and rate can be enhanced with surgical intervention [12, 26]. However, the risks of neurologic complication and infection come into prominence with surgery. Therefore, surgery seems to be an appropriate option when the components are unstable and are not in an acceptable position [12]. Wright and Cofield [26] divided the humerus fractures following the total SAs into three types.

Type A; The fracture line starts from the distal tip pf the humeral stem and lies proximally.

Type B; The fracture line starts from the distal tip of the humeral stem and lies distally.

Type C; The fracture line starts further distally from the distal tip of the humeral stem and lies distally.

The management of Type C fractures are recommended to treat as other humerus fractures, and 66–80% of these fractures are reported to heal with conservative methods [26, 27]. The union rate diminishes when the fracture area includes cement. On the other hand, sufficient fixation may not be constituted if there exists osteoporosis. Type A and Type B fractures have a less chance of healing. For this reason, an internal fixation or a revision total SA is recommended for these types. Total SAs are pronounced to be more appropriate in periprosthetic fractures if the union chance is low, if it is an osteoporotic fracture, and if the prosthesis is loose [26].

Humeral Component Problems Other Than Fractures

These problems are less commonly encountered than glenoid component problems. The points to pay attention in the revisions of humeral components are;

The condition of rotator cuff.

The centralisation of the humeral head.

The design of the prosthesis, regarding whether it is modular or not.

Whether the prosthesis is loose or not.

Loose Stems

Before the removal process, the bone stock to be lost and potential tubercular or corporal fractures should be taken into account.

Unimpaired Stems

It can be a well-integrated stem to the bone and also can be a poor-cemented stem. The removal of a loose stem usually does not pose trouble during the procedure, but the removal of a stem that is not loose may be quite challenging. Especially, the fractures of the humerus may occur with 12% chance in anatomic stems and with 30% chance in revision stems [1].

In general, steps to be performed for removal of humeral stems are; [1]

- The head is removed in modular stems.
- The soft tissue and cement in the metaphyseal region are removed.
- If the second step becomes unsuccessful, the metaphysis and the diaphysis is osteotomized along the stem, thus constituted a window to the prosthesis. This cleavage is then opened out and removal process is reiterated.
- If the third step becomes unsuccessful, the window on the humeral diaphysis is opened out and the stem, cement, and plug are removed.
- The cement should be removed completely if possible. Completely removal of the cement is not obligatory unless there exists infection. Removing down to allow placement of a new implant is sufficient.

Implantation of New Humeral Stem

The amount of bone loss and region is important factors in determining the reimplantation. Uncemented components are not used generally [1]. In the existence of bony defects, cancellous autografts or allografts are used while massive allografts are used in the existence of diaphyseal defects. During the removal process, if an osteotomy is performed, then the osteotomized part should be fixated by cerclage wires, and the leakage of the cement out of the humeral medulla must be prevented to protect the radial nerve from thermal damage during the cementing process.

Implantation of the New Glenoid Component

Removal of the Glenoid Component

If the glenoid component is loose, one can easily remove it. Especially, the removal of cemented components is quite difficult, and procedures may result in a significant bone loss.

Reconstruction

A new implant can be placed if there is no significant bone loss. If there is a significant bone loss and a new implant reimplantation is not planned, an uncemented implant design suitable for graft insertion is the preferred option. Shaped tricortical iliac wing grafts passed through the glenoid pegs are recommended for the attachment to the defected glenoid area [28].

Questions

1. What is the most common complication after reverse shoulder arthroplasty?
   A. Infection
   B. Humeral stem loosening
   C. Notching
   D. Nerve injury
   E. Periprosthetic fractures

   C.

2. Which type of humeral periprosthetic fracture has the highest chance of union?
   A. Type A
   B. Type B
   C. Type C
   D. Type D
   E. Type E

   C. Type D and E do not exist.

3. 72 year old male patient who underwent a total shoulder arthroplasty 6 months ago, came to the clinic with active fistula, and he had been offered a two stage revision. After 1 year of revision, he admitted to hospital with

another fistula and loss of shoulder function and pain. You do not want to try another two stage revision because of the little amount of bone stock although he has no other serious health problems. What would you recommend to relieve his pain and gain some range of motion?

A. One stage revision
B. Debridement
C. Antibiotic suppression
D. Resection arthroplasty
E. Antibiotic loaded cement spacers

What is new?

Glenoid bone loss is a challenging problem both in primary and revision arthroplasty. A useful review can be found in Journal of Shoulder and Elbow Surgery, 2016:

Glenoid Bone Loss in Primary and Revision Shoulder Arthroplasty, Malhas A et al.

References

1. Favard L. Revision of total shoulder arthroplasty. Orthop Traumatol Surg Res. 2013;99(1 Suppl):12–21.
2. Sperling JW, Cofield RH, Rowland CM. Minimum fifteen-year follow-up of Neer hemiarthroplasty and total shoulder arthroplasty in patients aged fifty years or younger. J Shoulder Elb Surg. 2004; 13(6):604–13.
3. Torchia ME, Cofield RH, Settergren CR. Total shoulder arthroplasty with the Neer prosthesis: long-term results. J Shoulder Elb Surg. 1997;6(6):495–505.
4. Wirth MA, Rockwood Jr CA. Complications of total shoulder replacement arthroplasty. J Bone Joint Surg. 1996;78:603–16.
5. Singh JA, Sperling JW, Cofield RH. Revision surgery following total shoulder arthroplasty: analysis of 2588 shoulders over three decades (1976 to 2008). J Bone Joint Surg Br. 2011;93(11):1513–7.
6. Bohsali KI, Wirth MA, Rockwood Jr CA. Complications of total shoulder arthroplasty. J Bone Joint Surg Am. 2006;88(10):2279–92.
7. Sajadi KR, Kwon YW, Zuckerman JD. Revision shoulder arthroplasty: an analysis of indications and outcomes. J Shoulder Elb Surg. 2010;19(2):308–13.
8. Zaval JA, Clark JC, Kissenberth MJ, Tolan SJ, Hawkins RJ. Management of deep infection after revers total shoulder arthroplasty: a case series. J Shoulder Elb Surg. 2012;21(10):1310–5.
9. Coffey MJ, Ely EE, Crosby LA. Treatment of glenohumeral sepsis with a commercially produced antibiotic-impregnated cement spacer. J Shoulder Elb Surg. 2010;19(6):868–73.
10. Myer D, Bell RH. Instability after total shoulder arthroplasty. Semin Arthroplast. 2010;21:191–4.
11. Sanchez-Sotelo J, Sperling JW, Rowland CM, Cofield RHJ. Instability after shoulder arthroplasty: results of surgical treatment. J Bone Joint Surg Am. 2003;85-A(4):622–31.
12. Gonzalez JF, Alami GB, Baque F, Walch G, Boileau P. Complications of unconstrained shoulder prostheses. J Shoulder Elb Surg. 2011;20(4):666–82. doi:10.1016/j.jse.2010.11.017.
13. Antuna SA, Sperling JW, Cofield RH, Rowland CM. Glenoid revision surgery after total shoulder arthroplasty. J Shoulder Elb Surg. 2001;10(3):217–24.
14. Walch G, Young AA, Boileau P, Loew M, Gazielly D, Molé D. Patterns of loosening of polyethylene keeled glenoid components after shoulder arthroplasty for primary osteoarthritis: results of a multicenter study with more than five years of follow-up. J Bone Joint Surg Am. 2012;94(2):145–50.
15. Young A, Walch G, Boileau P, Favard L, Gohlke F, Loew M, Molé D. A multicentre study of the long-term results of using a flat-back polyethylene glenoid component in shoulder replacement for primary osteoarthritis. J Bone Joint Surg Br. 2011;93(2):210–6.
16. Walch G, Mottier F, Wall B, Boileau P, Molé D, Favard L. Acromial insufficiency in reverse shoulder arthroplasties. J Shoulder Elb Surg. 2009;18(3):495–502.
17. Sanchez-Sotello J, Sperling JW, Rowland CM, Cofield RH. Intability after shoulder arthroplasty: results of surgical treatment. J Bone Joint Surg Am. 2003;85A:622–31.
18. Romanò CL, Borens O, Monti L, Meani E, Stuyck J. What treatment for periprosthetic shoulder infection? Results from a multicentre retrospective series. Int Orthop. 2012;36(5):1011–7.
19. Sabesan VJ, Ho JC, Kovacevic D, Iannotti JP. Two-stage reimplantation for treating prosthetic shoulder infections. Clin Orthop Relat Res. 2011;469(9):2538–43.
20. Klatte TO, Junghans K, Al-Khateeb H, Rueger JM, Gehrke T, Kendoff D, Neumann J. Single-stage revision for peri-prosthetic shoulder infection: outcomes and results. Bone Joint J. 2013;95-B(3):391–5.
21. Ince A, Seemann K, Frommelt L, Katzer A, Loehr JF. One-stage exchange shoulder arthroplasty for peri-prosthetic infection. J Bone Joint Surg Br. 2005;87(6):814–8.
22. Themistocleous G, Zalavras C, Stine I, Zachos V, Itamura J. Prolonged implantation of an antibiotic cement spacer for management of shoulder sepsis in compromised patients. J Shoulder Elb Surg. 2007;16(6):701–5.

23. Braman JP, Sprague M, Bishop J, Lo IK, Lee EW, Flatow EL. The outcome of resection shoulder arthroplasty for recalcitrant shoulder infections. J Shoulder Elb Surg. 2006;15(5):549–53.
24. Neyton L, Walch G, Nové-Josserand L, Edwards TB. Glenoid corticocancellous bone grafting after glenoid component removal in the treatment of glenoid loosening. J Shoulder Elb Surg. 2006;15(2):173–9.
25. Melis B, Bonnevialle N, Neyton L, Lévigne C, Favard L, Walch G, Boileau P. Glenoid loosening and failure in anatomical total shoulder arthroplasty: is revision with a reverse shoulder arthroplasty a reliable option? J Shoulder Elb Surg. 2012;21(3):342–9.
26. Sewell MD, Kang SN, Al-Hadithy N, Higgs DS, Bayley I, Falworth M, Lambert SM. Management of peri-prosthetic fracture of the humerus with severe bone loss and loosening of the humeral component after total shoulder replacement. J Bone Joint Surg Br. 2012;94(10):1382–9.
27. Wright TW, Cofield RH. Humeral fractures after shoulder arthroplasty. J Bone Joint Surg Am. 1995;77(9):1340–6.
28. Norris TR, Kelly II JD, Humphrey CS. Management of glenoid bone defects in revision shoulder arthroplasty: a new application of the reverse total shoulder prosthesis. Tech Shoulder Elbow Surg. 2007;8(1):37–46.

Shoulder Arthrodesis

25

Ehud Atoun, Zachary T. Sharfman, Ehud Rath, and Ofer Levy

Introduction

Arthrodesis is the creation of a bony union across a joint, it is a radical procedure that contradicts the primary function of the joint, which is to provide motion. The shoulder has the largest range of motion of any ball-and-socket joint in the body, movement that is crucial for the upper limb function. The term shoulder arthrodesis is frequently used to describe what is actually humero-scapular arthrodesis in which the humerus is fused to the glenoid and/or acromion, a procedure that limits shoulder movement.

For most of the past century, shoulder arthrodesis was a relatively common procedure but its indications have been diminishing, largely due to lower prevalence of poliomyelitis, tuberculosis, and good outcomes with shoulder arthroplasty. More specifically, reverse shoulder arthroplasty offered a solution for patients with non-functioning rotator cuff muscles. Nevertheless, arthrodesis has stood the test of time and can be a reliable method of restoring a limited range of pain-free motion to the shoulder, which is retained at the scapulothoracic joint by the scapulothoracic, trapezius and serratus anterior muscles.

Currently glenohumeral arthrodesis is still considered an end-stage salvage procedure for shoulder pain, weakness, and instability not suitable for soft-tissue or prosthetic reconstruction. The objective of shoulder arthrodesis is to create a painless, functional extremity, sufficient for most activities of daily living (ADLs) [3, 13, 14].

Indications

Paralytic Disorders

Until recent decades poliomyelitis was a major cause of flail shoulder, worldwide, this is still the case in developing countries, where poliomyelitis is prevalent. In the modern western world, the most common cause of paralytic shoulder is brachial plexus injury. Motor vehicle accidents account for most traumatic brachial plexus injuries, which affect young patients in most cases. When spontaneous recovery of the deltoid and rotator cuff muscles does not occur, shoulder arthrodesis may be considered in the presence of severely restricted, painful range of motion, and/or failed prior reconstructive measures such as neurolysis, nerve grafting, and muscle transfer.

E. Atoun (✉)
Faculty of Health Science, Ben Gurion University, Barzilai Medical Center Campus, Ashkelon, Israel

Z.T. Sharfman • E. Rath
Department of Orthopaedic Surgery, Tel Aviv Soursky Medical Center and the Sackler Faculty of Medicine at Tel Aviv University, Tel Aviv, Israel
e-mail: udirath@hotmail.com

O. Levy
Shoulder and Elbow Centre Reading Shoulder Unit, Berkshire Independent Hospital, Reading, UK

G. Huri, N.K. Paschos (eds.), *The Shoulder*, Orthopaedic Study Guide Series,
DOI 10.1007/978-3-319-51979-1_25

These patients usually have good elbow and hand function as well as good seratus anterior and trapezius function but are unable to optimize their upper extremity due to their inability to "place their hand in space." The goal of arthrodesis in this case is to create a stable platform for good elbow and hand function and active arm abduction through the scapulothoracic articulation. This allows patients to utilize their upper extremity and work effectively at bench level.

Failed Prosthetic Arthroplasty

The number of shoulder arthroplasties performed worldwide has exponentially increased during the last decade. The overall ten-year survival of shoulder arthroplasties has been reported to be 88%. Therefore, as the frequency of primary shoulder arthroplasty increases, the number of failures is expected to increase substantially.

Arthrodesis can be considered for selected patients with failed shoulder arthroplasty, when revision is impossible due to severe humeral and glenoid bone loss, poor deltoid and rotator cuff function, iatrogenic axillary nerve injury and refractory instability. When arthrodesis is considered for these patients, special techniques are needed to compensate for the significant glenoid and humeral bone loss, scarring and fibrosis (Fig. 25.1a, b) [1, 7].

Reconstruction After Tumor Resection

Limb-salvage surgeries have become the first-line treatment for malignant bone and soft tissue tumors of the shoulder girdle. In light of the reduction in the surgical margin achieved by refinements of imaging modalities and radiotherapy as well as improvements in adjuvant chemotherapy, patients are often able to retain limb function after these procedures.

Functional reconstruction of the shoulder joint after wide excision of a malignant bone tumor of the proximal humerus is clinically challenging, particularly because wide excision may result in deficits of the deltoid, rotator cuff, joint capsule, and bony elements. This makes arthroplastic reconstruction difficult. In these cases, arthrodesis is a useful technique to bridge bony defects using bone grafts, vascularized bone grafts, and massive allografts. Patient satisfaction was found to be higher than that for artificial prostheses in this patient population [11, 15].

Chronic Infection

Bacterial or tubercular infections uncontrolled with medication or debridement often result in pain and joint incongruency. In the past, arthritis due to tubercular infections was a major indication for shoulder arthrodesis. Although this is

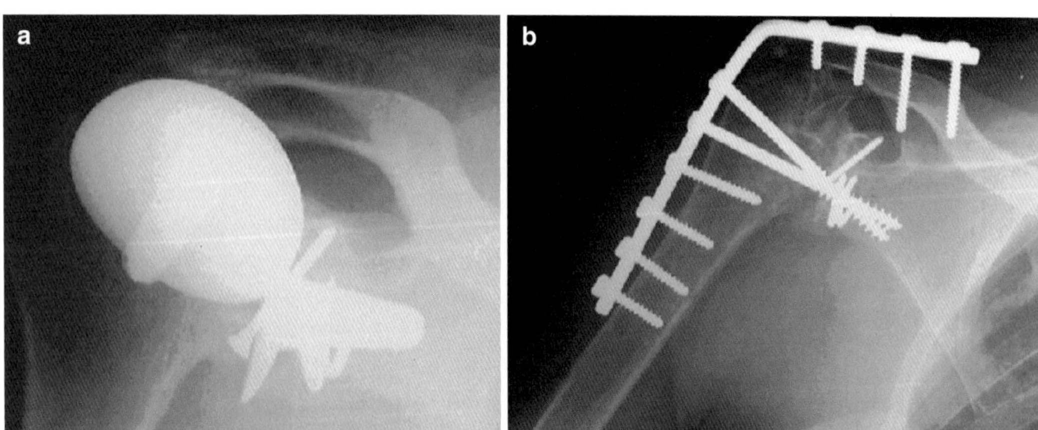

Fig. 25.1 Shoulder arthrodesis for failed prosthetic arthroplasty. (**a**) Pre operative radiograph with failed shoulder arthroplasty. (**b**) Post operative radiograph following shoulder arthrodesis with multiple screws and a 4.5-mm AO plate

still a problem worldwide, in the Western world, it has become rare.

Shoulder infection is one of the most feared complications after shoulder injections, arthroplasty or osteosynthesis for fracture. The diagnosis of septic arthritis of the shoulder represents an absolute indication for urgent surgical intervention, and if it is not undertaken, there is a high risk of irreversible local changes, severe morbidity and possible mortality.

In patients with persistent chronic infection, arthroplasty is contraindicated, and arthrodesis with limited internal fixation, with or without external fixation, often is the preferred salvage option [16].

Refractory Instability

Shoulder instability is usually managed through soft-tissue stabilisation and bone block procedures. With persistent refractory instability after multiple failed stabilization procedures, patients may be left with a painful, dysfunctional shoulder devoid of competent soft-tissue or bony restraints.

These patients are often young or seeking work, and find the prospect of living with a painful unstable shoulder untenable. In this setting, glenohumeral arthrodesis may be considered a salvage procedure [4].

Contraindications

Scapulothoracic motion is crucial for function after shoulder arthrodesis. Therefore severe dysfunction of the scapular stabilizing muscles, trapezius, levator scapulae, serratus anterior and latissimus dorsi is considered a contraindication for glenohumeral arthrodesis.

Charcot arthropathy has also been reported as a contraindication to shoulder arthrodesis. The rates of pseudoarthrosis and infection are stated to be higher in these patients, and thus shoulder arthrodesis is discouraged.

Bilateral arthrodesis is contraindicated because it severely inhibits the patient's functional abilities, including the ability to perform activities of daily living.

Patients who are believed to be unable to cooperate with the extensive course of rehabilitation after surgery, those who are unable to wear a shoulder spica or brace, and patients with severe skin problems or progressive neurologic disorders are contraindicated for glenohumeral arthrodesis as well.

Shoulder Positioning

The ideal position for shoulder arthrodesis remains controversial. When the position of the arm is being determined, the trunk is commonly used as the point of reference, with the scapula held in the anatomic position.

Currently, most authors prefer 10–20° of abduction and flexion and 35–45° of internal rotation. In addition, the patient's arm should be able to rest at the side without excessive scapular winging. This position allows the patient to reach the mouth, waist, back pocket, and contralateral shoulder, facilitating activities of daily living including dressing and self hygiene. The position of rotation is the most crucial factor in obtaining optimal function (Fig. 25.2).

It is difficult to objectively and accurately measure the different angles in various planes during surgery, and the ideal position depends on patient body, size and should be individually tailored intra operatively.

Abduction can be determined by measuring the angle formed by the body and the humerus, clinically or by obtaining an anteroposterior radiographic view using the spine rather than the border of the scapula as a landmark. Flexion is determined by observing the angle that the humerus forms with the horizontal plane in a supine patient. In order to determine the desired amount of internal rotation, the elbow is flexed to 90°, the hand is positioned over the ipsilateral area of the chest between the sternum and axilla so that further flexion of the elbow allows the top of the thumb to touch the chin.

The joint is then temporarily stabilized with two threaded Steinmann.

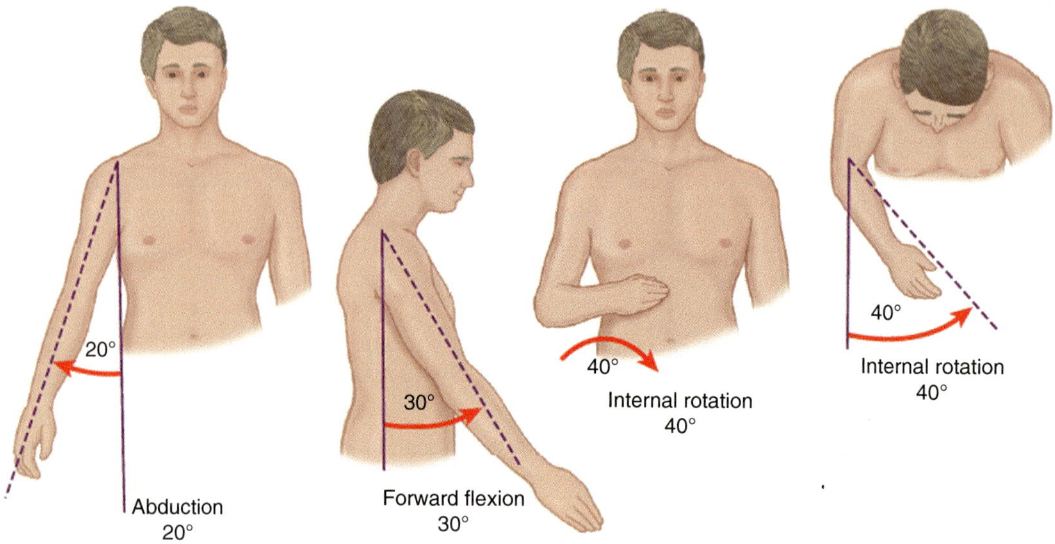

Fig. 25.2 Position of arm for arthrodesis of shoulder as recommended by Rowe: 20° of abduction (clinical measurement), 30° of forward flexion, and 40–50° of internal rotation. Reprinted with permission from Campbell's operative orthopaedics, 12th ed., S. Terry Canale, editor, Mosby, 2013. Chapter 13

Pins and the position is checked to ensure that the patient's hand can reach the mouth, the front of the abdomen, and perineal area before definitive fixation is applied.

Surgical Technique

Extra-Articular Technique

Shoulder arthrodesis is classified as extra-articular (acromiohumeral), intra-articular (glenohumeral), or a combination of extra-articular and intra-articular.

Extra-articular fusion is obtained by bringing the proximal humerus into maximal contact with the undersurface of the acromion, spine of scapula, and clavicle without entering the glenohumeral joint. This technique was performed early in the twentieth century, primarily in treating tuberculosis and is rarely performed as isolated procedure today.

Intra-Articular Technique

Intra-articular fusion involves a thorough decortication of the humerus and glenoid in an open or arthroscopically assisted technique, creating maximal bone to bone contact, preserving the anatomical height of the humeral head and preserving the rotator cuff tendons [12].

Currently, combined extra- and intra-articular fusion techniques are most commonly used.

External Fixation

Charnley originally described a procedure to accomplish shoulder arthrodesis by applying external fixation (Fig. 25.3b). Postoperatively, spica casts were used for additional stability in all patients. Although the supplementation of compression screws (Fig. 25.3c) reduced the length of postoperative immobilization, most patients still required relatively prolonged peri-

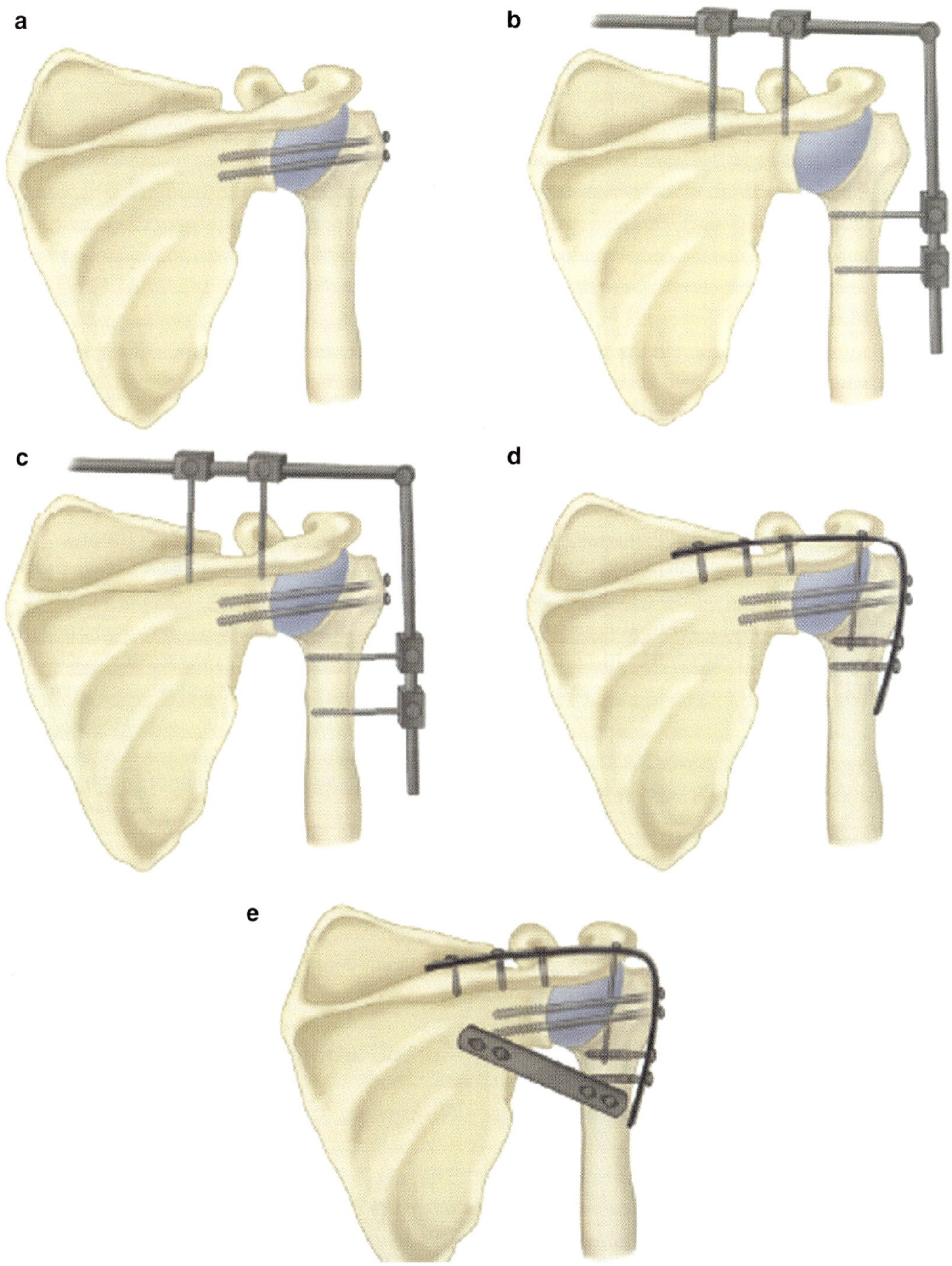

Fig. 25.3 Fixation techniques for shoulder arthrodesis (posterior view). (**a**) Screws alone. (**b**) External fixation alone. (**c**) External fixation with screws. (**d**) Single-plate fixation. (**e**) Double-plate fixation. Reprinted with permission from Miller BS, Harper WP, Gillies RM, et al.: Biomechanical analysis of five fixation techniques used in glenohumeral arthrodesis, Aust N Z J Surg 73:1015, 2003

ods of postoperative spica cast. External fixation should be considered in patients with significant soft tissue loss or deficiency, excessive scar tissue and in patients with recalcitrant infections.

Screw Fixation

A combination of horizontal screws compressing the humerus to the glenoid and vertical screws fixating the acromion to the humeral head are usually used for screw fixation shoulder arthrodesis (Fig. 25.3a). The number of humerus-glenoid screws varies from 0 to 4, and the number of acromion–humerus screws varies from 0 to 3. A partial osteotomy of the acromion can be performed near its junction with the scapular spine, and the acromion displaced downward, hinging through the acromioclavicular joint and attached to the humeral head or alternatively the humerus is displaced superiorly to contact the acromion [8].

Plate Fixation

Various techniques have been described for plate fixation in shoulder arthrodesis. Dynamic compression plates (DCP), pelvic reconstruction plates, and single or double plates (superior and posterior) can be used (Fig. 25.3e). The procedure includes decortication of the glenoid fossa, the undersurface of the acromion, and the head of the humerus, displacing humerus proximally to appose the undersurface of the acromion. Acromial osteotomy can be added to improve plate bone contact, horizontal compression screws are passed through the plate, traversing the humeral head and into the glenoid.

The combination of plates and traversing compression screws and has minimized the need for strict postoperative immobilization without a concurrent increase in nonunion rates (Fig. 25.3d); this has become the accepted standard of care for glenohumeral arthrodesis [2, 5, 6, 9, 10].

Bone Graft

In the presence of bone stock deficiency (arthrodesis after failed prosthetic arthroplasty or tumor resection), augmentation of the bone stock may be necessary. When the deficiency is <6 cm, the bone contact can be improved using a vascularized clavicular or tuberosity autograft, tricortical iliac bone, or an allograft reinforced with plate fixation. When >6 cm of the proximal humeral shaft is missing, single or double-barrel vascularized fibular grafts are recommended.

Postoperative Management

After surgery, the shoulder is immobilized using shoulder spica cast or a premade custom orthosis in the desired position. Stable internal fixation can reduce the need for spica casting since the use of orthosis is generally better tolerated. Spica cast is added post operatively in cases of external fixation, and pins are usually removed at 6 weeks.

The extent of immobilization depends on the quality and quantity of bone as well as the stability of the fixation. The length of immobilization may range from 8 to 16 weeks. Radiographs are used to assess bony fusion and in selected cases computed tomography may be necessary. Scapular exercises for range of motion and strength are started after radiographic signs of fusion are confirmed.

Complications

Nonunion

The incidence of nonunion has been reported to range from 0 to 20%. Nonunion rate largely depend on fixation technique, bone quality, bone quantity and soft tissue condition. Higher nonunion rates were found after screw fixation arthrodesis.

Patients should be encouraged to abstain from tobacco use because of the association of smoking with an increased risk for nonunion. Optimal operative technique includes careful attention to elimination of all cartilage, maximal bone contact, and solid positioning of all implants.

With modern fixation methods the nonunion rate is closer to 10%, however, in the presence of infection and bone loss, nonunion rates increase accordingly. Most reported non-unions are symptomatic, painful, and required further treatment. Revision surgery with bone grafting and re fixation achieves union in most patients.

Malposition

Excessive abduction and flexion produce mal-rotation or winging of the scapula, which results in a dull, painful ache in the shoulder. In addition, excessive abduction can cause traction neuritis of the brachial plexus.

If too much internal rotation has been incorporated, the patient cannot easily bring his hand to his mouth or reach his front or back pocket. When the malposition causes scapular pain or leads to dysfunction in ADLs, reconstructive osteotomy should be considered.

Fractures

Elimination of motion at the glenohumeral joint combined with local osteopenia increases the probability that relatively minor trauma will cause fracture around the arthrodesis.

Fracture may occur in association with hardware failure or distal to the site of the arthrodesis. Distal fractures are more common, these fractures are usually treated non-operatively with high union rates. Fractures in association with fixation failure have been successfully treated with removal of the devices and repeat plate application and bone grafting.

Prominence of Internal Fixation Device

The superficial location of internal fixation devices, particularly compression screws and plates, may cause local skin problems and skin penetration. Typically, this occurs over the spine of the scapula and acromion due to gross muscle wasting and atrophy around the shoulder in addition to excessive scar tissue due to multiple surgeries. In many cases, removal of the fixation device after consolidation of the fusion mass is necessary.

Postoperative infection, fractures of the humerus, and removal of material due to persistent pain are more frequent complications in plate arthrodesis whereas the rate of nonunion is higher after screw arthrodesis. In comparison with plate arthrodesis, screw arthrodesis reduces the need for extensive dissection and soft tissue damage. This may help to explain the lower infection rate after screw arthrodesis.

Overview

Shoulder arthrodesis has become a relatively rare surgical procedure after the introduction of shoulder arthroplasty and the reduced frequency of objective indications. Shoulder arthrodesis is currently indicated for selected patients with paralytic disorders, failed prosthetic arthroplasty, reconstruction after tumor resection, chronic infection and refractory instability.

The objective of shoulder arthrodesis is to create a painless, functional extremity, sufficient for most ADLs. The ideal position for shoulder arthrodesis remains controversial. Currently, most authors prefer 10–20° of abduction and flexion and 35–45° of internal rotation. In addition, the patient's arm should be able to rest at the side without excessive scapular winging.

Shoulder arthrodesis can be stabilized with external fixators, compression screws, DCPs and reconstruction plates. Patients are immobilized after surgery a shoulder spica cast or prefabricated brace for a period of 8–16 weeks until radiographic union is observed.

Complications of shoulder arthrodesis include nonunion, malposition, fractures, infection and prominence of the internal fixation device. Postoperative infection, fractures of the humerus, and hardware removal due to persistent pain are more frequent complications in plate arthrodesis, whereas the rate of nonunion is higher after screw arthrodesis. In comparison with plate arthrodesis, screw arthrodesis reduces the need for extensive dissection and soft tissue damage.

As a salvage procedure for patients with recalcitrant shoulder issues, arthrodesis can provide patients with a slable, functional and painless shoulder.

Questions

1. Which one of the circumstances is not an indication for shoulder arthrodesis?
   A. Inadequate soft and bone tissue after tumor resection
   B. Subacute infection
   C. Paralytic disorders
   D. Failed arthroplasty
   E. Refractory instability
   B

2. What would you consider intra-operatively as the most important criteria(s) for postoperative range of motion?
   A. Ability to reach and comb hair
   B. Ability to reach lumbosacral area
   C. Ability to reach the mouth
   D. Ability to reach the sternum
   E. Ability to reach the waist
   C and E

3. Despite of decreasing frequency, an orthopaedic surgeon should be aware of shoulder arthrodesis as a salvage option. Which method has the best postoperative outcomes for arthrodesis?
   A. External fixation
   B. Screw fixation
   C. Plate fixation
   D. Screw + plate fixation
   D

What's new?

A new technique is described by Boretto et al. by using both compression screws and locking plate without decreasing union rates and allowing early postoperative scapulothoracic motion

Glenohumeral Arthrodesis with Locking Compression Plate, J Hand Surg Am 2016 June, Boretto JG, Gallucci GL, De Carli P

References

1. Alta TD, Willems WJ. Once an arthrodesis, always an arthrodesis? J Shoulder Elb Surg. 2015;25(2):232–7.
2. Chun JM, Byeon HK. Shoulder arthrodesis with a reconstruction plate. Int Orthop. 2009;33(4):1025–30.
3. Clare DJ, Wirth MA, Groh GI, Rockwood Jr CA. Shoulder arthrodesis. J Bone Joint Surg Am. 2001;83-A(4):593–600.
4. Diaz JA, Cohen SB, Warren RF, Craig EV, Allen AA. Arthrodesis as a salvage procedure for recurrent instability of the shoulder. J Shoulder Elb Surg. 2003;12(3):237–41.
5. Dimmen S, Madsen JE. Long-term outcome of shoulder arthrodesis performed with plate fixation: 18 patients examined after 3–15 years. Acta Orthop. 2007;78(6):827–33.
6. Esenyel CZ, Ozturk K, Imren Y, Ayanoglu S. Shoulder arthrodesis with plate fixation. Acta Orthop Traumatol Turc. 2011;45(6):412–20.
7. Gadea F, Alami G, Pape G, Boileau P, Favard L. Shoulder hemiarthroplasty: outcomes and long-term survival analysis according to etiology. Orthop Traumatol Surg Res. 2012;98(6):659–65.
8. Lerch S, Berndt T, Lipka W, Ruhmann O. Screw arthrodesis of the shoulder. Oper Orthop Traumatol. 2011;23(3):215–26.
9. Lerch S, Keller S, Kirsch L, Berndt T, Ruhmann O. Biomechanical analysis for primary stability of shoulder arthrodesis in different resection situations. Clin Biomech (Bristol, Avon). 2013;28(6):618–25.
10. Miller BS, Harper WP, Gillies RM, Sonnabend DH, Walsh WR. Biomechanical analysis of five fixation techniques used in glenohumeral arthrodesis. ANZ J Surg. 2003;73(12):1015–7.
11. Mimata Y, Nishida J, Sato K, Suzuki Y, Doita M. Glenohumeral arthrodesis for malignant tumor of the shoulder girdle. J Shoulder Elb Surg. 2015;24(2):174–8.
12. Porcellini G, Savoie 3rd FH, Campi F, Merolla G, Paladini P. Arthroscopically assisted shoulder arthrodesis: is it an effective technique? Arthroscopy. 2014;30(12):1550–6.
13. Ruhmann O, Schmolke S, Bohnsack M, Flamme C, Wirth CJ. Shoulder arthrodesis: indications, technique, results, and complications. J Shoulder Elb Surg. 2005;14(1):38–50.
14. Safran O, Iannotti JP. Arthrodesis of the shoulder. J Am Acad Orthop Surg. 2006;14(3):145–53.
15. Tsukushi S, Nishida Y, Yamada Y, Hosono K, Ishiguro N. Vascularized clavicular rotation graft for revised shoulder arthrodesis after tumor resection of the proximal humerus: a case report. J Shoulder Elb Surg. 2009;18(3):e13–6.
16. Wick M, Muller EJ, Ambacher T, Hebler U, Muhr G, Kutscha-Lissberg F. Arthrodesis of the shoulder after septic arthritis. Long-term results. J Bone Joint Surg Br. 2003;85(5):666–70.

Anatomy, Assesment, and Surgery of the Biceps Tendon

26

Zachary T. Sharfman, Ran Atzmon, Eyal Amar, and Ehud Rath

Functional Anatomy

The long head of the biceps (LHB) attaches to its origin at the supraglenoid tubercle of the scapula where it meets the glenoid labrum [1–3]. This origin is fairly broad with a mean diameter of 6.6 mm (range 4.5–12) [4]. The insertion point is located medial to the articular rim of the glenoid and creates a subsynovial recess, which may be positioned variably [2]. Although multiple anatomic variants exist 86% of patients possess typical anatomy [5].

There are four large groups of anatomic variation in the intraarticular portion of the LHB, which are determined by LHB migration during embryonic growth [6]. The Meso group has free movement beneath the rotator cuff, the adherent group has a LHB adherent to the rotator cuff (Fig. 26.1), the split group has a LHB divided intraarticularly, and there is also an absence of the LHB [7].

Z.T. Sharfman, M.D. • E. Amar, M.D. • E. Rath, M.D. (✉)
Department of Orthopaedic Surgery,
Tel Aviv Soursky Medical Center and the Sackler Faculty of Medicine at Tel Aviv University,
Tel Aviv, Israel
e-mail: udirath@hotmail.com

R. Atzmon, M.D.
Department of Orthopaedic Surgery, Assaf Harofe Medical Center and the Sackler Faculty of Medicine,
Tzrifin, Israel

The complex vascularization of the proximal LHB is composed of ascending vessels of the anterior humeral circumflex artery [8, 9]. Branches of the brachial and deep brachial arteries supply the more distal aspects of the LHB [8, 9]. In the region where the tendon slides in the groove, 1.2–3 cm from the origin, the tissue is poorly supplied which may contribute to tendon rupture pathology [10].

The intraarticular portion of the LHBTs diameter is 5.1 mm on average (range 3–7 mm) [4] and distally the tendons slide 18 mm inside the

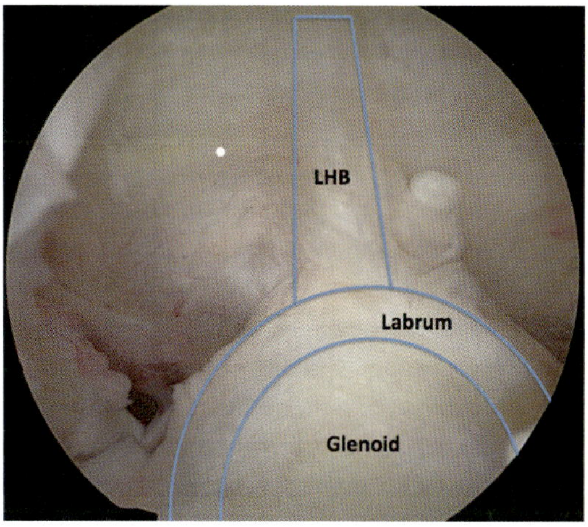

Fig. 26.1 Adherent long head of the biceps tendon pathology demonstrated in an arthroscopic image

G. Huri, N.K. Paschos (eds.), *The Shoulder*, Orthopaedic Study Guide Series,
DOI 10.1007/978-3-319-51979-1_26

joint to achieve anterior flexion and internal rotation movements [11]. Once the tendon enters the bicipital groove of the hummers, the LHBT twists 30–40° [12]. The bicipital groove is located between the greater and lesser tuberosity of the anterior humerus. The grooves 4 mm depth and opening angle stabilize the LHBT in collaboration with the transvers ligament and biceps pulley [13]. The biceps pulley is composed of the superior glenoid humeral ligament and coracohumeral ligament, which are associated with subscapularis and supraspinatus tendons.

The coracoid apophysis serves as the origin of the short head of the biceps (SHB) as well as other structures. The SHB contributes the medial aspect of the bicep mass. Distally the short and long heads combine to create one muscle belly and they insert in two layers to the radial tuberosity and to the bicipital aponeurosis fanning out over the medial aspect of the forearm flexors. The muscle mass of the biceps confers the flexion function of the elbow as well as supination [14, 15]. As the arm progresses from external to internal rotation, the tendon is displaced medially and superiorly, contacting the lesser tubercle and the transverse ligament [13]. The innervation of the biceps if derived from the musculocutaneous nerve.

Clinical Presentation and Physical Examination

The clinical presentation and physical examination of LHBT pathology is challenging even for experienced clinicians. The physical exam should begin with a detail history followed by a focused and systematic physical examination. A detailed patient history documenting the type of pain, catching, snapping, deformity, weakness and other complaints is key. Understanding mechanism of injury and acuity of injury may offer insight into both acute and chronic pathologies. Many patients with biceps pathology describe anterior shoulder pain that is exacerbated by lifting and or elevated pulling motions. This pain will most often localize to the anterior arm in line with the bicipital groove and intensify with movement. Anterior pain may help to delineate shoulder pathology specific to LHBT pathology. Overhead sports activities are likely in the history of patients we LBHT pathology. Understanding aggravating motions and unstable positions also help to differentiate LBHT pathology from other causes of shoulder pain.

Inspection of the upper extremity with comparison of the contralateral limb should be conducted first during the physical examination. It is crucial to maintain a high index of suspicion for subtle atrophy, deformity, swelling and ecchymosis while comparing the injured limb to the pain free extremity. In the case of marked deformity such as a "Popeye's" deformity inspection alone may be sufficient to diagnose complete rupture of the LHBT.

The patient's limbs should then be palpated for tenderness. Tenderness of the LHBT is best palpated with the patients arm placed in 10° of external rotation so the bicipital groove faces anteriorly (Fig. 26.2). Tendinitis localized to the bicipital groove is not typical in patients presenting with acute injury. However, partial rupture or full rupture of the biceps tendon may be suspected in patients with preexisting tendinitis. Structures adjacent to the bicipital groove should be palpated for tenderness as well, as the differential diagnosis for anterior shoulder pain includes acromioclavicular joint pathologies (Fig. 26.3), adhesive

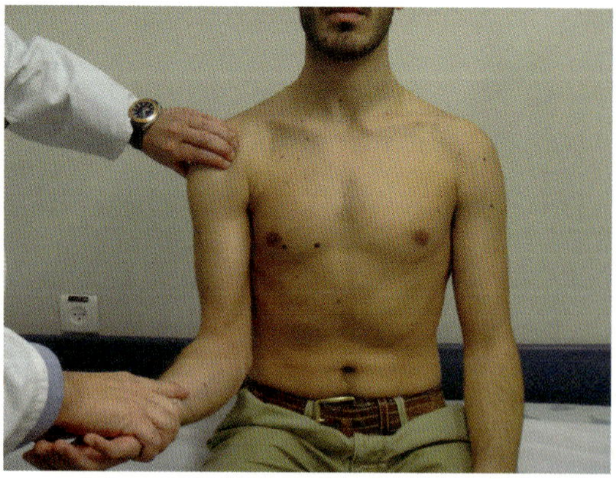

Fig. 26.2 Tenderness of the long head of the biceps tendon can be palpated with the patients arm placed in 10 degrees of external rotation so the bicipital groove faces anteriorly

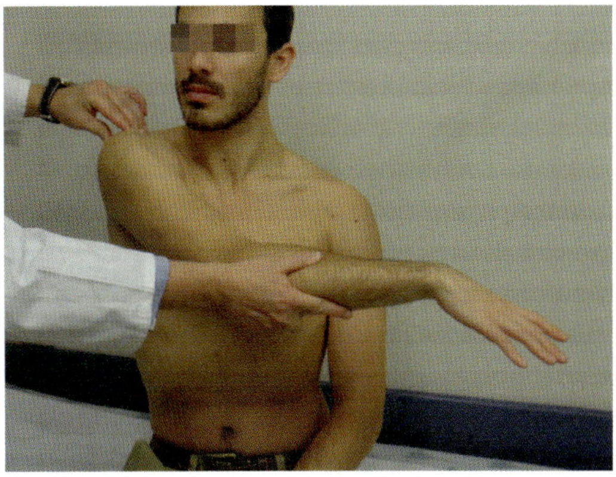

Fig. 26.3 Physical examination manuver demonstrating test to illicit pain in acromioclavicular joint pathologies

capsulitis, subacromial impingement, and coracoid impingement.

The neurovascular examination bilaterally of the upper extremities should be employed to assess motor strength, movement, and sensation. Both active and passive range of motion should be measured and recorded.

The structures above and below the area of pain should be inspected and palpated as the source of pain may be referred from the cervical spine or the elbow.

Pathologies

Biceps Tendonitis

Biceps tendonitis is characterized by anterior shoulder pain. Patients who regularly participate in repetitive lifting, pulling, reaching, and throwing motions in their work or during sport activities are likely to develop biceps tendonitis. Biceps tendonitis is more common in older individuals and may be associated with comorbid shoulder pathologies. Inflammation and painful motions in the shoulder are common and pain should be elicited on palpation of the bicipital groove with the patients arm held in 10° of internal rotation.

Rupture and Tears

Proximal rupture of the biceps may cause a sudden and painful popping sensation that the patient reports on examination. A retraced muscle belly may be clearly visible bulging over the anterior proximal portion of the arm, commonly known as the "Popeye" deformity. In patients without acute traumatic injuries, the biceps tendon rupture is usually preceded by a history of shoulder pain that quickly resolves after a painful audible snap occurs. Partial tears do not present with Popeye deformity but a patient may report a traumatic injury during motion followed by pain and even bruising. It may be difficult to differentiate biceps tendon tear from tendonitis based on history and physical examination alone.

Distal biceps avulsions are another rare pathology more commonly seen in older individuals. These injuries are most often acute traumatic injuries where the biceps is torn form its distal insertion on the radial tuberosity. Most often this is caused by eccentric overload in the dominant extremity and the patient may report pain in the anticubital fossa. There may be an audible pop at the time of injury. Distal biceps avulsions may present with proximal displacement of the biceps muscle belly that has been referred to as the "Reverse Popeye" sign.

Entrapment of the Biceps Tendon

Entrapment of the LHBT occurs due to inflammation and hypertrophy of the LHBT inside the joint. The increased biceps tendon diameter prevents the tendon from sliding in the bicipital groove due to physical blockade caused by the transverse ligament and or biceps pulley [16] who's functions are to stabilize the biceps in the bicipital groove thereby preventing a bowstring effect. Patients present with anterior shoulder pain and pain on forward motion of the shoulder especially with elbow extension. This pathology is often associated with rotator cuff rupture [16].

Superior Labral Anterior to Posterior Tears (SLAP)

SLAP tears are a common pathology in effecting the integrity of the glenoid labrum and the LHBT at their attachment point overlying the glenoid labrum. These injuries are often caused by repetitive overhead activities such as in throwing athletes. The presenting symptoms include but are not limited to non-specific deep shoulder pain, anterior shoulder pain, popping or clicking, weakness or muscle fatigue. The culprit traumatic injury associated with SLAP tears is often asymptomatic for a period of time know as the "Lag Time".

Instability

Shoulder instability and subluxation is associated with biceps degeneration due to chronic tendinitis. Instability or subluxation may cause palpable snapping of the tendon felt during painful arcs of motion such as during the throwing motion. Superior Labrum Anterior to Posterior (SLAP) tears can present with a similar clinical picture, however SLAP tears are prone to locking and catching symptoms over snapping.

Calcific Tendonitis

This condition is more common in women and mainly affects patients ages 30–60. It is associated with subacromial impingement. Risk factors include hypothyroidism and diabetes. The history will most generally show atraumatic pain, with catching and crepitus in addition to a decreased range of motion and mechanical blocking.

The differential diagnosis of shoulder complaints incudes the various conditions mentioned above as well as many others. Pathology of the biceps can be secondary to acute traumatic injury, overuse, vascular disruptions, impingement and other causes. There are many maneuvers that are sensitive for detecting pathology in the shoulder joint but due to overlapping elicitation of pain with similar maneuvers the tests are not specific [17, 18].

Tests

Although, many physical exam maneuvers are available to the experienced clinician, this chapter focuses on those that are common and most contributory to general examination of the LHBT. No maneuver has been shown to dependably diagnose LHBT pathology alone and they should be used in cohort with a detailed anamnesis of the patient and imaging studies. Generally the biceps tendon may be ruptured in three locations, both the proximal and distal insertions as well as in the muscle belly. Full rupture of the distal insertion of the biceps tendon is a relatively strait forward diagnosis as it most often presents with "Popeye" sign, ecchymosis, positive uppercut test (pain on flexion and supination against resistance) with associated radiological findings. However, diagnosing rupture of the proximal insertion of the LHBT becomes a challenging diagnosis, as it is an intra-articular pathology that articulates directly with the glenoid labrum and is encompassed by many surrounding tissues. These challenging diagnoses and the diagnosis of other LHBT pathology require the use of the maneuvers described below in order to direct the use of imaging technologies and patient treatment.

Yergasons Test

This test provokes pain and tenderness over the bicipital groove with forearm supination against resistance. The examiner "shakes the patients hand" with the forearm in neutral position, the elbow is flexed 90° and tight to the body. The patient resists supination, while the examiner palpates the bicipital groove [19] (Fig. 26.4). Pain elicited by this test indicates either a LHBT tear, Labral tear or both, but may be more suggestive of a biceps tear as the biceps is the primary flexor of the forearm and is also a supinator. This test

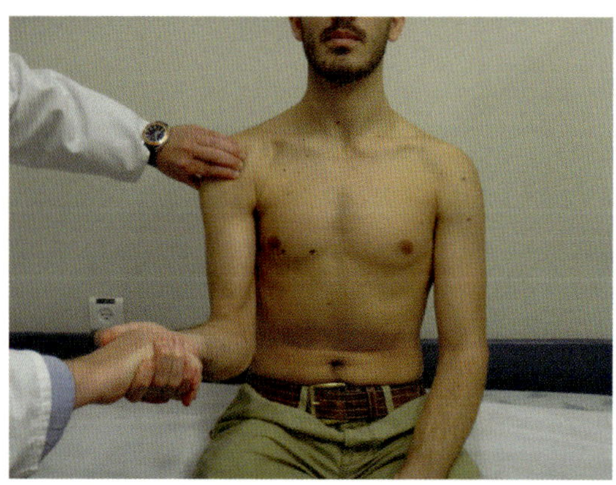

Fig. 26.4 The examiner is performing Yergason's test

may also illicit pain due to tendinopathy or tendinitis of the LHBT [20].

O'Brien's Test

This test is provocative of pain originating at the attachment of the superior labrum. With the elbow fully extended and the arm adducted to cross the midline, the patient raises their arm against resistance with their thumb pointing upwards and then downwards (Fig. 26.5a, b). Pain elicited with the thumb in the upwards position is more specific to LHBT pathology while the downward position may be more specific for labral tears. These maneuvers are sensitive for SLAP tear, biceps tendinitis and rupture but are not specific [20].

Speed's Test

Pain elicited in the bicipital groove by Speed's test indicates a LHBT tear, Labral tear or both [21]. With the hand extended in full supination and 90° flexion of the shoulder with a strait elbow the patient resists forward flexion (Fig. 26.6).

Upper Cut Test

The elbow is flexed to 90°, the shoulder is neutral and the forearm is supinated. The patient raises their fist to their chin against resistance (Fig. 26.7). Shoulder pain or anterior pop indicates a positive test. Utilization of the speed and upper cut tests in together was shown to be superior to either test alone [20, 22].

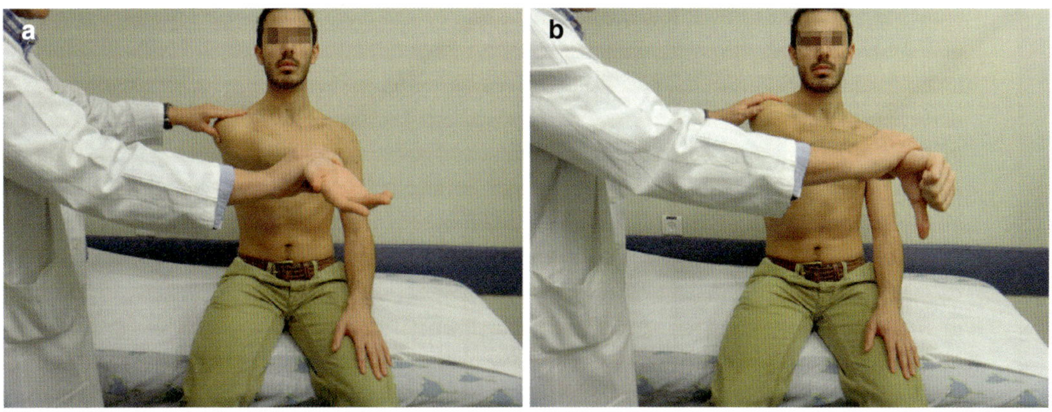

Fig. 26.5 (**a**) The examiner is performing O'Brien's test first with the upward position and then in the (b) downward position

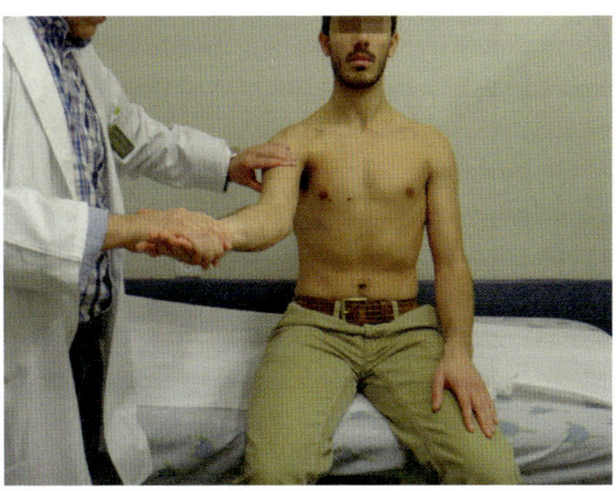

Fig. 26.6 The examiner is performing Speed's test

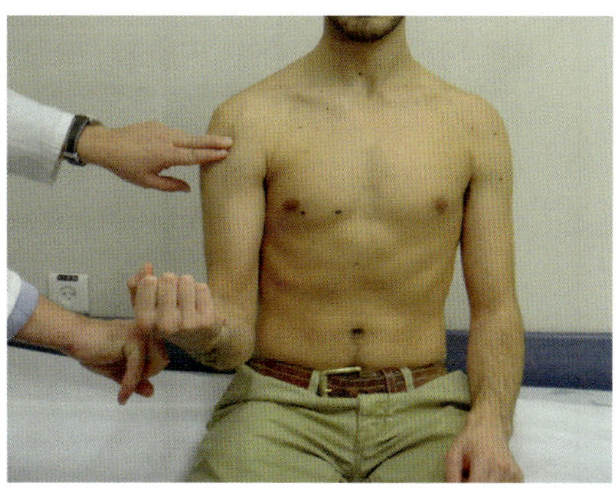

Fig. 26.7 The examiner is performing the uppercut test

Jobe's Empty Can Test

Due to its intimate location at the rotator cuff interval the long head of the biceps may be involved in impingement and rotator cuff pathologies. Impingement and rotator cuff tests can be positive in the presence of biceps pathology. The empty can test [23] evaluates the strength of the supraspinatus tendon. It is performed with each shoulder in 90° of abduction and 30° of forward flexion and internal rotation so the thumb is pointed to the floor (Fig. 26.8). This test is performed both passively and against active resistance. Weakness or inability to maintain this position passively may demonstrate supraspinatus tear or rotator cuff impingement [24].

Dislocation and subluxation of the medial biceps tendon are caused by disturbance to the biceps pulley anatomy. This pathology is often seen together with subscapularis tears [25]. A click may be palpated with the arm abducted at 90° and guided into external rotation. Palpation may demonstrate full dislocation of the tendon with the tendon displaced and located anterior to the lesser tuberosity [26, 27].

Horn Blowers Sign

This test evaluates the infraspinatus and teres minor [28]. The patient's arm is abducted to 90°, with external rotation of the shoulder to 90° and the palm facing forward. If the patient can maintain the position passively the examiner adds active resistance to the dorsal aspect of the hand anteriorly and caudally [29].

Lift Off Test and Belly Press Test

To examine the subscapularis muscle two main tests are employed. In the lift off test [30] the patient places the dorsal aspect of their hand in the small of the back or on their buttock and try to lift their hand against resistance without breaking their wrist. In the belly press test [31] the patient places their palm on their umbilicus and try to lift their arm off their abdomen against the examiners resistance without breaking their wrist or internally rotating their shoulder [32] (Fig. 26.9).

Biceps Load Test

The patient's arm is held in 90° abduction of the shoulder with 90° flexion of the elbow and external rotation [33, 34]. Then the patient draws the arm into external rotation until the end of their range of motion. The patient flexes against resistance in this position. Pain elicited by this test may indicate a LHBT tear, Labral tear or both [33, 35].

Hawkins-Kennedy Test

The patient's humerus is flexed forward to 90° and the examiner internally rotates the shoulder

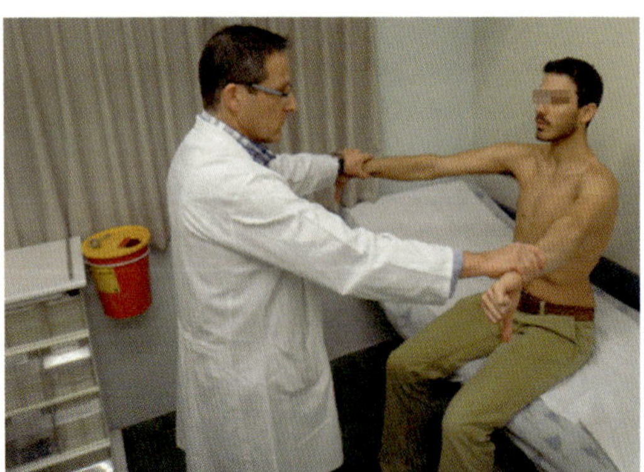

Fig. 26.8 The examiner is performing Jobe's empty can test

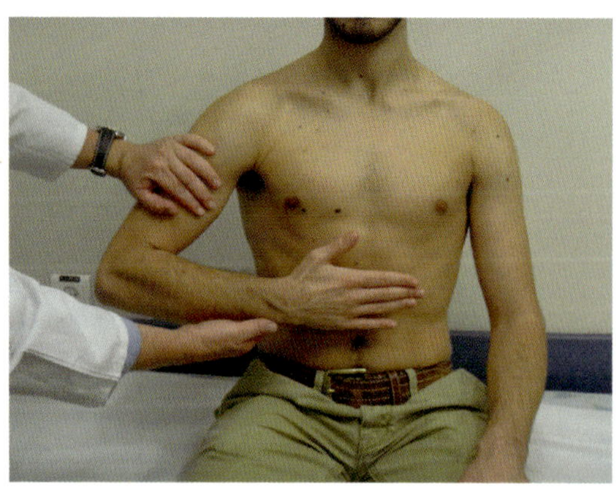

Fig. 26.9 The examiner is performing the belly press test

[36]. This test may reproduce pain due to impingement and has relatively high sensitivities for bursitis and rotator cuff abnormalities [36–38]. The bicipital groove is also provoked in this test as it becomes in direct contact with the acromion.

Selective Injection

The use of selective injections in cohort with the various maneuvers described above may clarify the clinical picture of a patient presenting with LHBT pathology [39]. Selective injections help to differentiate LHBT pathology from other causes of shoulder pain as well as pain referred from surrounding structures such as the cervical spine [40]. Ultrasound (US) guided injection is essential to ensuring accurate delivery of the analgesic to the proper location and to ensure the safety of the injection, preventing rupture of the LHBT. The injection can be delivered to the subacromial reign to alleviate the symptoms of impingement. If impingement is ruled out after subacromial injection and anterior pain remains, injection to the bicipital groove can further clarify pathology. If reduction of pain is seen after bicipital groove injection, this suggests LHB pathology. An examiner can further perform intra-articular injection when evaluating a suspected intra-articular origin of pain including SLAP tear or adhesive capsulitis.

Imaging

The use of imaging studies in relation to the physical exam can help in the evaluation and treatment of biceps tendon pathology. As with the use of all imaging technologies it is important to consider the advantages, exposure risks, costs, and accessibility of each imaging modality. Plain radiographs are ubiquitous, easily accessible and supply immediate results. Therefore, it essential that the clinician adopt a systemic approach in order to fully evaluate and utilize the plain film in the assessment and evaluation of each patient. Shoulder pain is often evaluated with three orthogonal plane film views. The anteroposterior (AP), scapular Y view (Trans scapular view), and axillary views are commonly taken. The bicipital groove view [13] (Fig. 26.10) can be useful in specific circumstances. This view serves to measure the depth and width of the groove as well as the slope of its medial wall in degenerative cases and instability of the LHB [13].

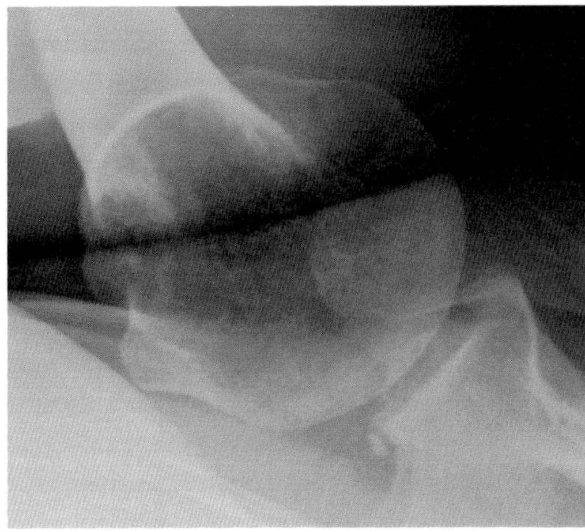

Fig. 26.10 This image is an X-ray demonstrating the bicipital groove view

Additional films in alternate radiographic views can be taken based on an examiners clinical suspicion. Though the majority of pathologies in the shoulder are related to soft tissue injuries, CT scans can be employed to obtain superior imaging of the bony anatomy as well as auxiliary testing for those patients with contraindications to MRI. Ultrasound (US) imaging plays a role in the diagnosis of shoulder pathologies, as it is a non-invasive, low cost, and low exposure technique. Specifically, US can demonstrate tendon or muscle rupture and inflammation in addition to assistance in localizing the LHBT in the humeral groove (Fig. 26.11a, b).

US can be used a tool to help excluded pathology as it can show the rotator cuff musculature dynamically. US aids in localization of pain by giving real time feedback upon palpation of underling anatomical structures with the US probe. The viewer can visualize subluxation and dislocation of the biceps tendon with external rotation in real time. US can help to diagnose rupture or partial rupture as well as hourglass

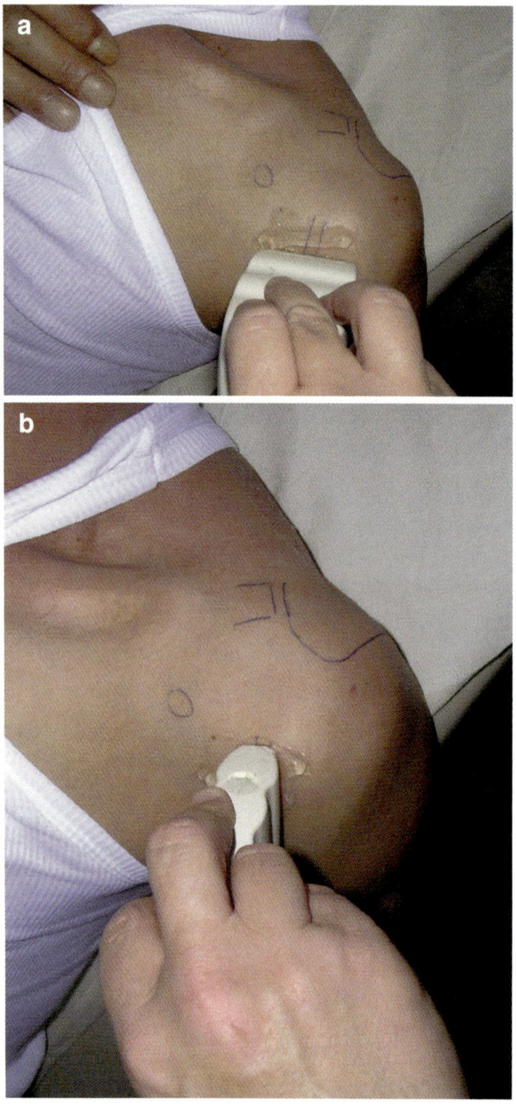

Fig. 26.11 The examiner is demonstrating ultra sound imaging technique for viewing the long head of the biceps tendon

appearance of the biceps tendon where the tendon is entrapped and cannot slide freely in the bicipital groove. Fluid can be seen on US around the biceps tendon, which may be secondary to primary bicipital biceps tendonitis or secondary to adhesive capsulitis, osteoarthritis, rotator cuff pathology or other mechanisms [41, 42].

Both Magnetic Resonance Imaging (MRI) and MRI arteriogram are regularly employed to visualize the biceps tendon and pathology of the shoulder joint. Axial and sagittal oblique views may provide superior visualization of the biceps tendon to other views. Unfortunately, even though MRI is a useful tool for non-invasive soft tissue inspection, the findings often correlated poorly with those seen directly by arthroscopy [43, 44]. Contrast materials improve the sensitivity and specificity of biceps pathology diagnoses aided by MRI [45, 46].

Classification

To the best of our knowledge there are no widely used classification systems solely employed for the description of isolated biceps tendon tears. Tears may be described according to the severity of the tear, location in relation to surrounding structures, and with regard to the length, width, and thickness. Multiple classification systems exit to classify SLAP tears, which include LHBT involvement. These classification systems include the original Snyder Classification [47] (types 1–4) and the Maffet Sub-Classification [48] (which adds types 5–7) as described below.

Type 1: Degenerative fraying of the superior labrum with intact biceps anchor.

Type 2: Detachment of the superior labrum and biceps tendon from the glenoid rim.

Type 3: Bucket-handle tear of labrum with intact biceps anchor.

Type 4: Bucket-handle tear of labrum extended into the biceps tendon.

Type 5: SLAP tear with anterior inferior extension.

Type 6: Anterior or posterior flap tear with the bucket handle tear.

Type 7: SLAP with extension to the glenohumeral ligament.

Nonsurgical Treatment

Although outcomes of operative procedures may be very good and reliable, nonsurgical treatment of biceps tendon pathology is the first and preferred treatment modality [49]. Tendinitis of the biceps tendon should first be treated with rest, modification of activity, non-steroidal anti-inflammatory medication and physical therapy. Physical therapy should be targeted at both the biceps tendon pathology and contaminant pathologies. Bicipital sheath steroid injections may offer adequate pain relief for symptomatic patients. This procedure can be performed under US [50]. Once a patient has failed a comprehensive course of conservative management or if a patient presents with marked injury requiring surgical interventions, invasive procedures may be considered.

Surgical Treatment

There are many effective procedures available for treatment of biceps pathology. In order to choose the optimal procedure a patients age, activity level, and expectations must always be taken into account. Decompression and or debridement are often suitable to treat minor tendon tears or fraying of the biceps tendon [51]. Biceps tenotomy usually consists of intra-articular dissection of the LHBT. Tenotomy of the biceps is more suitable of patients without physical demands or when an athlete requires a hasty return to activity [52]. The advantages and disadvantages of tenotomy must also be considered. Although tenotomy is a relatively simple surgical technique and does not require immobilization the procedure causes distal displacement of the muscle belly often with fatigue and muscle cramping [53, 54].

Tenodesis is a popular treatment for young active patients with tearing, subluxation, dislocation, or hourglass deformity [55]. However tenodesis is not a preferred procedure in individuals with full thickness biceps tendon rupture unless the patient prefers tenodesis due to cosmetic reasons, such as in a body builder. This procedure begins with detachment of the LHBT followed by reattachment of the tendon on the humerus. Tenodesis is often performed simultaneously with procedures to remedy concurrent shoulder pathology such as rotator cuff tears. Biceps tenodesis often is able to prevent atrophy while preserving muscle strength, function and cosmetic appearance [56, 57]. This technique does not require significant post surgical immobilization or prolonged rehabilitation. However, compared to tenotomy, tenodesis is a more challenging procedure and necessitates longer rehabilitation and immobilization for the patient. Fixation failure is a possible complication [12].

Procedures for SLAP tears include debridement, SLAP repair, and tenotomy or tenodesis. The optimal procedure for SLAP repair is most often chosen based on the classification of the SLAP tear. Type I lesions are most often treated with debridement. In patients with Type II SLAP tears arthroscopic debridement and reattachment of the biceps tendon to the superior glenoid rim is common. In type III SLAP tears the bucket handle tear is excised and the biceps anchor may be repaired in the case of anchor instability. Surgical intervention for type IV SLAP tears depends upon the degree of biceps tendon involvement. In cases with minimal biceps involvement the biceps anchor may be left intact and the pathological portion resected. In cases of extensive biceps tendon involvement age is an important factor in considering reattachment of the labrum and biceps tendon to the glenoid rim or biceps tenodesis. However, arthroscopic biceps screw arthrodesis performed at the articular margin is the preferred procedure and results in a low surgical revision rate, a low rate of residual pain, and significant improvement in objective shoulder outcome scores [58].

LHBT entrapment resulting in hourglass deformity of the biceps tendon is usually treated with isolated biceps tenotomy or tenodesis. Choosing the optimal operative procedure is based on a patient's age, expectations, contaminant pathology, surgeon preference and skills. In both tenotomy and tenodesis it is important that the intraarticular area of hypertrophy of the biceps tendon is excised to resolve the mechanical block. Tenodesis is the preferred technique in LHBT entrapment with hourglass deformity [16].

Postoperative Rehabilitation

The postoperative rehabilitation protocols for biceps tenodesis begin with immediate initiation of pendulum exercises. Both active and passive exercises are begun 7–10 days postoperatively.

Finally, active exercises are begun 6 weeks post surgery with regular rehabilitation follow up visits. All rehabilitation protocols should be individualized to fit the needs, recovery trajectory, range of motion progress and pain level of the patient. However, in the case of biceps tenodesis the patient often has undergone simultaneous procedures for contaminant pathology. The additional surgical procedures should be taken into account when designing postoperative rehabilitation protocols and goals for each patient.

In biceps tenotomy care must be taken not to extend the elbow beyond 45° for the first 3 weeks. It is also important to exclude active biceps flexion for the first 6 weeks. As always, managing patient expectations and encouraging communication between the patient and clinician is vital to successful surgical procedures and postoperative rehabilitation.

Questions

1. Please find the false statement about biceps tendon pathologies
   A. Distal tendon rupture of biceps is less common than proximal rupture
   B. Biceps tendonitis is characterized by anterior shoulder pain
   C. 'Reverse Popeye sign' is specific for proximal tendon avulsions
   D. It may be difficult to differentiate partial biceps tendon tear from tendonitis based on history and physical examination alone
   E. Entrapment of the biceps tendon is usually associated with rotator cuff tendon rupture
   C.

2. In which patients do the authors recommend tenodesis instead of tenotomy only?
   A. Elderly patients with rotator cuff tear
   B. Patients with shoulder pain due to arthritis
   C. Adhesive capsulitis
   D. Rotator cuff rupture
   E. Young athletic patients
      E. Although studies do not show any superiority of tenodesis vs tenotomy, tenodesis is recommended in young patients who participate in sports. The incidence of muscle spasm and cramping may be reduced in tenodesis patients as compared to tenotomy patients. Cosmetic appearance is another indication for tenodesis.

What is new?

What if a patient does not pursue any treatment for his/her biceps tendon rupture?

Chronic rupture of the long head of the biceps tendon: comparison of 2-year results following primary versus revision open subpectoral biceps tenodesis, Archives of Orthopaedic and Trauma Surgery, May 2016, Euler SA.

References

1. Sarmento M. Long head of biceps: from anatomy to treatment. Acta Reumatol Port. 2015;40:26–33.
2. Tuoheti Y, Itoi E, Minagawa H, et al. Attachment types of the long head of the biceps tendon to the glenoid labrum and their relationships with the glenohumeral ligaments. Arthroscopy. 2005;21:1242–9.
3. Cooper DE, Arnoczky SP, O'Brien SJ, et al. Anatomy, histology, and vascularity of the glenoid labrum. An anatomical study. J Bone Joint Surg Am. 1992;74:46–52.
4. Denard PJ, Dai X, Hanypsiak BT, et al. Anatomy of the biceps tendon: implications for restoring physiological length-tension relation during biceps tenodesis with interference screw fixation. Arthroscopy. 2012;28:1352–8.
5. Rao AG, Kim TK, Chronopoulos E, et al. Anatomical variants in the anterosuperior aspect of the glenoid labrum: a statistical analysis of seventy-three cases. J Bone Joint Surg Am. 2003;85-A:653–9.
6. Tena-Arregui J, Barrio-Asensio C, Puerta-Fonollá J, et al. Arthroscopic study of the shoulder joint in fetuses. Arthroscopy. 2005;21:1114–9.
7. Dierickx C, Ceccarelli E, Conti M, et al. Variations of the intra-articular portion of the long head of the biceps tendon: a classification of embryologically explained variations. J Shoulder Elbow Surg. 2009;18:556–65.
8. Becker DA, Cofield RH. Tenodesis of the long head of the biceps brachii for chronic bicipital tendinitis. Long-term results. J Bone Joint Surg Am. 1989;71:376–81.
9. Boesmueller S, Fialka C, Pretterklieber ML. The arterial supply of the tendon of the long head of the biceps brachii in the human: a combined anatomical and radiological study. Ann Anat. 2014;196:449–55.
10. Cheng NM, Pan WR, Vally F, et al. The arterial supply of the long head of biceps tendon: anatomical study with implications for tendon rupture. Clin Anat. 2010;23:683–92.

11. Braun S, Millett PJ, Yongpravat C, et al. Biomechanical evaluation of shear force vectors leading to injury of the biceps reflection pulley: a biplane fluoroscopy study on cadaveric shoulders. Am J Sports Med. 2010;38:1015–24.
12. Habermeyer P, Magosch P, Pritsch M, et al. Anterosuperior impingement of the shoulder as a result of pulley lesions: a prospective arthroscopic study. J Shoulder Elbow Surg. 2004;13:5–12.
13. Cone RO, Danzig L, Resnick D, et al. The bicipital groove: radiographic, anatomic, and pathologic study. AJR Am J Roentgenol. 1983;141:781–8.
14. Athwal GS, Steinmann SP, Rispoli DM. The distal biceps tendon: footprint and relevant clinical anatomy. J Hand Surg. 2007;32:1225–9.
15. Hutchinson HL, Gloystein D, Gillespie M. Distal biceps tendon insertion: an anatomic study. J Shoulder Elbow Surg. 2008;17:342–6.
16. Boileau P, Ahrens PM, Hatzidakis AM. Entrapment of the long head of the biceps tendon: the hourglass biceps—a cause of pain and locking of the shoulder. J Shoulder Elbow Surg. 2004;13:249–57.
17. Hegedus EJ, Goode A, Campbell S, et al. Physical examination tests of the shoulder: a systematic review with meta-analysis of individual tests. Br J Sports Med. 2008;42:80–92; discussion.
18. Hegedus EJ, Goode AP, Cook CE, et al. Which physical examination tests provide clinicians with the most value when examining the shoulder? Update of a systematic review with meta-analysis of individual tests. Br J Sports Med. 2012;46:964–78.
19. Yergason RM. Supination sign. J Bone Joint Surg. 1931;13:160.
20. Holtby R, Razmjou H. Accuracy of the Speed's and Yergason's tests in detecting biceps pathology and SLAP lesions: comparison with arthroscopic findings. Arthroscopy. 2004;20:231–6.
21. Gilcreest EL. Dislocation and elongation of the long head of the biceps brachii: an analysis of six cases. Ann Surg. 1936;104:118–38.
22. Ben Kibler W, Sciascia AD, Hester P, et al. Clinical utility of traditional and new tests in the diagnosis of biceps tendon injuries and superior labrum anterior and posterior lesions in the shoulder. Am J Sports Med. 2009;37:1840–7.
23. Jobe FW, Moynes DR. Delineation of diagnostic criteria and a rehabilitation program for rotator cuff injuries. Am J Sports Med. 1982;10:336–9.
24. Pandya NK, Colton A, Webner D, et al. Physical examination and magnetic resonance imaging in the diagnosis of superior labrum anterior-posterior lesions of the shoulder: a sensitivity analysis. Arthroscopy. 2008;24:311–7.
25. Christopher Patton W, McCluskey III GM. Biceps tendinitis and subluxation. Clin Sports Med. 2001;20:505–29.
26. Rokito AS, Bilgen OF, Zuckerman JD, et al. Medial dislocation of the long head of the biceps tendon. Magnetic resonance imaging evaluation. Am J Orthop (Belle Mead NJ). 1996;25:314, 8–23.
27. Slatis P, Aalto K. Medial dislocation of the tendon of the long head of the biceps brachii. Acta Orthop Scand. 1979;50:73–7.
28. Leroux JL, Thomas E, Bonnel F, et al. Diagnostic value of clinical tests for shoulder impingement syndrome. Rev Rhum Engl Ed. 1995;62:423–8.
29. Walch G, Boulahia A, Calderone S, et al. The 'dropping' and 'hornblower's' signs in evaluation of rotator-cuff tears. J Bone Joint Surg. 1998;80:624–8.
30. Gerber C, Krushell RJ. Isolated rupture of the tendon of the subscapularis muscle. Clinical features in 16 cases. J Bone Joint Surg. 1991;73:389–94.
31. Gerber C, Hersche O, Farron A. Isolated rupture of the subscapularis tendon. J Bone Joint Surg Am. 1996;78:1015–23.
32. Tokish JM, Decker MJ, Ellis HB, et al. The belly-press test for the physical examination of the subscapularis muscle: electromyographic validation and comparison to the lift-off test. J Shoulder Elbow Surg. 2003;12:427–30.
33. Kim SH, Ha KI, Ahn JH, et al. Biceps load test II: a clinical test for SLAP lesions of the shoulder. Arthroscopy. 2001;17:160–4.
34. Kim SH, Ha KI, Han KY. Biceps load test: a clinical test for superior labrum anterior and posterior lesions in shoulders with recurrent anterior dislocations. Am J Sports Med. 1999;27:300–3.
35. Hanchard NC, Lenza M, Handoll HH, et al. Physical tests for shoulder impingements and local lesions of bursa, tendon or labrum that may accompany impingement. Cochrane Database Syst Rev. 2013;4:CD007427.
36. Hawkins RJ, Kennedy JC. Impingement syndrome in athletes. Am J Sports Med. 1980;8:151–8.
37. Michener LA, Walsworth MK, Doukas WC, et al. Reliability and diagnostic accuracy of 5 physical examination tests and combination of tests for subacromial impingement. Arch Phys Med Rehabil. 2009;90:1898–903.
38. Hughes P. The Neer sign and Hawkins-Kennedy test for shoulder impingement. J Physiother. 2011;57:260.
39. Barber FA, Field LD, Ryu RKN. Biceps tendon and superior labrum injuries: decision-making. J Bone Joint Surg. 2007;89:1844–55.
40. Tallia AF, Cardone DA. Diagnostic and therapeutic injection of the shoulder region. Am Fam Physician. 2003;67:1271–8.
41. Huang S-W, Wang W-T. Quantitative diagnostic method for biceps long head tendinitis by using ultrasound. Sci World J. 2013;2013:7.
42. Nho SJ, Strauss EJ, Lenart BA, et al. Long head of the biceps tendinopathy: diagnosis and management. J Am Acad Orthop Surg. 2010;18:645–56.
43. Mohtadi NG, Vellet AD, Clark ML, et al. A prospective, double-blind comparison of magnetic resonance imaging and arthroscopy in the evaluation of patients presenting with shoulder pain. J Shoulder Elbow Surg. 2004;13:258–65.

44. Taylor SA, Newman AM, Nguyen J, et al. Magnetic resonance imaging currently fails to fully evaluate the biceps-labrum complex and bicipital tunnel. Arthroscopy. 2016;32:238–44.
45. Zanetti M, Weishaupt D, Gerber C, et al. Tendinopathy and rupture of the tendon of the long head of the biceps brachii muscle: evaluation with MR arthrography. Am J Roentgenol. 1998;170:1557–61.
46. Pfirrmann CWA, Zanetti M, Weishaupt D, et al. Subscapularis tendon tears: detection and grading at MR arthrography. Radiology. 1999;213:709–14.
47. Snyder SJ, Karzel RP, Del Pizzo W, et al. SLAP lesions of the shoulder. Arthroscopy. 1990;6:274–9.
48. Maffet MW, Gartsman GM, Moseley B. Superior labrum-biceps tendon complex lesions of the shoulder. Am J Sports Med. 1995;23:93–8.
49. Mazzocca AD, Rios CG, Romeo AA, et al. Subpectoral biceps tenodesis with interference screw fixation. Arthroscopy. 2005;21:896.
50. Messina C, Banfi G, Orlandi D, et al. Ultrasound-guided interventional procedures around the shoulder. Br J Radiol. 2016;89:20150372.
51. Mazzocca AD, Romeo AA. Arthroscopic biceps tenodesis in the beach chair position. Oper Tech Sports Med. 2003;11:6–14.
52. Sethi PM, Rajaram A, Beitzel K, et al. Biomechanical performance of subpectoral biceps tenodesis: a comparison of interference screw fixation, cortical button fixation, and interference screw diameter. J Shoulder Elbow Surg. 2013;22:451–7.
53. Kelly AM, Drakos MC, Fealy S, et al. Arthroscopic release of the long head of the biceps tendon: functional outcome and clinical results. Am J Sports Med. 2005;33:208–13.
54. Romeo AA, Mazzocca AD, Tauro JC. Arthroscopic biceps tenodesis. Arthroscopy. 2004;20:206–13.
55. Lo IKY, Burkhart SS. Arthroscopic biceps tenodesis using a bioabsorbable interference screw. Arthroscopy. 2004;20:85–95.
56. Provencher MT, LeClere LE, Romeo AA. Subpectoral biceps tenodesis. Sports Med Arthrosc Rev. 2008;16:170–6.
57. Gombera MM, Kahlenberg CA, Nair R, et al. All-arthroscopic suprapectoral versus open subpectoral tenodesis of the long head of the biceps brachii. Am J Sports Med. 2015;43:1077–83.
58. Brady PC, Narbona P, Adams CR, et al. Arthroscopic proximal biceps tenodesis at the articular margin: evaluation of outcomes, complications, and revision rate. Arthroscopy. 2015;31:470–6.

Rotator Cuff Surgery

27

Gazi Huri and Saygin Kamaci

Introduction

Rotator cuff pathology is one of the most common pathologies all around the globe treated by the upper extremity surgeon. Prognosis and approach to the rotator cuff lesions varies upon the type and the nature of the lesion. Several classification systems have been proposed in this manner. History, physical examination and imaging are crucial in the diagnosis of the torn cuff. Clinical management of these lesions varies from conservative treatment to arthroscopic and open cuff repair and even glenohumeral arthroplasty. Surgical procedure is driven by numerous factors including; the amount of the cuff tear, quality of the cuff, number of the tendons affected, patient age and coinciding glenohumeral osteoarthritis.

G. Huri, M.D. (✉)
Department of Orthopaedics and Traumatology, Hacettepe University School of Medicine, Ankara, Turkey
e-mail: Gazihuri@Hacettepe.Edu.Tr

S. Kamaci, M.D.
Department of Orthopaedic Surgery, University of Louisville Hospital, Kentucky, USA

Diagnosis and Classification

Diagnostic Tests

When evaluating the patient with shoulder complaints, a wide spectrum of test is available for diagnosis. Diagnostic test should be accurate and precise. However, the gold standard is often the appearance of the cuff during the rotator cuff surgery. Additionally, positive and negative likelihood ratio of the test is important that estimates the probability of having the diagnosis that the given test could change.

History

How a rotator cuff tear could precisely and accurately be diagnosed? History gives us important information. Acute rotator cuff tears are often manifested by acute onset pain accompanied with limited range of motion. Chronic tears might be related with activity pain and weakness, crepitus and night pain. A study of 518 patients diagnosed with rotator cuff tear presented that night pain had a sensitivity of 0.88 and specificity of 0.2 with a positive likelihood ratio of 1.1 (does not change the probability of disease when finding is present) and negative likelihood ratio of 0.6 (when absent in the history the probability that the patient has a rotator tear is somewhat less likely) in diagnosing

G. Huri, N.K. Paschos (eds.), *The Shoulder*, Orthopaedic Study Guide Series,
DOI 10.1007/978-3-319-51979-1_27

rotator cuff tear. Additionally, history of trauma had a sensitivity of 0.36 and specificity of 0.73; positive likelihood ratio of 1.33 and negative likelihood ratio of 0.88 (Litaker D, 2000 #1).

Tests

It has been widely studied whether physical examination tests are capable of diagnosing a full thickness rotator cuff tear. Interestingly, many tests had a positive likelihood ratio of near 1 which means a positive test does not change the probability of have rotator cuff tear. Best tests would have high likelihood ratios. Lag signs, have a high likelihood ratio, are the most useful tests for the diagnosis of rotator cuff tear (Table 27.1). Lag sign tests, in which the arm is positioned in a certain position and the patient is asked to hold the arm in the determined position. Lag signs require a functional rotator cuff otherwise the patient is unable to prevent the position of the arm and lags back in starting position. Lag sings for supraspinatus and infraspinatus tears are drop arm test, external rotation of the arm at the side and external rotation of the abducted arm. Lag sign for the subscapularis tear could be done by internally rotating the arm at the back. Lag signs have a positive high likelihood ratio, which means the patient had a high probability of rotator cuff tear when the test is positive. However, lag signs have a negative likelihood ratio close to 1.0 that means the probability of the patient has a rotator cuff tear is not changed much.

Accuracy and precision for a useful physical examination test is mandatory. The precision is determined by inter and intra-observer agreement studies. According to a study, painful arch and resisted external rotation tests had a fair to substantial inter-observer agreement while empty can test and lift-off test had lower levels of agreement (Il, 1990 #2). Great variation occurs in how physical examination tests for the shoulder are performed and how the findings are interpreted.

Imaging

MRI

Many studies have been done in order to assess the role of MRI in diagnosis of rotator cuff tears. According to a metaanalysis of 65 studies by Jesus et al. MRI was found to be highly sensitive and specific for diagnosing cuff tears (0.93 and 0.92, respectively). Additionally, MRI has positive likelihood ratio of 13.14 and negative likelihood ratio of 0.09. Otherwise MRI was found to have a

Table 27.1 Physical examination tests used to diagnose rotator cuff tears

Test	Author	*N*	Sensitivity	Specificity	PPV	NPV	+LR	−LR
Lag signs								
Drop arm test	Park (2005)	913	0.35	0.88	0.65	0.67	2.79	0.74
Lift off	Hertel (1996)	100	0.62	1.00	1.00	0.69	30.80	0.40
Belly off sign	Bartsch (2010)	50	0.86	0.91	0.81	0.94	9.56	10.15
Internal rotation lag	Hertel (1996)	100	0.7	1.00	1.00	0.56	34.8	0.3
External rotation lag	Miller (2008)	37	1.00	0.84	0.28	1.00	6.2	0.0
Physical examination								
Jobe (empty can)—pain	Itoi (1999)	143	0.63	0.55	0.31	0.82	1.4	0.7
Jobe (empty can)—weakness	Kim (2006)	200	0.76	0.71	0.56	0.86	2.6	0.34
Full can—pain	Itio (1999)	143	0.66	0.64	0.37	0.85	1.8	0.5
Full can—weakness	Kim (2006)	200	0.77	0.68	0.54	0.86	2.41	0.33
Neer	Park (2005)	913	0.59	0.47	0.41	0.65	1.12	0.86
Hawkins	Park (2005)	913	0.69	0.48	0.45	0.71	1.33	0.65
Painful Arc	Litaker (2000)	448	0.97	0.10	0.67	0.69	1.1	0.3
Belly Press Test	Barth (2006)	68	0.40	0.98	0.89	0.80	20.00	0.61
Napoleon Test	Barth (2006)	68	0.25	0.98	0.83	0.76	2.08	0.77

N number of patients, *PPV* positive predictive value, *NPV* negative predictive value, *+LR* positive likelihood ratio, *−LR* negative likelihood ratio sensitivity of 0.64 and specificity of 0.92 in diagnosing partial cuff tears (de Jesus JO, 2009 #3). This data shows that MRI is not only useful to detect cuff tears when present but also is very effective in ruling out cuff tears when absent. Which means that MRI is better than physical examination tests for ruling out the rotator cuff tears. (de Jesus JO, 2009 #3) (Balich SM, 1997 #4).

USG

Ultrasonography is a useful diagnostic tool for diagnosis full thickness rotator cuff tears with a sensitivity of 0.92, specificity of 0.94 and positive likelihood ratio of 15.33 and negative likelihood ratio of 0.08. Major drawbacks of USG are; the lower sensitivity and specificity for partial thickness rotator cuff tears and the need for an experienced ultrasonographist are the drawbacks. Indeed, non-invasive USG is still one of the most powerful tools in diagnosis. (de Jesus JO, 2009 #3).

MR Arthrography

Gadolinium injected magnetic resonance arthrography is the most powerful tool for diagnosing both full thickness and partial rotator cuff tears. MR arthrography had a sensitivity of 0.95, specificity of 0.99, positive likelihood ratio of 95 and negative likely hood ratio of 0.05 (Snyder SJ, 1991 #5). These values are much better than MRI and ultrasonography. Additionally, MR arthrography has an excellent inter-observer (k: 0.91) and moderate intra-observer (k: 0.49) agreement. However, risk of infection or reaction to gadolinium and higher cost of this imaging are major drawbacks.

Classification Systems for Rotator Cuff Tears

Rotator cuff tears includes a wide spectrum of pathologies from tendinosis, to partial cuff tears, to full thickness cuff tears and cuff tear arthropathy. It is relatively easy to distinguish these pathologies and each portion has its own classification system. The best classification system should (1) Be unambiguous in how patients are differentiated, (2) Have high inter and intra-observer agreement, (3) Give insight into prognosis and influence the treatment.

Tendinosis requisites an intact rotator cuff. Rotator cuff tear arthropathy is seen with arthritic changes in glenohumeral joint. Partial and full thickness rotator cuff tears could be easily diagnosed and differentiated from each other using MRI (Spencer EE, 2008 #6). However, distinguishing the type and the severity of partial thickness rotator cuff tear is challenging.

Partial Thickness Tears of Rotator Cuff

Charles Neer II recognized that the severity of rotator cuff tear is associated with patient's age. (II, 1983 #7) He classified partial rotator cuff tears into three stages; Stage I: reversible edema and hemorrhage stage with the patient <25 years of age, Stage 2: Fibrosis and tendinitis stage with the patient 25–40 years of age, Stage 3: Bone spurs and tendon ruptures stage (>40 years of age).

Fukuda modified the Neer's classification based on the integrity of the tendon (Fukuda H, 1982 #8). Additionally, Fukuda stated that partial thickness rotator cuff tears may present on articular surface, bursal surface and may be the delamination of the tendon.

Ellman classified partial rotator cuff tears based on location and grade (H, 1990 #9). Location of the tear was either on the articular surface, bursal surface or interstitial and grading was the deepness of the tear.

Snyder reported their results of arthroscopic treatment and proposed a classification system based on location, size and severity. He defined the letter "A" for articular surface, "B" for bursal tears, "C" for complete tears. Size and severity of tear is classified upon arthroscopic examination of the tendon from Grade 0 (normal rotator cuff) to Grade 4 (flap formation and retraction of partial-thickness flap >3 cm) (Snyder SJ, 1991 #10).

In summary, there is no ideal classification system for partial-thickness rotator cuff tears. Imaging studies could precisely distinguish full-thickness rotator cuff tears from partial-thickness cuff tears but could not easily differentiate partial-thickness cuff tears.

Full Thickness Tears of Rotator Cuff

Several classification systems were proposed for differentiating the full-thickness rotator cuff tears. Various features were described including chronicity, size, shape or the geometry, number of the tendons involved, quality of the muscle and quality of the tendon.

Chronicity

Chronicity may have profound influence on the outcome, yet not many classification systems include this entity. Neer (ll, 1990 #2) considered chronicity in his classification system as impingement (chronic and progressive) and traumatic. Ellmen (H, 1991 #11) described rotator cuff tears as acute (<6 weeks), subacute (6 weeks to 6 months), chronic (6 months to 1 year) and old tears (>1 year). Sallay (Sallay PI, 2007 #12) mentioned acute on chronic full thickness rotator cuff tears in his classification system.

Size

DeOrio and Cofield (DeOrio JK, 1984 #13) classified full thickness rotator cuff lesions based on the greatest length as small (<1 cm), medium (1–3 cm), large (3–5 cm) and massive (>5 cm).

Geometric Classifications

Invention of MRI has resurrected interest on the geometry of the full thickness rotator cuff tears. Buckhart recognized that the geometric pattern of the rotator cuff tear might influence the way that the surgeon mobilizes tendon during repair. He proposed a geometric classification and suggested optimal treatment for the different types (Davidson J, 2010 #14). Type I: Crescent tear is best treated with end to bone repair, Type II: Longitudinal, L-shaped, U-shaped tears are best treated with margin convergence, Type III: Massive and retracted tears are best treated with interval slides and partial repair, Type IV: Rotator cuff tear arthropathy is best treated with arthroplasty.

Number of Tendons Torn

First classification system described by Ellman based on the tendon involved, the classification is lacking that there is no way the describe rupture of two or more tendons that often occurs. Several classification systems described in this manner. Patte's offered a complex classification system for full thickness rotator cuff tear, that included information of the extend of the tear, topography in the sagittal and frontal planes, the trophic quality of the muscle, and the integrity of the long head of biceps (D, 1990 #15) (Table 27.2).

Table 27.2 Patte's classification for full-thickness rotator cuff tears

Extend of tear
Group 1: Partial tears. Full tears <1 cm in sagittal plane at bony detachment
(a) Deep, partial tears
(b) Superficial tears
(c) Small, full-substance tears
Group 2: Full substance tears of entire supraspinatus
Group 3: Full substance tears of more than one tendon
Group 4: Massive tears with glenohumeral arthritis
Topography of tear in sagittal plane
Segment 1: Subscapularis tears
Segment 2: Coracohumeral ligament tear
Segment 3: Isolated supraspinatus tear
Segment 4: Entire supraspinatus and 1/2 of infraspinatus tear
Segment 5: Entire supraspinatus and infraspinatus tear
Segment 6: Subscapularis, supraspinatus, infraspinatus tear
Topography of tear in frontal plane
Stage 1: Proximal stump close to bony insertion
Stage 2: Proximal stump at level of humeral head
Stage 3: Proximal stump at level of glenoid
Quality of muscle
State of long head of biceps

From Patte D. Classification of rotator cuff Iesions. Clin Orthop and Relat Res 1990;254:81–86

Mobility of the Tendon and Tissue Quality

In addition to the features described above, Sallay proposed a classification system based on mobility and tissue quality. Mobility of the tendon is defined as excursion and elasticity of the tendon (subjectively described as excellent, moderate, poor). Tissue quality is defined as tendon thickness, and ability to hold suture (excellent, moderate, poor) (Sallay PI, 2007 #12).

Quality of Muscle—Atrophy and Fatty Infiltration

Atrophy and fatty infiltration of the rotator cuff muscles had been classified by various classification systems. The most widely known classification system proposed by Goutallier used computed tomography (CT) to assess muscle atrophy associated with rotator cuff tears (Goutallier D, 1994 #16). On the CT image, the tip of the coracoid process and the inferior margin of the glenoid are noted and measurements are made. Stage 0 = completely normal muscle, Stage 1 = muscle contains some fatty streaks, Stage 2 = Muscle more than fatty infiltration, Stage 3 = Muscle equal to fat, Stage 4 = More fat than muscle. Goutallier classification was found to have moderate inter-observer agreement (Goutallier D, 1994 #16).

Thomazeau described fatty infiltration using MRI in the oblique sagittal plane to produce a Y-shaped view (Thomazeau H, 1996 #18). An "occupation ratio" is calculated as the cross-sectional area of the supraspinatus muscle over the cross-sectional area of the entire supraspinatus fossa.

Subscapularis Tears

Tears of the subscapularis deserves special attention as the often occur independently and may be associated with glenohumeral instability and biceps instability. Lafosse proposed a classification system based on increased severity. Type I: partial lesions of the superior third, Type II: complete lesions of the superior third, Type III: complete lesions of superior two-thirds, Type IV: complete lesions of the tendon with humeral head centered and fatty degeneration as less than or equal to Gautallier stage III, Type V: Complete lesion of the tendon with eccentric head with coracoid impingement and fatty degeneration of greater than Goutallier stage III.

Rotator Cuff Tear Arthropathy

Glenohumeral joint stability might be interfered with large rotator cuff tears. Deltoid over powers following the rotator cuff deficiency and the humeral head migrates superiorly resulting in articulation of humeral head with the acromion. Abnormal joint kinematics leads cartilage degradation and ends with arthritis. Neer described this pathology as " Rotator cuff tear arthropathy" (Neer CS II, 1977 #19).

Visotsky-Seebauer described rotator cuff tear arthropathy into four radiological grades; Hamada proposed a classification system based on the radiologic severity of gleohumeral arthritis into five grades; and Sirviaux classified glenohumeral arthritis based on glenoid erosion into four grades (Table 27.3).

Kappe et al. studied the reliability of Favard, Visotksy-Seebauer, Hamada and Siveroux radiologic classification systems for rotator cuff tear arthropathy (Kappe T, 2011 #20). Sirveaux classification system was found to have the best reliability but it classifies only the glenoid (Sirveaux F, 2004 #21). The Favard system was not reliable and the Visotsky-Seebauer systems were found to have similar intra- and inter-observer agreement.

Table 27.3 Sirveaux classification of cuff tear arthropathy

Type	Description
E0	Upward migration of humeral head without erosion of glenoid
E1	Concentric erosion of glenoid
E2	Erosion of superior part of the glenoid
E3	Erosion extends to inferior part of the glenoid

From Sirveaux F, Favard l, Oudet D, Huquet D, Walch G, Mole D. Grammont inverted total shoulder arthroplasty in the treatment of glenohumeral osteo-arthritis with massive rupture of the cuff. Results of a multicentre study of 80 shoulders. J Bone Joint Surg Br 2004;86:388–395

Rotator Cuff Repair; Open Approach

Rotator cuff repair surgery is evaluating gradually since the first rotator cuff repair reported by Codman in 1911 (EA, 1911 #23). Long-term clinical studies showed a success rate of 83% for avoiding further surgery in patients with rotator cuff tears (Cofield RH, 2001 #24). There has been a significant evolution with the introduction of arthroscopic techniques and understanding the rotator cuff surgery principles in the past two decades. To best of our knowledge, almost all of the rotator cuff tears could be treated arthroscopically. The main principles of rotator cuff repair that were derived from open surgery remain the same. The fundamental principles include; tear identification, debridement, proper mobilization and tension-free repair, individualized and surgeon driven physical therapy. Understanding the principles of open surgery is crucial for the upper extremity surgeon. Additionally, open approaches are still in use of some revision surgeries and massive tear surgery with tendon transfer.

Approach

Many approaches were identified for rotator cuff surgeries. Posterior approach was identified by Norwood et al. (Norwood LA, 1989 #25) and anterior delto-pectoral approach for subscapularis tears was Leffert and Rowe (CR, 1988 #26). Some authors preferred an anterior-superior approach through a split down or take down proximal deltoid while others use anterior deltoid splitting approach. Various modifications of these approaches were published regarding the additional procedures included like acromionectomy and distal clavicle resection.

Decompression

Traditional decompression consists of anterior acromioplasty, resection of coracoacromial ligament, and resection of the osteophytes of the acromion projecting inferiorly (2nd, 1972 #27). Coracoacromial arch is believed to have a buffering affect in resisting superior translation of the humeral head especially when the rotator cuff stability is absent due to rupture. Superior subluxation of the humeral head can be seen after decompression without repairing massive rotator cuff repair. Furthermore, it could be seen after decompression in the setting of failed massive cuff repair (AM, 1991 #29). Watson reported better results with acromioclavicular ligament incision rather than resection in his cases of rotator cuff repair (M, 1985 #28). The coracoacromial arch was conjectured to be a stabilizing factor during arthroplasty in patients with end stage rheumatoid arthritis and cuff tear arthropathy (Arntz CT, 1993 #30).

Tendon Mobilization and Repair

Tendon mobilization is an essential factor not only to allow tendon repair but also to free muscle-tendon units and glide for avoiding stiffness (CS, 1990 #31). Muscle tendon unit should be freed from adhesions so that it could glide provide tension-free repair. Without optimal mobilization, the repair might end with stiff shoulder. Then the stretching exercises could pull out the repair. Intraoperatively, the repair should always be done with arm at the side to ensure adequate mobilization.

Repair done arm positioned in abduction would likely fail. Even though, the abduction brace relieves the tension on the construct. Removing the brace would create a gap between two ends of the repair.

It has been emphasized that the underlying biology of the tendon has superior effect on healing an outcome than the small amount of difference in biomechanical strength between different fixation methods (2nd, 1972 #32). None of the specific reattachment methods was shown to be superior to the others.

Creating a cancellous bone surface by removing the cortical bone from the tuberosity is unnecessary and might reduce the fixation of anchors. Additionally, healing capacity of cancellous bone has not been shown to be significantly superior to the cortical bone (St Pierre P, 1995 #39). It is widely believed that removing non-healing bursal tissue and scar freshens the repair site. Most surgeons remove cortical bone surface simply without interpreting the repair site.

An inexpensive method for osseous fixation is to create bone tunnels through the greater tuberosity. Several conventional methods and implants were identified in this manner.

With popularization of arthroscopic rotator cuff surgery, suture anchors were invented which also could be used in open surgery. Double row constructs was found to have better contact area, initial mechanical strength and reduced gap formation compared to single row constructs, biomechanically (Ahmad CS, 2008 #33) (Ahmad CS, 2009 #34) (Baums MH, 2010 #35) (Baums MH, 2008 #36) (KimDH, 2006 #37) (Ma CB, 2006 #38). However, several level 1 studies failed to show the effect of fixation method on the outcome (Burks RT, 2009 #40) (Franceschi F, 2007 #41) (Grasso A, 2009 #42). A meta-analysis show reduced re-tear rates with double row repair but is clinical benefits of the double row is small (Pennington WT, 2010 #43). The optimal fixation should be determined and individualized, intra-operatively. It is worthless to over tension a tendon with double row construct instead of using a single row.

Deltoid Repair

Deltoid must be securely repaired during open surgery. Damage to the deltoid origin or detachment of deltoid might cause serious complications. Deltoid origin should be reattached with heavy (2-0) non-absorbable sutures. Preserving the deltoid origin is the major advantage of arthroscopic rotator cuff surgery. However, subperiosteal elevation of deltoid origin during arthroscopic acromioplasty might cause damage, which might cause weakness of the deltoid muscle (Rockwood CA Jr., 1995 #44). Is of paramount importance to keep the anterior-superior origin of the deltoid during arthroscopic acromioplasty.

Rehabilitation

Delayed rehabilitation after arthroscopic rotator cuff repair is found to allow tendon healing without impairing the motion (Parsons BO, 2010 #45). However, wide soft tissue dissection performed in open surgery might cause extensive scarring if the rehabilitation is delayed. Many surgeons start passive range of motion immediately after the surgery and delay active range of motion for tissue healing. The secure limit of motion is best assessed depending on the strength of fixation and tissue quality during surgery.

Stiffness most likely occurs after massive rotator cuff repair. Gradual passive range of motion exercises without pulling out the repair is the keystone of rehabilitation protocol. Otherwise in patients with small tears dehiscence of the repair is uncommon and more aggressive rehabilitation program could be started after surgery. Close communication with physical therapists is crucial and the surgeon should lead the rehabilitation.

Open Management; Mini-Open Rotator Cuff Repair

Mini open approaches are performed with splitting the deltoid without any take down of the origin. Skin incision ranges 3 cm from portal extensions in a longitudinal fashion. Mini-open approach is best suited for small (0–1 cm) to medium sized (1–3 cm) tears. The retraction of the tendon should not exceed mid-humeral head.

Arthroscopy assisted mini-open approach starts with diagnostic arthroscopy of the glenohumeral joint following diagnostic arthroscopy of subacromial space. Than arthroscopic bursectomy, soft tissue debridement and acromioplasty is performed. Tendon is mobilized and greater tuberosity is prepared. Suture anchor is placed and sutures are passed into the tendon. Finally, the knots are tied. These steps could also be performed in a full arthroscopic approach. If the case becomes more challenging for the skill of the surgeon, the procedure could easily be changed to mini-open approach.

This technique is recommended for isolated supraspinatus tears only. Retracted, large tears could be repaired easier with a full open or full arthroscopic technique. Because of the limited exposure of mini-open technique, a complete visualization of the tear configuration for anchor placement, tendon-to-tendon repair, or tying the sutures might be challenging.

Rotator Cuff Repair; Arthroscopic Approach

Arthroscopic rotator cuff repair had enormously evolved in the past two decades. With the advancements of the surgical principles, techniques and instrumentation almost all patterns and sizes of rotator cuff tears can now be repaired arthroscopically. Biologic healing could be achieved with a biomechanically stable construct. The ideal repair construct must optimize the suture-to-bone fixation, suture-to-tendon fixation, abrasion resistance of suture, suture strength, suture strength, loop security, knot security and restoration of anatomic footprint.

The arthroscopic management of the cuff begins with understanding the basic and arthroscopic principles. There is a strict relationship between normal anatomy and biomechanics. Thus, repairing the torn cuff, restoring the anatomy is like solving the puzzle. Restored anatomy and normal biomechanics with appropriate repair pattern brings the function.

Balance of Forced Couples

The rotator cuff and extrinsic muscles create moments to produce specific rotational motion.

Surrounding muscles are positioned to create balance thus shoulder can maintain a stable fulcrum of motion (Inman VT, 1944 #46) (SS, 1993 #47) (SS, 1991 #48). This mechanical system is called forced couples. When force couples are disrupted with a massive cuff tear active shoulder motion will be lost. The main principle of rotator cuff repair is to rebalance forced couples.

Rotator Cable

The intact rotator cuff demonstrates an arching, cable like thickening surrounding a thinner crescent of tissue that inserts into the greater tuberosity of humerus. This is known as cable-crescent complex. The cable like structured is located medial to the avascular cuff insertion. This cable might function as a load bearing bridge, which transmits the force to the avascular zone. That could cause stress-shielding effect and protect the cuff insertion from excessive loading forces.

Load distribution in rotator cuff tear could be explained with a suspension bridge model. The free margins of the tear corresponds the supports at each end.

Seeing and Reaching the Pathology

Any tear that is visualized and reached by the instruments could be repaired arthroscopically. Visualization is directly related with bleeding control, which is achieved by controlling the factors below.

Hypotensive anesthesia during arthroscopic rotator cuff repair is widely used. Unless contraindicated, patients' systolic blood pressure is maintained between 90 and 100 mmHg. Arthroscopic pump pressure is generally maintained at 60 mmHg. If the bleeding impairs vision, it can be temporarily increased to 75 mmHg up to 10–15 min. A separate 8 mm inflow cannula is used to maximize inflow. It is better not to use inflow cannula for instruments because it might cause turbulence.

The most important factor for bleeding control is fluid turbulence. Turbulence result from rapid inflow from the portal incision, which does not have cannula, inserted. If the turbulence occurs it could be stopped by applying digital pressure to the portal. Increasing pump pressure worsens the bleeding.

Surgeon must be familiar to all standard and accessory arthroscopic portals to reach and treat different types of tears.

Tear Pattern

Tear patterns are classified based on the shape and mobility of the tendon. Four different types of rotator cuff tears were described. These are; (1) Crescent Shaped, (2) U-Shaped, (3) L-Shaped, and (4) Massive retracted immobile tears.

Crescent shaped tears are classic tears and have excellent medial to lateral mobility. These tears can be directly fixed bone with minimal tension.

U-shaped tears are retracted more medial than crescent shaped tears. The apex of the tear is located close to the medial glenoid rim. The repair of U-shaped tear deserves special attention. The apex of the tear has minimal mobility and cannot be fixed to the bone without over tensioning. Over tensioning the repair site causes failure. Margin convergence method described to repair U-shaped tears. The tear is sequentially sutured in a side-to-side fashion from medial to lateral. This creates a free lateral edge. Lateral free edge is then fixed to the bone with minimal tension.

L-shaped and reverse L-shaped tears are similar to U-shaped tears however; in L-shaped tears one leaf is more mobile than the other. Mobile leaf could easily reach the bone. Sequential side-to-side suturing is performed longitudinally. Converged margin is then attached to the tuberosity. In chronic L-shaped tears the posterior retraction of the tendon is prominent and the tear assumes as a more U-shaped. During repair the point facing the corner is pulled via a traction suture than longitudinal side-to-side suturing is performed from medial to laterally. Than converged margin is attached to the bone.

Massive, contracted, irreparable tears could be repaired with more sophisticated techniques. These tears represent 9.6% of all massive cuff tears (Lo IK, 2004 #49). Neither medial-lateral nor anterior-posterior mobility can be obtained. These tears cannot be repaired with margin convergence or direct repair. Management of these tears is challenging and simple debridement has no affect on pain relieve and motion restoration (Ellman H, 1993 #50).

Massive tears represents is two different types; massive contracted longitudinal and massive contracted crescent. In massive contracted longitudinal tears the "tongue" of supraspinatus at the anterior origin is useful during repair after adequate mobilization. Massive contracted crescent tears are wider in anterior-posterior direction than longitudinal are that makes them difficult to repair.

Arthroscopic anterior interval sliding technique described by Tauro is performed through accessory lateral portal with cutting instrument by releasing the anterior interval between supraspinatus and the rotator interval (JC, 1999 #51). Supraspinatus gains 1–2 cm of lateral excursion by effectively incising the coracohumeral ligaments with anterior interval releasing. It is generally enough to repair massive contracted longitudinal tears. Supraspinatus is directly fixed to the bone and infraspinatus is repaired with side-to-side sutures plus advancement of infraspinatus on the bone bed if possible.

For massive contracted crescent tear, 1–2 cm lateral excursion is usually not enough for tendon-to-bone repair. Double interval sliding by releasing the posterior interval in addition to the anterior interval provides up to 5 cm lateral excursion for supraspinatus and infraspinatus. With posterior interval releasing infraspinatus can be fixed to the bone. Repairing at least inferior 1/2 of infraspinatus important because the anterior moment should be balanced according to the force couples principle.

Posterior interval slide could be performed through lateral viewing portal. Scapular spine is cleared from surrounding fibroadipose soft tissue. Great care should be taken not to harm suprascapular nerve, which curves tightly around scapular spine and its junction to posterior glenoid neck (Warner JJP, 1992 #52). Single and double interval slides significantly improves motion and relieves pain (SS, 1997 #53).

Biomechanics of Cuff Fixation

In the light of the recent biomechanical studies, cuff fixation constructs are much more superior to those of past decade. However, recognizing the tear pattern and using an appropriate technique must be considered. Using in appropriate repair techniques will result extensive tensioning at the tear margin and cause fixation failure. For example, a secure fixation could not be obtained in a U-shaped tear repaired with medial-to-lateral sutures without using margin convergence.

Transosseous rotator cuff repairs are prone to failure under cyclic loads because of the bone cut by the sutures (Burkhart SS, 1997 #59) (Burkhart SS, 1997 #60). This type of failure usually occurs when the distal holes were drilled in metaphyseal bone rather than thick cortical bone.

Suture anchor repair has a unique failure pattern. The weak link is transferred to tendon-suture interface and the failure is a result of sutures cutting through the tendon. Even so, the failure pattern occurs at higher cycles then similar transosseous repairs (Burkhart SS, 1997 #60). Double loading the number of fixation points of suture to the tendon would reduce the load by 50% in each suture (Burkhart SS, 2000 #61).

Arthroscopic knot tying is the final component optimizing the rotator cuff repair. The optimal knot should provide knot security and loop security. Knot security, is effectiveness of the knot resisting slippage, depends of friction interference and slack between throws. Loop security is achieved by tight know and protecting the fixation. Therefore, it is important to achieve a balance between loop security and knot security.

Cuff foot print restoration is another important issue, which determines the tendon-bone contact area. Increasing the tendon-bone contact area will more effectively transmit forces and might improve the potential for complete healing. Rotator cuff print could be completely be reconstructed with double-row repair technique. Therefore, adequate lateral excursion should be maintained for repair (Liu SH, 1994 #62).

Subscapularis Tendon Tears

Arthroscopic repair of the subscapularis deserves special attention. The technique has the following difficulties; (1) the available working space for the instruments is limited and it is recommended to repair subscapularis first. (2) Subscapularis tears are usually associated with coracoid impingement and subcoracoid stenosis that often necessitates arthroscopic coracoplasty (Lo IK, 2003 #54) (Lo IK, 2003 #55) (Lo IK, 2003 #56) (3) Medial subluxation of biceps tendon may be accompanied with subscapularis tears, necessitating tenotomy or tenodesis (Lo IK, 2004 #57).

In chronic retracted tears of subscapularis, it is difficult to identify the tendon. A "comma shaped" arc of ligamentous tissue was identified located in the superolateral border of subscapularis. That might help locating the superolateral border. Comma sign is superior glenohumeral ligament-coracohumeral ligament complex torn from the humerus (Lo IK, 2003 #58). Comma sign functions as the medial sling for the biceps tendon serves as a guide to subscapularis tear.

Massive Contracted Immobile Anterosuperior Rotator Cuff Tears

Arthroscopic management of massive contracted immobile tears is different when subscapularis is chronically torn along with supraspinatus and infraspinatus. Coracohumeral ligament has a tendency to rigidly retract and pull the cuff medially. Interval slides is helpful to gain lateral excursion. Coracohumeral ligament is incised from the base of the coracoid, preserving an intact bridge of rotator interval tissue containing comma sign. Usually better tendon repair is possible. Lateral portion of the rotator interval could be used if margin convergence is needed.

Questions

1. Which rotator cuff tear is associated mostly with glenohumeral and biceps instability?
   A. Supraspinatus
   B. Infraspinatus
   C. Subscapularis
   D. Teres minor

   C

2. Please find the false statement…
   A. Crescent type tears can be fixed directly to the bone
   B. Rotator cable might function as a load bearing bridge, which transmits the force to the avascular zone
   C. The failure pattern of suture anchors occurs at lower cycles then similar transosseous repairs
   D. Mini open technique can be applied at isolated supraspinatus tears
   E. Arthroscopic pump pressure is generally maintained at 60 mmHg

   C

3. Which imaging technique has a lower sensitivity to partial thickness rotator cuff ruptures?
   A. USG
   B. MRI
   C. MR arthrography
   D. Arthroscopy

   A

What is new?

Some people lives asymptomatic with rotator cuff tears. We do not exactly know why and when the rotator cuff tear becomes symptomatic. This review gives us a clue about this unlighted topic.

'A Prospective Evaluation of Survivorship of Asymptomatic Degenerative Rotator Cuff Tears' JBJS 2015 January, Keener JD et al.

Surgical Management of Stiff Shoulder

28

Ahmet Yildirim and Mustafa Özer

Introduction

Stiffness problem in the shoulder, is a symptom that can be caused by many pathologies. It can be seen in different clinical presentations like primary or secondary simple stiffness, adhesive capsulitis, frozen shoulder or algodystrophy. The etiology is intricate and multifactorial, so that treatment of stiff shoulder is often empirical and confederated [1].

The stiff shoulder is also frequent and affects daily life in the middle aged population. It is an idiopathic problem which has a privative impact on the routine activities of many middle-aged people. The prevalence of stiff shoulder is about more than 5% in the general population and seen in females more than males [1]. The clinical symptoms help us to diagnose stiff shoulder; especially pain (night pain) and limited motion in all planes.

The pictures were taken from the personal archive of Prof Dr. Ulunay Kanatlı with his permission.

A. Yildirim, M.D. (✉)
Department of Orthopaedics and Traumatology, Selcuk University Medical School, Konya, Turkey
e-mail: drorto@yandex.com

M. Özer, M.D.
Department of Orthopaedics and Traumatology, Necmettin Erbakan University Medical School, Konya, Turkey

The pathology was first defined by Duplay in 1872, and later literature; this illness was named as "adhesive capsulitis" by Neviaser [2]. Codman had used the name "frozen shoulder" in 1934. It is caused by inflammation of the synovial lining and capsule, leading to dense adhesion formation within the joint [2].

Stiff shoulder is subdivided into two groups as idiopathic (primary) frozen shoulder and acquired (secondary) stiff shoulder (2.4) Capsular contracture without prior trauma or surgery causes idiopathic (primary) frozen shoulder; if the stiffness occurs after trauma or surgery it will be named as acquired (secondary) stiff shoulder [3].

Phases of stiff shoulder can be divided into the freezing, frozen, and thawing phases, or stage 1, 2, 3, and 4 [4].

In stage 1, the patients have pain and restricted motion that can be restored under anesthesia.

In stage 2 (freezing phase), patients have pain with restricted motion that can not be restored under anesthesia.

In stage 3 (frozen phase) patients have mild or minimal pain with marked loss of motion.

In stage 4 (thawing phase) patients exhibit advancing improvement in restricted motion.

According to the old literature; some cases cure itself by own resolution for the duration about 1–3 years. The "no touch" behavior may be the optimal treatment for them [5] most of them also treated with a supervised multimodal non-operative treatment schedule; but for

G. Huri, N.K. Paschos (eds.), *The Shoulder*, Orthopaedic Study Guide Series,
DOI 10.1007/978-3-319-51979-1_28

selected cases surgery is the only option for the treatment [6]. Recent literature is pessimistic about the conservative treatment of stiff shoulder, and suggests selection of early surgery Identification and detailed analyze of the different stages of development is main purpose to establish successful strategies for prevention and treatment of this condition.

Stage progression is thoroughly associated to anatomical impairment, and standardized conservative treatment schedules are easy, cheap and useful alternative to surgery in most patients. As usual, conservative treatment of stiff shoulder is recommended for a minimum of 6–12 months before choosing surgical option.

By the way, surgical treatment would be the best option in patients with risk factors such as diabetes mellitus, or the patients who are affected bilaterally or have chronic symptoms [7].

Shaffer et al. declared persistence of symptoms and range of motion limitation especially in external rotation in over 50% of cases at a 7-year follow-up [8]. Non operative treatment modality for stiff shoulder walks through many steps including medication with non-steroidal anti-inflammatory drugs or oral administration of corticosteroid, intra-articular injection of corticosteroid, and physiotherapy. [9] During these treatment modalities, the efficacy of intra-articular injection of corticosteroid for patients in the freezing phase and that of physiotherapy for patients in the frozen phase are well described [9]. Bulgen et al. demonstrated ineffectiveness of non-steroidal anti-inflammatory drugs for the freezing phase patients [1]. Approximately 90% of patients with stiff shoulder respond well to intra-articular injection of corticosteroid and physiotherapy, and accordingly, surgical treatment is required in approximately 10% of patients [10, 11]. The treatment options as hydrodilation and suprascapular nerve blocks would be added nearby physiotherapy in the latter stages and these might ensure varying degrees of success for frozen shoulder with respect to restoring range of motion [11].

If patients can't success above-described conservative measures, additional invasive procedures might be needed. Closed manipulation under anaesthesia has been reported to be an easy and effective approach for frozen shoulder. On the other hand some intra-articular soft tissue lesions and problems of rotator cuff may occur during closed forceful manipulation and also quite a few severe catastrophic injuries as dislocations of shoulder, humeral fractures, brachial plexus injuries and rarely glenoid fracture could make intricate this technique. So closed manipulation under anaesthesia is contraindicated for osteoporotic patients [9].

Prognostic factors for the conservative treatment of stiff shoulder are diabetes mellitus, trauma at onset, duration of symptoms before treatment, sex, age, and severity of restricted joint motion [11]. The stiff shoulder incidence and bilateral involvement are higher in patients with diabetes mellitus, and this kind is refractory to the conservative treatment compared to the type in nondiabetic patients [9]. Although corticosteroid injections may be beneficial, increased risk of bacterial infection and osteonecrosis of the humeral head should be considered.

Many samples in the literature have shown that; conservative treatment fails and patients suffer from residual pain and limitation of motion which is called refractory shoulder stiffness [12]. This type of patient needs surgery.

Surgery

Indications/Contraindications

Primarily, patients with shoulder stiffness should have conservative treatment include physical therapy, stretching exercises, intra-articular injections, and pain medications. In each case affected anatomical structures must be evaluated carefully and treatment should be planned accordingly. In addition to diagnosis; patient's age, activity level, co-morbidities, and complaints should be considered in the decision for surgical treatment. There is no consensus on duration of physical therapy before deciding the surgical treatment in the Literature. In general, if the patient has constant pain and stiffness after 6 months of proper conservative treatment, surgical management can be planed [13]. Surgical management is indicated when the conservative treatment modalities have failed to restore motion and relieve pain.

Gartsman define severe stiffness as 0° of external rotation and less than 30° of abduction; moderate stiffness is defined as a degree of 30° in external rotation and abduction compared with the contralateral shoulder. Loss of internal rotation is not considered as a parameter for surgical management except throwing athletes by Gartsman. Throwing athletes may have only posterior contracture and decreased internal rotation. He reported that the degree of external rotation is the most important predictor for conservative management success [13].

In adhesive capsulitis, the capsular inflammation, hypertrophy and contracture causes restriction of active and passive glenohumeral motion. The most common reason of acquired (secondary) shoulder stiffness are trauma and surgery. Acquired shoulder stiffness occurs because of the intra-articular (capsular contracture, tendon shortening) and/or extra-articular (subacromial or subdeltoid scarring, scarring of the subscapularis and conjoined tendon) pathologies, but primary adhesive capsulitis occurs with only intra-articular pathologies. Acquired shoulder stiffness are frequently refractory to conservative management. Therefore the differentiation of primary and acquired adhesive capsulitis is important [14].

Surgical management in the presence of degenerative joint disease is controversial. Capsular release can reduce pain in patient with moderate degenerative joint disease (humeral head congruent to the glenoid) [15]. In patients who has rotator cuff tears, there is some degree of total range of motion deficit (mostly less than 75°). Usually stiffness progressively improve after cuff repair with proper physical therapy. If the patient has more than 75° of total range of motion deficit, the incidence of concomitant adhesive capsulitis is 50% [16]. In patients with rotator cuff tears and concomitant adhesive capsulitis, adhesive capsulitis treatment should be planned before the rotator cuff repair.

Arthroscopic release is contraindicated in posttraumatic and postoperative shoulder stiffness due to the presence of the extra-articular pathologies. The regions of extra-articular pathologies are subdeltoid, subacromial, rotator interval, and subcoracoid [17]. Proximal humerus malunions should be treated open surgery for good results. Stiffness after open instability surgery typically related with contracture between subscapularis and conjoint tendon and this area can not be visualized well with arthroscopy [13]. Less soft tissue damage and early mobilization is important for reduction of the posttraumatic and postoperative stiffness [18, 19]. Intracapsular and slight extracapsular adhesions can be treated with arthroscopically. Extracapsular adhesions are treated with limited open approach.

Surgical management is contraindicated in the inflammatory (acute) phase of idiopathic adhesive capsulitis, because the surgery may exacerbate the pain level, adhesions, and motion loss with additional injury to the capsule [13, 19]. The differentiation of the phase (acute and chronic) of the adhesive capsulitis is important.

Arthroscopic capsular release is contraindicated in the stiffness with instability [14] and myositis ossificans [13]. Severe degenerative joint disease, and cuff tear arthropathy are contraindications for capsular release. In this patients shoulder arthroplasty is a treatment option.

Detailed history and physical examination are very important in the selection of appropriate treatment. In the surgical management of stiff shoulder there are some modalities include closed manipulation under anesthesia, open surgical release and arthroscopic capsular release.

Anesthesia

General anesthesia with or without interscalene block is our preference like in other shoulder procedures. Required complete muscle paralysis can be provided with only general anesthesia for entrance to contracted joint. Intra-artricular catheters can be used for early pain control and mobilization.

After the anesthesia, firstly both shoulder are examined for range of motion in flexion, abduction, and external rotation and internal rotation in adduction.

Manipulation

After the anesthesia, firstly the shoulder forced to abduction and flexion. If the shoulder manipulation can be achieved to this directions, than external rotation and internal rotation forces applied. Rotation force is applied in both abduction and abduction positions. If the shoulder does not respond to flexion and abduction forces, the applying of internal and external rotational forces may cause fractures. After manipulation, if full range of motion is not obtained, remaining contractures must be released arthroscopically (Fig. 28.1).

In a study, closed manipulation under anesthesia and arthroscopic capsular release are compared. In patients undergoing arthroscopic capsular release had superior pain relief and functional restoration [20].

There are some complications, such as proximal humerus fracture, glenohumeral dislocations, osteochondral defects, bleeding, and rotator cuff rupture. Therefore closed manipulation under anesthesia is not performed by some surgeons.

Arthroscopic Release

Arthroscopic surgery is performed in the lateral decubitus position and the arm of the patient in 45° abduction and 15° flexion under 10 lbs of longitudinal traction on a shoulder holder (Fig. 28.2). Some surgeons perform this procedure in the beach-chair position, but entrance of joint more difficult without traction. After the positioning of patient and before the surgery, shoulder is examined for passive range of motion to compare with last range of motion. After the preparation of the patient, landmarks are outlined (acromion, spine of scapula, clavicle, and coracoid) (Fig. 28.3). Standard posterior portal is used for the initial view of the shoulder but entry into the stiff shoulder is quite difficult. The contraction of glenohumeral joint increasing the risk of glenoid and humeral head cartilage injury during the trocar insertion. This portal is made more superiorly than usual for decreasing the risk of injury, where the joint space is wider than usual soft spot. Additional portals are constituted according to the planned intervention. In glenohumeral joint, arthroscope is directed to rotator interval. For the true portal orientation, using of a spinal needle is critical. The anterior working portal is used for intra-articular releases in the rotator interval and this portal is made more medially than usual for better exposure when releasing the contractures. Before the anterior portal placement, the direction of the cannula should be checked with a spinal needle under arthroscopic visualization. Hypertrophic synovial tissue may prevent arthroscopic visualization and electrocautery can be used to improve it (Fig. 28.4). Firstly, thick, contracted, and hemorrhagic capsule is seen and for other pathologies, the glenohumeral joint is evaluated arthroscopically. The standard lateral portal is used for subacromial decompression.

There are some complications, such as instability, axillary nerve injury, osteochondral defects, and infection.

Systematic release of the contracted tissues in stiff shoulder is important for success.

Rotator Interval

We release the rotator interval as a first step in arthroscopy (Fig. 28.5). Posterior portal is created, and the 30° arthroscope is introduced into the glenohumeral joint. We use a radiofrequency electrode for release, this device is inserted into the joint through the anterior portal. Rotator interval is excised from biceps to superior border of the subscapularis tendon. Rotator interval capsule is released until the tip of the coracoid becomes visible. Then contractures are released around the coracoid and between subscapularis and conjoint tendon. The release of rotator interval should increase external rotation because it releases the anterior capsule, coracohumeral ligament, and superior glenohumeral ligament [21]. After the rotator interval has been released, closed manipulation can be tested and if full range of motion is achieved, the procedure may be ended. If full range of motion is not achieved, proceed to the next step.

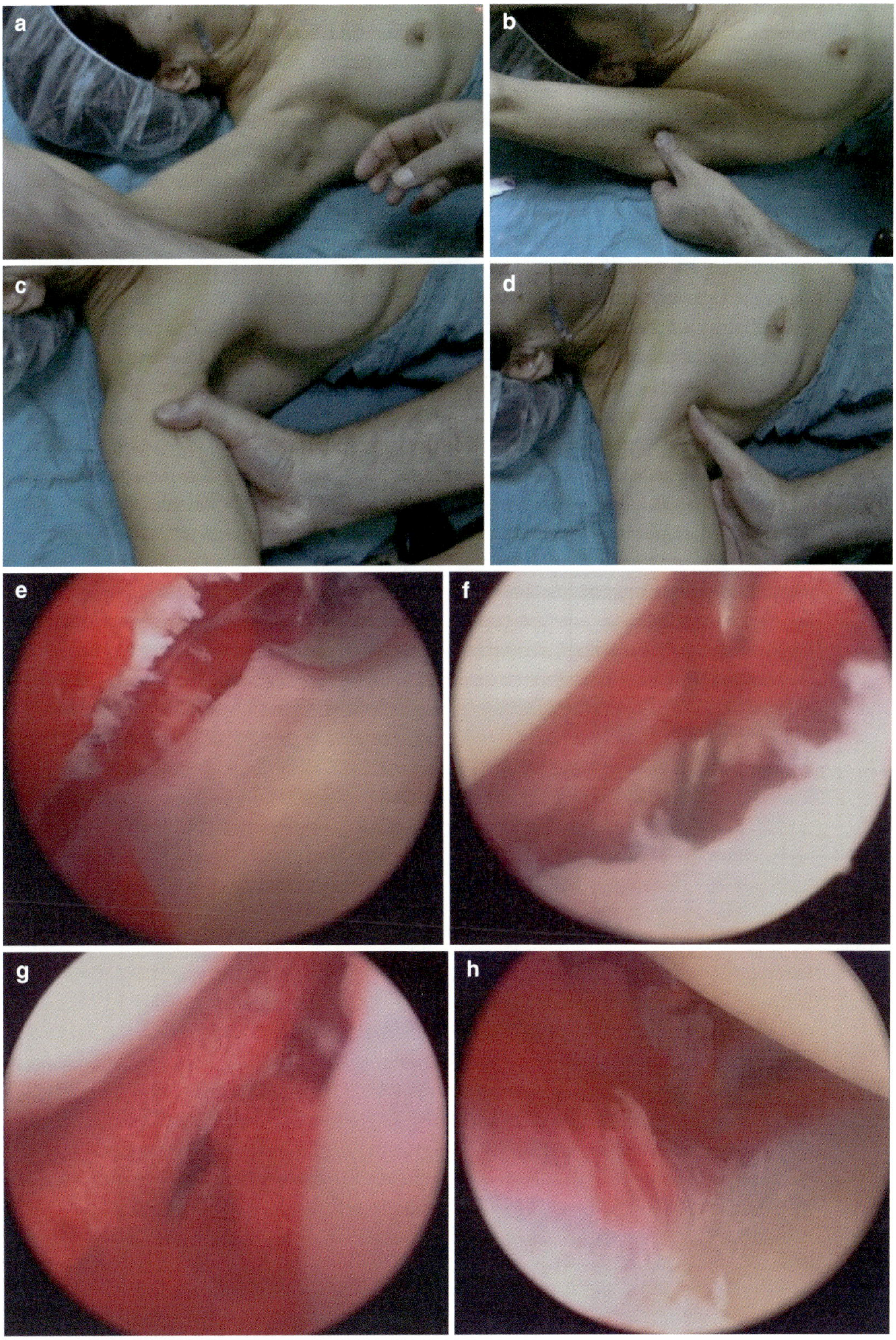

Fig. 28.1 The maneuvers of closed manipulation under anesthesia and torn capsule views. (**a**) Abduction. (**b**) Flexion. (**c**) Internal rotation. (**d**) External rotation. (**e**) Anterior capsular tear. (**f**) Anterior-inferior capsular tear. (**g**) Inferior capsular tear. (**h**) Posterior capsular tear

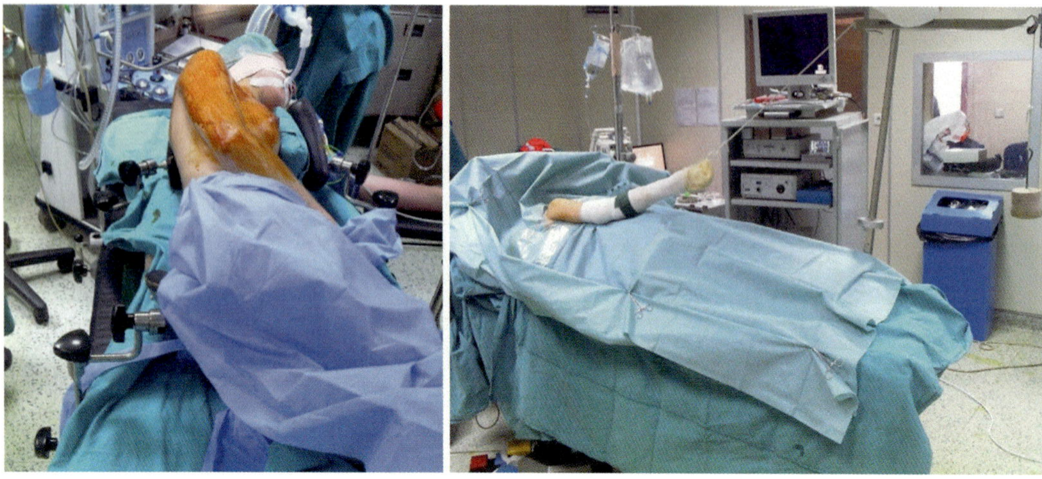

Fig. 28.2 Position of the patients

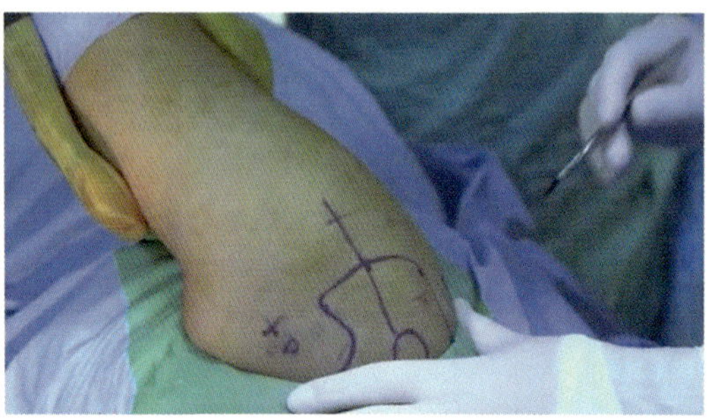

Fig. 28.3 Landmarks

Table 28.2 The complications of arthroscopic capsular release

Complications
Stiffness recurrence
Instability
Axillary nerve injury
Glenoid and humeral head cartilage injury
Infection
Anesthesia related
Interscalene catheter placement related

Table 28.1 The pattern of stiffness indicates where the capsule must be released

Stiffness pattern	Pathology
Flexion	Inferior capsule
Abduction	Inferior capsule
External rotation in abduction	Anterior-inferior capsule
External rotation in adduction	Anterior-superior capsule
Internal rotation in abduction	Posterior-inferior capsule
Internal rotation in adduction	Posterior-superior capsule

Anterior Capsule

Middle glenohumeral ligament, anterior inferior glenohumeral ligament, and anterior capsule are released with radiofrequency probe until the underlying subscapularis muscle tendon is exposed (Figs. 28.6 and 28.7) (Tables 28.1 and 28.2). The subscapularis muscle tendon must be protected against iatrogenic injury during releasing. The anterior capsular release is stopped at the level of anterior inferior border of glenoid, because of the risk of the iatrogenic injury of the axillary nerve.

Posterior Capsule

Posterior capsular release is important for limitation of internal rotation. The arthroscope is removed from posterior portal and inserted to anterior portal (Fig. 28.8). Posterior capsular release is started almost 1 cm posterior to biceps tendon and continues superior to inferior direction until the teres minor muscle tendon becomes visible. The posterior capsular release is stopped at the level of posterior inferior border of glenoid, because of the risk of the iatrogenic injury of the axillary nerve.

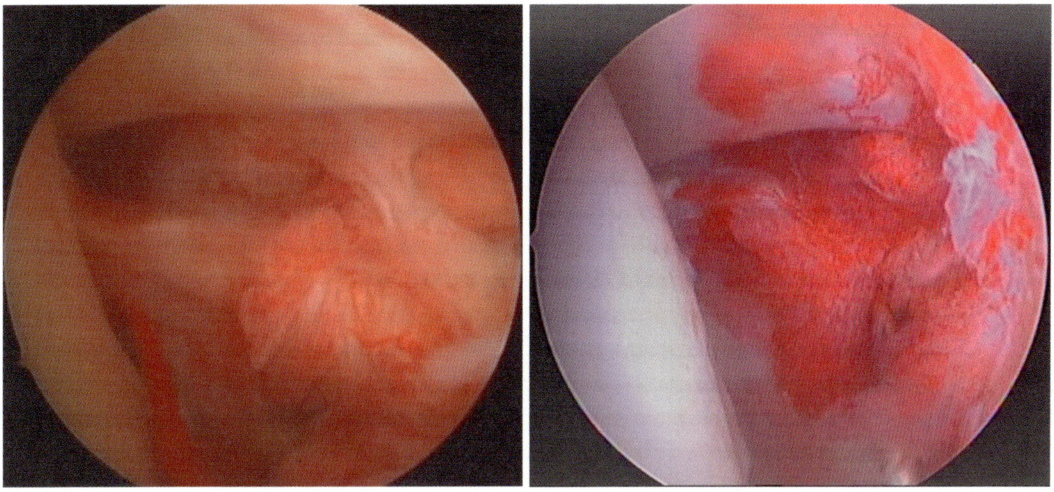

Fig. 28.4 Synovitis of the rotator interval

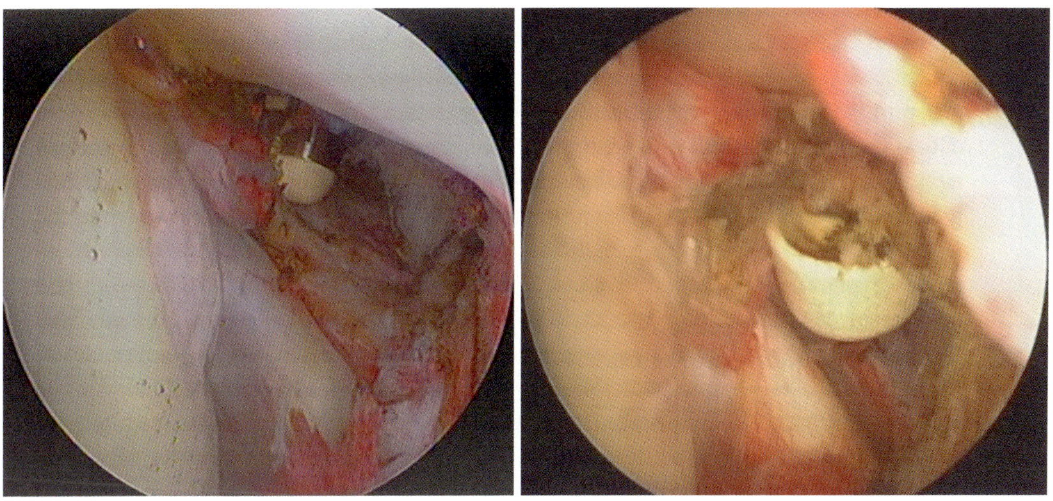

Fig. 28.5 Rotator interval release

Inferior Capsule

After the rotator interval, anterior, and posterior releases have been performed, closed manipulation (inferior capsule can be torn through manipulation) can be tested and if full range of motion is achieved, the procedure may be ended. If full range of motion is not achieved, the arthroscope is inserted posterior portal and inferior capsule is released adjacent to the glenoid labrum to avoid the iatrogenic injury of the axillary nerve (Fig. 28.9). Minimal abduction and external rotation of the arm can also reduce the risk of iatrogenic injury. The release of inferior capsule should increase forward elevation [21].

Subacromial Space

After the intra-articular capsular release, the arthroscope is inserted into the subacromial space through the posterior subacromial portal. The subacromial space is evaluated for adhesions and other pathologies. Bursectomy and subacromial debridement are performed. After the subacromial decompression, rotator cuff is evaluated. Supraspinatus and infraspinatus tendons are checked with a probe. If rotator cuff pathology is detected, rotator cuff repair should not be performed in the same session. After the arthroscopic capsular release immediate stretching exercise is needed for improvement. But after the rotator cuff repair immobilization is needed and this may cause postoperative adhesions [22]. Because of the risk of postoperative adhesions, acromioplasty should not be performed. Some surgeons perform acromioplasty and repair small tears of rotator cuff in the same session [14]. Radiofrequency probe should be used for control of bleeding that causes adhesions.

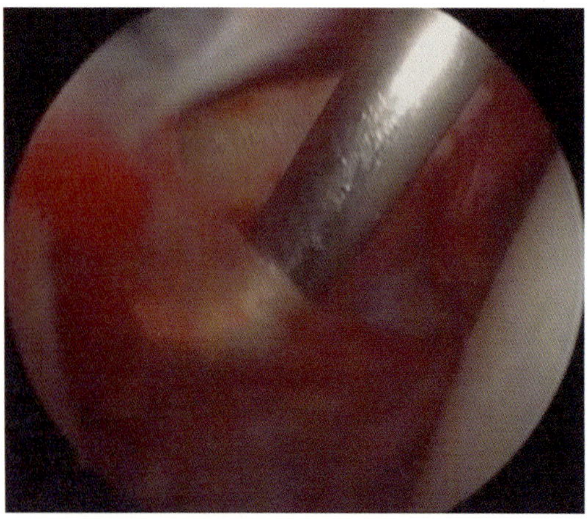

Fig. 28.6 Middle glenohumeral ligament on the subscapularis tendon

After all procedures, last closed manipulation is performed and then the joint is controlled arthroscopically. If there is no problem, the procedure is completed.

There are four basic conditions defined by Gartsman that produce shoulder stiffness and are amenable to arthroscopic treatment: idiopathic adhesive capsulitis, diabetic stiff shoulder, and posttraumatic and postoperative stiffness [13].

Idiopathic Adhesive Capsulitis

Patients with idiopathic adhesive capsulitis have global limitation of active and passive range of motion without causative etiology. In idiopathic adhesive capsulitis, the intra-articular volume decreases depending on capsular inflammation, thickening, and shortening (pathognomonic). Idiopathic adhesive capsulitis is a painful but self-limited condition that resolves with time (after 1–2 years).

Diabetic Stiffness

Diabetic stiff shoulder causes more pain and is more refractory to non-operative treatment than idiopathic stiffness. Diabetic patients may be more prone to stiffness after trauma and surgery [23].

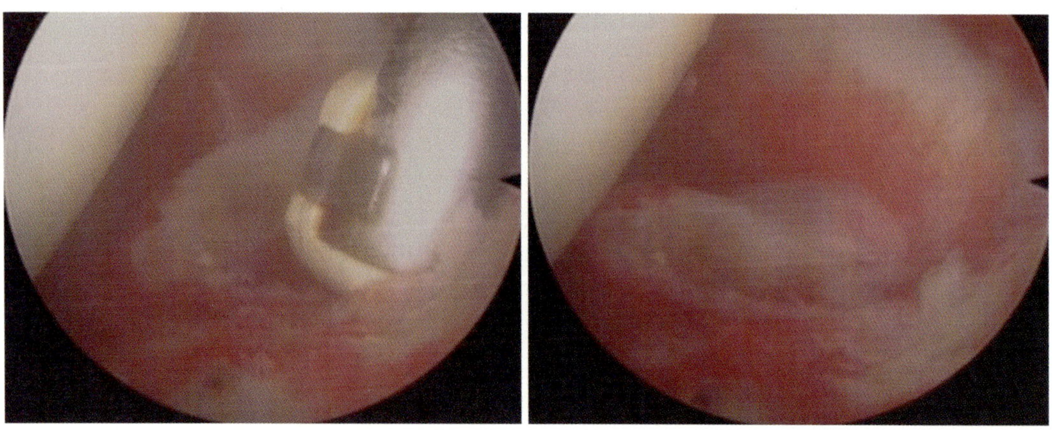

Fig. 28.7 Anterior capsular release

Postoperative Stiffness

Postoperative stiffness can be the result of excessive scarring in the area of surgery. Limitation of active and passive range of motion in a single direction occurs in the postoperative and posttraumatic stiffness unlike idiopathic form. Fracture malalignment, excessive soft tissue injury, repaired rotator cuff, and instability repairs can cause postoperative stiffness [24].

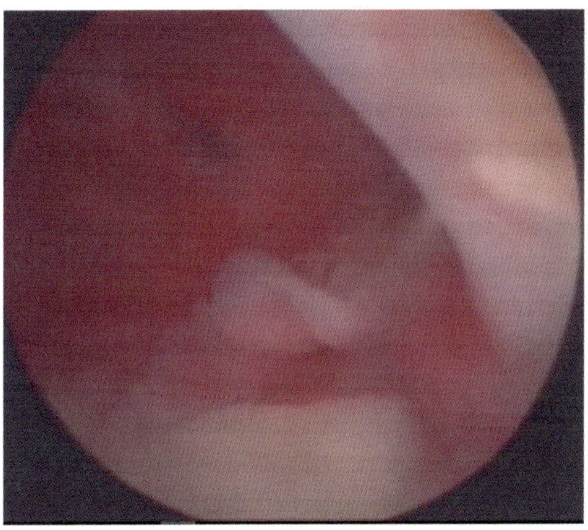

Fig. 28.8 Posterior capsular release

Posttraumatic Stiffness

Fracture, dislocation, and soft tissue trauma related scar tissue may cause posttraumatic stiffness. The mechanism of posttraumatic stiffness is firstly inflammations, and then shortening and thickening of capsular structures. The severity of posttraumatic stiffness is directly related to the severity of the trauma. In the published literature, patients with proximal humerus fracture there is a wide correlation with posttraumatic stiffness [25, 26]. Older patients more prone to posttraumatic stiffness than younger patients.

Degenerative Arthritis

In patients with degenerative arthritis, osteophytes, synovial hypertrophy, and capsular contractures may cause loss of range of motion. Arthroscopic capsular release and debridement may improve range of motion in patients with stiffness and degenerative arthritis [27]. Before the shoulder replacement surgery, patients should be evaluated for stiffness. Because of the most common cause of failure of shoulder arthroplasty is stiffness [28]. Patients with degenerative arthritis related shoulder stiffness can be initially treated with physical therapy.

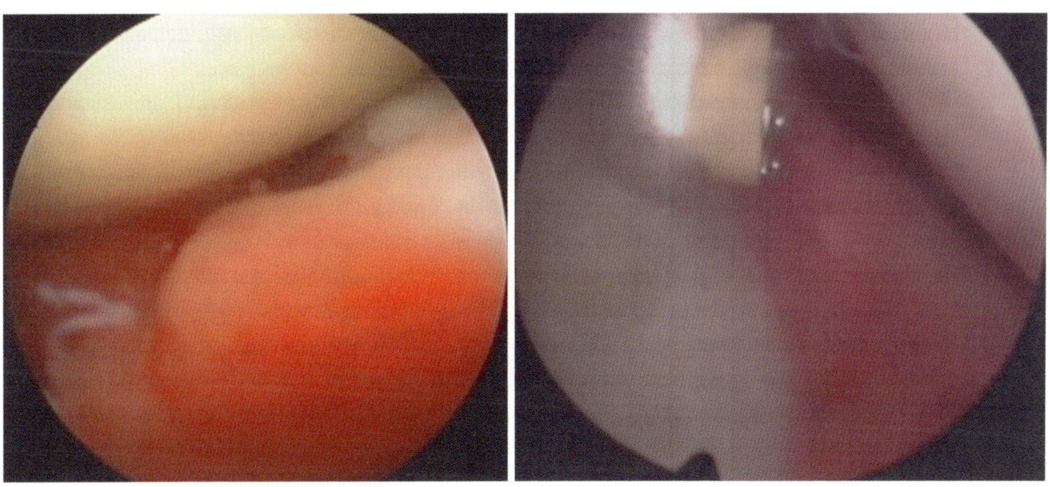

Fig. 28.9 Inferior capsular release

Most studies related with arthroscopic capsular release of stiff shoulder have found no significant difference among idiopathic, diabetic, postoperative, and posttraumatic groups [29, 30]. In a study, the results of arthroscopic capsular release in patients with shoulder stiffness were reported. The patients were divided into three groups: idiopathic, postoperative, and post-traumatic. All patients reported an improvement of pain and range of motion. However, the outcome was better after surgery of idiopathic group compared to postoperative and posttraumatic groups. Patients with posttraumatic shoulder stiffness had lower improvement than the other patients [29]. In a study, the results of arthroscopic capsular release in patients with shoulder stiffness was reported. The patients were divided into five groups: idiopathic, postoperative, posttraumatic, diabetic, and subacromial impingement syndrome. All patients reported a considerable improvement of pain and shoulder function. For all groups of patients similar results were reported [30]. In another study, the results of arthroscopic capsular release and closed manipulation under general anesthesia in patients with shoulder stiffness were reported. The patients were divided into two groups: idiopathic and posttraumatic. There was a significant improvement of range of motions and pain relief after arthroscopic shoulder capsular release and manipulation under anesthesia. Patients with posttraumatic shoulder stiffness had higher level of satisfaction with their shoulder function than the idiopathic stiff shoulder patients [12].

Rotator Cuff Tears and Stiffness

Shoulder Stiffness with Rotator Cuff Tear

The presence of trauma history, bursal pathologies, and systemic diseases such as diabetes and hypothyroidism are significantly associated with the development of shoulder stiffness concomitant with rotator cuff tear [31]. There is no association between stiffness development concomitant with rotator cuff tear and age, gender, type and size of the rotator cuff tear [10, 32]. In patients who has rotator cuff tears, there is some degree of total range of motion deficit (mostly less than 75°). Usually stiffness progressively improve after cuff repair with proper physical therapy. If the patient has more than 75° of total range of motion deficit, the incidence of concomitant adhesive capsulitis is 50% [16, 31]. In patients with rotator cuff tears and concomitant shoulder stiffness. Arthroscopic capsular release should be planned before the rotator cuff repair. Rotator cuff repair should be planned as a second procedure after proper rehabilitation program, if necessary. Shoulder range of motion should be completely restored before rotator cuff repair.

Shoulder Stiffness After Repair of Rotator Cuff Tear

Shoulder stiffness is frequent complication of repair of rotator cuff. Moderate stiffness may occurs after rotator cuff repairs and it usually recover with convenient physical therapies. Subacromial inflammation, adhesion and contracture, and muscle atrophy are possible causative factors for the development of shoulder stiffness after the surgery of rotator cuff repair. There are some factors associated with risk of stiffness development: open repair, limited preoperative range of motion, size and type of tear, presence of diabetes and hypothyroidism, subacromial and intra-articular other pathologies, immobilization time, and compliance of the patient to postoperative rehabilitation program. Aggressive physical therapy despite pain should be avoided because it can cause shoulder stiffness. Pain management is as important as physical therapy. Surgical management is indicated when the conservative treatment modalities have failed to restore motion and relieve pain. Extra-articular adhesions must be treated with a combined arthroscopic and limited open approach. This procedure is performed after closed manipulation under anesthesia and arthroscopic intra-articular release.

Questions

1. A 50 year old female patient with an insidious onset of right shoulder pain admitted to your clinic. You examine that she has a restricted passive external rotation and abduction. Your pre-diagnosis is stiff shoulder secondary to adhesive capsulitis. What would be your first treatment option?

A. NSAİD
B. NSAİD + corticosteroid injection
C. Corticosteroid injection + physical therapy
D. Arthroscopic capsular release + manipulation
E. Reverse shoulder arthroplasty

C. Conservative treatment with PT and corticosteroid injection has a success rate of nearly 90%. Surgical option can be brought into question for other 10% after conservative treatment.

2. Which of the following statements is false about arthroscopic surgery of frozen shoulder?
A. Care should be taken when entering into joint space because of the risk for injury to cartilage.
B. The anterior working portal is used for intra-articular releases in the rotator interval
C. The anterior capsular release is stopped at the level of anterior inferior border of glenoid, because of the risk of the iatrogenic injury of the axillary nerve
D. The posterior capsular release is stopped at the level of posterior inferior border of glenoid, because of the risk of the iatrogenic injury of the suprascapular nerve
E. Subacromial decompression should be performed before manipulation.

D. Axillary nerve is in danger if the level of posterior inferior border of glenoid is passed with radiofrequency

3. Please find the true statement about stiff shoulder.
A. Patients with both stiffness and glenohumeral arthritis should be treated first for their stiffness of the shoulder in order to avoid failure of shoulder replacement surgery
B. Diabetic patients has less tendency for stiff shoulder after shoulder surgery
C. In stiff shoulder patients with concomitant rotator cuff tear, arthroscopic capsular release should be planned after the rotator cuff repair
D. Shoulder stiffness is a rare complication after repair of rotator cuff

A.

What is new?

A new review is released at 'Arthroscopy' by Itoi E et al. Itoi summarized new trends at stiff shoulder management. This review will be a good repetition for our readers.

Shoulder Stiffness: Current Concepts and Concerns. Arthroscopy 2016 July, Itoi et al.

References

1. Gleyze P, et al. Management of the stiff shoulder. A prospective multicenter comparative study of the six main techniques in use: 235 cases. Orthop Traumatol Surg Res. 2011;97(8):S167–81.
2. Neviaser JS. Adhesive capsulitis of the shoulder: study of pathological findings in periarthritis of the shoulder. J Bone Joint Surg Am. 1945;27:211.
3. Goldberg BA, Scarlat MM, Harryman 2nd DT. Management of the stiff shoulder. J Orthop Sci. 1999;4:462–71.
4. Neviaser RJ, Neviaser TJ. The frozen shoulder. Diagnosis and management. Clin Orthop Relat Res. 1987;223:59–64.
5. Diercks RL, Stevens M. Gentle thawing of the frozen shoulder: a prospective study of supervised neglect versus intensive physical therapy in seventy-seven patients with frozen shoulder syndrome followed up for two years. J Shoulder Elbow Surg. 2004;13(5):499–502.
6. Bunker TD, Anthony PP. The pathology of frozen shoulder. A Dupuytren-like disease. J Bone Joint Surg Br. 1995;77(5):677–83.
7. Eljabu W, Klinger HM, von Knoch M. Prognostic factors and therapeutic options for treatment of frozen shoulder: a systematic review. Arch Orthop Trauma Surg. 2016;136(1):1–7.
8. Shaffer B, Tibone JE, Kerlan RK. Frozen shoulder. A longterm follow-up. J Bone Joint Surg Am. 1992;74:738–46.
9. Ando A, et al. Identification of prognostic factors for the nonoperative treatment of stiff shoulder. Int Orthop. 2013;37(5):859–64.
10. Papalia R, et al. Shoulder stiffness and rotator cuff repair. Br Med Bull. 2012;104(1):163–74.
11. Xu J, et al. All arthroscopic release of the glenohumeral joint for severe frozen shoulder: initial glenohumeral visualization through trans-cuff portal. Arch Orthop Trauma Surg. 2013;133(11):1549–56.
12. Trsek D, et al. Functional results and patient satisfaction after arthroscopic capsular release of idiopathic and post-traumatic stiff shoulder. Int Orthop. 2014;38(6):1205–11.
13. Gartsman GM. Shoulder arthroscopy. 2nd ed. Philadelphia: Saunders Elsevier; 2009. p. 380.
14. Craig EV. The shoulder. 3rd ed. Philadelphia: Lippincott Williams & Wilkins; 2013. p. 690.
15. MacDonald P, Hawkins R, Fowler P, et al. Release of the subscapularis for internal rotation contracture and pain after anterior repair for recurrent anterior dislocation of the shoulder. J Bone Joint Surg Am. 1992;74:734–7.

16. Angelo RL, Esch JC, Ryu RKN. The shoulder. Philadelphia: Saunders Elsevier; 2010. p. 320.
17. Ozaki J, Nakagawa Y, Sakurai G. Recalcitrant chronic adhesive capsulitis of the shoulder. Role of contracture of the coracohumeral ligament and rotator interval in pathogenesis and treatment. J Bone Joint Surg Am. 1989;71:1511–5.
18. Holloway G, Schenk T, Williams G, et al. Arthroscopic capsular release for the treatment of refractory postoperative or post-fracture shoulder stiffness. J Bone Joint Surg Am. 2001;83:1682–7.
19. Warner J. Frozen shoulder: diagnosis and management. J Am Acad Orthop Surg. 1997;5:130–40.
20. Fredrickson MJ, Ball CM, Dalgleish AJ. Successful continuous interscalene analgesia for ambulatory shoulder surgery in a private practice setting. Reg Anesth Pain Med. 2008;33:122–8.
21. Burkhart SS, Lo IKY, Brady PC. Burkhart's view of the shoulder: a cowboy's guide to advanced shoulder arthroscopy. Philadelphia: Lippincott Williams & Wilkins; 2006. p. 245–6.
22. Weber SC, Abrams JS, Nottage WM. Complications associated with arthroscopic shoulder surgery. Arthroscopy. 2002;18:88–95.
23. Chen AL, Shapiro JA, Ahn AK, et al. Rotator cuff repair in patients with type I diabetes mellitus. J Shoulder Elb Surg. 2003;12:416–21.
24. Pelet S, Jolles BM, Farron A. Bankart repair for recurrent anterior glenohumeral instability: results at twenty-nine years' follow-up. J Shoulder Elb Surg. 2006;15:203–7.
25. Pevny T, Hunter RE, Freeman JR. Primary traumatic anterior shoulder dislocation in patients 40 years of age and older. Arthroscopy. 1998;14:289–94.
26. Platzer P, Thalhammer G, Oberleitner G, et al. Displaced fractures of the greater tuberosity: a comparison of operative and nonoperative treatment. J Trauma. 2008;65:843–8.
27. Weinstein DM, Bucchieri JS, Pollock RG, et al. Arthroscopic débridement of the shoulder for osteoarthritis. Arthroscopy. 2000;16:471–6.
28. Hasan SS, Leith JM, Campbell B, et al. Characteristics of unsatisfactory shoulder arthroplasties. J Shoulder Elb Surg. 2002;11:431–41.
29. Gerber C, Espinosa N, Perren TG. Arthroscopic treatment of shoulder stiffness. Clin Orthop Relat Res. 2001;390:119–28.
30. Nicholson GP. Arthroscopic capsular release for stiff shoulders: effect of etiology on outcomes. Arthroscopy. 2003;19:40–9.
31. Tauro JC. Stiffness and rotator cuff tears: incidence, arthroscopic findings, and treatment results. Arthroscopy. 2006;22:581–6.
32. Oh JH, Kim SH, Lee HK, et al. Moderate preoperative shoulder stiffness does not alter the clinical outcome of rotator cuff repair with arthroscopic release and manipulation. Arthroscopy. 2008;24:983–91.

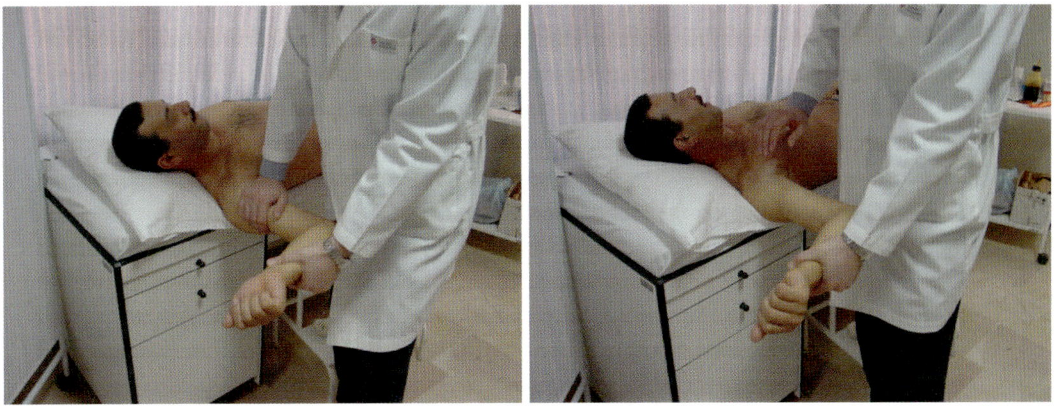

Fig. 29.3 Relocation test to evaluate anteroinferior shoulder instability

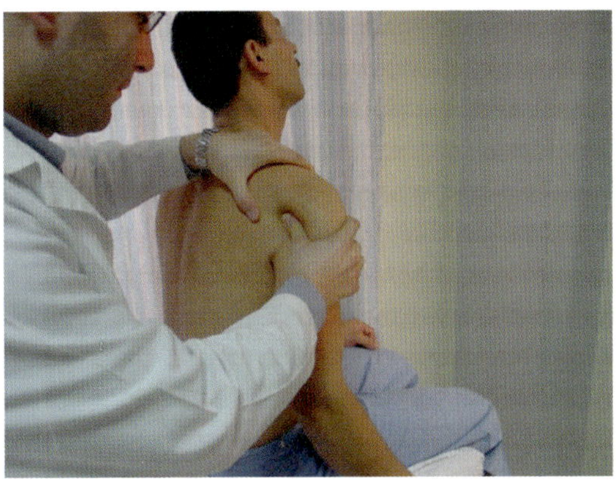

Fig. 29.4 Load and Shift test

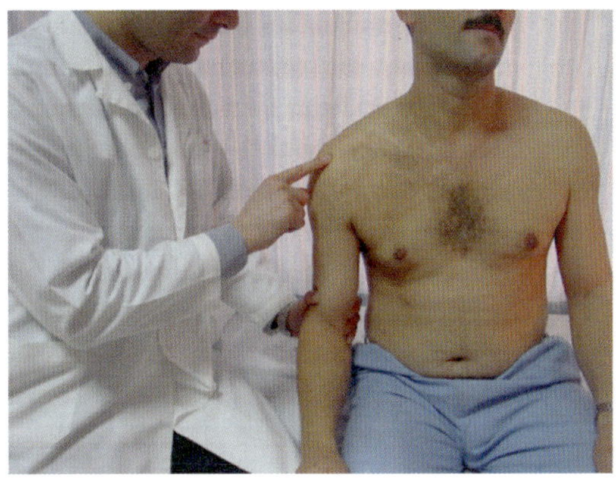

Fig. 29.5 Sulcus test

- By hooking his/her arm around the patient's elbow to achieve the above position or using the load application technique by grasping the lower arm
- Apply drawer-test (anterior/posterior) with the patient's freehand (Fig. 29.4)

Sulcus Sign Test

To perform a sulcus sign test, in order to detect the inferior glenohumeral instability [70],

- The patient's injured arm is held straight and relaxed, elbow supported by the surgeon and inferior directed traction is applied
- Severe inferior translation and a depression creating a visible sulcus appearance just below the acromion is a positive sign (Fig. 29.5)
- It is also utilized to detect multidirectional instability

Rotary Stress Test

To perform a rotatory stress test, to detect the intactness of the anterior shoulder stabilizers begin the test on the normal side [70] the following is to be done:

- Translate the shoulder while using their auxiliary space to stabilize the motion as they use one hand to do this anteriorly (Anterior Shift Test) (Fig. 29.6)
- Externally rotate the arm after abducting it
- Translate the shoulder anteriorly

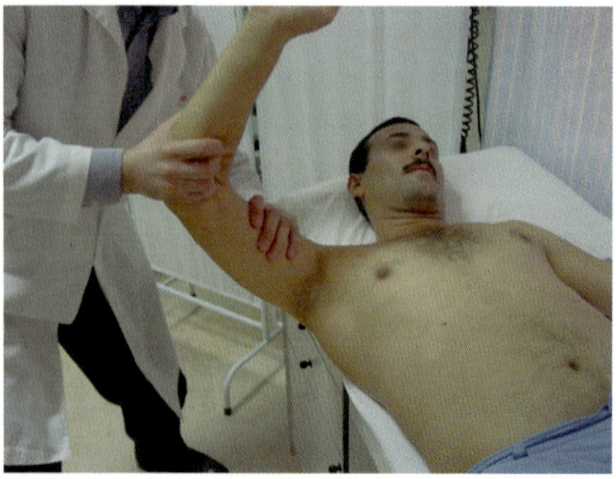

Fig. 29.6 Anterior Shift test

Humeral head translation and anterior shifting decreases significantly when glenohumeral ligament is normal and intact. Shoulder joints, sometimes, experience anterior dislocations sustaining subscapularis muscle injury furthering shoulder instability. The surgeon should promptly remember this and not overlook subscapularis muscle examination.

Neurologic and Vascular Evaluations

Neurovascular tissue injuries, during the reduction maneuvers and tractions, may occur. Before such an intervention, the orthopaedic surgeon should evaluate the neurovascular structures initially to confirm that they have not been injured during the trauma and dislocation. This is common among the elderly population. Neurovascular injury usually may occur during the prolonged, difficult or overpowered reduction closed attempts. The damaged artery might not withstand tractional forces which are necessary in reducing aged dislocation. The most commonly affected nerve during an anterior dislocation is the axillary nerve and the most commonly affected artery is the axillary artery [67, 68]. Transient neuropraxias are the most common axillar nerve lesions with 5% reported rate, incidence or prevalence [68].

Imaging

After the careful history and physical examination of the shoulder instability patients, orthopaedic surgeon should look for imaging data to confirm and prove his diagnoses. Effective diagnosis and treatment of shoulder injuries depends, in part, on effective radiography. Accurate and strategic planning of the imaging studies specifically for the suspected pathologies warrants a high incidence of accurate diagnosis and accurate treatment leading to satisfactory healing.

Radiography

A thorough diagnostic workup will consider the following elements [71]:

- Apical oblique view
- Axillary view
- True AP (35° oblique to the body)
- Transcapular view
- Stryker notch view for detecting a Hill–Sachs lesion
- West Point axillary view to detect osseous Bankart defect on the anteroinferior glenoid rim

Radiographic changes on anterior shoulder instability correspond to Hill–Sachs lesion, hardening in areas surrounding the glenoid rim, as well as fractures, erosions and blunting occurring in the anteroinferior region.

Ultrasonography, Computerized Tomography and Magnetic Resonance Imaging

Surgeons conducting further imaging studies to determine the ethiology and type of shoulder injury may proceed with the following:

- Ultrasonography (USG) [79]; optimal for evaluating the practical dynamic evaluation of the shoulder joint and related rotatory cuff and capsuloligamentous structures.
- Computerized tomography (CT) [71]; optimal for evaluating the quality of reduction and bony lesions and the affected glenoid surface area (Fig. 29.7). Also involves the

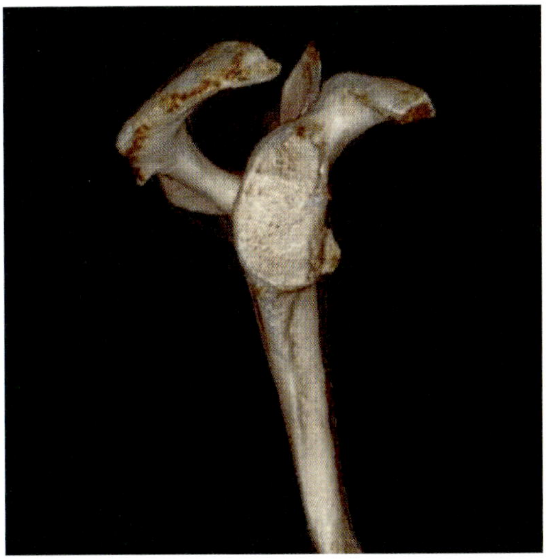

Fig. 29.7 Three-dimensional CT evaluation of the glenoid bony defect

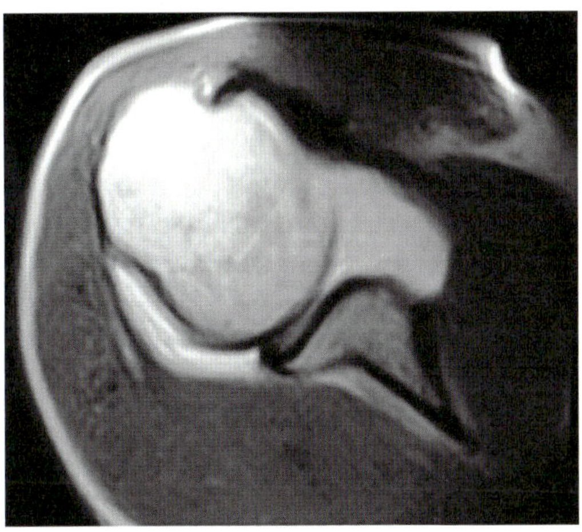

Fig. 29.8 Three dimensional CT scan evaluation of the anteroinferior glenoid rim bony defect

optimal evaluation and quantification of the degree of glenoid and humeral head bony compromisations.

- Magnetic resonance imaging (MRI) [72]; optimal for evaluating muscle, labrum, and ligamentous tears (Figs. 29.8 and 29.9). MRI arthrogram has a higher rate of specificity and sensitivity compared to a conventional MRI scan [72]. Bankart, HAGL, ALPSA, GLAD, Hill–Sachs and Perthes lesions can be detected via MRI scans.

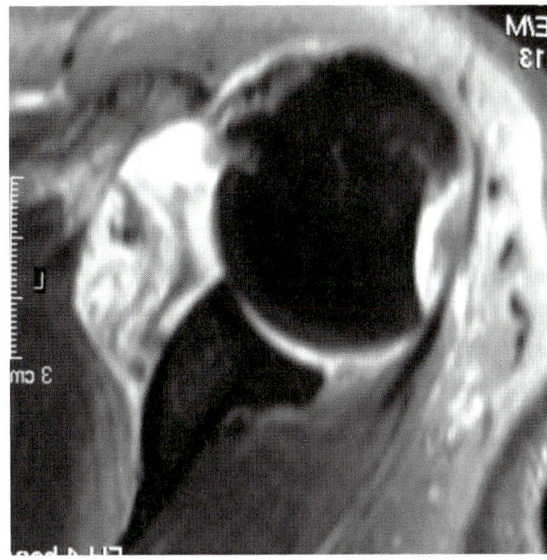

Fig. 29.9 Glenoid insufficiency CT scan view in an anteroinferior should instability patient

Arthroscopic Findings

Arthroscopic findings indicating anteroinferior glenohumeral instability may include:

- Bankart lesion [73–78]
- Humeral avulsion of glenohumeral ligament lesion (HAGL lesion) [75]
- Glenoid labrum articular defect lesion (GLAD lesion) [75]
- Anterior labral periosteal sleeve avulsion lesion (ALPSA lesion) [75]
- Glenoid rim and tuberosity fractures [75]
- Glenoid fracture with Bankart [75] and Hill–Sachs lesions [75] and rotator cuff tears [75]

According to a prospective study by Hintermann et al. [75], the incidences of associated arthroscopic findings were as follows:

- 87% labrum tears occurring anteroinferior
- 79% capsule insufficiencies
- Hill–Sachs lesions at 68%
- 55% glenohumeral ligament insufficiencies
- 14% complete tendon tears in rotatory cuff regions
- 12% labral tears in the posterior glenoid region
- 7% superior labrum anteroinferior lesions

Robinson et al., in a prospective case series study, reported the incidences of associated arthroscopic findings as follows [76]:

- 64% rotatory cuff tears
- 64% Bankart lesions
- 32% rotatory cuff tears with presence of Bankart lesions
- 11% HAGL lesions
- 7% ALPSA lesions
- 100% Hill–Sachs lesions

Differential Diagnosis

When evaluating shoulder injuries, differential diagnoses should be considered. Differential diagnosis is the final key point for a shoulder surgeon to guarantee and accurate treatment modality specific to the patient's clinical profile. Since possible differential diagnoses, such as neurologic disorder has the potential to lead inferior outcomes, surgeon should keep in mind the potential differentials of their diagnoses.

- Plastic deformation which is located at the capsular joint
- Rotator interval deficiency
- Multidirectional Instability
- Neurologic disorders with muscular dysfunction

Variations of Anterior Dislocation

The orthopaedic surgeons should be aware of the different types of anterior dislocations before attempting to treat an anterior instability diagnosis since these may include different underlining pathologies. These variations of the anterior dislocations of the shoulder are subcoracoid, subglenoid, subclavicular dislocations.

Treatment

Treatment of anterior shoulder instability may be nonoperative or operative. Nonoperative treatment options are usually preferred for light to moderate cases without involvement of severe functional bony, ligamentous or muscular injuries, while operative treatments involve reconstruction and restoration of the functional key anatomical structures and such treatment are the Bankart, Hill–Sachs, HAGL lesions, glenoid fractures and rotatory cuff ruptures. In summary, surgical treatment of anterior instabilities is inclusive of joint capsule stretching repairs when they are loosened, Bankart and Hill–Sachs lesion repairs, rectification of the glenoid bony defects by reconstructing all erosions which are anteroinferior and removal of loose bodies.

The following needs to be looked for while deciding the most appropriate treatment strategy

- The level and degree of the instability
- atraumatic, recurrent and traumatic instability due to different treatment modalities
- The presentation of different forms of anterior instabilities
- Presence of associated injuries prior to any treatment attempt

Initial Field Treatment

An acute shoulder dislocation, either anterior or posterior, should be treated in accordance with the most common orthopaedic rules. A shoulder dislocation is an emergency condition that requires immediate reduction as soon as it has been diagnosed. For field treatment, consider intra-articular lidocaine (4 mg/kg with [<200 mg] or 20 cc of lidocaine [1%] [77]. This anesthesia has the advantage of saving time and eliminating the need for conscious sedation protocol.

Non-operative Treatment

A patient history should be considered before surgical intervention. Non-operative treatment may be indicated for patients with [78, 79]:

- Multidirectional instability
- Voluntary instability
- Posterior glenohumeral instability
- Need for a supranormal joint range of motion

Non-operative treatment includes immediate reduction, immobilization, and physical therapy and rehabilitation with subscapularis muscle strengthening exercises. This method is usually the treatment of choice for first-time dislocations. Recent studies have shown superior outcomes and lower recurrence rates with external rotation immobilization [47, 80, 81].

Chahal et al. [82], in a systematic review of randomized controlled trials, reported the results of the efficacy of repair versus arthroscopic lavage surgery and versus nonoperative sling immobilization in first-time dislocations. The results revealed lower recurrence rates and superior Western Ontario shoulder scores in the repair group versus sling and sham surgery groups.

Operative Treatment

Historically, many operative procedures have been prescribed for treating anteroinferior shoulder instability, such as the Putti–Platt, Magnuson–Stack, and Boyd–Sisk procedures. The Putti–Platt procedure is a combination of shoulder capsule's advancement, medially and subscapularis muscle's advancement, laterally. The Magnuson–Stack procedure is the subscapularis muscle's advancement laterally to the lateral edge of the bicipital groove or greater tuberosity. The Boyd–Sisk procedure is the transfer of biceps muscle tendon posterolateral. Comprehensive reports of confirmed joint stiffness, severe loss of joint range-of-motion and capsulorrhaphy arthropathy have led to the abandonment of these techniques.

In some cases, a reduction and conservative treatment may not be an effective treatment for anterior shoulder instability. Surgery, however arthroscopic or open, may be indicated when the following set of indications emerge:

- Soft tissue interposition
- Rotatory cuff tendon ruptures
- Biceps tendons that are trapped and joint capsule preventing the reduction
- Displaced great tuberosity fracture
- Glenoid rim fractures [83]

Immediate Arthroscopic Bankart Repair With or Without Capsular Shift Procedure

Arthroscopic Bankart repair with or without capsular shift procedure is the optimal treatment of choice for first-time anterior shoulder dislocations in athletes younger than 25 years. Patients with a history of high demand activity, positive physical examination findings and whose MRIs' confirm the presence of a Bankart lesion are optimal candidates for this procedure. Based on the intraoperative injury evaluation and the state of Bankart repairs, inferior capsular shift also may be performed via an arthroscopic approach by utilizing the anterior and anteroinferior portals. A diagnostic exam to confirm the presence of a *drive-through sign* is required when performing the Bankart repair and capsular shift procedures. When performing the inferior capsular shift technique, the inferior portion of the joint capsule is shifted and stabilized superiorly, thus decreasing the amount of the anterior capsular and shoulder joint volume (Fig. 29.10). This technique may lead to iatrogenic subscapularis tendon injury, joint stiffness by the overtightened capsule, arthritis by chondral injury and axillary nerve injury [84].

Open/Arthroscopic Repair for Capsular Shift and Bankart's Lesion

Open/arthroscopic procedure for Bankart can be performed in combination or otherwise without the capsular shift procedure. The optimal treatment when there is a confirmed loss in glenoid bony beyond 25%, Hill–Sachs lesion (locking and engaging), and HAGL lesion's, usually includes the repair of the Bankart lesion together with the capsular shifting procedure. This is the technique typically performed via utilizing a deltopectoral approach, subscapularis split or tenotomy exposure, Bankart lesion repair with suture anchors, and the capsulorraphy with inferior capsular shifting procedure (Fig. 29.11) [84–87].

Selective Capsular Shift

The selective capsular shift is the optimal modification of the inferior capsular shifting procedure

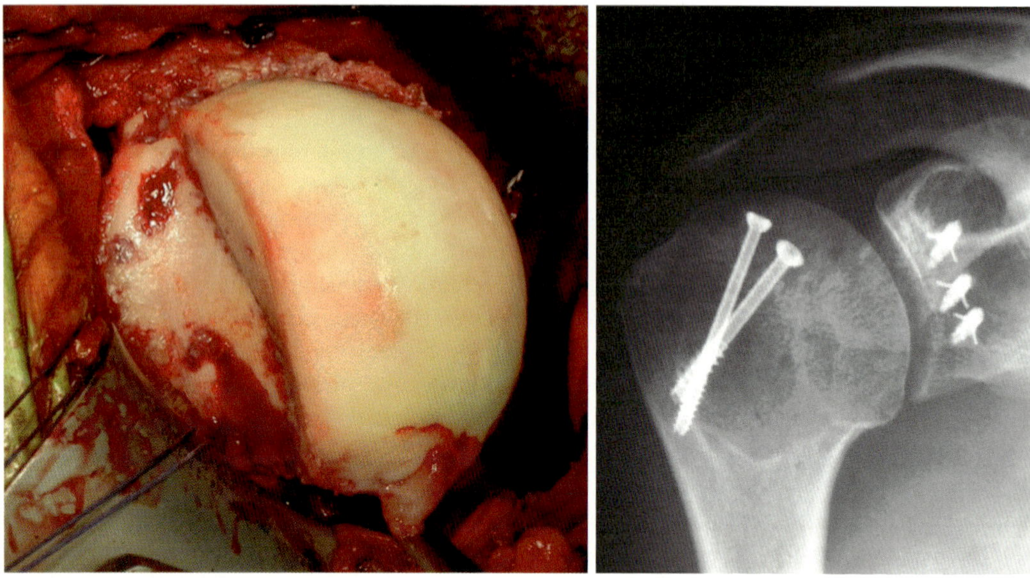

Fig. 29.10 Capsular Shift with grafting for Hill–Sachs lesions

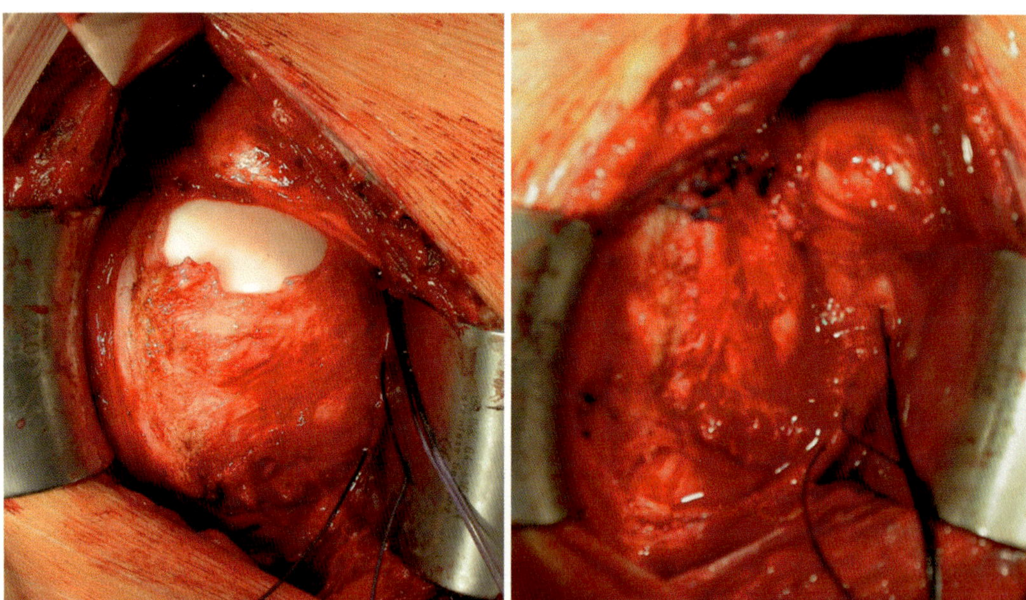

Fig. 29.11 Rotator interval defect leading to anterior instability and rotator interval closure

described by Neer et al. [85] and Bigliani et al. [86], which offers a potential advantage of controlling the amount of capsule involved in the shift, thus the surgeon can prevent the overtightening of the joint capsule, on the other hand having been preserving the normal shoulder joint capsular anatomy, range of motion and functioning [84–86].

Bristow and Latarjet Procedure

The Bristow and Latarjet procedure is the optimal treatment of choice when the anterior dislocation exhibits chronic, habitual, and bony deficiency of the glenoid greater than 20%. This procedure includes the transfer of coracoid bone with the conjoint tendon, thus creating an anterior sling effect during abduction and external rotation (Figs. 29.13, 29.14, and 29.15). It is performed using a deltopectoral approach which includes split or tenotomized exposure of the subscapularis muscle. The Bristow and the modified Bristow procedures include the transfer of the coracoid's tip alongside any conjoint tendon beneath the subscapularis muscle creating an anterior stabilizing effect [88]. The Latarjet procedure has a "triple effect," known as superiority has been described by Patte [89]. This procedure increases the glenoid contact surface area, the conjoint tendon anterior stabilization sling effect during arm abduction and external rotation [90, 91]. It supports the inferior subscapularis. antero-inferior capsular functioning and enabling the accurate darning of the compromised joint capsule (Figs. 29.12, 29.13, and 29.14). Common complications of this procedure include no union, hardware failures, and musculocutaneous nerve injury [92].

Arthroscopic Latarjet procedure is another recent innovation to treat this condition as described by Lafosse et al. [93] in 2007. This technique demands advanced arthroscopic skills and experience to work on within the proximity of the main neurovascular tissues such as the brachial plexus and the axillary artery [92].

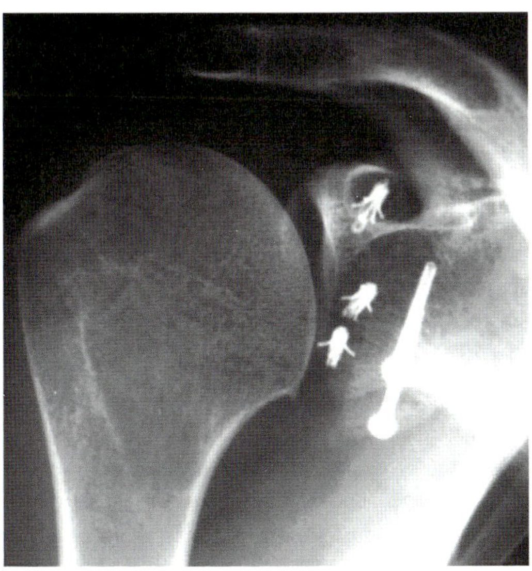

Fig. 29.12 Glenoid deficiency reconstruction: Bristow Latarjet procedure

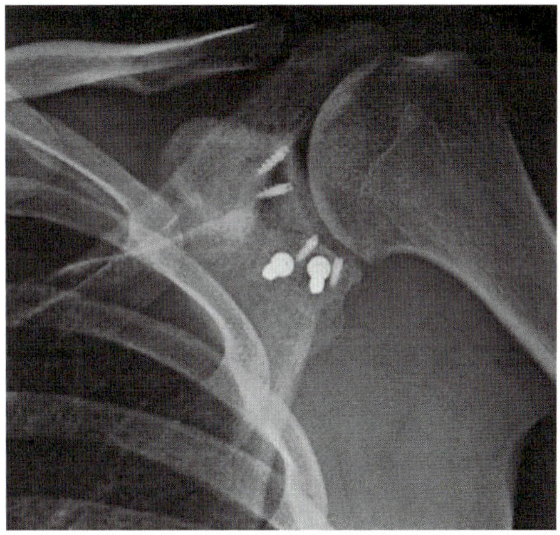

Fig. 29.13 Revision Bristow Latarjet surgery

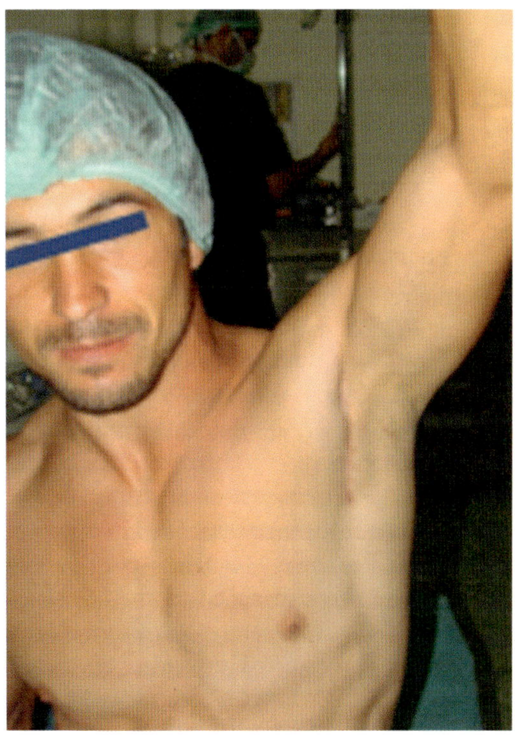

Fig. 29.14 Outcomes following a revision Bristow Latarjet surgery

Remplissage Technique

The Remplissage technique is the optimal treatment of choice for decreasing the rate of recurrence when combined with the arthroscopic anterior Bankart repair procedures. In French, "remplissage" means "filling in." This procedure was initially described by Wolf et al. in 2007 [94]. It addresses a large, engaging Hill–Sachs bony defect at the posterosuperior humeral head region including the filling of the defect by the suture anchor knots tied over the infraspinatus tendon and posterior joint capsule to decrease the shoulder joint/humeral head volume ratio. Thus, the accurate stabilization of the shoulder anteroinferior instability would have been guaranteed. Traumatic anterior instability patients treated with the Remplissage procedure reveal significantly outstanding recurrence rates around 10% when compared to an arthroscopic Bankart repair alone with a recurrence rate of 67% [94, 95].

Bony Reconstruction of the Hill–Sachs Lesion

Bony reconstruction is the optimal treatment of choice for large engaging Hill–Sachs lesions, failed Remplissage procedures and unsatisfactory stability post Remplissage technique. Other possible treatment options for large bony defects include allograft reconstructions, arthroplasty and rotational osteotomies. If a Hill–Sachs lesion is present in isolation with no bony defects, a humeral defect can be augmented either with bone plugs (autograft, allograft) or synthetic augmentation (metal, plastic plugs). The disimpaction of the lesion through a cortical window and osteochondral bone grafting may also be performed [96].

Shoulder Arthroplasty

When there are large Hill–Sachs bony lesions that are hard to be managed by the aforementioned techniques, humeral head resurfacing or replacement is considered to stabilize a recurrent instability [97]. However, definitive indications for this procedure have not been defined. Currently, these options are reserved as salvage procedures for advanced habitual dislocation and severe bony compromisation cases [98–100].

Posterior Shoulder Instability

Posterior shoulder dislocations leading to posterior shoulder instabilities are rarely seen but usually commonly missed under emergency care conditions. On the other hand, they are also a major concern for seizures, electric shocks, or ECT without muscle relaxants. Posterior shoulder instability accounts for 2–5% of unstable shoulders joints presented [101–103].

Mechanism

The most common mechanism that leads to posterior shoulder disability is anteroposterior directed force when the arm is flexed, adducted, and internally rotated. Common etiology is trauma, fall from heights, motor vehicle accidents, seizure, and electric shocks. Posterior anatomical structures of the glenohumeral joint enabling the posterior shoulder stability are glenoid, labral tissue, posterior joint capsule, inferior glenohumeral ligament (especially posterior band of the IGHL), coracohumeral ligament, rotatory interval subscapular, rotatory cuff and biceps muscles [104]. Also, anterior capsular tightness and the contracture of the anterior tissues may contribute to posterior instability [104].

Risk Factors

The following conditions contributes this type of instability [104]:

- Fully abducted and rotated arm when loaded axially
- Recurrent glenohumeral subluxation posteriorly which is involuntary, possibly associated with forces resulting from sports activities such as weightlifting, Calisthenics and push-ups

- Development of injury in flexion, internal rotation and abduction
- Anterior deltoid, or subscapularis deficiency and contractures
- Voluntary dislocations

Associated Injuries

In the physical examination, inspection reveals a prominent shoulder from the posterior view and a prominent coracoid process from the anterior view. Patients usually have painful and limited external rotation with their shoulder locked in an abducted, internally rotated position. Posterior dislocation is different than the recurrent posterior instability. Posterior instability usually accompanies laxity and only occurs in 23% of documented posterior dislocation cases [104]. Associated conditions may include, humeral head's anterior portion defect (reverse Hill–Sachs lesion), the glenoid humeral head increased retroversion, posterior glenoid deficiency, posterior labral tears and multidirectional instability.

Classification and Grading of Posterior Shoulder Instability

Types of posterior shoulder dislocation and instability can be also summarized as acute and chronic, voluntarily and involuntarily, uni or bidirectional in the inferior and posterior directions and multidirectional (inferiorly, anteriorly or posteriorly) at the time of the physical examination [104]. Various classification and grading attempts in the current literature have been focussed on the posterior humeral head translation classification and grading. Historic focus has been on the posterior instability evaluation of the shoulder joint [69, 105–108].

Currently, the posterior drawer test grading system for posterior instability of the glenohumeral joint is quantified in percentages and been represented by four grades [108]. The percentage amount of posterior translation of humeral head on the glenoid by the posterior drawer test is considered to reveal a deficient rotatory interval capsular tissue, severe muscular patterning, or a severe glenoid retroversion as the percentage of posterior translation increases.

Posterior drawer test grading system [108]:

- 1+: apparent translation but not to rim
- 2+: translation to glenolabral rim
- 3+: translation over glenolabral rim
- 4+: translation with complete dislocation

Physical Examination of Posterior Shoulder Instability

Posterior Apprehension Sign Test

The posterior apprehension test is considered positive when posterior dislocation or apprehension occurs during patient endeavors to touch the lower region of his/her thoracic spine. The surgeon abducts and places the arm in internal rotation and applies the posterior drawer test on the shoulder joint. Another similar test is performed while the shoulder maintains an internal rotation in flexion and adduction. To apply the stress posteriorly on the translation of a shoulder, the arm is positioned into internal rotation, flexion, and adduction (Fig. 29.15). The test is recommended when findings include shoulder pain with prominent coracoid process in addition to patient's inability to perform arm supination [107].

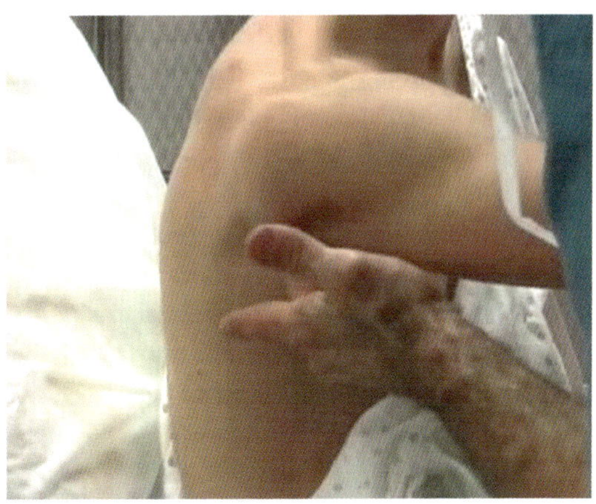

Fig. 29.15 Posterior dislocation

Posterior Load-Shift Test

In order to conduct a posterior load and shift test, the humeral head is forced anteroposteriorly while the patient is supine and the arm is abducted at 40–60° of rotation and forward flexion.

Jerk Test

For the Jerk test, a "clunk" feeling should be looked for when:

- The arm is at 90° abduction and the elbow is at flexion and internal rotation
- A force is applied parallel to the humerus in a state of abduction and in a position of forward-flexion
- A 'clunk' feeling is positive for posterior subluxation
- Along with Kim test 97% sensitivity is presented for labral tears occurring posteriorly [123]

Kim Test

The Kim test is performed and considered positive when:

- In a seated posture, an abduction of 90% is performed
- At a forward shoulder flexion of 45°
- Applying an axial load to the elbow and humeral head posteroinferior, the feeling of pain is reported by the patient.

Posterior Stress Test

The posterior stress test is performed by stabilizing the scapula as looking for posterior translation with applying a posteriorly directed force and when pain is usually triggered and in the absence of a root cause (Fig. 29.16).

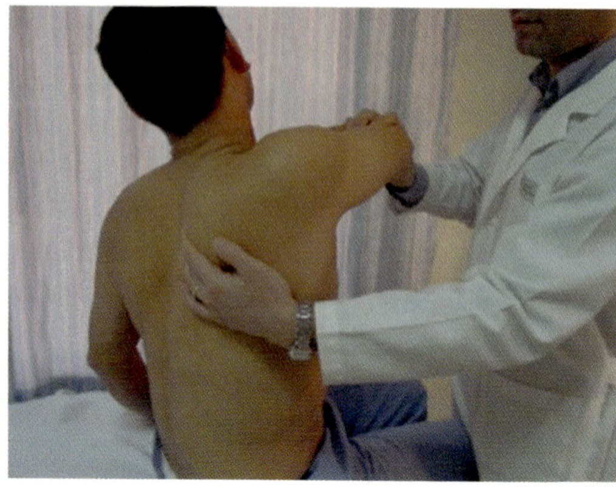

Fig. 29.16 Posterior stress test

Imaging

Radiography

Radiography is the first step on the road to diagnosing a posterior shoulder dislocation. According to the physicians' suspicion and experience, the following views may be taken [104]:

- Apical oblique view
- Axillary view–this view is the most diagnostic view for posterior shoulder instability (Fig. 29.18)
- True AP (35° oblique to the body)
- Transcapular view
- West Point axillary view to detect any reverse osseous Bankart defects on the posteroinferior glenoid rim

Computerized Tomography and Magnetic Resonance Imaging

Surgeons should also look for reverse Hill–Sachs lesion and compression fracture at the humeral head's anteromedial aspect [71]. Additional imaging includes ultrasonography, CT, MRI, arthrograms and diagnostic arthroscopy (Figs. 29.17, 29.18, and 29.19). CT scans are useful for evaluating the retroversion and bony structure of the glenoid and humeral head while MRI is a reliable tool to evaluate the patulous capsule, labral integrity, posterior glenoid chondral injuries and Kim lesion [71].

Arthroscopic Findings

In cases of posterior shoulder instability, arthroscopically, a Kim lesion at the posteroinferior region of the glenohumeral joint, including a marginal bony lesion with the degeneration of chondrolabral tissues may be detected [104, 108].

Differential Diagnosis

The following conditions which may lead to posterior shoulder instability are congenital anatomical glenoid abnormalities, glenoid retroversion deformities or hypoplasia, hypermobility syndromes leading to ligamentous laxities, and neurologic disorders leading to imbalanced muscle functioning and contractions triggered by seizures.

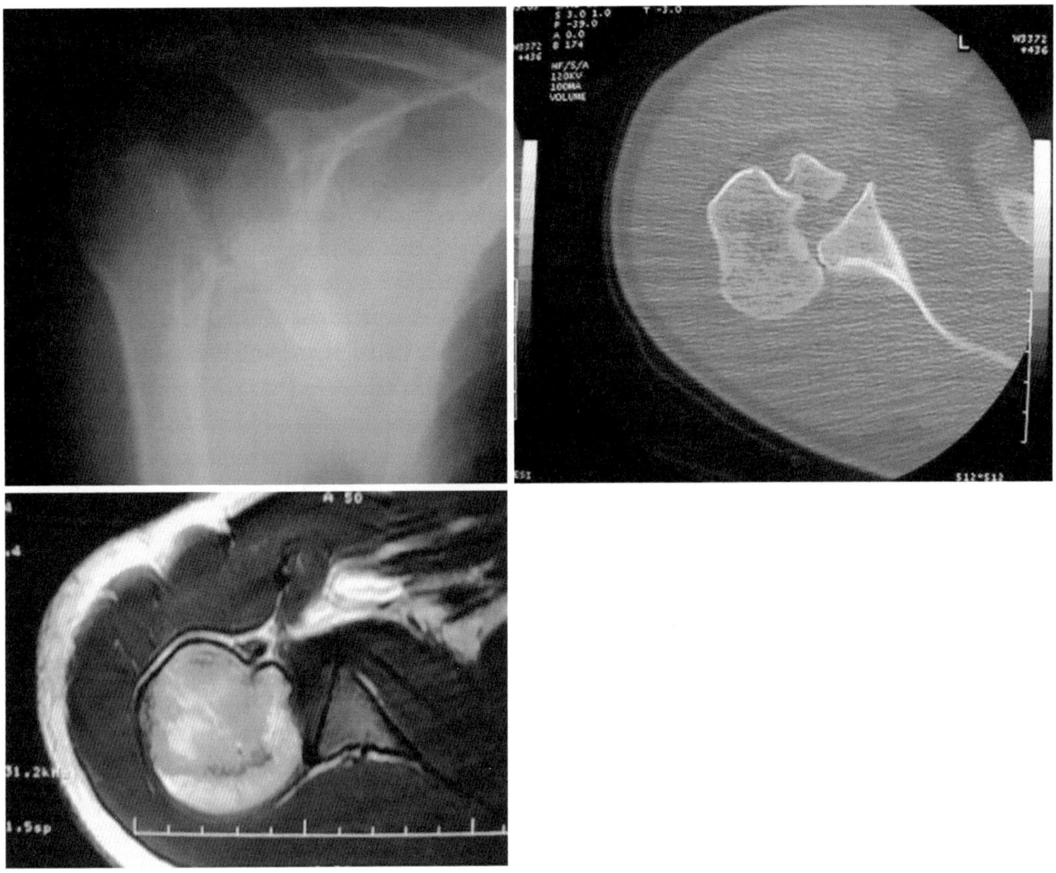

Fig. 29.17 Posterior shoulder dislocation as seen on X-ray, CT and MRI scans

Treatment

Non-operative Treatment

There are various treatment options that have been proposed for the posterior shoulder instability. Following the closed reduction of the first time posterior shoulder dislocation, the primary nonoperative treatment to prevent a posterior instability involves the strengthening of the external rotatory infraspinatus muscle. This technique is indicated for first time dislocations or recurrent dislocations with defects resulting in less than 20% loss of stability [109]. Following, rotator cuff and parascapular muscle strengthening programs to compensate the compromised static structures, external rotation exercises to strengthen these structures collaborated with an effective scapulohumerothoracic synchronisation rehabilitation is essential for a successful nonoperative treatment [110–112].

Operative Treatment

Patients with recurrent posterior instabilities, failed nonoperative treatments, grade +II and more, professional athletes with severe posterior glenohumeral instability lesions such as glenoid erosion, labral rupture, reverse Hill–Sachs lesion and multiple dislocation histories may require operative treatment. The patient's neurological and psychological condition is also a significant concern when choosing the most appropriate treatment for the posterior shoulder instability. Operative procedures for the posterior shoulder instability can be summarized under bony or soft-tissue deformities, open or arthroscopical procedures [103, 104, 113–115].

Bone block procedures, glenoid/humerus or versional/rotational correction procedures may require open approaches. Commonly, operative procedures for the instabilities purely arisen by soft tissue abnormalities may be summarized under posterior capsular shift/thermal shrinkage,

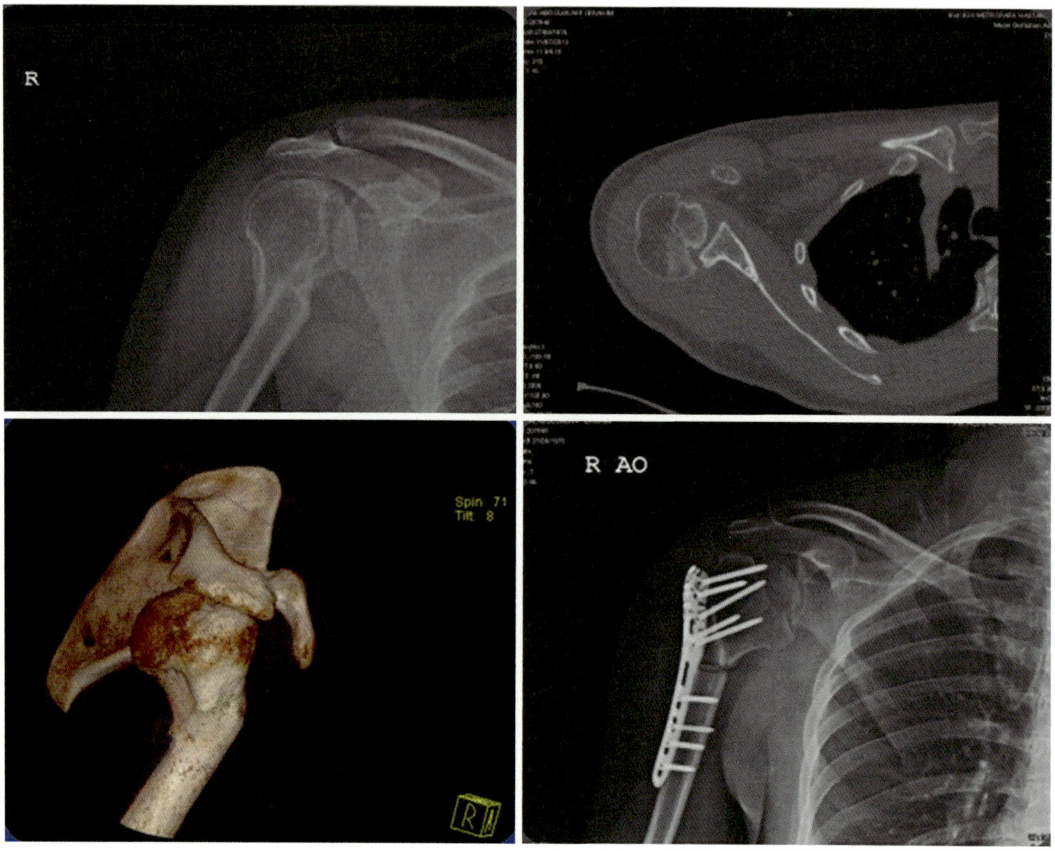

Fig. 29.18 Posterior shoulder fracture-dislocation

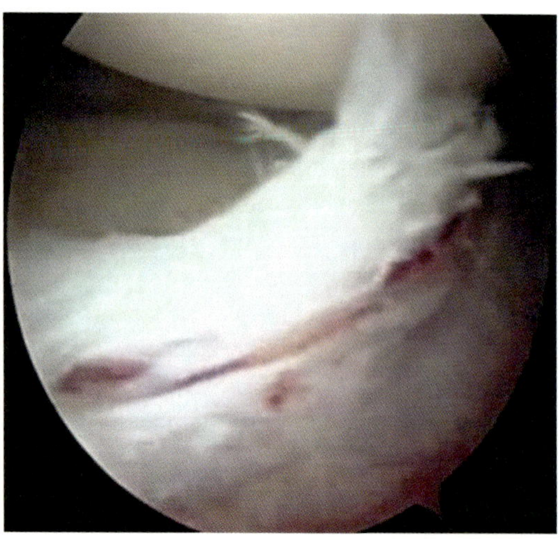

Fig. 29.19 Posterior capsulolabral lesion following posterior shoulder dislocation

subscapularis tendon transfers, posterior capsular plication, infraspinatus advancement reverse Putti–Platt plication, reverse Bankart repair, Boyd–Sisk procedure and biceps tendon transposition, rotatory interval closure [103, 104, 113–115].

Posteroinferior Capsular Shift Procedure

The posteroinferior capsular shift procedure is the most commonly utilized treatment modality regarding to the posterior shoulder instability [104, 117]. It can be performed both open and arthroscopically. A multi centric study by Bottoni et al. compared the outcomes of open versus arthroscopic posterior shoulder instability treatments and reported superior outcomes with the arthroscopic treatment over open treatment [104, 116].

Open procedure is performed via an oblique, posterior, infraspinatus split approach of choice. Incision usually begins over the scapular spine at the acromion's posterolateral aspect. Deltoid muscle is split not more than 5 cm below the acromion.

This approach utilizes the intermission existing between teres minor and infraspinatus muscles. In this approach, the infraspinatus muscle is transected and tagged for utilization during the final closure session of the surgery [104, 116].

Also, the deltoid muscle may be split off the scapular spinous process to improve the surgical exposure. Regardless of the method, especially when an open surgical intervention is being performed, surgeons must be careful when approaching within the proximity of the axillary nerve trajectory.

Arthroscopic posteroinferior capsular shift procedure is the most common posterior instability treatment procedure. It involves the shifting of the posteroinferior joint capsule superiorly in order to reduce the posterior capsule and the glenohumeral joint volume. Performed with a lateral decubitus position usually via high lateral portals. The failure rate is reported around 50% in the current literature [104]. When the posterior labral tissue is significantly compromised, it can be performed together with the posterior labral repair. Rotatory interval closure procedure performed together with a capsular shift or thermal shrinkage can be another reliable treatment option instead of a posteroinferior capsular shift procedure only. In patients with a persistent Sulcus test at 45° of external rotation, rotatory interval closure may be indicated [104].

Post operative care involves the following:

- 30° arm sling immobilizer with the arm neutral internal rotation
- Early passive range-of-motion followed by an initiation for strengthening based on patient's compliance for the initiation
- Unrestricted return to normal activities with the full heavy labor after 4 weeks and contact sports after 6 weeks [104, 117]

McLaughlin Procedure

This procedure is composed of the humeral head's open reduction with the transfer of lesser tuberosity and subscapularis [116]. Modified McLauglin procedure is the most commonly utilized open operative technique for posterior should instability. It's performed via a deltopectoral approach. Technically the aim is to repair the defect. Subscapularis tendon and lesser tuberosity is transferred (Fig. 29.19). Iliac crest bone grafting may be utilized to compensate the glenoid bony loss. When the injury is three weeks or earlier preoperatively, disaimpaction and bone grafting of the defect may be performed. Opening wedge glenoplasty may be preferred for glenoid hypoplasia (Fig. 29.20).

Post operative care involves the following [117]:

- Arm sling immobilization with external rotation brace for 6 weeks
- Internal rotation of the arm should be strictly avoided
- Functional hand, wrist exercises, passive, active-assisted and progressively active and rotatory cuff strengthening may be initiated respectively
- Unrestricted return to sports and full heavy labor can be initiated after 12 weeks

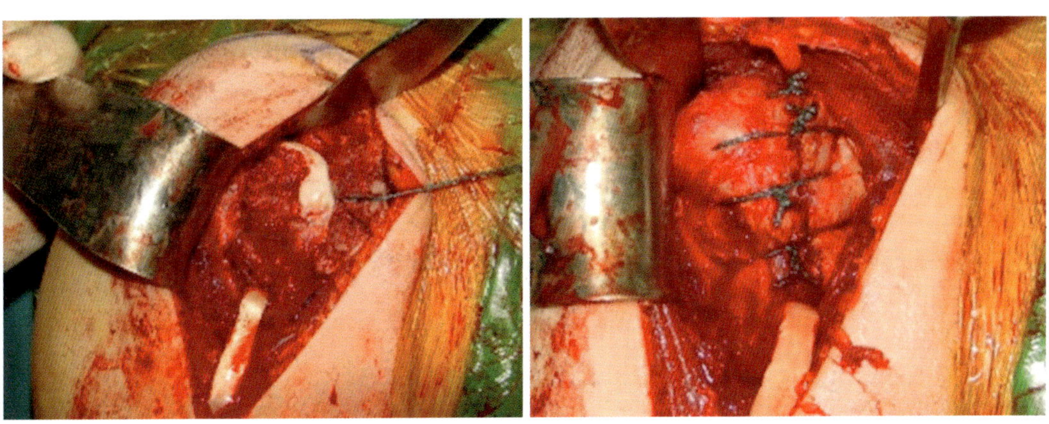

Fig. 29.20 Modified McLaughlin procedure for posterior shoulder instability treatment

Allograft Reconstruction for Posterior Shoulder İnstability

Posterior shoulder joint allograft reconstruction by utilizing bone allograft which is uniquely shaped to fill the bony defect higher than a 40% in the humeral head is indicated when there is a recurrent glenohumeral instability [118]. Reconstruction has the advantage of preventing posterior dislocation without limiting internal rotation. It utilizes an anterior approach to the shoulder. Specially shaped bone allograft is fitted into the humeral head defect and the spherical outer surface should be congruent with the joint surface.

Complications

Posterior shoulder instability surgery have been reported to reveal failure rates about 30–40% [116]. The most common complication following posterior shoulder instability surgeries is the recurrence. Capsular necrosis, axillary and suprascapular nerve injuries have been reported [104].

Surgeons should be also aware of the following potential complications [116, 117]:

- Stiffness
- Avascular necrosis
- Osteoarthritis
- Adhesive capsulitis
- Overtightening of posterior capsule

Multidirectional Shoulder Instability

Multidirectional shoulder instabilities (MDI) are rarely seen but are still a major point of concern for the shoulder surgery and sports medicine practice. Commonly defined as an atraumatic, multidirectional or bilateral condition, it often exhibits superior outcomes with physical therapy and rehabilitation. Multidirectional instability refers to a subluxation or dislocations which occur posteriorly, anteriorly or inferiorly. Patients who are experiencing multidirectional instability usually do not have Bankart lesions, but may have capacious axillary pouches. This injury usually affects overhead throwing athletes, gymnasts and swimmers.

Mechanism

This instability is generally presented as a bilateral and atraumatic condition affecting shoulder function [107]. It is caused by insufficiency of the static ligament constraints of the glenohumeral joint (GHJ) also known as capsular laxity. Also a degenerative condition leading to acquired ligamentous laxity or congenital ligamentous laxity syndromes such as Marfan's and Ehler's Danlos syndromes, scurvy, and Lathyrism may be underlying. Associated conditions may include inferior capsule laxity, rotator interval deficiency, Bankart (anteroinferior), and Kim's (posteroinferior) lesions [107].

Risk Factors

The most common risk factors for multidirectional shoulder instability are the presence of the congenital or acquired conditions; Marfan's and Ehlers–Danlos syndrome, Osteogenesis Imperfecta, Lathyrism, Scurvy and similar associated conditions [107]. The prevalence of generalized joint laxity in patients with MDI ranges between 40 and 70% [119–122].

Classification and Grading of Multidirectional Shoulder Dislocation

Multidirectional shoulder instability may also be referred as belonging to the AMBRI (atraumatic-multidirectional-bilateral-rehabilitation-inferior capsular shift) classification group. Key to classifying the MDI is to define the etiology (traumatic, atraumatic, microtraumatic), the degree of symptomatic translation and the presence volitional control (voluntary and involuntary). We do also advise to perform a Beighton hyperlaxity grading to evaluate the presence of an underlying hyperlaxity condition. MDI can be classified as [14]:

- Multidirectional Instability without hyperlaxity
- Multidirectional Instability with hyperlaxity
- Voluntary Multidirectional Instability with hyperlaxity

Physical Examination of Multidirectional Shoulder instability

Physical examination may reveal bilateral, atraumatic compromise mainly on the soft tissue and secondarily, on the bony tissues of the glenohumeral joint. Mainly, the presence of the generalized capsular laxity leads to the multidirectional pattern of the condition.

Symptoms may include:

- Pain
- Instability
- Weakness
- Paresthesias
- Crepitus and shoulder instability during sleep
- Hyperlaxity

The physical exam can be summarized as the following:

- Sulcus sign test; for rotator interval pathologies
- Apprehension/relocation test
- Load and shift test
- Neer and Hawkins test
- Beighton hyperlaxity grading

Other signs to look for include generalized hyperlaxity such as genu recurvatum, elbow hyperextension, metacarpophalangeal backwards hyperextension, hyperabduction of the thumb about the distal radius [14].

Imaging

Radiography

- AP-External rotation
- Axillary
- AP-True
- AP-Internal rotation
- Scapular notch views may be obtained

Computerized Tomography and Magnetic Resonance Imaging

- Possible glenoid dysplasia conditions should be eliminated on CT scans.
- Inferior joint capsule is seen slacked between the bands of IGHL on MRI
- Also Kim's lesion, Bankart lesion, Glenoid cartilage erosions may be evaluated on MRI scans.

Arthroscopic Findings

- Drive-through sign

Treatment

Non-operative

Multidirectional instability is not well-suited for operative treatment. Thus, physicians should consider options in consultation with the patient [108]. Based on the surgeon's physical examination of the severity of the multidirectional instability, the treatment should consist of rotator cuff strengthening and intensive rehabilitation for at least one year. Dynamic stabilization together with physical therapy is the trivial first step that applies to majority of multidirectional instabilities of the shoulder. The technique involves a 3–6 month strengthening of dynamic stabilizers and closed kinetic chain exercises. Success rates with the nonoperative treatment modalities between 30 and 80% have been reported [16, 123, 124]. Unresponsive cases may be treated with arthroscopic inferior capsular shift procedures.

Operative

Open or arthroscopic capsular procedures focused to produce a shifting and stabilizing effect. Indications of operative treatment in multidirectional shoulder instability are:

- Failure to respond treatment
- Severe pain
- Evident disabling instability [107].

Contraindications of operative treatment in multidirectional shoulder instability are specifically for voluntary dislocations [107].

In selected cases, such as refractory and collagen disorders, capsular reconstruction via allografts may be performed.

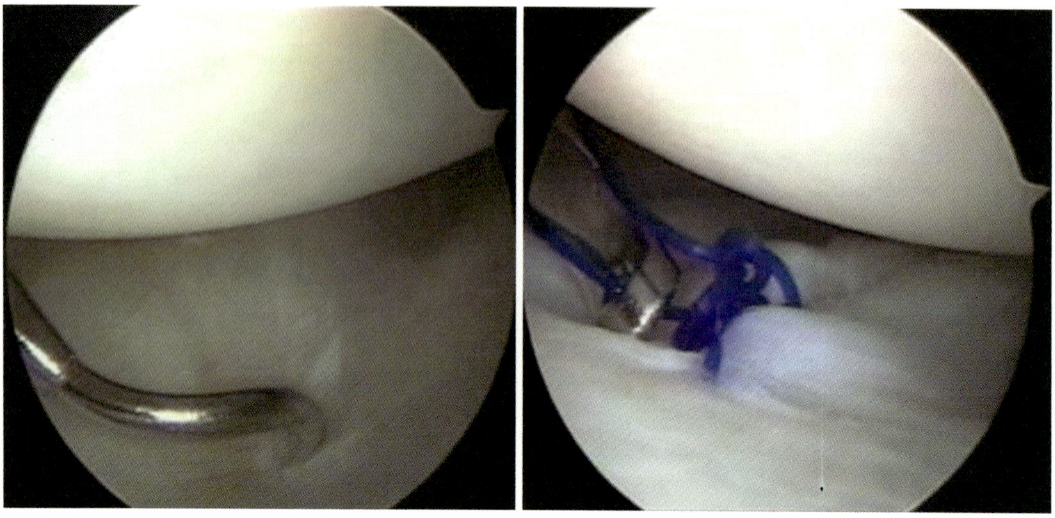

Fig. 29.21 Arthroscopic capsular plication for multidirectional instability treatment

Subsequent operative treatment options include: Open or Arthroscopic techniques with inferior capsule posteroanterior plications, rotator interval plication, thermal capsulorrhaphy joint capsule imbrication (Fig. 29.21), anterior reconstruction plus inferior capsule vertical shifting.

Inferior Capsular Shift Procedure

Approach may be performed via either open or arthroscopic. Usually arthroscopic approach is preferred (Fig. 29.21). Surgeons should note that sometimes the humeral head posterior subluxation sometimes may occur according to the overtightened anterior joint capsule with arthroscopic inferior capsular shifting. This technique includes carefully and adequately shifting of the capsule with plication suturation while reducing the joint volume (Fig. 29.21).

Several studies have reported successful results with both open and arthroscopic techniques, specially for the open T-plasty modification of the Bankart procedure for multidirectional instability of the anterior and inferior types [120, 121, 125–127].

Choi et al. reported promising outcomes among 92% of their open anterior surgical repairs and in 81% of their posterior ones [128]. Also, they reported outstanding return to contact sports among 82% of their anterior repairs, among 75% of their posterior repairs, and among 17% of their bilateral repairs. Throughout their follow-up, 96% of their repairs remained stable [128]. On the other hand, Hamada et al. reported recurring anteroinferior joint subluxations according to the later onset of posterolateral humeral bony defects among the posteriorly approached patients [125]. On the other hand, Baker et al., in 2009 have reported a rate 91% full range of motion and satisfaction following arthroscopic repair outcomes among athletes, together with a rate of 98% slight decrease in strength, and with a 86% rate of return to sports with no limitations [129].

Complications

- Recurrence
- Subscapularis deficiency
- Loss of motion
- Axillary nerve injury
- Capsular thinning/insufficiency and chondrolysis
- Late arthritis [128]
- Post-operative rehabilitation includes:
- Initial 4–6 weeks, the shoulder is immobilized by sling or immobilizer
- 6–10 weeks, according to the stiffness status of the shoulder abduction brace with limit of 45° on abduction as well as external rotation
- 6–14 weeks, progressive range of motion and isometric exercises

- By 10th week, as soon as the full range of motion has been established, progressive isotonic exercises
- After 16 weeks, strengthening
- After 10 months, full return to activities and contact sports [128]

References

1. Cutts S, Prempeh M, Drew S. Anterior shoulder dislocation. Ann R Coll Surg Engl. 2009;91(1):2–7. doi:10.1308/003588409X359123.
2. Bankart ASB. The pathology and treatment of recurrent dislocations of the shoulder joint. Br J Surg. 1938;26:23–9.
3. Dumont GD, Russell RD, Robertson WJ. Anterior shoulder instability: a review of pathoanatomy, diagnosis and treatment. Curr Rev Musculoskelet Med. 2011;4(4):200–7. doi:10.1007/s12178-011-9092-9 PMCID: PMC3261242.
4. Robinson CM, Seah M, Akhtar MA. The epidemiology, risk of recurrence, and functional outcome after an acute traumatic posterior dislocation of the shoulder. J Bone Joint Surg Am. 2011;93(17):1605–13. doi:10.2106/JBJS.J.00973.
5. Kim SH, Ha KI, Yoo JC, Noh KC. Kim's lesion: an incomplete and concealed avulsion of the posteroinferior labrum in posterior or multidirectional posteroinferior instability of the shoulder. Arthroscopy. 2004;20(7):712–20.
6. Maltz SB, Fantus RJ, Mellett MM, et al. Surgical complication of Ehlers-Danlos syndrome type IV: case report and review of the literature. J Trauma. 2001;51:387–90.
7. Zweers MC, Hakim AJ, Grahame R, et al. Joint hypermobility syndromes: the pathophysiologic role of tenascin-X gene defects. Arthritis Rheum. 2004;5:2742–9.
8. Voos JE, Livermore RW, Feeley BT, et al. Prospective evaluation of arthroscopic Bankart repairs for anterior instability. Am J Sports Med. 2010;38:302–7.
9. Boileau P, Richou J, Lisai A, et al. The role of arthroscopy in revision of failed open anterior stabilization of the shoulder. Arthroscopy. 2009;25:1075–84.
10. Petrera M, Patella V, Patella S, et al. A meta-analysis of open versus arthroscopic Bankart repair using suture anchors. Knee Surg Sports Traumatol Arthrosc. 2010;18:1742–7.
11. Zabinski SJ, Callaway GH, Cohen S, et al. Revision shoulder stabilization: 2- to 10-year results. J Shoulder Elbow Surg. 1999;8:58–65.
12. Levine WN, Arroyo JS, Pollock RG, et al. Open revision stabilization surgery for recurrent anterior glenohumeral instability. Am J Sports Med. 2000;28:156–60.
13. Meehan RE, Peterson SA. Results and factors affecting outcome of revision surgery for shoulder instability. J Shoulder Elbow Surg. 2005;14:31–7.
14. Saccomanno MF, Fodale M, Capasso L, Cazzato G, Milano G. Generalized joint laxity and multidirectional instability of the shoulder. Joints. 2013;1(4):171–9.
15. RichardsR,DelaneyJ.Syringomyeliapresentingasshoulder instability. J Shoulder Elbow Surg. 1992;1(3):155–61. doi:10.1016/1058-2746(92)90094-j.
16. Misamore GW. A longitudinal study of patients with multidirectional instability of the shoulder with seven- to ten-year follow-up. Shoulder Elbow Surg. 2015;14(5):466–70. doi:10.1016/j.jse.2004.11.006.
17. Cooper D, O'Brien S, Arnoczky S, Warren R. The structure and function of the coracohumeral ligament: An anatomic and microscopic study. J Shoulder Elbow Surg. 1993;2(2):70–7. doi:10.1016/1058-2746(93)90003-y.
18. Yang HF, Tang KL, Dong SW, et al. An anatomic and histologic study of the coracohumeral ligament. 2009;18(2):305-310.
19. O'Brien SJ, Schwartz RS, Warren RF, Torzilli PA. Capsular restraints to anterior-posterior motion of the abducted shoulder: a biomechanical study. J Shoulder Elbow Surg. 1995;4(4):298–308. doi:10.1016/S1058-2746(05)80024-2.
20. Harryman DR 2nd, Sidles JA, Harris SL, Matsend FA 3rd. The role of the rotator interval capsule in passive motion and stability of the shoulder. J Bone Joint Surg Am. 1992;74(1):53–66.
21. Tetro AM, Bauer G, Hollstien SB, Yamaguchi K. Arthroscopic release of the rotator interval and coracohumeral ligament: An anatomic study in cadavers. Arthroscopy. 2015;18(2):145–50.
22. Bennett WF. Subscapularis, medial, and lateral head coracohumeral ligament insertion anatomy. Arthroscopic appearance and incidence of "hidden" rotator interval lesions. Arthroscopy. 2001;17(2):173–80.
23. Williams MM, Snyder SJ, Buford D Jr. The Buford complex--the "cord-like" middle glenohumeral ligament and absent anterosuperior labrum complex: a normal anatomic capsulolabral variant. Arthroscopy. 1995;10(3):241–7.
24. Ferrari DA. Capsular ligaments of the shoulder. Anatomical and functional study of the anterior superior capsule. Am J Sports Med. 1990;18(1):20–4.
25. Labriola JE, Lee TQ, Debski RE, McMahon PJ. Stability and instability of the glenohumeral joint: the role of the shoulder muscles. J Shoulder Elbow Surg. 2005;14(1 Suppl S):32S–8S.
26. Saha AK. Dynamic stability of the glenohumeral joint. Acta Orthop Scand. 1971;42(6):491–505.
27. Warner J, Caborn D, Berger R, Fu F, Seel M. Dynamic capsuloligamentous anatomy of the glenohumeral joint. J Shoulder Elbow Surg. 1993;2(3):115–33. doi:10.1016/s1058-2746(09)80048-7.
28. Rockwood CA. Subluxation of the shoulder: the classification, diagnosis and treatment. Orthop Trans. 1979;4:306.

29. Farrar NG, Malal JJ, Fischer J, Waseem M. An overview of shoulder instability and its management. Open Orthop J. 2013:338–46. doi:10.2174/1874325001307010338.
30. Schneeberger AG. C Gerber. Classification and therapy of the unstable shoulder. Ther Umsch. 1998;55(3):187–91.
31. Thomas SC, Matsen FA. An approach to the repair of avulsion of the glenohumeral ligaments ın the management of traumatic anterior glenohumeral ınstability. J Bone Joint Surg Am. 1989;71(4):506–13.
32. Kessel L, Bayley JIL. Clinical Disorders of the Shoulder. Churchill Livingstone. 1986;2:189–97.
33. Lewis A. T Kitamura, and JIL Bayley. "The Classification of Shoulder Instability: New Light Through Old Windows!". Curr Orthop. 2004;18(2):97–108.
34. Cofield RH, Nessler JP, Weinstabl R. Diagnosis of shoulder instability by examination under anesthesia. Clin Orthop Relat Res. 1993;(291)45–53.
35. Farrar NG. An overview of shoulder instability and its management. Open Orthop J. 2013;7:338–46. doi:10.2174/187432500130010338.
36. Lee SB, Kim KJ, O'Driscoll SW, Morrey BF, An KN. Dynamic glenohumeral stability provided by the rotator cuff muscles in the mid-range and end-range of motion. A study in cadavera. J Bone Joint Surg Am. 2000;82(6):849–57.
37. Lippitt S, Matsen F. Mechanisms of glenohumeral joint stability. Clin Orthop Relat Res. 1993;291:20–8.
38. Willemot L, Thoreson A. Ryan Breighner, Hooke A, Verborgt O, An KN. Mid-range shoulder instability modeled as a cam-follower mechanism. J Biomech. 2015;48(10):2227–31. doi:10.1016/j.jbiomech.2015.02.053.
39. Pouliart N, Gagey O. Reconciling arthroscopic and anatomic morphology of the humeral insertion of the inferior glenohumeral ligament. Arthroscopy. 2005;21(8):979–84.
40. O'Brien SJ, Neves MC, Arnoczky SP, Rozbruck SR, Dicarlo EF, Warren RF, Schwartz R, Wickiewicz TL. The anatomy and histology of the inferior glenohumeral ligament complex of the shoulder. Am J Sports Med. 1990;18(5):449–56.
41. Bayley JIL, Fischer K, Tsutsui H, Matthews J. Functional biofeedback in the management of habitual shoulder instability: a pilot study. In: Takagishi N, editor. The shoulder proceedings of the third international conference of the shoulder, Fukusica, 1986. p. 312–7.
42. Wang VM, Flatow EL. Pathomechanics of acquired shoulder instability: a basic science perspective. J Shoulder Elbow Surg. 2005;14(1 Suppl S):2S–11S.
43. Owens BD. Pathoanatomy of first-time, traumatic, anterior glenohumeral subluxation events. J Bone Joint Surg Am. 2010;92(7):1605–11. doi:10.2106/JBJS.I.00851.
44. Hovelius L, Augustini GB, Fredin H, Johansson O, Norlin R, Throling J. Primary anterior dislocation of the shoulder in young patients. A ten-year prospective study. J Bone Joint Surg Am. 1996;78:167701684.
45. Gamulin A, Dayer R, Lübbeke A, Miozzari H, Hoffmeyer P. Primary open anterior shoulder stabilization: a long-term, retrospective cohort study on the impact of subscapularis muscle alterations on recurrence. BMC Musculoskelet Disord. 2014;15:45. doi:10.1186/1471-2474-15-45.
46. Burkhart SS, De Beer JF. Traumatic glenohumeral bone defects and their relationship to failure of arthroscopic Bankart repairs: significance of the inverted-pear glenoid and the humeral engaging Hill-Sachs lesion. Arthroscopy. 2000;16:677–94.
47. Robinson CM, Kelly M, Wakefield AE. Redislocation of the shoulder during the first six weeks after a primary anterior dislocation: risk factors and results of treatment. J Bone Joint Surg Am. 2002;84-A:1552–9.
48. Hawkins RH, Hawkins RJ. Failed anterior reconstruction for shoulder instability. J Bone Joint Surg Br. 1985;67:709–14.
49. Pagnani MJ, Dome DC. Surgical treatment of traumatic anterior shoulder instability in American football players. J Bone Joint Surg Am. 2002;84-A:711–5.
50. Bacilla P, Field LD, Savoie FH. Arthroscopic Bankart repair in a high demand patient population. Arthroscopy. 1997;13:51–60.
51. Zaffagnini S, Marcheggiani M, Uccioli GM, Giordano G, Bonanzinga T, Grassi A, Nitri M, Bruni D, Ravazzolo G, Marcacci M. Long-term outcomes after repair of recurrent post-traumatic anterior shoulder instability: comparison of arthroscopic transglenoid suture and open Bankart reconstruction. Knee Surg Sports Traumatol Arthrosc. 2012;20:816–21.
52. O'Neill DB. Arhroscopic Bankart repair of anterior detachments of the glenoid labrum. A prospective study. J Bone Joint Surg Am. 1999;81:1357–66.
53. Cameron KL, Mountcastle SB, Nelson BJ. History of shoulder instability and subsequent injury during four years of follow-up: a survival analysis. J Bone Joint Surg Am. 2013;95(5):439–45.
54. Cameron KL, Duffey ML, DeBerardino TM, Stoneman PD, Jones CJ, Owens BD. Association of generalized joint hypermobility with a history of glenohumeral joint instability. J Athl Train. 2010;45(3):253–8.
55. Owens BD, Agel J, Mountcastle SB, Cameron KL, Nelson BJ. Incidence of glenohumeral instability in collegiate athletics. Am J Sports Med. 2009;37(9):1750–4.
56. Owens BD, Campbell SE, Cameron KL. Risk factors for anterior glenohumeral instability. Am J Sports Med. 2014;42(1):2591–8.
57. Roach CJ, Cameron KL, Westrick RB, Posner MA, Owens BD. Rotator cuff weakness is not a risk factor for first-time anterior glenohumeral instability. Orthop J Sports Med. 2013;1(1).
58. Groh GI, Rockwood CA Jr. The terrible triad: anterior dislocation of the shoulder associated with rupture of the rotator cuff and injury to the brachial plexus. J Shoulder Elbow Surg. 1995;4(1 Pt 1):51–3.
59. Ovesen J, Sojbjerg JO. Lesions in different types of anterior glenohumeral joint dislocation. An experimental study. Arch Orthop Trauma Surg. 1986;105(4):216–8.

60. Tasto JP, Roberts WO. Shoulder stability testing using the lateral decubitus position. Phys Sportsmed. 1998;26(12):75–6.
61. Hovelius L, Augustini BG, Fredin H, Johansson O, Norlin R, Thorling J. Primary anterior dislocation of the shoulder in young patients. A ten-year prospective study. J Bone Joint Surg Am. 1996;78:1677–84.
62. UG L, Loppini M, Rizzello G, Romeo G, Huijsmans PE, Denaro V. Glenoid and humeral head bone loss in traumatic anterior glenohumeral instability: a systematic review. Knee Surg Sports Traumatol Arthrosc. 2014;22(2):392–414. doi:10.1007/s00167-013-2403-5.
63. Tirman PF, Steinbach LS, Feller JF, Stauffer AE. Humeral avulsion of the anterior shoulder stabilizing structures after anterior shoulder dislocation: demonstration by MRI and MR arthrography. Skeletal Radiol. 1996;25:743–8.
64. Wolf EM, Cheng JC, Dickson K. Humeral avulsion of glenohumeral ligaments as a cause of anterior shoulder instability. Arthroscopy. 1995;11:600–7.
65. Neviaser TJ. The GLAD lesion: another cause of anterior shoulder pain. Arthroscopy. 1993;9(1):22–3.
66. Neviaser TJ. The anterior labroligamentous periosteal sleeve avulsion lesion: a cause of anterior instability of the shoulder. Arthroscopy. 1993;9(1):17–21.
67. Visser CP, Coene LN, Brand R, Tavy DL. The incidence of nerve injury in anterior dislocation of the shoulder and its influence on functional recovery. A prospective clinical and EMG study. J Bone Joint Surg Br. 1999;81(4):679–85.
68. Stayner LR, Cummings J, Andersen J, Review JCM. Shoulder dislocations in patients older than 40 years of age. Orthop Clin North Am. 2000;31(2):231–9.
69. Gerber C, Ganz R. Clinical assessment of instability of the shoulder with special reference to anterior and posterior drawer tests. J Bone Joint Surg Br. 1984;66:551–6.
70. King J, Wright T. Physical examination of the shoulder. J Hand Surg. 2014;39(10):2103–12. doi:10.1016/j.jhsa.2014.04.024.
71. Babacan M, Kesmezacar H, Ogut T, Cansu E, Erginer R. Radiologic evaluation of shoulder instability: conventional radiography, computed tomography and magnetic resonance imaging. Acta Orthop Traumatol Turc. 2005;39(1):24–33.
72. Cook TS, Stein JM, Simonson S, Kim W. Normal and variant anatomy of the shoulder on MRI. Magn Reson Imaging Clin N Am. 2011;19(3):581–94.
73. Rasmussen OS. Anterior shoulder instability: Sonographic evaluation. J Clin Ultrasound. 2004;32:430–7. doi:10.1002/jcu.20064.
74. Ozbaydar M, et al. Results of arthroscopic capsulolabral repair: Bankart lesion versus anterior labroligamentous periosteal sleeve avulsion lesion. Arthroscopy. 2008;24(11):1277–83.
75. Hintermann B, Gächter A. Arthroscopic findings after shoulder dislocation. Am J Sports Med. 1995;23(5):545.
76. Robinson EC, Thangamani VB, Kuhn MA, Ross G. Arthroscopic Findings After Traumatic Shoulder Instability in Patients Older Than 35 Years. Orthop J Sports Med. 2015;3(5):2325967115584318. doi:10.1177/2325967115584318.
77. Kosnik J, Shamsa F, Raphael E, et al. Anesthetic methods for reduction of acute shoulder dislocations: a prospective randomized study comparing intraarticular lidocaine with intravenous analgesia and sedation. Am J Emerg Med. 1999;17(6):566–70.
78. Young TB, Wallace WA. Conservative treatment of fractures and fracture-dislocations of the upper end of the humerus. J Bone Joint Surg Br. 1985;67(3):373–7.
79. Sonnabend DH. Treatment of primary anterior shoulder dislocation in patients older than 40 years of age. Conservative versus operative. Clin Orthop Relat Res. 1994;304:74–7.
80. Itoi E, Hatakeyama Y, Sato T, et al. Immobilization in external rotation after shoulder dislocation reduces the risk of recurrence. A randomized controlled trial. J Bone Joint Surg Am. 2007;89(10):2124–31.
81. Paterson WH, Throckmorton TW, Koester M, et al. Position and duration of immobilization after primary anterior shoulder dislocation: a systematic review and meta-analysis of the literature. J Bone Joint Surg Am. 2010;92(18):2924–33. doi:10.2106/JBJS.J.00631.
82. Chahal J, Marks PH, Macdonald PB, et al. Anatomic Bankart repair compared with nonoperative treatment and/or arthroscopic lavage for first-time traumatic shoulder dislocation. Arthroscopy. 2012;28(4):565–75. doi:10.1016/j.arthro.2011.11.012.
83. Arciero RA, St Pierre P. Acute shoulder dislocation. Indications and techniques for operative management. Clin Sports Med. 1995;14(4):937–53.
84. Neer CS 2nd, Foster CR. Inferior capsular shift for involuntary inferior and multidirectional instability of the shoulder. A preliminary report. J Bone Joint Surg Am. 1980;62:897–907.
85. Neer CS, Fithian TE, Hansen PE, et al. Reinforced cruciate repair for anterior dislocation of the shoulder. Orthop Trans. 1985;9:44–5.
86. Bigliani LU, Kurzweil PR, Schwartzbach CC, Wolfe IN, Flatow EL. Inferior capsular shift procedure for anterior-inferior shoulder instability in athletes. Am J Sports Med. 1994;22(5):578–84.
87. Cole BJ, Warner JJ. Arthroscopic versus open Bankart repair for traumatic anterior shoulder instability. Clin Sports Med. 2000;19(1):19–48.
88. Cowling PD, Akhtar MA, Liow RY. What is a Bristow-Latarjet procedure? A review of the described operative techniques and outcomes. Bone Joint J. 2016;98-B(9):1028–14.
89. Patte D, Debeyre J. Luxations recidivantes de l'e paule. Encycl Med Chir Paris-Technique Chirugicale Orthope'die. 1980;44265:44–52.
90. Joshi MA, Young AA, Balestro JC, Walch G. The Latarjet-Patte procedure for recurrent anterior shoulder instability in contact athletes. Orthop Clin North Am. 2015;46(1):105–11.
91. Bhatia S, Frank RM, Ghodadra NS, Hsu AR, Romeo AA, Bach BR Jr, Boileau P, Provencher MT. The

outcomes and surgical techniques of the latarjet procedure. Arthroscopy. 2014;30(2):227–35.
92. Gartsman GM, Waggenspack WN <>Jr, O'Connor DP, Elkousy HA, Edwards TB. Immediate and early complications of the open Latarjet procedure: a retrospective review of a large consecutive case series. J Shoulder Elbow Surg 2017;26(1)68-72. doi: 10.1016/j.jse.2016.05.029.
93. Agneskirchner JD, Lafosse L. Transfer of the coracoid process in recurrent anterior instability of the shoulder joint. The arthroscopic Latajert procedure. Oper Orthop Traumatol. 2014;26(3):296–306.
94. Wolf EM, Pollack M, Smalley C. Hill-Sachs "Remplissage:" An arthroscopic solution for engaging Hill-Sachs Lesion. Arthroscopy. 2007;23(6):e1–2.
95. Purchase RJ, Wolf EM, Hobgood ER, Pollock ME, Smalley CC. Hill-Sachs "remplissage": an arthroscopic solution for the engaging Hill-Sachs lesion. Arthroscopy. 2008;24(6):723–6.
96. Kropf EJ, Sekiya JK. Osteoarticular allograft transplantation for large humeral head defects in glenohumeral instability. Athroscopy. 2007;23(3):322.e1-e5.
97. Ramhamadany R, Modi CS. Current concepts in the management of recurrent anterior gleno-humeral joint instability with bone loss. World J Orthop. 2016;17(6):343–54.
98. Raiss P, Aldinger PR, Kastern P, Rickert M, Loew M. Humeral head resurfacing for fixed anterior glenohumeral dislocation. Int Orthop. 2009;33:451–6.
99. Grondin P, Leith J. Combined large Hill-Sachs and bony Bankart lesions treated by Latarjet and partial humeral head resurfacing: a report of 2 cases. Can J Surg. 2009;52(3):249–54.
100. Moors C, Ahmad CS. Partial humeral head resurfacing and Latarjet coracoid transfer for treatment of recurrent anterior glenohumeral instability. Orthopedics 2009. 32(8). doi: 10.3928/01477447-20090624-21.
101. Antoniou J, Harryman DT. Posterior instability. Orthop Clin North Am. 2001;32:463–73.
102. Boyd HB, Sisk TD. Recurrent posterior dislocation of the shoulder. J Bone Joint Surg Am. 1972;54:779–86.
103. McLaughlin HL. Posterior dislocation of the shoulder. J Bone Joint Surg Am. 1952;34:584–90.
104. Provencher MT, King S, Solomon DJ, Bell J, Mologne TS. Recurrent Posterior Shoulder Instability: Diagnosis and Management. Am J Sports Med. 2011;39(4):874–86. doi:10.1177/0363546510384232.
105. Hawkins RJ, Schutte JP, Janda DH, Huckell GH. Translation of the glenohumeral joint with the patient under anesthesia. J Shoulder Elbow Surg. 1996;5:286–92.
106. Krishnan SG, Hawkins RJ, Bokor DJ. Clinical evaluation of shoulder problems. In: Rockwood Jr CA, Matsen III FA, Wirth MA, Lippitt SB, editors. The shoulder. 3rd ed. Philadelphia, PA: WB Saunders; 2004. p. 145–85.
107. McFarland EG, Kim TK. Laxity and instability. In: McFarland EG, editor. Examination of the shoulder: a complete guide. New York: Thieme; 2006. p. 179.
108. Cheatham SA, Mair SD. Arthroscopic technique for the evaluation and treatment of posterior shoulder instability. Orthopedics. 2009;32(3):194.
109. Tibone JW, Bradley JP. The treatment of posterior subluxation in athletes. Clin Orthop. 1993;291:124–47.
110. Pollock RG, Bigliani LU. Recurrent posterior shoulder instability. Diagnosis and treatment. Clin Orthop. 1993;(291):85–96.
111. Moseley JB, Jobe FW, Perry J, et al. EMG analysis of the scapular rotator muscles during a baseball rehabilitation program. Orthop Trans. 1990;14:252.
112. Rowe C, Yee L. A posterior approach to the shoulder joint. J Bone Joint Surg. 1944;26:580–4.
113. Goss TP. Recurrent symptomatic posterior glenohumeral subluxation. Orthop Rev. 1988; 1024-1028(1032):17.
114. Rowe C, Zarins B. Chronic unreduced dislocation of the shoulder. J Bone Joint Surg Am. 1982;64494–505.
115. Hawkins RJ, Janda DH. Posterior instability of the glenohumeral joint: A technique of repair. Am J Sports Med. 1996;24:275–8.
116. Savoie FH. 3RD, Holt MS, Field LD, Bell J, Ramsey JR. Arthroscopic management of posterior instability: evolution of technique and results. Arthroscopy. 2008;24(4):389–96.
117. Bottoni CR, Franks BR, Moore JH, et al. Operative stabilization of posterior shoulder instability. Am J Sports Med. 2005;33:996–1002.
118. Gerber C, Lambert SM. Allograft reconstruction of segmental defects of the humeral head for the treatment of chronic locked posterior dislocation of the shoulder. J Bone Surg Am. 1996;78(3):376–82.
119. Provencher MT, Romeo AA. Posterior and multidirectional instability of the shoulder: challenges associated with diagnosis and management. Instr Course Lect. 2008;57:133–52.
120. Neer CS 2nd, Foster CR. Inferior capsular shift for involuntary inferior and multidirectional instability of the shoulder. A preliminary report. 1980. J Bone Joint Surg Am. 2001;62(6):897–908.
121. Altchek DW, Warren RF, Skyhar MG, et al. T-plasty modification of the Bankart procedure for multidirectional instability of the anterior and inferior types. J Bone Joint Surg Am. 1991;73:105–12.
122. Cooper RA, Brems JJ. The inferior capsular-shift procedure for multidirectional instability of the shoulder. J Bone Joint Surg Am. 1992;74:1516–21.
123. Burkhead WZ Jr, Rockwood CA Jr. Treatment of instability of the shoulder with an exercise program. J Bone Joint Surg Am. 1992;74(6):890–6.
124. Kiss J, Damrel D, Mackie A, et al. Non-operative treatment of multidirectional shoulder instability. Int Orthop. 2001;24:354–7.
125. Hamada K, Fukuda H, Nakajima T, et al. The inferior capsular shift operation for instability of the shoulder: long-term results in 34 shoulders. J Bone Joint Surg. 1999;81(2):218–25.
126. Beighton PH, Horan F. Orthopedic aspects of the Ehlers-Daplos Syndrome. J Bone Joint Surg. 1969;51:444–453x.

127. Pollock RG, Wang VM, Buchieri JS, et al. Effects of repetitive subfailure strains on the mechanical behavior of the inferior glenohumeral ligament. Joint Shoulder Elbow Surg. 2000;9(5):427–35.
128. Choi C, Ogilvie-Harris DJ. Inferior capsular shift operation for multidirectional instability of the shoulder in players of contact sports. Br J Sports Med. 2002;36:290–4.
129. Baker LC, Mascarenhas R, Kline JA, Chhabra A, Pombo MW, Bradley JP. Arthroscopic Treatment of Multidirectional Shoulder Instability in Athletes. Am J Sports Med. 2009;37(9):1712–20. doi:10.1177/0363546509335464.

Index

G. Huri, N.K. Paschos (eds.), *The Shoulder*, Orthopaedic Study Guide Series,
DOI 10.1007/978-3-319-51979-1

Printed by Printforce, the Netherlands